Recommended Dietary Allowances,[a] Revised 1989

Designed for the maintenance of good nutrition of practically all healthy people in the United States

Category	Age (years) or Condition	Weight[b] (kg)	Weight[b] (lb)	Height[b] (cm)	Height[b] (in)	Protein (g)	Vitamin A (μg RE)[c]	Vitamin D (μg)[d]	Vitamin E (mg α-TE)[e]	Vitamin K (μg)
Infants	0.0–0.5	6	13	60	24	13	375	7.5	3	5
	0.5–1.0	9	20	71	28	14	375	10	4	10
Children	1–3	13	29	90	35	16	400	10	6	15
	4–6	20	44	112	44	24	500	10	7	20
	7–10	28	62	132	52	28	700	10	7	30
Males	11–14	45	99	157	62	45	1,000	10	10	45
	15–18	66	145	176	69	59	1,000	10	10	65
	19–24	72	160	177	70	58	1,000	10	10	70
	25–50	79	174	176	70	63	1,000	5	10	80
	51+	77	170	173	68	63	1,000	5	10	80
Females	11–14	46	101	157	62	46	800	10	8	45
	15–18	55	120	163	64	44	800	10	8	55
	19–24	58	128	164	65	46	800	10	8	60
	25–50	63	138	163	64	50	800	5	8	65
	51+	65	143	160	63	50	800	5	8	65
Pregnant						60	800	10	10	65
Lactating	1st 6 months					65	1,300	10	12	65
	2nd 6 months					62	1,200	10	11	65

[a] The allowances, expressed as average daily intakes over time, are intended to provide for individual variations among most normal persons as they live in the United States under usual environmental stresses. Diets should be based on a variety of common foods in order to provide other nutrients for which human requirements have been less well defined.

[b] Weights and heights of Reference Adults are actual medians for the U.S. population of the designated age, as reported by NHANES II. The median weights and heights of those under 19 years of age were taken from Hamill et al. (1979). The use of these figures does not imply that the height-to-weight ratios are ideal.

Median Heights and Weights and Recommended Energy Intake from the RDA

Category	Age (years) or Condition	Weight (kg)	Weight (lb)	Height (cm)	Height (in)	REE[a] (kcal/day)	Average Energy Allowance (kcal)[b] Multiples of REE	Average Energy Allowance (kcal)[b] Per kg	Average Energy Allowance (kcal)[b] Per day[c]
Infants	0.0–0.5	6	13	60	24	320		108	650
	0.5–1.0	9	20	71	28	500		98	850
Children	1–3	13	29	90	35	740		102	1,300
	4–6	20	44	112	44	950		90	1,800
	7–10	28	62	132	52	1,130		70	2,000
Males	11–14	45	99	157	62	1,440	1.70	55	2,500
	15–18	66	145	176	69	1,760	1.67	45	3,000
	19–24	72	160	177	70	1,780	1.67	40	2,900
	25–50	79	174	176	70	1,800	1.60	37	2,900
	51+	77	170	173	68	1,530	1.50	30	2,300
Females	11–14	46	101	157	62	1,310	1.67	47	2,200
	15–18	55	120	163	64	1,370	1.60	40	2,200
	19–24	58	128	164	65	1,350	1.60	38	2,200
	25–50	63	138	163	64	1,380	1.55	36	2,200
	51+	65	143	160	63	1,280	1.50	30	1,900
Pregnant	1st trimester								+0
	2nd trimester								+300
	3rd trimester								+300
Lactating	1st 6 months								+500
	2nd 6 months								+500

[a] Calculation based on FAO equations, then rounded.

[b] In the range of light to moderate activity the coefficient of variation is ±20%.

[c] Figure is rounded.

Recommended Dietary Allowances,[a] Revised 1989 (continued)

Designed for the maintenance of good nutrition of practically all healthy people in the United States

Category	Water-Soluble Vitamins							Minerals						
	Vita-min C (mg)	Thia-min (mg)	Ribo-flavin (mg)	Niacin (mg NE)[f]	Vita-min B$_6$ (mg)	Fol-ate (µg)	Vita-min B$_{12}$ (µg)	Cal-cium (mg)	Phos-phorus (mg)	Mag-nesium (mg)	Iron (mg)	Zinc (mg)	Io-dine (µg)	Sele-nium (µg)
Infants	30	0.3	0.4	5	0.3	25	0.3	400	300	40	6	5	40	10
	35	0.4	0.5	6	0.6	35	0.5	600	500	60	10	5	50	15
Children	40	0.7	0.8	9	1.0	50	0.7	800	800	80	10	10	70	20
	45	0.9	1.1	12	1.1	75	1.0	800	800	120	10	10	90	20
	45	1.0	1.2	13	1.4	100	1.4	800	800	170	10	10	120	30
Males	50	1.3	1.5	17	1.7	150	2.0	1,200	1,200	270	12	15	150	40
	60	1.5	1.8	20	2.0	200	2.0	1,200	1,200	400	12	15	150	50
	60	1.5	1.7	19	2.0	200	2.0	1,200	1,200	350	10	15	150	70
	60	1.5	1.7	19	2.0	200	2.0	800	800	350	10	15	150	70
	60	1.2	1.4	15	2.0	200	2.0	800	800	350	10	15	150	70
Females	50	1.1	1.3	15	1.4	150	2.0	1,200	1,200	280	15	12	150	45
	60	1.1	1.3	15	1.5	180	2.0	1,200	1,200	300	15	12	150	50
	60	1.1	1.3	15	1.6	180	2.0	1,200	1,200	280	15	12	150	55
	60	1.1	1.3	15	1.6	180	2.0	800	800	280	15	12	150	55
	60	1.0	1.2	13	1.6	180	2.0	800	800	280	10	12	150	55
Pregnant	70	1.5	1.6	17	2.2	400	2.2	1,200	1,200	320	30	15	175	65
Lactating	95	1.6	1.8	20	2.1	280	2.6	1,200	1,200	355	15	19	200	75
	90	1.6	1.7	20	2.1	260	2.6	1,200	1,200	340	15	16	200	75

[a] Retinol equivalents. 1 retinol equivalent = 1 µg retinol or 6 µg β-carotene.

[b] As cholecalciferol. 10 µg cholecalciferol = 400 IU of vitamin D.

[c] α-Tocopherol equivalents. 1 mg d-α tocopherol = 1 α-TE.

[d] NE (niacin equivalent) is equal to 1 mg of niacin or 50 mg of dietary tryptophan.

Food Guide Pyramid
A Guide to Daily Food Choices

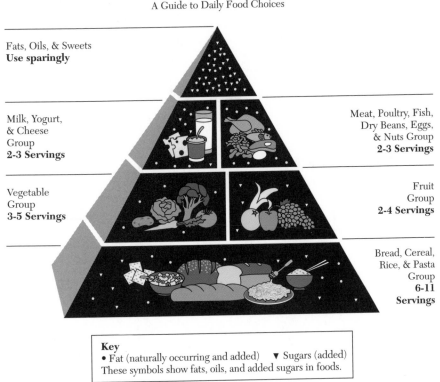

Fats, Oils, & Sweets
Use sparingly

Milk, Yogurt, & Cheese Group
2-3 Servings

Meat, Poultry, Fish, Dry Beans, Eggs, & Nuts Group
2-3 Servings

Vegetable Group
3-5 Servings

Fruit Group
2-4 Servings

Bread, Cereal, Rice, & Pasta Group
6-11 Servings

Key
• Fat (naturally occurring and added)   ▼ Sugars (added)
These symbols show fats, oils, and added sugars in foods.

USDA, 1992

NUTRITION
SCIENCE AND APPLICATIONS

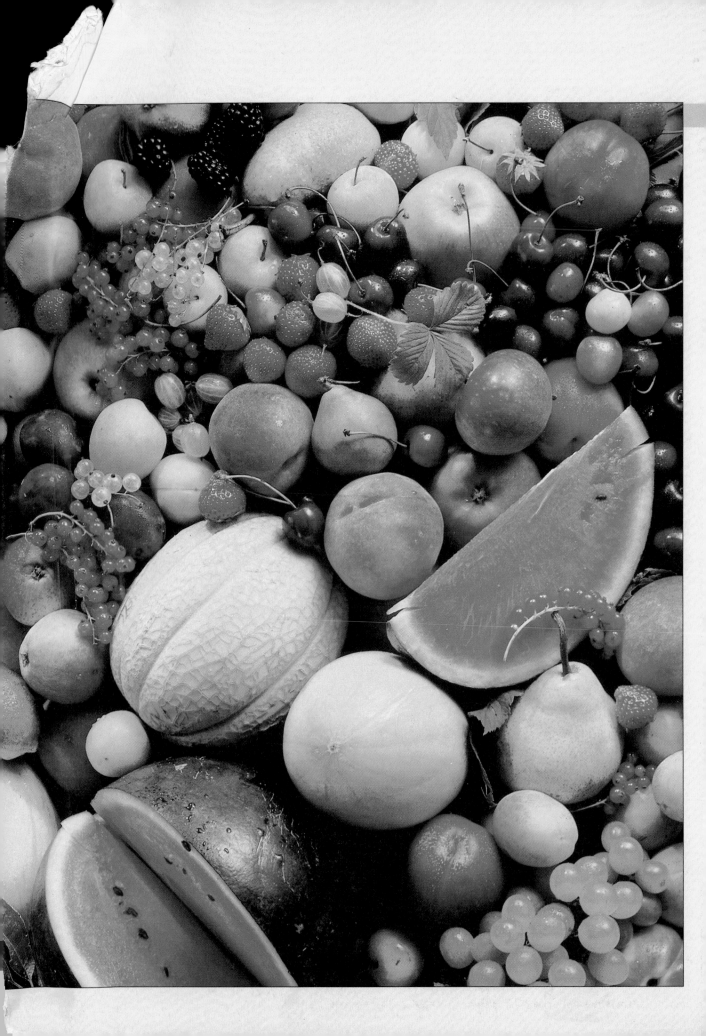

NUTRITION
SCIENCE AND APPLICATIONS

second edition

Lori A. Smolin
University of Connecticut

Mary B. Grosvenor
Harbor–UCLA Medical Center
Western Wyoming Community College

Saunders College Publishing

Harcourt Brace College Publishers

FORT WORTH   PHILADELPHIA   SAN DIEGO   NEW YORK   ORLANDO   AUSTIN

SAN ANTONIO   TORONTO   MONTREAL   LONDON   SYDNEY   TOKYO

Text Typeface: New Caledonia
Compositor: University Graphics, Inc.
Acquisitions Editors: Julie Levin Alexander, Edith Beard Brady
Developmental Editor: Christine Connelly
Photo Editor: Jane Sanders Wood
Managing Editor: Carol Field
Project Editor: Bonnie Boehme
Copy Editor: Maureen Iannuzzi
Manager of Art and Design: Carol Bleistine
Art Director: Caroline McGowan
Illustration Supervisor: Sue Kinney
Art and Design Coordinator: Kathleen Flanagan
Text Designer: Caroline McGowan
Cover Designer: Ruth A. Hoover
Text Artwork: Rolin Graphics
Director of EDP: Tim Frelick
Manager of Production: Joanne Cassetti
Marketing Manager: Sue Westmoreland

Cover Credit: Cover photograph by John Williams, courtesy of Ben & Jerry's Homemade, Inc.
Frontispiece: Christel Rosenfeld/Tony Stone Images

Frontmatter Photo Credits: p. vii, © Bill Margerin/FPG International; p. xvi, © Pickerell-Weber 1986/FPG International; p. xvii, M. Nelson/FPG International; p. xviii, Will & Deni McIntyre/Tony Stone Images; p. xix, Matthew Klein/Photo Researchers, Inc.; p. xxi, Thomas Brase/Tony Stone Images; p. xxii, Tony Craddock/Tony Stone Images; p. xxiv, Trevor Wood/Tony Stone Images

Part Opening Photo Credits: Part I, Rosemary Weller/Tony Stone Images; Part II, Trevor Wood/Tony Stone Images; Part III, Laurie Evans/Tony Stone Images; Part IV, © Ken Reid/FPG International; Part V, © Tim Beddow/Tony Stone Images

Backmatter Photo Credits: Appendix, © Victor Scocozza/FPG International; Glossary, Charles Thatcher/Tony Stone Worldwide; Index, Simon Yeo/Tony Stone Images

Printed in the United States of America

NUTRITION: SCIENCE AND APPLICATIONS
Second Edition

ISBN 0-03-017708-1
Library of Congress Catalog Card Number: 95-072725

789012345   032   10 9876543

To our husbands for their patience and understanding.

To Zachary, David, John, and Max for surviving with part-time mothers.

To Julie Levin Alexander for her faith in us and her vision for this text; and to Christine Connelly for going beyond the call of duty to make all of our efforts come together. We wish them both the best in their new choices.

ABOUT THE AUTHORS

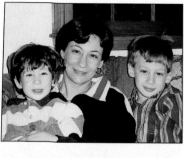

Lori A. Smolin Received her B.S. at Cornell University, where she studied human nutrition and food science, and her doctorate in Nutritional Sciences at the University of Wisconsin at Madison. She completed postdoctoral research at the Harbor–UCLA Medical Center as well as the University of California at San Diego. She has done research and published in peer-reviewed journals in the areas of protein and amino acid metabolism, genetic diseases of amino acid metabolism, and human obesity. Lori has extensive teaching experience and is currently an instructor at the University of Connecticut, where she teaches courses in introductory nutrition, lifecycle nutrition, biology, and biochemistry.

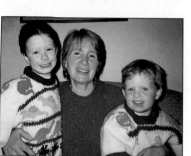

Mary B. Grosvenor Received a B.A. in English from Georgetown University and her Masters in Nutrition Science from the University of California at Davis. She worked for many years managing human nutrition research studies in the General Clinical Research Center at Harbor–UCLA Medical Center and has published extensively in nutrition and cancer and nutrition and HIV infection. She is currently living with her family in a small town in Wyoming, where she is continuing her work in nutrition research via the electronic superhighway and teaching introductory nutrition at Western Wyoming Community College.

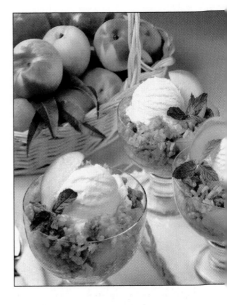

Life is full of choices. Whether you choose plain vanilla or rocky road ice cream depends on many factors. How these choices affect you and your nutritional health depends on the other choices you make. No one choice can make or break the overall diet. What is important is the combination of the foods and nutrients that make up the total diet. The theme of this book is choice because we believe that the key to applying nutrition knowledge lies in comprehending how to make wise choices. By emphasizing choices, we have focused on the total diet. For example, choosing a healthy diet doesn't just mean reducing your fat intake. Fat is only one component of a healthy diet. Similarly, the benefits of increasing complex carbohydrates come not only from the carbohydrate itself but also from the increase in phytochemicals and micronutrients, the reduction in fat, and other changes in the total diet that result when wise high-carbohydrate choices are made.

As nutritionists, we are frequently asked questions about which nutrition choices are best. A student may ask, is this food good for me or bad for me? Should I be eating a lowfat diet? Should I take a protein supplement to improve my athletic performance? How can I lose 10 pounds? The answers to all these questions involve choices. And it is these personal concerns that trigger student interest in nutrition. When introductory nutrition classes and textbooks present the basics—what is carbohydrate, protein, fat?—but fail to prepare students to make choices about foods and popular nutrition issues, students cannot apply what they have learned. *Nutrition: Science and Applications* presents complete nutrition information and can be used to teach both major and nonmajor nutrition students how to use a scientific approach in making decisions about the nutrition issues they face every day.

APPROACH

The approach of this second edition is an integrated one. No nutrition decision is made in isolation but, rather, depends on our individual preferences, cultural and genetic background, the risks and benefits of these choices, and other nutrition and lifestyle choices we have made. Discussions of all of these issues are integrated throughout the text rather than isolated in separate chapters.

When discussing nutrients and dietary habits, we have integrated foods and examples from many cultures. In addition, we have included topics relevant to individuals of different ages, of both sexes, and in many stages and circumstances of life. This lifecycle information is highlighted by lifecycle icons throughout the text and is expanded on in separate chapters. Thus, students are repeatedly exposed to the important differences in nutrition during various stages and circumstances of life. For instance, the importance of growth in determining protein needs is highlighted by discussing the protein needs of infants, children, and adolescents along with those of adults. This integration of lifecycle material provides students with information that often cannot be covered due to the time constraints of a one-semester course. Human diversity is further emphasized in the Critical

Thinking Exercises in each chapter. These present the common nutrition challenges faced by people from many cultures and in many times and circumstances of life—young college students, working parents with children, athletes, pregnant women, and older adults.

The relationships between nutrition, health, and disease are discussed with each nutrient rather than being presented in an isolated section at the end of a chapter or in an entirely separate chapter. For example, the role of fiber in gastrointestinal health and cancer is discussed with carbohydrates, heart disease and cancer are covered along with dietary fat, osteoporosis is discussed with calcium, and hypertension is presented with sodium. Likewise, this text has integrated metabolism by including, in appropriate chapters, an explanation of how each nutrient is used by the body. This allows information about metabolism to be applied to discussions that are of interest to the student and reinforces the concept of metabolism by presenting related information and building on existing knowledge in subsequent chapters.

We have also included discussions of environmental issues where they tie in with each chapter because they can have an impact on nutrient composition of foods as well as on food choices. The amounts of certain nutrients, such as iodine and selenium, depend on the environmental conditions where the food was produced. And, the foods we choose are often affected by concern for the environment. For instance, the recent increase in vegetarianism may be attributed to the perception that meatless diets have less impact on the environment.

A scientific approach is employed throughout the text. Our goal is to teach students how to apply the logic of science to their own nutrition concerns. We present the process of scientific inquiry and demonstrate how it is used to evaluate the role of nutrition in health. The text contains all of the information students need to analyze and modify their own diets in order to promote health and reduce the risk of deficiency and chronic diseases related to nutrition. A critical thinking approach is used in each chapter to help students logically evaluate their diets and other aspects of nutrition science. These exercises are unique to this text. They introduce real-world nutrition problems and guide students step by step through a logical process to arrive at potential solutions to the problems. This approach is reinforced at the end of each chapter in application exercises that ask students to follow the model of the Critical Thinking Exercises to answer questions about their own diets and lifestyles.

Information provided by diet planning tools such as food labels, the *Dietary Guidelines*, and the Food Guide Pyramid is included with the presentation of each nutrient so that students can apply this information to their daily choices. The information provided by these three tools is integrated throughout the text. The art program supports this integration by using analogous figures to explain key concepts throughout. For example, when sugar is discussed, a *Dietary Guidelines* figure highlighting sugar is included, as is a figure of the Food Guide Pyramid highlighting the food groups high in added sugars. Because all of these sources can be used to make food choices, they are integrated throughout the text teaching nutrition science and its applications.

The integrated approach extends to the writing and the art program. The writing style is consistent, engaging, and easy to read. The organization from chapter to chapter is uniform, each chapter starting with a "friendly" or familiar topic to capture students' interest. The food composition information given throughout the chapters is in agreement with that in the appendix and the food composition data base. Analogous figures illustrating the metabolism of carbohydrate, fat, and protein; the carbohydrate, fat, and protein content of foods; the nutrients provided by the recommendations of The Food Guide Pyramid and the *Dietary Guidelines* appear throughout the chapters. Colors are also used consistently to represent carbohydrate, fat, and protein and to identify certain steps in metabolism.

NEW TO THIS EDITION

In addition to the theme of choice, the second edition of *Nutrition: Science and Applications* has a number of new and improved features and expanded coverage of topics that are of current interest.

- A focus on the importance of the total diet and not just single nutrients helps students understand that one choice doesn't make or break a diet. Just reducing fat intake without other changes doesn't provide a healthy diet. Traditional diets such as Asian and Mediterranean diets are used to help illustrate this.

- A stronger focus on ethnic diversity increases student awareness of the diversity of the modern world. Examples and sample menus throughout use diverse diets from a variety of ethnic groups, and an appendix presents tools designed for specific populations, such as Samoan and Mexican American exchange lists.

- More information on phytochemicals helps promote the message that nutrients should be consumed in foods, not supplements, and supports an emphasis on basing the diet on foods of plant origin such as grains, vegetables, and fruits.

- Expanded coverage of the role genetics play in obesity helps students understand the most recent thinking on the relationship of obesity to genetics and how this is related to energy balance and the potential for treatment of obesity.

- The latest tools for diet planning and analysis are presented. The 1995 Diabetic Exchange lists are included. The 1995 *Dietary Guidelines* provide the most up-to-date national nutrition recommendations for health and disease prevention. The information found in the nutrition messages of the *Dietary Guidelines*, the Food Guide Pyramid, and food labels has been linked to help students better understand how all of these tools help build a better diet.

- A focus on environmental concerns related to nutrition helps students have a more global view of foods and nutrition. For example, Chapter 6 contains a discussion of the environmental impact of vegetarianism, and Chapters 16 and 17 have a strong environmental focus.

- Expanded coverage of biotechnology and genetic engineering and how these relate to environmental concerns helps students better comprehend the technology behind consumer and world issues related to genetic engineering.

- More focus on risk-benefit analysis helps students to see that most choices have both risks and benefits.

- References have been updated, and the latest research has been presented. Almost all references are from 1990 or later, providing students with the most up-to-date information. New population studies such as NHANES III are included.

- Critical Thinking Exercises have been revised to incorporate more student participation. Some questions are answered to provide a model for students, and others require students to think critically and answer on their own. There are one or two Critical Thinking Exercises in each chapter. The exercises have been slightly shortened and placed in the chapter in such a way as not to interrupt the text flow.

- Application exercises have been expanded to provide a more stepwise approach to diet analysis and modification. These exercises are designed to help students apply the critical thinking skills learned throughout the chapter to their own diets.

- New "Off the Shelf" and "Off the Label" boxes have been included. Off the Shelf boxes present updated information related to items that can be obtained off the shelves of stores, such as books, supplements, and foods. Off the Label boxes provide an updated discussion of the uses of the standard food labels.

- Just a Taste questions, which have been added at the beginning of each chapter, feature common nutrition issues and misconceptions and serve to spark interest and provide a student pretest.
- Much of the existing line art has been revised to improve clarity and to match the level of the text, and new art has been added where appropriate.
- An integrated package of nutrient information in the software, Appendix A, and all tables in the book have been developed from the same source in order to provide consistent information on the nutrient content of foods.

LEARNING AIDS

Just a Taste   These questions provide a simple self-test to pique interest before starting the chapter.

Chapter Outline   This provides student and teacher with an outline of all material presented in the chapter.

Chapter Concepts   Each chapter opens with a list of the concepts to be explored in that chapter. These aid students in understanding up front how the material will be covered and serve as a study guide once the chapter is completed.

Easy-to-Understand Metabolism Information   Coverage of metabolism is integrated with discussion of the macronutrients. This prevents students from being overwhelmed because new metabolism information builds on and reinforces what they learned in the previous chapter. For example, the information on fat metabolism in Chapter 5 builds on that presented about carbohydrates in Chapter 4. Chapter 7 integrates all of the information on energy production, and Chapter 12 applies this knowledge to the exercising body.

Critical Thinking Exercises   The highly acclaimed Critical Thinking Exercises used in the first edition have been revised to incorporate more student participation. These exercises use case histories to direct student thinking and solve nutrition problems by leading students through the logical thought processes needed to answer nutrition questions. Some questions are answered to provide a model for students, and others require students to think critically. They provide a guide for students to use when answering application exercises at the end of the chapter. Answers are included in Appendix M.

Lifecycle Icon   In each chapter lifecycle icons highlight issues and recommendations that apply to specific stages and circumstances of life. The diversity of the material contained in each chapter is thereby increased, offering information relevant to students in all phases of life.

"Off the Shelf" Boxes   "Off the Shelf" boxes discuss issues that relate to items that can be obtained off the shelves of stores, such as foods, books, and supplements. They focus on consumer issues and choices and on evaluating nutrition information. These boxes are a unique aspect of this text, briefly highlighting topics of special interest that deserve more explanation than the scope of a one-semester course allows. These can be read separately or in conjunction with the body of the text.

"Off the Label" Boxes   "Off the Label" boxes present in-depth information on food labels as they apply to specific nutrients or issues. The most up-to-date information is included.

Updated References and Resources   Since knowledge of nutrition science is expanding so quickly, new information is continually coming to light. In response to this, we have added the most recent findings and references even during the production of the text, providing the most up-to-date information and interpretations available in the science. Most references are more recent than 1990. The authors would be happy to provide references for information that is not referenced in the text.

Ethnic Diversity   The use of ethnic foods in text examples and Critical Thinking Exercises throughout the text makes the book more appealing to a diverse audience. These examples expose students to the foods and eating patterns of other cultures. For example, in Chapter 5 Asian and Mediterranean diets are discussed in relation to the risk of heart disease.

Bold-faced Terms and Margin Definitions   Bold-faced terms are used throughout the text to identify important terms and concepts. All bold-faced terms are defined in the margin as an easy reference glossary and a study aid. These terms and many others are included in the glossary.

Art   The illustrations are geared to the level of understanding of the students using the text. Some students learn better from visual examples. The illustrations avoid using terminology that has not been explained. Many of these are also reproduced as overhead transparencies to accompany the text. The photographs were carefully chosen to enhance the student's understanding of and interest in the material.

Chapter Summary   A summary at the end of each chapter parallels the concepts used to introduce each chapter but provides more detail. This summary of important material covered in the chapter can be used by students as a study tool.

Self-Test   These brief questions direct students to the most important concepts covered in the chapter. They are designed to review in a simple manner the key points of each chapter and serve as a study review.

Applications   These exercises help students apply the critical thinking skills developed in Critical Thinking Exercises and the knowledge gained throughout the chapter to their own diets and lifestyles.

Appendices   Extensive appendices are found at the end of the text. These include a comprehensive food composition table including fast foods and convenience foods; standards for nutritional indices, such as height and weight for infants through the elderly; normal blood values; dietary recommendations from the United States, Canada, and other countries; food labeling information for the United States and Canada; food exchange lists; energy expenditure values; and answers to Critical Thinking Exercises.

Glossary   An extensive glossary of terms is included at the end of the text to provide a quick reference for terminology with which students are unfamiliar or for which they require review.

Index   The text is well indexed to allow students to easily cross-reference material of interest.

ORGANIZATION

The book is divided into five parts. The material is presented in a consistent and logical order that will capture the student's interest, but the chapters and sections can be taught in any order.

The first part, *Nutrition: Sorting Fact From Fantasy*, introduces the reader to the basic concepts in nutrition and the science necessary for understanding issues presented throughout the book. Chapter 1, "Nutrition: Everyday Choices," introduces the theme of choice and the important point that no one choice is good or bad but must be made within the context of the total diet and lifestyle. It also discusses factors that determine food choices. Chapter 1 provides an overview of the nutrients and their roles in the body, introduces nutritional assessment, and suggests sources of nutrition information, such as food labels, that are available to help consumers make informed decisions. Chapter 2, "Nutrition Science: The Basis for Nutrition Sense," focuses on identifying accurate nutrition information and distinguishing between factual and fictional nutrition information. It begins with the scientific method and demonstrates how this process is applied to nutrition research studies. It then discusses the types of nutrition research studies used and how the results of these studies are used to develop dietary standards, such as the RDAs, and guidelines for health and disease prevention, such as the *Dietary Guidelines for Americans*. Tools for diet planning, such as the Food Guide Pyramid and 1995 Exchange Lists, are also presented so that students can begin applying these to their own diets. The integrated message of the *Dietary Guidelines*, the Food Guide Pyramid, and food labels is stressed. Chapter 3, "The Human Body: From Meals to Molecules," explains digestion and absorption by showing how a particular meal is digested, absorbed into the body, and transported to the cells, where metabolism takes place.

Part II, *Energy-Containing Nutrients*, includes chapters on carbohydrates, lipids, and proteins as well as a chapter that covers energy balance, weight control, and eating disorders. For each of the energy-providing nutrients, the respective chapter begins with information on the types of foods that contain these nutrients, followed by discussion of the role of the nutrient in the body—nutrient function and metabolism, the role of that nutrient in health and disease, nutrient requirements and how they vary through life, and information on the use of that nutrient in the manufacture and processing of food. To teach students how to select a healthy diet, the recommendations of the *Dietary Guidelines* are integrated with the information provided by food labels and the Food Guide Pyramid. The health and disease topics in these chapters include the role of fiber in gastrointestinal health in Chapter 4, dietary fat and heart disease and dietary fat and cancer in Chapter 5, and protein deficiency and excess and the risks and benefits of vegetarian diets in Chapter 6. In each chapter, energy production is summarized using a consistent metabolism figure that illustrates how the metabolism of each nutrient interfaces with others. Chapter 7, "Energy Balance and Weight Management," then discusses the concept of energy balance and applies it to weight management. The discussion of energy balance includes a discussion of the genetic determinants of body weight and how our growing understanding of obesity genes is leading toward improved treatment. The health risks of too much or too little body fat as well as of eating disorders are addressed in this chapter. This chapter reflects the newer view of obesity as a disease that can be treated in an individualized fashion with diet, exercise, behavior modification, and drugs.

Part III, *Water and the Micronutrients*, examines the non-energy-containing nutrients: water, vitamins, and minerals. Chapter 8, "A Vitamin Primer and the Water Soluble Vitamins," begins with a vitamin primer that introduces vitamins in general, where they are found in the diet, and how they function. It then discusses each of the water soluble vitamins in terms of sources in the diet, uses in the body, impact on health, recommended intakes, supplement use, and potential for toxicity. The water soluble vitamins are presented first because most function in energy production and students have just studied energy production in the previous section. Chapter 9, "Fat Soluble Vitamins and Meeting Your Vitamin Needs," presents each of the fat soluble vitamins, discussing sources in the diet, uses in the body, impact on health, recommended intakes, supplement use, and potential for toxicity. The chapter closes with a discussion of choices for meeting vitamin needs. It emphasizes that food sources of vitamins also provide other health-promoting substances such as phytochemicals that are not classified as essential. In Chapter 10, "The Internal Sea: Water and the Major Minerals," water and the major minerals are presented. Again, chapter organization is consistent, introducing the chapter with information on where these nutrients are found and then discussing their function in the body, their relationship to health and disease, and recommended intakes. Health and disease topics addressed here include sodium and hypertension and calcium and osteoporosis. Practical information on food sources helps students apply this knowledge to their own diets. Chapter 11, "The Trace Minerals: Our Elemental Needs," discusses the trace elements in a format similar to that in Chapter 10. The nutrients are presented in an order that emphasizes the similar functions and interactions that exist between elements, rather than the typical laundry list approach. To engage the student's interest, each section begins with the friendly topic of food. The sources of the nutrients and their metabolic role are then addressed. Again, health issues related to these nutrients help create interest, as do discussions of the pros and cons of vitamin and mineral supplements.

Part IV, *Applying Nutrition to Life*, applies the basics of nutrition to different lifestyles and stages of development. Exercise is presented in this section as a lifestyle factor that affects nutritional status and nutritional needs. Chapter 12, "Fueling Fitness: Nutrition and Exercise," reviews metabolism, which was introduced in Part II, in relation to energy production. It is included here to allow a complete discussion of both macro- and micronutrient needs for energy production, athletic performance, and fitness in general. Practical aspects of selecting meals to maintain fitness throughout life as well as meals for the competitive athlete are included. Chapter 13, "In the Beginning: Nutrition for Mothers and Infants," addresses the role of nutrition in development by discussing the nutritional needs of pregnancy, lactation, and the infant's first year of life. Current recommendations and practical information about feeding infants are given. Chapter 14, "The Growing Years: Toddlers to Teens," continues this discussion with issues relating to nutrition for toddlers through teens. A discussion of nutrition and alcohol consumption is included in this chapter because the decision to use alcohol or not is an important choice often made by adolescents. Chapter 15, "Nutrition and Aging: The Adult Years," addresses how nutrition affects aging and aging affects nutrition. Nutrient-drug interactions are discussed in this chapter. Nutrition policies that affect special groups, such as school lunch programs, Meals on Wheels, and WIC, are presented in appropriate chapters in this part.

The final part, *Nutrition in Today's World*, addresses issues of food safety, food policy, and food practice in North America and the world. Chapter 16, "How Safe Is Our Food Supply?," discusses the risks and benefits of our food supply and includes information on microbial hazards, chemical toxins, food additives, and genetically engineered foods and how each has an impact on the safety and availability of the food we eat. Chapter 17, "The Global View: Feeding the World," deals with global nutrition issues. The problems and causes of world hunger are examined, along with potential solutions. And the health impact of "Westernization" of the diet in many developing countries is discussed.

ANCILLARIES

New Diet Analysis Software   A new software package has been designed to incorporate the foods mentioned throughout the text, and the nutrient recommendations discussed in the text. It includes more foods, and more ethnically diverse foods, and has the capacity to add foods to meet the ever-growing market of available products. Using information from food labels, students will be able to enter foods they eat frequently into the database.

Overhead Transparencies   This is a set of full color overheads to help instructors illustrate the more complicated concepts in the classroom.

Instructor's Manual with Testbank   This manual includes key concepts, complete chapter outlines, new Critical Thinking Exercises, key terms, student self-assessment forms, and sources of supplementary materials including Web sites. The Testbank includes multiple choice and short answer questions.

Study Guide   This guide reinforces concepts from the text through study activities such as reviewing key terms and answering test questions. It has been reworked from the first edition to follow the approach of the current text.

ExaMaster™   This is a computerized version of the printed Testbank that makes preparing clear, concise tests quick and easy. It is available for both Macintosh and IBM computers in either 5″ or 3″ format.

RequesTest™   Instructors who do not have access to computers may request test masters through Saunders College Publishing RequesTest Call-in Testing Service.

ExamRecord™   This is a computerized gradebook program that enables instructors to record, curve, graph, and print grades.

Nutrition Videodisc

Nutrition MediaActive™ **CD-ROM**   For more information on electronic support for this text, please contact your local sales representative.

Saunders College Publishing may provide complimentary instructional aids and supplements or supplement packages to those adopters qualified under our adoption policy. Please contact your sales representative for more information. If as an adopter or potential user you receive supplements you do not need, please return them to your sales representative or send them to

Attn: Returns Department
Troy Warehouse
465 South Lincoln Drive
Troy, MO 63379

ACKNOWLEDGMENTS

The authors wish to thank the many professors and students who helped in the development of this text. Their endless hours of careful reading and divergent viewpoints helped to make this text the best available on today's market.

The reviewers, who offered comments and suggestions on both the presentation and the accuracy of this information, include the following: Reviewers for the second edition include Melody Anacker, Montana State University; Alan Avakian, Kings River Community College; Karen Balnicki, University of Tennessee–Knoxville; Jeffrey Backstrand, New York University; Beverly Benes, University of Nebraska–Lincoln; Kari Berg, Moorhead State University; Joan Bosworth, Shasta College; Pat Brown, Cuesta College; John Capeheart, University of Houston–Downtown; Gwen Chapman, University of British Columbia; Janet Colson, Middle Tennessee State University; Carol Costello, University of Tennessee–Knoxville; Rhonda Crackel, Michigan State University; Georgia Crews, South Dakota State University; Darcye Cuff, Simon Fraser University; Cara Ebbeling, University of Connecticut; Catherine Gilmore, Orange Coast College; Jan Goodwin, University of North Dakota; Deloy Hendricks, Utah State University; Carolyn Hollingshead, University of Utah; Michael Keenan, Louisiana State University; Roger Kelton, York University; Ruth Litchfield, Iowa State University; Nelda Malm, Seminole Community College; Frances Mathews, California State University–Fullerton; Nina Mercer, University of Guelph; Stella Miller, Mt. San Antonio College; Ruby Moore, Louisiana State University; Sharon Morcos, Kansas State University; Marcia Nahikian-Nelms, Southeast Missouri State University; Debra Pearce, Northern Kentucky University; Stanley Segall, Drexel University; Samuel Smith, University of New Hampshire; Diana Spillman, Miami University; Alison Stephen, University of Saskatchewan; Elaine Turner, Clemson University; Carol Underwood, East Stroudsburg University; Elise West, Cornell University; Adrienne White, University of Maine; and Wendy White, Iowa State University.

We would also like to acknowledge the participants of our focus group. Their enthusiasm and insights helped us refine our ideas. Student Focus Group participants from Lora Beth Brown's Nutrition class at Brigham Young University included Brent Cowan, Mindy Lei Gunn, Heather Huffaker, Stephanie Nuttall, Kirk Roberts, and Gina Schmoe. Student Focus Group participants from Karen Balnicki's Nutrition class at University of Tennessee–Knoxville included Stacy Appleton, Victoria Bowman, Keriann Dool, Emily Fielding, John Fitzwilliam, Shannon Hickman, Srimathi Kannan, Brian Keeton, Sara Larkins, Aida Manalac, Jyotsna Muthuswamy, Suzanne Perry, Daniel Russell, Greg Sharp, Ronald Tipper, Cynthia Tipton, Amy Tragesser, Anna Maria Welker, Laura Wills, and Kerri Williams.

We would also like to acknowledge the Price Chopper Grocery Store in Oneonta, New York, for providing locations for some of the original photos; Charles Winters, Dennis Drenner, and Gregory Smolin for shooting many of the stunning photographs throughout the book; David Knecht for technical assistance in keeping our computers and modems running; and Peter Ambrose for artistic and literary advice.

We are grateful to the editorial and production staff at Saunders College Publishing for their help and support. We thank our Acquisitions Editors Julie Levin Alexander and Edith Beard Brady for constant enthusiasm and support, and our Developmental Editor Christine Connelly for endless hours of expert advice, moral support, and general hand-holding. We also thank our Photo Editor Jane Sanders Wood for ensuring the outstanding quality of the photos in this text, our Art Director Caroline McGowan for delivering an attractively designed text with high-quality artwork, our Art Developmental Editor Leslie Ernst for translating our sketches into effective figures, and our Project Editor Bonnie Boehme for her limitless patience in guiding this project through production.

TO THE STUDENT

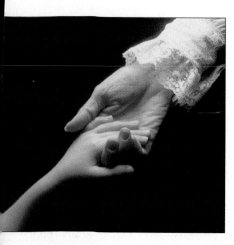

Most nutrition texts choose to put a photo of fruits, vegetables, or grain products on the cover. This is because these foods make up the basis of a healthy diet. We chose ice cream for our cover to emphasize that the total diet is more important than each individual food choice. Ice cream can be part of a healthy diet if your *total* diet is based on grains, vegetables, and fruits.

Good nutrition doesn't mean giving up all the foods you like; it means making wise choices to select an overall diet that promotes health, protects you from disease, and provides enjoyment. Each food and lifestyle choice you make depends on other choices you have made or intend to make. To help you with these nutrition choices we have provided a text that bridges the gap between popular nutrition and nutrition science. Our goal is not to say, for instance, that you should or should not eat potato chips. Instead, we have provided you with the information you need to make informed decisions for yourself. This text takes nutrition science out of the classroom and allows you to apply it to the decisions you make about foods, nutritional supplements, and diet and lifestyle factors important for your health. We have included the latest tools for selecting a healthy diet, including the Food Guide Pyramid, the *Dietary Guidelines*, and product food labels. We hope that the knowledge you gain from this book will help you choose a healthy diet while allowing you to enjoy the diversity of flavors, textures, and tastes that are available in today's food supply.

CONTENTS OVERVIEW

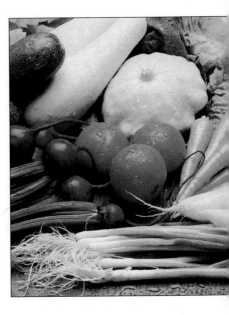

CONTENTS

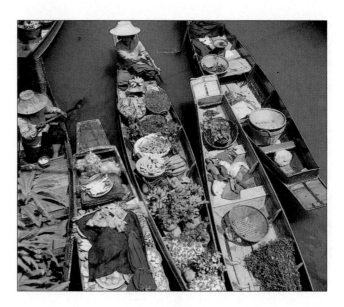

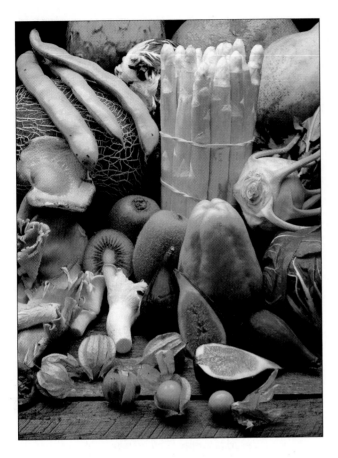

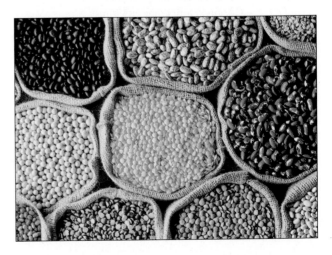

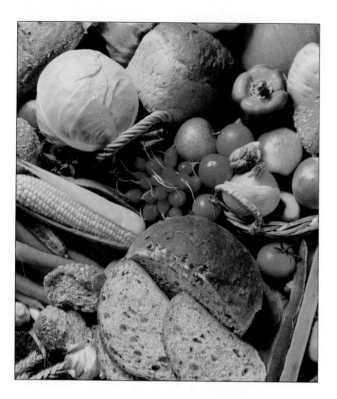

IV APPLYING NUTRITION TO LIFE 351

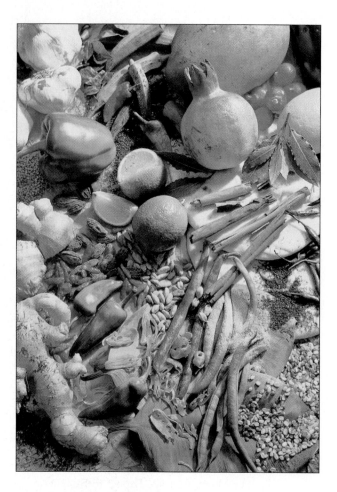

NUTRITION: SORTING FACT FROM FANTASY

I

LIFE CYCLE

Nutrition: Everyday Choices

CHAPTER CONCEPTS

1. Any food choice can be part of a healthy diet as long as it is balanced with other food choices.
2. The food choices we make are determined by what is available, what we like and are culturally conditioned to eat, as well as what we think we should be eating.
3. Most of us are not choosing the healthiest of diets.
4. The study of nutrition includes all the interactions of living organisms with food.
5. Nutrients are substances found in food that provide energy, structure, and regulation for the body processes of maintenance, growth, and reproduction.
6. Nutrients must be consumed in the proper proportions in order to meet our nutritional needs.
7. Too much, too little, or the wrong combination of nutrients can result in malnutrition.
8. Our nutritional status can be assessed by evaluating nutrient intake as well as by clinical and laboratory measures that reflect nutritional health.

JUST A TASTE

What foods can never be included in a healthy diet?

Can someone who is overweight be malnourished?

Is water a nutrient?

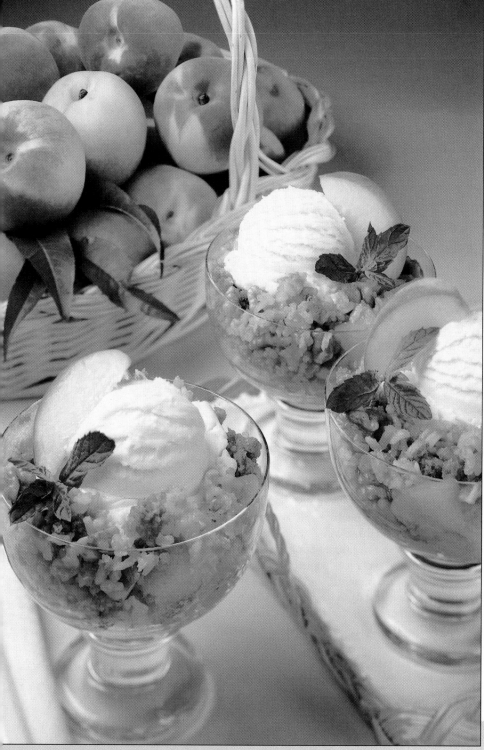

(© Bill Margerin/FPG International)

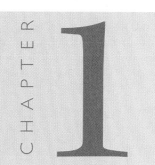

CHAPTER 1

Ice cream—cold, creamy, delicious—but is it nutritious? Should it be on the cover of a nutrition book? Can it be part of a healthy diet? The answer depends on the choices you make. Ice cream comes in many colors, flavors, and varieties: neopolitan, rainbow sherbet, heavenly hash, hot fudge, frozen yogurt, fat-free, sorbet, sugar-free . . . . Each tastes different, looks different, and makes a different contribution to the diet as a whole. Strawberry sorbet is low in fat and a good source of vitamin C, but it is high in sugar; premium fudge swirl ice cream tastes creamy, chocolatey, and rich, contains protein and calcium, but is high in fat, cholesterol, and sugar; nonfat peach frozen yogurt has pieces of fruit in it, has negligible fat, is a good source of protein and calcium, but is high in sugar. Any food choice can be a part of a nutritious diet as long as it is balanced with other choices throughout the day.

In order to choose foods that contribute to a healthy diet, you need information about what nutrients you need and what foods contain them. The purpose of this text is to provide an understanding of basic nutritional science in a way that will allow you to make everyday choices about the foods and nutrients you consume. In this introductory chapter, we will discuss:

- What are the nutrition choices we face each day?
- What are nutrients and what do they do?
- How do we assess our nutritional health?

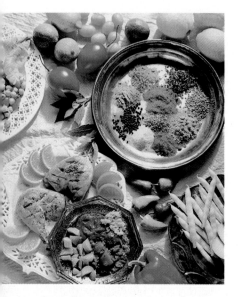

FIGURE 1-1
We make hundreds of food choices every day. (Trevor Wood/Tony Stone Images)

FOOD CHOICES

We make many food choices daily (Figure 1-1). And there are many reasons for our choices: a food tastes good, it's good for us, it isn't bad for us, it costs less, it comes in an appealing package, it's kosher, it's the kind you always buy, or even because the manufacturer is environmentally responsible and promotes minorities and women. There are hundreds of choices and hundred of reasons for making them. Each of these choices contributes to our total nutrient intake. Some foods contribute vitamins, minerals, and protein. Others may provide just energy. Some may be very high in fat and others contain no fat at all. None of the foods we choose are good or bad in and of themselves, but combined they make up a healthy or a not-so-healthy diet.

WHAT ARE WE CHOOSING?

Currently the American diet is not as healthy as it could be. As a population, we don't eat enough fruits and vegetables.[1] We eat too few whole grains and too much sugar.[2] We eat more energy than we expend and we consume more fat than is recommended (Figure 1-2).[3] These dietary patterns increase the risk of developing chronic diseases, such as diabetes, obesity, heart disease, and cancer, which are the major causes of death in our nation. In the United States today, 13 million people have diabetes, and a disproportionate number of these cases are in minorities and women.[4] One in every four adults is obese; approximately 7 million people suffer from heart disease;[1] and one third of cancer cases can be attributed to dietary and nutritional factors.[5]

Then why do people choose to eat this way? Most of us want to eat a healthy diet.[6] In a recent survey of adults in the United States, 54% of individuals surveyed

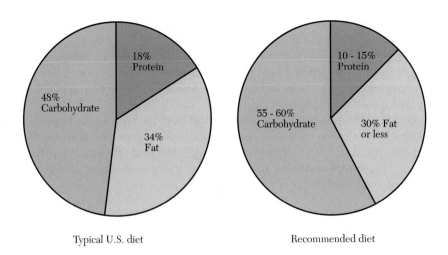

Typical U.S. diet

Recommended diet

FIGURE 1-2
The typical American diet contains more fat and less carbohydrate than is recommended.

said eating a healthy diet was important to them; however, only 37% of these said they were careful to choose a balanced nutritious diet.[6] The reasons for this are varied. Thirty-nine percent of those surveyed said they didn't want to give up the foods they liked. Twenty-two percent said it took too much time to eat well, and others said they ate in restaurants too often to choose a healthy diet. Many said they didn't know what was good for them, and others said they didn't know enough about the composition of foods to choose a healthy diet.

WHAT INFLUENCES OUR FOOD CHOICES?

The food choices we make affect our nutritional health, but nutrition is not the only factor determining food choice. What is available to us, where we live, what is within our budget and compatible with our lifestyle, what we like, what is culturally acceptable, as well as what we think we should eat all affect our choices and food intake.

Availability The availability of food is affected by geography, socioeconomics, and health status. In some parts of the world, the foods consumed are limited to those produced locally. Survival depends on making the correct choices from a limited selection of foods. Nutrients that are lacking in local foods will be lacking in the population's diet. In developed nations, the ability to store, transport, and process food allows year-round access to seasonal foods and foods grown and produced at distant locations. Grocery stores stock thousands of items from all over the world. Pasta from Italy and chocolates from Switzerland are processed and packaged for sale in North America. Mexican, Chinese, and Japanese foods can be found in Denver and Toronto. Pacific salmon is available in Iowa, and Chilean grapes are sold in Wyoming grocery stores (Figure 1-3). We can make varied food choices, and if we are concerned about the nutrient content of our diet, we can take vitamin and mineral supplements.

Even if foods are available in the store, it doesn't mean that they are available to all individuals. Socioeconomic factors such as income level, living conditions, education, and lifestyle affect the types and amounts of foods that are available. Individuals living in poverty can choose only the types and amounts of foods that they can afford. Access to transportation can determine which grocery stores are available and how much food can be transported at one time. The availability of food storage and cooking facilities determines what foods can be stored and prepared at home. Knowledge of cooking and menu planning can also affect what

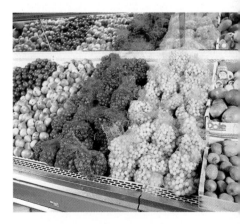

FIGURE 1-3
Modern processing and transportation allow foods from around the world to be available in local grocery stores. (Charles D. Winters)

foods are available. For example, if you don't know how to plan or cook a meal, you are limited to prepared meals and restaurants. Busy lifestyles and full schedules also affect the foods available to choose from. For example, individuals who travel for a living are often forced to eat in restaurants several times a day. Individuals with jobs and families and little time to cook must select foods that can be prepared quickly and simply.

Health status also dictates the availability of food. People who can't carry heavy packages are limited in what they can purchase. People with food allergies, digestive problems, and dental disease are limited in the foods they can consider for consumption. People following special diets for disease conditions are limited to foods that meet their dietary prescriptions.

Personal and Sociocultural Factors   Availability affects the foods we have to choose from; but individual palates and convictions determine what we actually consume, and tradition and social values may dictate what foods we consider appropriate. Personal preferences for taste, smell, appearance, and texture affect which foods we select. Presentation and packaging can also affect food choices. If a food doesn't appeal to us, we won't eat it, and if we like it, it is difficult to eliminate from the diet. This is demonstrated by the fact that not liking healthy foods is the number one reason people give for not choosing a healthier diet.[6]

Food preferences and eating habits are learned as part of each individual's cultural, national, and social background. They are among the oldest and most entrenched features of every culture.[7] An individual of Asian descent may consider rice the focus of the meal, whereas Italians may build a meal around pasta. The foods we are exposed to as children influence what foods we buy and cook as adults. We grow up eating turkey on Thanksgiving, eggs on Easter, or tamales at Christmas time. Religious background also affects food intake: Seventh-Day Adventists are vegetarians; Jews and Moslems do not eat pork. Even for those who choose not to observe religious dietary rules, habit may dictate many meal-time decisions. Jewish kosher laws prohibit the consumption of meat and milk in the same meal. Even Jews who do not follow kosher law may not serve milk at dinner because they never had it as children.

Food is a focus for social interaction and may be a determinant of social acceptance. Peer pressure exerts a tremendous influence on what foods we choose. For an adolescent, stopping for a cheeseburger or taco after school can be the basis for acceptance by one's peers. If all of your peers are choosing fish and chicken, you may not select the 16-ounce steak that you really want. These pressures change as society's values change and can influence food choices.

What We Think We Should Eat   Our attitudes about what foods we think are good for us also affect what we choose. We think that low fat is healthy for our hearts, high fiber protects us from cancer, eating less helps us live longer, antioxidants keep us young . . . . The health and nutrition information that shapes our attitudes about what we should and should not eat comes to us in a variety of ways. Some nutrition information comes from individual contact with physicians or nutrition professionals, some is printed on food labels and in educational pamphlets, but much of it reaches us through television, radio, newspapers, and magazines.

Government Agencies   In the interest of public health, many government agencies make recommendations regarding healthy dietary practices. These include recommendations on the amounts of specific nutrients needed to avoid nutrient deficiencies, guidelines on choosing a diet to avoid nutrient excesses, and recommendations on food safety. These recommendations are published in pamphlets and brochures as well as incorporated into food-labeling regulations.

The Power of the Media   Mass media are very powerful tools in promoting health and nutrition messages. Information that would take individual health-care workers years to disseminate can reach millions of individuals in a matter of hours or days. However, using the mass media to promote nutrition messages can also be misleading. Magazines and newspapers are trying to present stories that will sell subscriptions, and television news programs are interested in improving their ratings. Because of these motives, information may be reported prematurely or with a different emphasis than was intended by the scientists who did the research (Figure 1-4).

Food Marketing and Advertising   When nutrition and health information originates from food manufacturers it is in the form of marketing and advertising. Food manufacturers will often key in on research discoveries and use them to sell existing products or target new ones. This promotional information can be confusing to the consumer, who may not know what to believe. For instance, in the 1980s, oat bran, a high-fiber product, was headlined by the media as a preventive of high blood cholesterol levels and heart disease. In response, food manufacturers produced and advertised products containing oat bran, and consumers emphasized oat bran in their diets. They bought oat bran muffins, sprinkled oat bran onto their cereals, and ate oatmeal. Over a two-year period, the touted cholesterol-lowering properties of oat bran boosted breakfast cereals to a $7.5 billion industry. Then, a report that oat bran was ineffective at lowering blood cholesterol hit the news. The oat bran bubble burst, and every evening news network featured the story. The scientific reality is that many studies have shown that oat bran can be helpful in lowering cholesterol. However, it is not a cure-all. Reports on both the benefits and the lack of benefits of oat bran have been exaggerated. The fiber in oat bran is an important dietary component needed to ensure health, but it is not the only dietary component needed for good health. This kind of contradictory information bombards us daily, making it difficult to know which choices are healthy and which are not.

   In order to make wise food choices, whether you want to reduce your consumption of animal products, lower your fat intake, lose a few pounds, optimize your athletic performance, or simply consume a diet of safe, nutritious foods, it is necessary to understand the principles of nutrition. (See *Off the Shelf*: Do We Have Too Many Choices?)

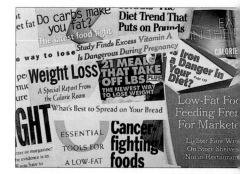

FIGURE I-4
Nutrition information often makes the headlines but does not always provide an accurate presentation of new discoveries. (Dennis Drenner)

WHAT IS NUTRITION?

Nutrition is more than just the food we choose to eat. It is a science that encompasses all the interactions that occur between living organisms and food. These interactions include the physiological processes by which an organism ingests, digests, absorbs, transports, and uses food. Nutrition includes the biological actions and interactions of food with the body and their consequences for health and disease. It also includes the psychological, social, cultural, economic, and technological factors that influence which foods we choose to eat. The biological importance of food is dictated by the nutrients it contains.

Nutrition–A science that studies the interactions that occur between living organisms and food.

WHAT ARE NUTRIENTS?

Nutrients are substances in food that are required by the body for growth, maintenance, and reproduction. They provide energy, contribute to structure, and regulate biological processes. To date, approximately 45 nutrients are considered essential to human life. There are many ways to classify nutrients—by their

Nutrients–Chemical substances in foods that provide energy, structure, and regulation of body processes.

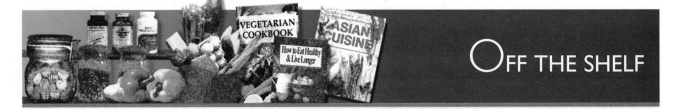

OFF THE SHELF

Do We Have Too Many Choices?

Availability is not a problem for most of modern America. The variety of foods, diet and nutrition information, and nutritional supplements available off the shelves of grocery stores, bookstores, and drug stores is staggering. Choosing from this supply can be challenging. Would we be better off without all these choices?

A modern supermarket may carry 15,000 different items.[1] Some are fresh, some are canned, some come in boxes and bags, and some are frozen. Some items are complete meals, some are main courses, and some are appetizers or desserts. For those with concerns about pesticide residues, the use of drugs in the meat and poultry industry, or the safety of chemicals used in processed foods, you can choose "natural" and "organic" foods. In the fresh produce section you can choose peas, carrots, and broccoli, or you can buy cherimoya, chayote, and bok choy. Many of these foods have names we can't pronounce and are prepared and used in ways that are not familiar to us.

For those who want to go beyond peas and carrots, cookbooks abound. They teach you how to make Indian, Chinese, Vietnamese, Thai, Italian, Mexican, and Japanese food. If you are interested in changing your eating habits, there are hundreds of diet books that purport to help you lose weight, lower your cholesterol, and even live longer. In addition to the nutrition information in books, newspapers, magazines, and on television, there are also computer programs available for diet planning and diet analysis, and a wealth of information is appearing through the Internet.

If you are concerned about getting enough nutrients from your food, supermarkets, drug stores, and health-food stores offer a wide selection of conventional and unconventional nutritional supplements. About half of all adults in the United States take some kind of vitamin or mineral supplement and over a quarter take some kind of supplement daily. A review of the market showed that there are about 3400 types of vitamin and mineral supplements to choose from.[2]

Is all this too much? Too many foods, too much information, too many decisions? For one individual, yes; but for the population as a whole, this variety is necessary. This sea of availability must exist to satisfy the diverse needs and desires of the population as a whole. Our population is made up of Native Americans, African Americans, people of Asian descent, Hispanic descent, people whose family came from India, Japan, Indonesia, Vietnam, Thailand, Italy, and every other country and culture around the world. There are people who are old, young, middle-aged, people with food allergies, heart disease, diabetes, and a host of other special needs. To meet the needs of this diverse population, foods from around the world, foods produced and packaged in many ways, information on diet and food preparation, and even nutritional supplements are necessary. To meet your individual needs, you must have a knowledge of your personal nutritional status and the ability to choose from this sea of availability.

[1] *Standards and Labeling Policy Book.* Washington, DC: U.S. Department of Agriculture, Standards and Labeling Division, 1990.

[2] American Dietetic Association Position of the American Dietetic Association. Vitamin mineral supplementation. J. Am. Diet. Assoc. 96:73–77, 1996.

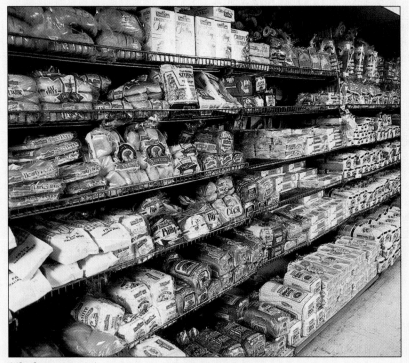

(Charles D. Winters)

essentiality, by their chemistry, by whether they provide energy, by the amounts required to meet needs. **Essential nutrients** are those substances that must be supplied in the diet because they either cannot be made by the body or cannot be made in large enough quantities to meet needs. Food also contains many substances classified as nonessential. Some have health-promoting properties. For example, sulforaphane found in broccoli may reduce the risk of cancer. Others can be produced in sufficient amounts by the body. For example, Lecithin, which is needed for nerve function, is not an essential nutrient because it can be made in the body from other substances.

Chemically, there are six classes of nutrients: carbohydrates, lipids, proteins, water, vitamins, and minerals. Carbohydrates, lipids, and proteins provide energy to the body and along with water constitute the major portion of most foods. These are referred to as **macronutrients** because they are required in relatively large amounts ("macro" means large). Their requirements are measured in kilograms (kg) or grams (g) (see Table 1-1 and the back cover for metric conversions). Alcohol also provides energy but is not considered a nutrient because it can interfere with body functions like growth, maintenance, and reproduction.

Carbohydrates include sugars such as those in table sugar, fruit, and milk, and starches such as those in vegetables and grains. Sugars are the simplest form of carbohydrate, and starches are more complex carbohydrates made of many sugars linked together. Carbohydrates provide a readily available source of energy to the body. Fiber is also a form of carbohydrate. It cannot be completely broken down by the body, so it provides little energy. However, it is important for gastrointestinal health. Fiber is found in vegetables, fruits, and whole grains.

Lipids, commonly referred to as fats, provide a storage form of energy. Most lipids contain fatty acids, some of which are essential in the diet. Lipids in our diets come from foods that naturally contain fats, such as meat and whole milk, and from processed fats, such as vegetable oils and butter that we add to food.

Proteins, such as those in meat, milk, grains, and legumes, are needed for growth and maintenance of body structures and regulation of body processes. Protein is made up of units called amino acids. Some amino acids can be made

Essential nutrients–Nutrients that must be provided in the diet because the body either cannot make them or cannot make them in sufficient quantities to satisfy its needs.

Macronutrients–Nutrients needed by the body in large amounts. These include water, carbohydrates, lipids, and proteins.

TABLE I-1 Measures Used in Nutrition

Metric	English
Measures of weight	
1 kilogram (kg) = 1000 grams (g)	= 2.2 pounds (lb)
454 grams	= 1 pound = 16 ounces (oz)
28.4 grams	= 1 ounce
5 grams of sugar or salt	= about 1 teaspoon (tsp)
1 gram = 1000 milligrams (mg)	
1 milligram = 1000 micrograms (μg or mcg)	
Measures of volume	
1 liter = 1000 milliliters (ml)	= approximately 1 quart (qt) = 4 cups
240 milliliters	= 1 cup = 8 oz
5 milliliters	= 1 teaspoon
15 milliliters	= 1 tablespoon (Tbsp) = 3 teaspoons
Measures of length	
1 meter (m) = 100 centimeters (cm) = 1000 millimeters (mm)	= 39.4 inches (in.) = 1.09 yards (yd)
2.54 centimeters	= 1 inch

FIGURE 1-5
Starches are made of sugars linked together; most lipid such as the triglyceride shown here contain fatty acids; and proteins are made of amino acids linked together. (Photographs, Charles D. Winters)

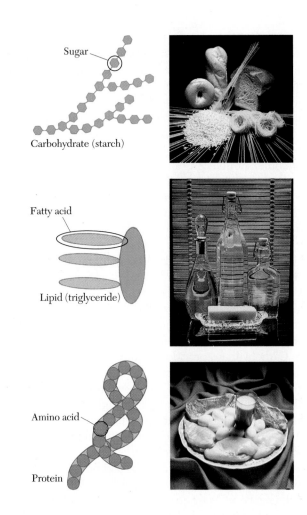

Sugar

Carbohydrate (starch)

Fatty acid

Lipid (triglyceride)

Amino acid

Protein

by the body, and others are essential in the diet. Dietary protein must meet the need for the essential amino acids (Figure 1-5).

Water is a nutrient in a class by itself. Water makes up about 60% of the human body and is required in kilogram amounts in the diet. It is a macronutrient that doesn't provide energy. Water serves many functions in the body, including acting as a lubricant, a transport medium, and a regulator of body temperature.

Vitamins and minerals are classified as **micronutrients** because they are needed in small amounts in the diet ("micro" means small). The amounts required are expressed in milligrams (1 mg = 1/1000 g) or micrograms (1 μg [mcg] = 1/1,000,000 g). They provide no energy, but many help regulate the production of energy from carbohydrate, lipid, and protein. Vitamins and minerals are found in most of the foods we eat. Fresh foods are generally the best sources of vitamins and minerals because storage, processing, and cooking often result in losses. However, many foods are high in micronutrients because they are added to food during processing. For example, breakfast cereals are a good source of iron because it is added during manufacture. Vitamin and mineral supplements are also a source of micronutrients in today's diet.

Micronutrients–Nutrients needed by the body in small amounts. These include vitamins and minerals.

WHAT DO NUTRIENTS DO?

Together, the macronutrients and micronutrients perform three basic functions: energy, structure, and regulation, which are needed for growth, maintenance, and reproduction. Nutrients provide the energy that is required to maintain life. If more energy is consumed than is needed, the extra is stored as body fat. If less energy is consumed than is needed, the body will burn its own fat as well as

TABLE I-2	Energy Content of Carbohydrate, Protein, Lipid, and Alcohol	
	Kcalories/gram	**Kjoules/gram**
Carbohydrate	4	16.7
Protein	4	16.7
Lipid	9	37.6
Alcohol	7	29.3

carbohydrate and protein to meet its energy needs. The energy needed for all body processes and activities is measured in **kilocalories** (abbreviated as *kcalories* or *kcals*) or in **kilojoules** (abbreviated as *kjoules*). The more common term "calorie" is technically 1/1000 of a kilocalorie, but when spelled with a capital "C" it is equivalent to a kilocalorie. For instance, the term "Calories" on food labels actually refers to kilocalories. One gram of carbohydrate or protein provides 4 kcalories. One gram of fat provides 9 kcalories. Alcohol contributes about 7 kcalories per gram (Table 1-2).

Nutrients are also needed for the formation and maintenance of body structures. Water, proteins, lipids, and minerals are important structural nutrients. For example, muscle is made up primarily of protein and water, and bone is composed of a protein core embedded with minerals. Nutrients also regulate biochemical reactions in the living body. Together all of the reactions that occur in the body are referred to as **metabolism**. Metabolic processes must be regulated to maintain a constant environment inside the body, referred to as **homeostasis**. Vitamins, minerals, water, and protein are important regulatory nutrients. For example, water helps to regulate body temperature. When body temperature increases, water lost through sweat helps to cool the body. Protein, vitamins, and minerals help to speed up or slow down the reactions of metabolism (see Table 1-3 for further examples).

Kilocalorie–A unit of heat that is used to express the amount of energy provided by foods.
Kilojoule–A measure of work that can be used to express energy intake and energy output. 4.18 kjoules = 1 kcalorie.

Metabolism–The sum of all the chemical reactions that take place in a living organism.
Homeostasis–The capacity to maintain a stable internal body environment.

TABLE I-3	Examples of How Nutrients Function in the Body	
Function	**Nutrient**	**Example**
Energy	Carbohydrate	Blood glucose is a carbohydrate that fuels body cells.
	Lipid	Fat is the most plentiful source of stored fuel in the body.
	Protein	Protein consumed in excess of protein needs will be used for energy.
Structure	Lipid	The membranes that surround each cell are primarily lipid.
	Protein	Connective tissue protein holds bones together and holds muscles to bones.
	Minerals	The minerals calcium and phosphorus make teeth and bones hard.
Regulation	Lipid	Estrogen is a lipid hormone that helps regulate the reproductive cycle in women.
	Protein	Transferrin is a protein that helps regulate iron transport.
	Water	Water lost as sweat helps cool the body to regulate body temperature.
	Vitamins	B vitamins regulate the use of macronutrients for energy.
	Minerals	Sodium helps regulate blood pressure.

HOW MUCH OF EACH NUTRIENT DO WE NEED?

To support life and maintain health nutrients must be supplied in the appropriate amounts and combinations. The amount of each nutrient needed by the body depends on the nutrient's function as well as on the needs of the individual. The amount an individual requires depends on many factors, including age, sex, body size, health status, and activity level. Both deficiencies and excesses of nutrients can affect health either in the short term or over a lifetime.

Effects of Too Little or Too Much   Conditions resulting from either too much or too little of one or more nutrients are referred to as **malnutrition** (Figure 1-6). We usually think of malnutrition as **undernutrition**, a deficiency of nutrients. Starvation, the most severe form of undernutrition, is a deficiency of energy that causes weight loss, poor growth, the inability to reproduce, and if severe enough, death. Deficiencies of specific nutrients also cause undernutrition. The symptoms of specific nutrient deficiencies often reflect the body functions that rely on the deficient nutrients. For example, vitamin A is necessary for vision; a deficiency of vitamin A can result in blindness.

Nutrient deficiencies may occur due to increased nutrient requirements, a deficient intake, or an inability to absorb or use nutrients. Young children and adolescents are at risk for iron deficiency because their rapid growth increases their need for iron. Individuals who consume a strict vegetarian diet with no animal products are at risk for vitamin B_{12} deficiency because the vitamin is primarily found in animal foods. Older adults are at risk for vitamin B_{12} deficiency because changes in the stomach that often occur with age decrease vitamin B_{12} absorption.

Overnutrition, an excess of nutrients, is also a form of malnutrition. When food is consumed in excess of energy need, the extra is stored as body fat. Some fat is necessary to insulate the body and store energy, but an excess of body fat, called obesity, increases the risk for many chronic diseases such as high blood pressure, heart disease, and diabetes. When excesses of specific nutrients are consumed, an adverse or **toxic** reaction may occur. For example, a large dose of vitamin A can cause liver, kidney, and bone damage. Nutrient toxicities rarely occur as a result of food consumption because most foods do not contain extremely large amounts of vitamins and minerals. In some rare cases, a toxic level of a nutrient can be obtained from food. For instance, polar bear liver, which has been consumed by Arctic explorers, is extremely high in vitamin A and can cause toxic reactions. Nutrient toxicities result more frequently from the overconsumption of vitamin and mineral supplements than from foods.

Malnutrition–Poor nutritional status resulting from a dietary intake either above or below that which is optimal.
Undernutrition–Poor nutritional status resulting from a dietary intake below that which meets nutritional needs.

Overnutrition–Poor nutritional status resulting from a dietary intake in excess of that which is optimal for health.

Toxic–The capacity to produce injury at some level of intake.

FIGURE 1-6
Malnutrition includes both undernutrition and overnutrition. (Left, Gamma Liaison/Camera Pix. Right, © Van Bucher/Photo Researchers, Inc.)

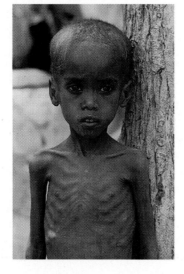
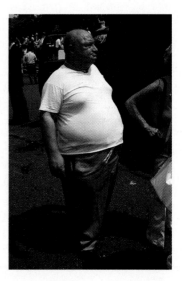

Short- and Long-Term Effects of Poor Nutrition   The symptoms of a nutritional excess or deficiency may appear rapidly or take a lifetime to develop. Both short-term and long-term nutritional effects have important health implications. For example, the symptoms associated with a lack of water occur rapidly. An athlete exercising in hot weather may become dehydrated in a matter of hours, developing symptoms such as headache and dizziness. Drinking water relieves the symptoms as rapidly as they appeared. The effects of other nutritional imbalances may take weeks or months to manifest themselves. For example, consumption of an iron-deficient diet for weeks or months will cause iron deficiency anemia and its symptoms of irritability and fatigue. An excess or deficiency of energy is another nutritional imbalance that takes a long time to manifest. When excess energy is consumed, body fat is deposited, but it may take months before a significant amount of weight is gained. Likewise, as anyone who has tried to lose weight knows, it can take months of consuming less energy to use up the excess fat.

Recently, nutritional effects that occur over a much longer time have become an important health focus. An individual's nutrient intake today may affect the development of cancer or heart disease 20, 30, or 40 years from now. The effects of nutrition on the development of chronic disease are difficult to determine because other variables or **risk factors**, such as age, heredity, and gender, are also often involved. Nutrition, however, has received a great deal of attention because it, along with smoking and exercise, is a lifestyle variable that individuals can change to decrease their risk of developing chronic disease.

Risk factor–A characteristic or circumstance that is associated with the occurrence of a particular disease.

ASSESSING OUR NUTRITIONAL HEALTH

The science of nutrition has developed a body of knowledge on the types and amounts of nutrients needed to maintain the health of the human population. However, nutritional health doesn't come from knowledge alone; it comes from the consumption of the right combination of foods in appropriate amounts. The term **nutritional status** is used to describe health condition as influenced by the intake and use of nutrients.[8] Group or individual nutritional status can be assessed for the purpose of identifying nutritional needs and goals and planning personal health care or community programs to meet these goals.

Nutritional status–The health of an individual as it is influenced by the intake and utilization of nutrients.

THE NUTRITIONAL HEALTH OF THE POPULATION

We know that there is enough food available in the United States to meet the needs of the population. We also know that poor nutritional choices from this food supply result in diets high in some nutrients and low in others. This kind of information is obtained by monitoring what foods are available and what is consumed. In the United States, the National Nutrition Monitoring and Related Research Program is responsible for providing an ongoing description of nutrition conditions in the population of the United States by collecting information about food availability and consumption; knowledge, attitudes, and behavior as they relate to food; food composition; and the health and nutritional status of the population.[9] This information is used for the purpose of planning nutrition-related policies and programs and predicting future trends of public health importance.

Monitoring the Food Supply   The amount of food available for consumption by the population is estimated using food disappearance surveys. Available food includes all that is grown, manufactured, or imported for sale in the country. Measuring what food is sold, or food disappearance from the food supply, gives

FIGURE 1-7
Food disappearance studies estimate food use by measuring what is available to the population. It doesn't account for losses that occur between production and consumption.

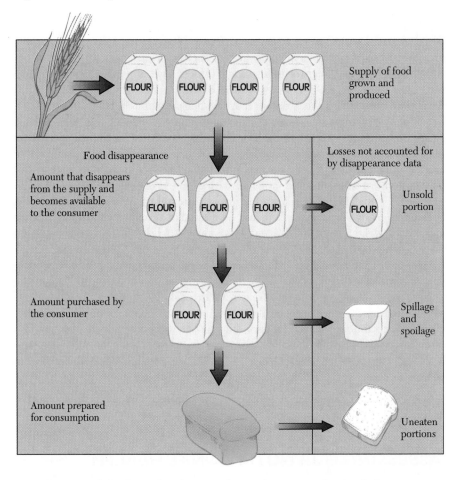

an indication of food use by the population (Figure 1-7). Food disappearance surveys estimate what is available to the population, provide year-to-year comparisons, and identify trends in the diet; but they tend to overestimate actual intake because they do not consider losses that occur during processing, marketing, and home use. Also, they do not assess food distribution throughout the population.

Monitoring Our Nutritional Status The nutritional status of the population is monitored by examining and comparing trends in food intake and health. This is done by interviewing individuals from within the population to determine what food is actually consumed, and collecting information on health and nutritional attitudes and status. One series of surveys conducted by the U.S. Department of Agriculture (USDA) is the Nationwide Food Consumption Surveys (NFCS), which collect information on the use of foods by households. The USDA also conducts the Continuing Surveys of Food Intakes of Individuals (CSFII), which collect data on intakes of individuals within households. Together, these monitor the adequacy of food and nutrient intake by the population. The Department of Health and Human Services conducts the National Health and Nutrition Examination Survey (NHANES), which combines information on food consumption with medical histories, physical examinations, and laboratory measurements to monitor both nutritional and health information. Data from the most recent survey, NHANES III, is currently being used to assess the nation's nutritional health.[9]

INDIVIDUAL NUTRITIONAL HEALTH

What is your nutritional status? Are you losing weight? Gaining weight? Do you have symptoms of a deficiency? Do you have a history of heart disease in your

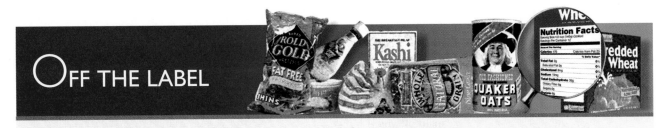

OFF THE LABEL

Know What You Are Choosing

Food labels are an important source of information for consumers. They let you know the nutrient content of foods as you are making choices. Food labels are also an important advertising tool for manufacturers. Products with eye-catching banners and headlines sell better. Although food labels must conform to federal guidelines and use standard definitions for most terms, they can still be misleading. Understanding food labels will help you know what you are choosing and how it fits into your diet.

The first thing that may catch your eye when shopping is a large print banner describing some nutritious feature of the product. Fat-free, high-fiber, and low-salt are all current big sellers. In order to carry these banners, foods must conform to the definitions of these terms. However, these descriptors highlight individual nutrients, and just as no single food determines the healthfulness of a diet, no single nutrient makes a food good or bad for you. Chocolate cookies labeled fat-free may not be your best choice if you are trying to reduce your sugar intake.

"Healthy" is an attractive byline that applies to more than a single nutrient. It implies that the product is wholesome and nutritious. In fact, to use the term "healthy" a food must be low in fat and saturated fat, contain no more than 480 mg of sodium and 60 mg of cholesterol per serving, and be a good source of one or more important nutrients. While all of these qualities are part of a healthy diet, foods that fit this definition are not necessarily the basis for a healthy diet. For instance, fat-free brownies fit the definition of healthy. They are low in fat, saturated fat, cholesterol, and sodium, and supply 10% of the recommended intake for iron. But they are only a good choice in limited quantities because they are not a nutrient-dense food—they are high in sugar and contain few other nutrients. Likewise, a food that doesn't meet the definition of healthy is not necessarily a poor choice. Vegetable soup, for example, contains more sodium than the definition of healthy will allow, but if the rest of the diet is not high in sodium, the soup can be a healthy choice.

Enticing product names can also be misleading. However, unless you have memorized the USDA and Food and Drug Administration (FDA) labeling regulations you can't tell exactly what you are buying. These standards determine how much beef is in a beef enchilada, how much chicken is in chicken soup, and how much fruit is in a Fruit Roll-Up. Product names must comply with legal definitions, but they don't have to make sense to consumers. For example, "lasagna with meat sauce" must be 6% meat, but "lasagna with meat *and* sauce" must be 12% meat.

To get the whole picture, you need to look beyond the headlines of the label. Since the nutrient content of foods must be listed, as well as information on how a food fits into the diet as a whole, reading beyond the banner will provide you with the information you need to make wise choices. (See Chapter 2 for more information on how to read food labels.)

---

family? Are you at risk for a deficiency because you can't get to the store or can't afford to buy food or you don't know what to eat or cook? An individual's nutritional status can be evaluated by an individual **nutritional assessment**. This requires a review of past and present dietary intake; assessment of medical history and clinical status; and laboratory measurements.

Estimating Dietary Intake   The first step in determining nutritional status is to evaluate an individual's typical dietary intake. This is done by having that person either record his current consumption or recall what was eaten previously. These techniques are not ideal, since they rely on the memory and reliability of the individual. For instance, overweight persons tend to report less food than is actually eaten, whereas underweight individuals tend to report more. Despite this problem, these commonly used methods are the best tools available for evaluating dietary intake to predict nutrient deficiencies or excesses.

Nutritional assessment—The process of determining the nutritional status of individuals or groups for the purpose of identifying nutritional needs and planning personal health care or community programs to meet these needs.

24-Hour Recall The most common method of assessing dietary intake is a 24-hour recall in which a trained interviewer asks individuals to recall exactly what they ate during the preceding 24-hour period. Detailed descriptions of all food and drink, including descriptions of cooking methods and brand names of products, are elicited from the individuals. Since food intake varies from day to day, repeated 24-hour recalls on the same individuals provides a more accurate estimate of typical intake.[8]

Food Diary or Food-Intake Record A food diary is a record of all food and drink consumed during a defined period. Most commonly used are three-, four-, or seven-day food records that include at least one weekend day, since most people eat differently on weekends than during the school or work week. The record is kept by the individual as the foods are consumed and should include meals and snacks, brand names, and cooking methods. Food records may involve weighing all foods consumed or just estimating portion sizes[10] (Figure 1-8).

Food Frequency A food frequency questionnaire is designed to obtain information about typical food-consumption patterns. Individuals are asked how often they eat specific foods or categories of food; for example, "How often do you drink milk?" Responses are recorded as the number of times the food is consumed per day, week, or month. This doesn't recall a specific day's intake, but it gives a general picture of nutrient intake.

Diet History A diet history is a less clearly defined procedure that collects information about dietary habits and patterns. It may include a history of nutritional habits: Do you skip lunch? Did you drink milk as an adolescent? It may also include a combination of other methods such as a 24-hour recall along with a food frequency. The combination of two or more methods often provides more complete information than one method alone. For instance, if an individual's 24-hour recall does not include milk, but a food frequency questionnaire suggests that the individual typically drinks milk once a day, the two can be combined to provide a more accurate picture of this individual's typical intake.

Analyzing Nutrient Intake Once information on food intake has been obtained, the nutrient content of the diet can be evaluated. This can be done in a number of ways. To get a general picture of dietary intake, an individual's food record can be compared with a guide for diet planning such as the Food Guide Pyramid (see

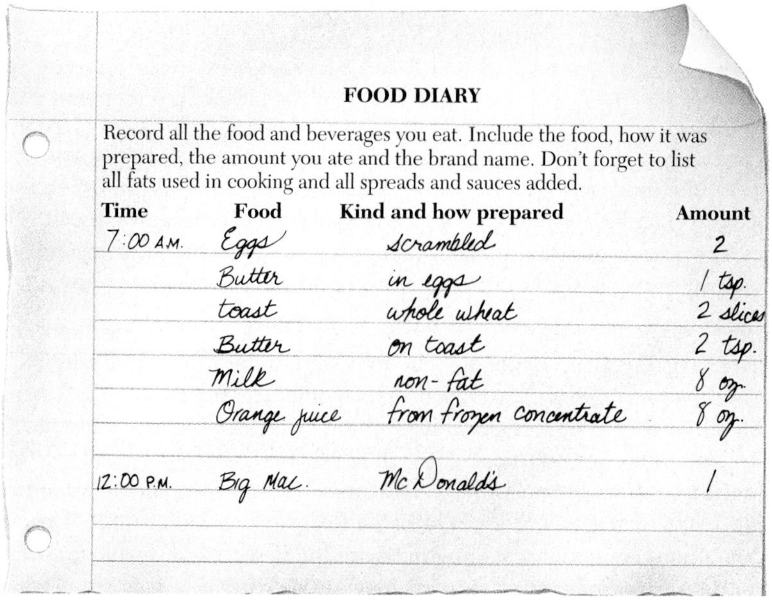

FIGURE 1-8
Accurate food diaries require the recording of all food and drink consumed.

FOOD DIARY

Record all the food and beverages you eat. Include the food, how it was prepared, the amount you ate and the brand name. Don't forget to list all fats used in cooking and all spreads and sauces added.

Time	Food	Kind and how prepared	Amount
7:00 A.M.	Eggs	Scrambled	2
	Butter	in eggs	1 tsp.
	toast	whole wheat	2 slices
	Butter	on toast	2 tsp.
	Milk	non-fat	8 oz.
	Orange juice	from frozen concentrate	8 oz.
12:00 P.M.	Big Mac	McDonald's	1

REFERENCES

1. *Healthy People 2000: National Health Promotion and Disease Prevention Objectives*. Washington, DC: U.S. Department of Health and Human Services, 1990.
2. Albertson, A.M. and Tobelmann, R.C. Consumption of grain and whole-grain products by an American population during 1900–1992. J. Am. Diet. Assoc. 95:703–704, 1995.
3. Crane, N.T., Lewis, C.J., and Yeltry, E.A. Do time trends in food supply levels of macronutrients reflect survey estimates of macronutrient intake? Am. J. Public Health 82:862–866, 1992.
4. Tinker, L.F. Diabetes mellitus—a priority health care issue for women. J. Am. Diet. Assoc. 94:976–985, 1994.
5. Diet and cancer: what can be done to reduce the carcinogenic effects of foods? Food Safety Notebook 4:47–48, 1993.
6. American Dietetic Association 1993 Survey of American Dietary Habits: Executive summary. Chicago: American Dietetic Association, 1993.
7. Pratt, E.L. Historical perspectives: food, feeding, and fancies. J. Am. Coll. Nutr. 3:115–121, 1984.
8. Gibson, R. *Principles of Nutritional Assessment*. New York: Oxford University Press, 1990.
9. Kuczmarski, M.F., Moshfegh, A., and Briefel, R. Update on nutrition monitoring activities in the United States. J. Am. Diet. Assoc. 94:753–760, 1994.
10. Poa, E.M. and Cypel, Y.S. Estimation of dietary intake. In *Present Knowledge in Nutrition*, 6th ed. Brown, M.L., ed. Washington, DC: International Life Sciences Institute—Nutrition Foundation, 1990, pp. 399–406.

Nutrition Science: The Basis for Nutrition Sense

CHAPTER CONCEPTS

1. Advances in the understanding of nutrition are made by using the scientific method. This involves making observations, formulating hypotheses, testing these by experimentation, and developing theories from the results.

2. Well-conducted experiments use controls to limit the variables tested, use the right group of subjects, and are carefully interpreted.

3. Judging nutrition claims involves applying the scientific method. Is the claim based on carefully designed experiments that are accurately interpreted and reported?

4. Many types of research are used in nutrition to study relationships among diet, health, and disease. Epidemiological observations can be used to formulate hypotheses. Laboratory studies are conducted to test hypotheses and develop theories.

5. The knowledge gained from nutrition research is used to establish dietary standards and guidelines for populations.

6. The Food Guide Pyramid and exchange lists are developed from dietary standards and guidelines and are used to help plan individual diets.

7. Food labels provide information on how foods fit into the diet as a whole.

JUST A TASTE

Is the nutrition information published in newspapers and magazines reliable?

If your diet doesn't meet the RDAs, will you develop a nutrient deficiency?

Is a diet that meets the serving recommendations of the Food Guide Pyramid necessarily low in fat?

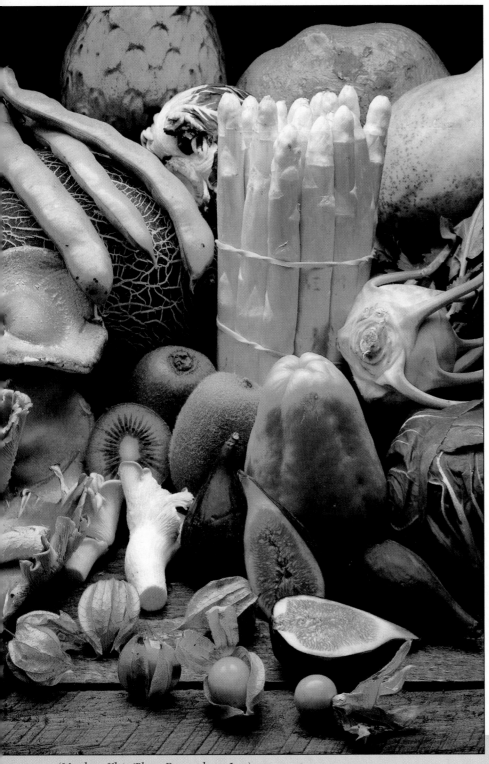

(*Matthew Klein/Photo Researchers, Inc.*)

CHAPTER **2**

To early humans, nutrition was not science—it was survival. The food that was available provided their nutrients, but food choices were limited and the safety and healthfulness of food were determined by trial and error. Today, we still need to eat to survive, but rather than doing our hunting and gathering on prairies and hillsides, we do it in huge supermarkets where food choices seem infinite. The science of nutrition has been used to develop guidelines for the safety and healthfulness of food. We are bombarded with this information from government recommendations as well as from product advertisements and news reports. Some of what we hear is accurate and based on well-conducted experiments, but some of it is incorrect or exaggerated to sell products or make news headlines more enticing: Oat bran lowers cholesterol, beta-carotene prevents cancer, obesity is genetic, vitamin C cures the common cold, vitamin E slows aging. Some of it is hype. Some of it carries important health promotion information. Filtering out the worthless and understanding the worthwhile can be a mind-boggling task. Only an understanding of the process of science and how it is used to understand the relationship between nutrition and health will allow you to develop the nutrition sense needed to judge the validity of nutrition claims.

In this chapter, we will discuss:

- How are nutrition discoveries made?
- How are nutrition experiments translated into nutrition recommendations for the population?
- What nutrition tools are available to help you choose a better diet?

THE SCIENCE OF NUTRITION

The science of nutrition strives to understand the process by which the food we eat is used to provide energy, regulation, and structure to the human body. It is a multidisciplinary science that draws methods and concepts from biochemistry, physiology, chemistry, physics, and other sciences. Like all science, nutrition continues to develop as new discoveries provide clues to the right combination of nutrients needed for optimal health. As knowledge and technology advance, new nutrition principles are developed. Sometimes, established beliefs and concepts must give way to new ideas. Yesterday's truths can be difficult to unlearn. Some of the nutrition principles we follow today would have seemed ridiculous to our great grandparents and someday may be a source of humor to our great grandchildren. One hundred and fifty years ago, fresh fruits and vegetables were thought to cause cholera; today, their use is promoted to reduce the risk of disease. As knowledge advances, recommendations change. The public may find this frustrating because the experts seem to change their minds so often. One day you are told margarine is better for you than butter; the next day a report says that it is just as bad. Why does this happen? Do scientists make that many mistakes? Nutrition, like all science, is evolving. The process that allows concepts to be developed and to continually change with the advancement of knowledge is the **scientific method**.

Scientific method—The general approach of science that is used to explain observations about the world around us.

THE SCIENTIFIC METHOD

Advances in the science of nutrition occur by following the systematic unbiased approach of the scientific method to evaluate the relationships between food and health. The first step of the scientific method is to make an observation and ask questions about the observation. The next step is to propose an explanation for the observation. This explanation is called a **hypothesis**. Once a hypothesis has been proposed, experiments can be designed to test it. The experiments must provide objective results that can be measured and repeated. If the experimental results do not prove the hypothesis to be wrong, a **theory**, or a scientific explanation based on experimentation, can be established (Figure 2-1). The scientific

Hypothesis–An educated guess made to explain an observation or to answer a question.

Theory–An explanation based on scientific study and reasoning.

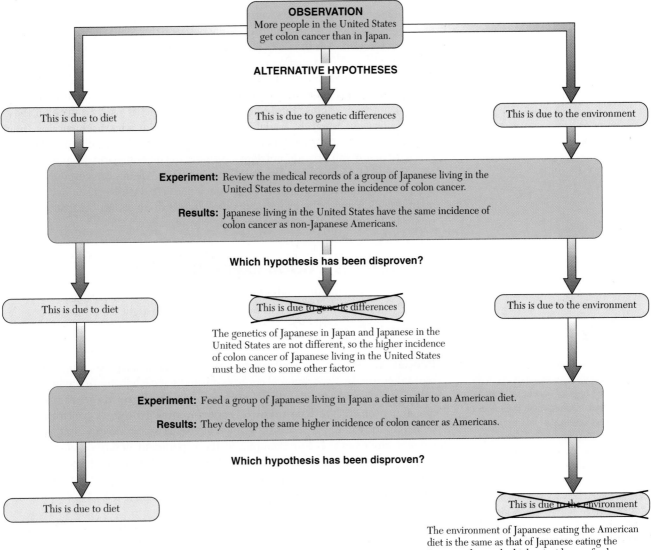

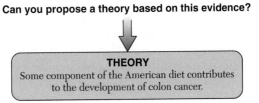

FIGURE 2-1

This example illustrates how the scientific method can be used to formulate hypotheses based on observations, design experiments to test these hypotheses, and interpret the results to support or disprove the hypotheses, helping establish a theory.

method dictates that we continue to view theories with skepticism. Thus a theory is accepted only as long as it cannot be disproved and continues to be supported by all new evidence that accumulates. Even a theory that has been accepted by the scientific community for years can be proved wrong. This flux allows the body of knowledge to increase, but it can be confusing as old theories give way to new ones.

The discovery of the relationship between nutrition and pellagra, a disease now known to be caused by a deficiency of the vitamin niacin, is an example of how the scientific method has been used in nutrition research. The events leading to this discovery began with the observation that prisoners suffered from pellagra, but their jailers did not. If pellagra was an infectious disease, both populations would be equally affected. The hypothesis proposed was that pellagra was due to a deficiency in the prisoners' diets. To test this hypothesis, nutritious foods such as fresh meats and vegetables were added to the diet of prisoners. The symptoms of pellagra disappeared, supporting the hypothesis that pellagra is due to a deficiency of something in the diet. This experiment and others led to the theory that pellagra is caused by a dietary deficiency. This theory, further developed by the discovery of the vitamin niacin, still holds today.

The same process of developing and testing hypotheses can be used to evaluate all nutrition claims. Information about experiments used to develop these claims, however, is rarely available. For example, the advertisement for Brain Power illustrated in Figure 2-2 claims that this product will revitalize and energize you, and that it will provide nutrients essential for mental clarity, memory retention, coordination, concentration, and stamina. These claims are certainly appealing, but are difficult to evaluate for accuracy because the advertisement provides no information about the experiments used to test these claims. Instead, the consumer is presented with information as if it were fact.

WHAT MAKES A GOOD EXPERIMENT?

Even when the scientific method is used, errors can occur if experiments are not carefully designed to include proper controls and the right experimental population, or if these experiments and their results are not properly interpreted.

Proper Controls   A well-conducted experiment must use proper **experimental controls**. Experimental controls ensure that each factor or **variable** studied can be compared with a known situation. **Control groups** act as a standard of comparison for the **treatment** or **experimental groups**. A control group is treated in the same way as the experimental groups except no experimental treatment is implemented. For example, in the experiment described above to test whether a change in diet would prevent pellagra, an appropriate control group would have been a group of prisoners whose diet did not change, and the experimental group would consist of those prisoners consuming fresh meats and vegetables in addition to the original prison diet.

A potential source of error in experiments is bias on the part of the experimental subjects or the investigators. For example, if a study were done to test the effect of Brain Power on memory, the experimental subjects receiving the supplement might believe that their memories were going to be improved by taking the supplement. This might cause them to concentrate more on a memory test and improve their scores. One way of avoiding this effect would be to create a control group with a **placebo**. This is a treatment that is identical in appearance to the actual treatment but has no therapeutic value. The use of a placebo prevents the subjects from knowing whether they are receiving the experimental treatment. When the subjects do not know which treatment they are receiving, the study is

Experimental controls–Factors included in an experimental design that limit the number of variables, allowing an investigator to examine the effect of only the parameters of interest.
Variable–A factor or condition that is changed in an experimental setting.
Control groups–Groups of participants in an experiment that are identical to the experimental group except that no experimental treatment is used. They are used as a basis of comparison.
Treatment or experimental groups–Groups of participants in an experiment who are subjected to an experimental treatment.

Placebo–A fake medicine or supplement that is indistinguishable in appearance from the real thing. It is used to disguise the control and experimental groups in an experiment.

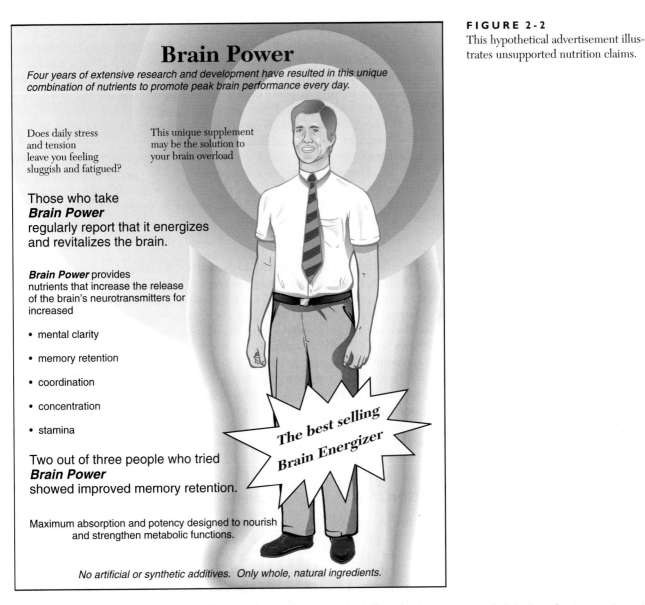

FIGURE 2-2
This hypothetical advertisement illustrates unsupported nutrition claims.

called a **single-blind study**. Errors can also occur if investigators allow their own desire for a specific result to affect the interpretation of the data. This type of error can be avoided by designing a **double-blind study**, in which neither the subjects nor the investigators know who is in which group until after the results have been analyzed. Blind studies help to prevent the expectations of subjects and investigators from biasing the results.

The Right Experimental Population   In addition to carefully using controls and controlling for bias, valid experiments must study the right population. Some studies of human nutrition use animals to model what may happen in people. As is discussed later, the right type of animal must be chosen in order to develop results that are meaningful in human nutrition. When studies are performed in humans, the right population must also be chosen. For example, if Brain Power claims to enhance memory in people with normal memories, it should be tested in that population. An improvement in memory in the normal group would indicate that normal memory had been enhanced, whereas an improvement in people with a memory disorder could mean that the supplement was reversing a disease process.

Single-blind study–An experiment in which either the study participants or the researchers are unaware of who is in a control or an experimental group.
Double-blind study–An experiment in which neither the study participants nor the researchers know who is in a control or an experimental group.

The number of subjects included in a study is also important. To be successful, an experiment must show that the treatment being tested causes a result to occur more frequently than it would occur by chance. Fewer subjects are needed to demonstrate an effect that rarely occurs by chance. For example, if only one person in a million can improve his score on a memory test by taking the test twice, then the experiment to see if Brain Power improves memory requires only a few subjects to demonstrate an effect. If one in four people can improve his scores by repeat testing, then many more subjects are needed. Statistical methods should be applied before a study is conducted to determine how many subjects are needed to show the effect of the experimental treatment. The number of subjects will depend on the type of study and the effect being tested. The fewer variables included in a study, the fewer experimental subjects needed to demonstrate an effect.

Interpretation of Experimental Results   In science, the interpretation of results is as important as the way studies are done. If Brain Power is tested in people with memory disorders, the results cannot claim that it will help people with normal memories. One way to ensure that experiments are correctly interpreted is to use a **peer-review** system. Most scientific journals require that reports of studies be reviewed by two or three experts in the field who did not take part in the research that is being evaluated. Before an article can be published in the journal, these scientists must agree that the experiments were well conducted and that the results were interpreted fairly. Nutrition articles can be found in peer-reviewed journals such as the *American Journal of Clinical Nutrition*, *Journal of Nutrition*, *Journal of the American Dietetic Association*, and *The New England Journal of Medicine*.

Peer-review–Review of the design and validity of a research experiment by experts in the field of study who did not participate in the research.

JUDGING NUTRITION CLAIMS

Every day we are presented with nutrition information that we use to make food choices. We get this information from many sources: health professionals, government guidelines, word of mouth, product advertisements, and news headlines. Some of this is valid information, some is slightly misinterpreted or exaggerated, and some is fraudulent. When deciding which information to believe, the first question to ask yourself is, Does the information make sense? (Table 2-1). Some claims are too outlandish to be true. If, for example, a weight-loss product claims that you can lose 20 pounds in one day with no exercise or change in food intake, common sense should tell you it is too good to be true.

If the claim seems reasonable, look to see where it came from. Was it a government recommendation, the result of a research study, or one person's opinion? Government recommendations are developed by committees of scientists who interpret the latest well-conducted research studies and use their conclusions to develop recommendations for the population as a whole. Research studies published in peer-reviewed journals are well scrutinized. But results presented at conferences or published in popular magazines, although they may be legitimate, have not been scrutinized by the scientific community to determine their quality and validity. Claims that come from individual testimonies or opinions, referred to as **anecdotal**, have not been measured objectively.

If the source of the information seems reliable, then ask if the study was well designed and if the results were interpreted accurately. Even well-designed, carefully executed, peer-reviewed experiments can be a source of misinformation if the experimental results are interpreted incorrectly or if the implications of the results are exaggerated. For example, a study that shows that rats fed a diet high in vitamin E live longer than those consuming less vitamin E could be the basis

Anecdotal–Information based on a story of personal experience.

TABLE 2-1	Questions to Ask When Judging Nutrition Claims

1. Does the information make sense?
   Is it too outlandish to believe?
   Is it based on a cultural or religious belief?

2. Where did the information come from?
   Is it based on a government recommendation?
   Is it based on a study in a peer-reviewed journal?
   Is it based on the opinions of individuals?

3. Were the experiments well designed?
   Were proper controls used?
   Were enough study subjects used to get reliable results?
   Were the experimental results interpreted correctly?
   Was the importance of the study exaggerated?

4. Can the information be applied to humans?
   Was the study done in animals?
   Was the level of food or nutrient used compatible with amounts in a human diet?
   Could the result be extrapolated to human health?

5. Who stands to benefit from the information?
   Is it helping to sell a product?
   Is it making a magazine cover or newspaper headline more appealing?
   Is it designed to improve public health?

of the headline, "Vitamin E Supplements Increase Longevity." The fact that a diet high in vitamin E increased longevity does not mean that supplements will have the same effect. In addition, this study was done in rats. Can the result be extrapolated to human health? Just because rats consuming diets high in vitamin E live longer does not mean that the same is true for humans.

The final question in judging nutrition claims is, Who stands to benefit from the information? Is it helping to sell a product? If a claim such as "lose 20 pounds in one day with no exercise or change in food intake" is part of an advertisement to increase sales, the company stands to profit from your believing the claim. Is it making a magazine cover or newspaper headline more appealing? If a claim is part of a news headline, it may be true but exaggerated to sell newspapers and magazines. Is it designed to improve public health? Most public health bulletins do not directly sell products. They are designed to improve the health of the population and, if followed, may reduce health-care costs to taxpayers.

Using these steps (see Table 2-1) can help in deciding what information to believe and what to reconsider. If you are still not sure, check with a nutrition professional such as a registered dietitian or nutrition research scientist at a reputable institution (see Appendix D).

TYPES OF NUTRITION STUDIES

Nutrition research studies are done to determine nutrient requirements, to learn more about the metabolism of nutrients, and to understand the role of nutrition in health and disease. Perfect tools do not exist for addressing all these questions. However, many types of research can be useful, including epidemiological observations and a variety of types of laboratory studies.

Epidemiological Observations   **Epidemiology** is the study of patterns that occur within populations. In nutrition, epidemiological studies are used to suggest relationships between diet and health. For instance, epidemiology can be used to estimate nutrient needs by examining the typical intake of a nutrient in a healthy

Epidemiology—The study of the inter-relationships between health and disease and other factors in the environment or lifestyle of different populations.

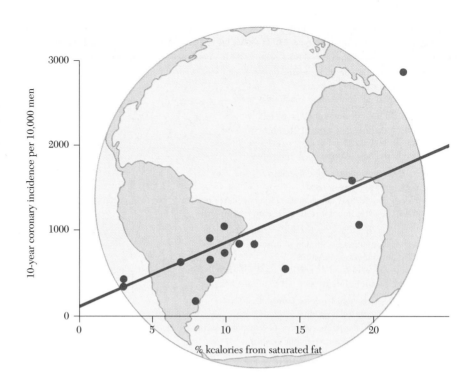

Cross-sectional data—Information obtained by a single broad sampling of many different individuals in a population.
Longitudinal data—Information obtained by repeatedly sampling the same individuals in a population over time.
Correlation—Two or more factors occurring together.

population. **Cross-sectional data** can be collected from a cross section of the population at one point in time or **longitudinal data** can be collected from the same group of individuals over a period of time.

Epidemiology does not determine cause and effect relationships—it just identifies patterns. For instance, epidemiology was used to identify the association, or **correlation**, between high-fat diets and heart disease by looking at the incidence of heart disease in different countries and then finding dietary factors that followed the same pattern (Figure 2-3). From the observation that populations with high dietary fat intakes also have high incidences of heart disease, one possible hypothesis is that a high intake of fat in the diet predisposes to cardiovascular disease. This hypothesis must then be tested by controlled laboratory studies.

Laboratory Studies   Laboratory nutrition studies are used to test hypotheses and verify relationships suggested by epidemiological and other observations. They may study nutrient requirements and functions in whole organisms, or they may focus on nutrient functions at the cellular level.

Depletion-repletion study—A study that feeds a diet devoid of a nutrient until signs of deficiency appear, and then adds the nutrient back to the diet to a level at which symptoms disappear.

Studies Using Whole Organisms   **Depletion-repletion studies** are a classic method for determining the requirement of a particular nutrient. They involve completely using up or depleting that nutrient by feeding a person or animal a diet devoid of that nutrient. After a period of time, if it is needed to maintain health, symptoms of a deficiency will develop. The nutrient is then added back to the diet, or repleted, until the symptoms are reversed. The requirement for that nutrient is determined by the amount needed to reverse the deficiency symptoms. The deficiency symptoms for a specific nutrient often reflect the functions of the nutrient, and the severity may vary when different amounts of a nutrient are consumed. For example, magnesium is needed for muscle contraction. Depletion of magnesium from the diet causes a lack of muscle coordination. When enough magnesium is again added to the diet, muscle control returns. The amount of magnesium needed to return muscle control to normal is concluded to be its requirement. Unfortunately, results from this type of study are often exaggerated to imply that if some of a nutrient is good, then more is better. For example, producers of magnesium supplements might claim that their product will improve

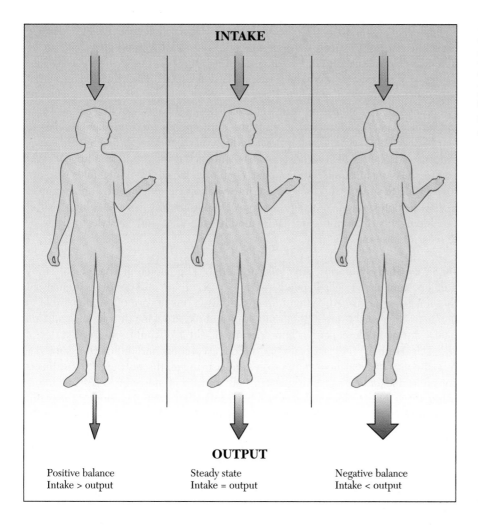

INTAKE

OUTPUT

Positive balance
Intake > output

Steady state
Intake = output

Negative balance
Intake < output

FIGURE 2-4
The concept of nutrient balance is illustrated here. If more of a nutrient is consumed than excreted, balance is positive; if the same amount is consumed and excreted, a steady state exists; and if less is consumed than excreted, balance is negative.

coordination. However, there are not sufficient data to make this claim. Magnesium supplements have been shown to improve coordination in individuals whose diet was deficient in magnesium, but not in individuals who are not suffering from a magnesium deficiency.

Another method for determining nutrient requirements is to compare the intake of a nutrient with its excretion. This type of study is known as a **balance study**. If more of a nutrient is consumed than is excreted, it is assumed that the nutrient is being used or stored by the body. If more of the nutrient is excreted than is consumed, some is being lost from body stores. When the amount consumed equals the amount lost, the body is neither gaining nor losing that nutrient and is said to be in a steady state, or in balance (Figure 2-4). By varying the amount of a nutrient consumed and then measuring the amount excreted, it is possible to determine the minimum amount of that nutrient needed to balance the body losses. This minimum amount is set as the requirement.

Balance study—A study that compares the total amount of a nutrient that enters the body with the total amount that leaves the body.

Studies Using Cells   Depletion-repletion and balance studies can estimate the nutrient requirements of an organism but tell little about nutrient function. To learn what nutrients do at the cellular level, biochemical and molecular biological techniques can be used to study cells extracted from humans or animals or grown in the laboratory. Biochemistry studies how nutrients are used for energy and how they regulate chemical reactions in cells. **Molecular biology** studies how **DNA (deoxyribonucleic acid)**, the genetic material in cells, dictates and regulates the functions of body cells. The types and amounts of nutrients available to cells can affect the action of DNA. Certain nutrients, such as vitamin A, can directly activate

Molecular biology—The study of cellular function at the molecular level.
DNA (deoxyribonucleic acid)—The genetic material that codes for the synthesis of proteins.

Gene—A length of DNA that provides instructions for heritable traits.

or inactivate segments of DNA called **genes**. Using molecular biology to study nutrition can help explain nutrient function and identify processes that can be influenced by inadequate or excessive nutrient supplies. For example, molecular biology can be used to study how vitamin A deficiency affects the destruction of the cornea of the eye.[1]

Knowledge gained from studying molecules and genes can be used to study nutrition-related conditions that affect the entire organism. For example, molecular biology helps us understand the hereditary basis of diseases like heart disease, cancer, and obesity. These advances are enhancing our understanding of diet-disease relationships and will someday enable us to identify individuals who are susceptible to specific diseases so that intervention can begin early. For example, if it were determined by analyzing your DNA that you were at a high risk of developing heart disease, you could modify your diet and lifestyle to delay or prevent disease onset.

When to Study Humans, Animals, or Cells The choice of whether to study humans, animals, or cells depends on time, cost, ethics, and the types of analyses that must be performed. When humans are used, results are often impossible to obtain in a reasonable amount of time. For example, studying the effect of calcium intake during adolescence on bone density in old age would require decades of research. Human studies are also costly for researchers and difficult for subjects. A well-controlled balance study involves measuring all the nutrients that subjects consume and collecting and analyzing all sources of nutrient losses, including urine, feces, sweat, sloughed skin and hair, and other body secretions. Study subjects must be housed under carefully controlled conditions for lengthy periods. Even if cost and time are not a limitation, ethically, studies that compromise the health of human subjects cannot be done. For example, much of what we know about the effects of starvation was determined during World War II by conducting depletion-repletion studies using conscientious objectors as experimental subjects. These subjects were monitored physically and psychologically while they were starved and then refed.

Today, the ethics of intentionally creating nutrient deficiencies in humans has been called into question. The federal government mandates that institutions conducting research on humans have committees of scientists and nonscientists review these studies before they are conducted. The committees are responsible for ensuring that the rights of the subjects are respected and that the risk of physical, social, and psychological injury is balanced against the potential benefit of the research. Ethics also limits the types of analyses that can be done. Analyses in humans are usually limited to measurement of nutrient levels in easily collected body fluids such as blood or to **noninvasive** measures such as blood pressure or body weight. When the determination of nutrient needs requires that the levels of a nutrient be measured in body tissue such as muscle or bone or that changes in nutrient content be observed in specific organs, animal studies can play an important role in understanding human nutrient metabolism and predicting human requirements.

Noninvasive—Methods that do not involve penetrating the body.

To effectively use animals to study human nutrient needs and functions, the type of animal must be carefully chosen. An ideal animal model is one about the same size as humans with similar metabolic and digestive processes. For example, cows are rarely used in human nutrition research because they digest their food in four stomach-like chambers as opposed to our single stomach. Pigs, on the other hand, are a good model because they digest food in a manner similar to that of humans. However, in addition to size and metabolism, factors such as cost and time must be considered. Pigs are expensive animals to use, and they take a long time to develop nutrient deficiencies. Because of these factors, smaller laboratory animals, such as rats and mice, are the most common experimental animals. They

Nutrition and Your Health:
Dietary Guidelines for Americans

Eat a variety of foods. Foods contain combinations of nutrients and other healthful substances. No single food can supply all nutrients in the amounts you need. Choose the recommended number of daily servings from each of the five food groups of the Food Guide Pyramid.

Balance the food you eat with physical activity; maintain or improve your weight. Being overweight and gaining weight as an adult are linked to high blood pressure, heart disease, stroke, diabetes, certain types of cancer, and other illnesses. Most adults should not gain weight and if you are overweight you should try to lose weight.

Choose a diet with plenty of grain products, vegetables, and fruits. These foods provide vitamins, minerals, complex carbohydrates, and other substances that are important for good health. They are low in fat and are associated with a lower risk of many chronic diseases including certain types of cancer.

Choose a diet low in fat, saturated fat, and cholesterol. Fat supplies energy and essential fatty acids, and promotes the absorption of fat soluble vitamins. However, high levels of saturated fat and cholesterol in the diet are linked to increased blood cholesterol and a greater risk of heart disease. Choose a diet that provides no more than 30 percent of total kcalories from fat.

Choose a diet moderate in sugars. Sugars occur naturally in many foods, including milk, fruits, and vegetables, that also supply other nutrients. Sugars added to food during processing add energy but no other essential nutrients. Both sugars and starch can promote tooth decay. Avoid excessive snacking and brush and floss teeth regularly.

Choose a diet moderate in salt and sodium. Salt and sodium are found mainly in processed and prepared foods. A high sodium intake is associated with high blood pressure. To reduce dietary sodium decrease the amount added in cooking and at the table and use the Nutrition Facts label to choose foods lower in sodium.

If you drink alcoholic beverages, do so in moderation. Alcoholic beverages supply kcalories but few or no nutrients. Alcohol alters judgment and can lead to dependency and other serious health problems including liver disease and birth defects.

FIGURE 2-7
The *Dietary Guidelines for Americans* promote healthful diets. (USDA, DHHS, 1995)

to the public. This rethinking has generated a variety of new dietary recommendations designed not only to prevent deficiencies but also to promote health and prevent chronic disease.

Dietary Goals and Guidelines   The first recommendation for health promotion rather than just deficiency prevention was the *Dietary Goals for the United States*, established in 1977 by the Senate Select Committee on Human Needs.[6] Since then, the dietary goals have been modified and are currently published as *Dietary Guidelines for Americans*, 1995[7] (Figure 2-7 and Appendix G). These guidelines are not meant to replace individual dietary prescriptions for disease conditions, but to recommend food choices that meet nutrient requirements, promote health, support active lives, and reduce chronic disease risks in the general population. They emphasize choices based on variety, balance, and moderation and suggest the use of the Food Guide Pyramid and food labels in planning diets to meet these guidelines. Similar public health concerns have been identified in Canada and addressed in *Canada's Guidelines for Healthy Eating*[8] and by the World Health Organization (see Appendices E and F).

Recommendations have been generated by other groups concerned with the nation's health. The *U.S. Surgeon General's Report on Nutrition and Health* released in 1988 included recommendations on body weight and the intake of fat, salt, sugar, and fruits and vegetables. It also gave advice for groups with special needs: Fluoride supplementation was recommended for those without fluoridated water; foods high in calcium were stressed for adolescent girls and women; foods high in iron were recommended for children, adolescents, and women of child-bearing age; and limiting sugar intake was suggested for children.[9]

The National Research Council issued *Diet and Health: Implications for Reducing Chronic Disease Risk* in 1989. The recommendations of this report are designed to reduce the incidence of chronic diseases such as atherosclerosis, high blood pressure, obesity, cancer, osteoporosis, diabetes, liver disease, and tooth decay.[10]

The U.S. Public Health Service along with 300 private and public organizations has also developed a set of public health objectives for the year 2000, called Healthy People 2000.[11] Many of these objectives are directed toward improving the nutritional status of the population (see Appendix H). For instance, Healthy People 2000 plans to work toward reducing the incidence of cancer and heart disease deaths and the prevalence of obesity in adults by promoting active lifestyles and diets low in fat and sodium and high in carbohydrate. It promotes a reduction in growth retardation in children by promoting healthy feeding practices, including breast feeding for infants. Other nutrition-related objectives are designed to improve the delivery of nutrition information and services.

Many of the most recent recommendations for health promotion and disease prevention have been incorporated into a set of standards used in food labeling.

Recommendations for Reducing Risks for Specific Diseases   In addition to guidelines for a healthy diet for the general population, recommendations to populations at risk for certain diseases have been published by groups such as the American Heart Association and the National Cancer Institute. These groups base their recommendations on sound scientific literature, but because of their special interest in preventing a specific disease, their recommendations may differ slightly from one another in emphasis and focus. For example, the guidelines developed by the American Heart Association recommend restricting dietary cholesterol to less than 300 mg per day, whereas the recommendations of the National Cancer Institute do not comment on cholesterol intake, since a correlation has not been established between cholesterol intake and cancer incidence. On the other hand, the National Cancer Institute recommends a reduction in the consumption of salt-cured and pickled foods because of a correlation with stomach cancer, but the American Heart Association guidelines don't include this (see Appendix G).

TOOLS FOR DIET PLANNING

Dietary standards and guidelines designed for the population as a whole can be used to plan and evaluate individual diets. A number of systems have been developed to translate the recommendations on specific nutrients into choices based on foods. The most commonly used tools are food group systems. These divide foods into groups based on the nutrients they supply most abundantly and then recommend the number of servings from each group needed to provide a healthy diet. The most recent version of a food group system used in the United States is the Food Guide Pyramid (Figure 2-8). In Canada, the Food Guide to Healthy Eating is used (Figure 2-9 and Appendix E). The exchange lists are another food

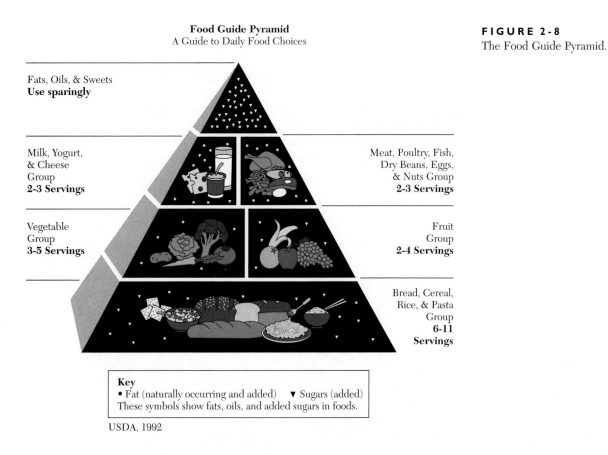

Food Guide Pyramid
A Guide to Daily Food Choices

Fats, Oils, & Sweets
Use sparingly

Milk, Yogurt,
& Cheese
Group
2-3 Servings

Meat, Poultry, Fish,
Dry Beans, Eggs,
& Nuts Group
2-3 Servings

Vegetable
Group
3-5 Servings

Fruit
Group
2-4 Servings

Bread, Cereal,
Rice, & Pasta
Group
**6-11
Servings**

Key
• Fat (naturally occurring and added)   ▼ Sugars (added)
These symbols show fats, oils, and added sugars in foods.

USDA, 1992

FIGURE 2-8
The Food Guide Pyramid.

group system that can be used for planning diets. Food labels provide information on the nutrient content of foods. They can help in the selection of individual foods within each group that are good sources of essential nutrients and meet the *Dietary Guidelines*.

THE FOOD GUIDE PYRAMID

The Food Guide Pyramid is a guide for planning diets that meet nutrient requirements and the recommendations for health and disease prevention. It proposes a diet plan based on servings from five food groups: bread, cereal, rice, and pasta; vegetables; fruits; milk, yogurt, and cheese; and meat, poultry, fish, dry beans, eggs, and nuts. The Pyramid also recommends that a sixth group—fats, oils, and sweets—be used sparingly in the diet. The serving sizes within each group of the Pyramid are fairly constant. For instance, 1 serving from the grain group is 1 slice of bread; 1 ounce of dry cereal; or ½ cup of cooked cereal, rice, or pasta. Foods within each food group supply similar nutrients. For example, foods in the milk, yogurt, and cheese group are good sources of protein, calcium, and riboflavin.

Why Use a Pyramid Shape?   The shape of the Pyramid helps emphasize the relative contribution each food group should make to the diet. The large base of the Pyramid is made up of foods that come from grains: bread, cereal, rice, and pasta. These high-carbohydrate foods are the foundation of a healthy diet; between 6 and 11 servings per day are recommended from this group. In the next level of the Pyramid are two groups of plant foods: the vegetable group, of which 3 to 5

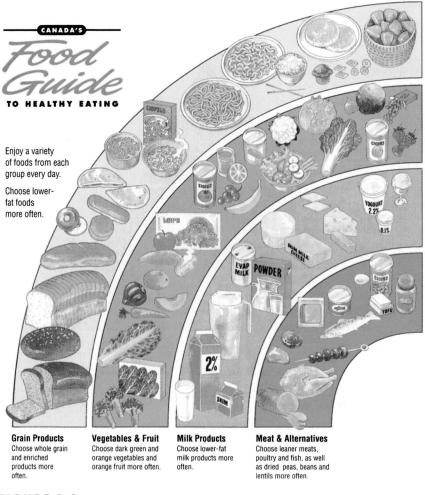

FIGURE 2-9
Canada's Food Guide to Healthy Eating. (Health and Welfare Canada, 1992)

Nutrient density–A measure of the nutrients provided by a food relative to the energy it contains.

servings per day are recommended, and the fruit group, of which 2 to 4 servings per day are recommended. The next level, where the decreasing size of the Pyramid boxes reflects the smaller number of recommended servings, comprises 2 groups of foods that come primarily from animals: the milk, yogurt, and cheese group, of which 2 to 3 servings are recommended, and the meat, poultry, fish, dry beans, eggs, and nuts group, of which 2 to 3 servings a day are recommended. At the narrow tip of the Pyramid are fats, oils, and sweets. These should be used sparingly after other nutrient needs have been met.

In addition to recommended serving sizes and numbers of servings, the Food Guide Pyramid makes recommendations on food choices from within each group. Many of these suggestions are based on the **nutrient density** of the foods within groups. Nutrient density refers to the amounts of essential nutrients in a food relative to the energy provided. For example, both skim milk and ice cream are in the milk group. However, a serving of skim milk provides 300 mg of calcium in 85 kcalories, whereas the ice cream provides 168 mg of calcium in 265 kcalories. High-nutrient-density foods such as whole grain products, fruits, and vegetables provide more nutrients per kcalorie than do low-nutrient-density foods like pastries and candy, which are high in energy relative to other nutrients. Selection tips for choices from the Food Guide Pyramid are listed in Table 2-2.

TABLE 2-2   Servings and Selections from the Food Guide Pyramid

Food Group/Serving Size	Nutrients Provided	Selection Tips
Bread, Cereal, Rice, and Pasta (6 to 11 servings) ½ cup cooked cereal · 1 ounce dry cereal · 1 slice bread · 2 cookies · ½ medium doughnut	B vitamins, fiber, iron, magnesium, zinc	Choose whole grain breads, cereals, and grains such as whole wheat or rye bread, oatmeal, and brown rice. Use high-fat, high-sugar baked goods such as cakes, cookies, and pastries in moderation. Limit fats and sugars added as spreads, sauces, or toppings.
Vegetable (3 to 5 servings) ½ cup cooked or raw chopped vegetables · 1 cup raw leafy vegetables · ¾ cup vegetable juice · 10 french fries	Vitamin A, vitamin C, folate, magnesium, iron, fiber	Eat a variety of vegetables, including dark-green leafy vegetables like spinach and broccoli, deep-yellow vegetables like carrots and sweet potatoes, starchy vegetables such as potatoes and corn, legumes like kidney beans, and other vegetables such as green beans and tomatoes. Cook by steaming or baking. Avoid frying, and limit high-fat spreads or dressings.
Fruit (2 to 4 servings) 1 medium apple, banana, or orange · ½ cup chopped, cooked, or canned fruit · ¾ cup fruit juice · ¼ cup dried fruit	Vitamin A, vitamin C, potassium, fiber	Choose fresh fruit, frozen without sugar, dried, or fruit canned in water or juice. If canned in heavy syrup, rinse with water before eating. Eat whole fruits more often than juices; they are higher in fiber. Regularly eat citrus fruits, melons, or berries rich in vitamin C. Only 100% fruit juice should be counted as fruit.
Milk, Yogurt, and Cheese (2 to 3 servings) 1 cup milk or yogurt · 1½ ounces natural cheese · 2 ounces process cheese · 2 cups cottage cheese · 1½ cups ice cream · 1 cup frozen yogurt	Protein, calcium, riboflavin	Use lowfat or skim milk for healthy people over 2 years of age. Choose lowfat and nonfat yogurt, "part skim" and lowfat cheeses, and lower-fat frozen desserts like ice milk and frozen yogurt. Limit high-fat cheeses and ice cream.
Meat, Poultry, Fish, Dry Beans, Eggs, and Nuts (2 to 3 servings) 2–3 ounces cooked lean meat, fish, or poultry · 2–3 eggs · 4–6 tablespoons peanut butter · 1½ cups cooked dry beans · 1 cup nuts	Protein, niacin, vitamin B_6, vitamin B_{12}, iron, zinc	Select lean meat, poultry without skin, fish, and dry beans often. Trim fat, and cook by broiling, roasting, grilling, or boiling rather than frying. Limit egg yolks, which are high in cholesterol, and nuts and seeds, which are high in fat. Be aware of serving size; 3 ounces of meat is the size of an average hamburger.
Fats, Oils, and Sweets (use sparingly) Butter, mayonnaise, salad dressing, cream cheese, sour cream, jam, jelly		These are high in energy and low in micronutrients. Substitute lowfat dressings and spreads.

Human Nutrition Information Service. *The Food Guide Pyramid.* Home and Garden Bulletin No. 252. Hyattsville, MD: U.S. Department of Agriculture, 1992.

Planning Diets Using the Food Guide Pyramid   The Food Guide Pyramid is designed to be flexible enough to suit the needs and preferences of a wide variety of people from a spectrum of cultures. The Pyramid can be used by people with different energy requirements. Someone who needs 1600 kcalories per day could meet their needs by using the low end of the range of servings, for instance, 6 bread servings per day. Someone who needs 2800 kcalories per day should choose from the high end of the range for each food group, for instance, 11 breads, 5 vegetables, 4 fruits, and so on.

The Pyramid can also be modified for groups with special needs. Pregnant and lactating women, children, adolescents, and adults under 25 years of age should consume 3 servings from the milk group. Small children can follow the Pyramid guidelines by using smaller serving sizes (see Chapter 14). Vegetarians can use the Food Guide Pyramid by choosing meat alternatives like legumes and nuts from the meat group (see Chapter 6).

To plan a diet that satisfies the recommendations of the Pyramid, several servings of breads and grains and fruits or vegetables should be included at each meal. From this base, servings from the milk and meat groups can be added. Mixed dishes can be planned with the Pyramid by considering the component parts. For example, a chicken taco consists of tortillas (a bread), chicken (a meat), and lettuce and tomatoes (vegetables). A beef with broccoli stir-fry consists of beef (a meat), broccoli (a vegetable), and rice (a grain).

EXCHANGE LISTS

Exchange lists are a modification of a food group system. The exchange system was first developed in 1950 by the American Dietetic Association and the American Diabetes Association as a meal-planning tool for individuals with diabetes. Since then, its use has been expanded to weight-loss diets and diets in general. The latest revision of the exchange system divides foods into three main groups: the carbohydrate group, the meat and meat substitute group, and the fat group. The carbohydrate group includes exchange lists for starches, fruits, milk (subgroups of skim/very lowfat, lowfat, and whole), and vegetables. It also defines a group of other high-carbohydrate foods and indicates how to fit these foods into a diet based on exchanges. The meat and meat substitutes group includes an exchange list with four subgroups: very lean, lean, medium-fat, and high-fat meat. The fat group includes an exchange list with subgroups of monounsaturated, polyunsaturated, and saturated fats[12] (see Appendix I) (Figure 2-10). The serving sizes for foods within each exchange list are set so that each food within an exchange list contains approximately the same amount of energy, carbohydrate, protein, and fat. For instance, each fruit in the fruit exchange list provides about 60 kcalories, 15 grams of carbohydrate, no protein, and no fat, whereas foods in the starch list provide about 80 kcalories, 15 grams of carbohydrate, 3 grams of protein, and 0 to 1 gram of fat. The exchanges differ from the Food Guide Pyramid groups because the lists are designed to meet macronutrient criteria, whereas the Pyramid groups are designed to be good sources of certain nutrients regardless of their energy content. For example, a potato is included in the starch exchange list because it contains about the same amount of energy, carbohydrate, protein, and fat as breads and grains, but in the Food Guide Pyramid a potato is in the vegetable group because it is a good source of vitamins, minerals, and fiber.

The exchange system can be used to design diets at specific energy levels. However, this requires a thorough knowledge of the system and of food composition. These diets are usually calculated by a dietitian or other health professional. The consumer is then instructed to select a specific number of foods from each exchange list. For example, a 1500-kcalorie diet providing 75 grams of protein and less than 30% fat could be designed and then the consumer would be instructed to choose 6 starch exchanges, 2 milk exchanges, 3 vegetable exchanges, and so on.

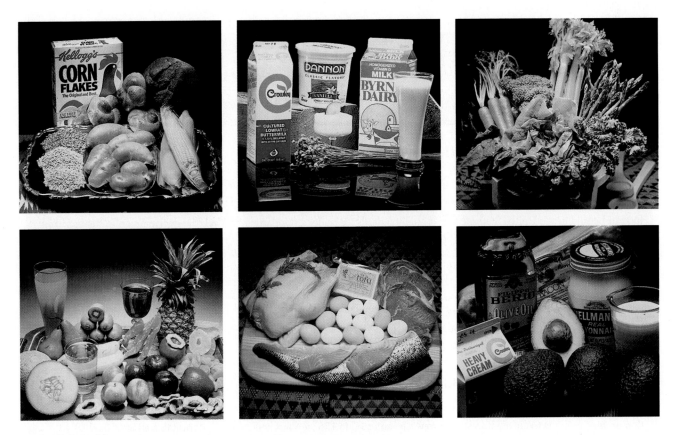

FIGURE 2-10
These are examples of foods included in different exchange lists. Starches, milk, vegetables, and fruits are high-carbohydrate foods. Meat, fish, eggs, and tofu are in the meat and meat substitute group. Fats and oils are in the fat group. (Charles D. Winters)

Although the calculations are not simple, diets can be designed to meet individual tastes and preferences. Exchange lists have been developed to include the traditional foods of different ethnic groups (see Appendix J).

FOOD LABELS

Food labels are another tool that can be used in diet planning. They are designed to help consumers make food choices by providing information about the nutrient composition of foods and about how a food fits into the overall diet. To make this information uniform and easy to use, food labeling standards are specified by the Nutrition Labeling and Education Act of 1990.[13] The format of food labels and serving sizes has been standardized to allow comparisons between products. For example, comparing the energy content of different types of crackers is simplified by the fact that all labels present information for a serving size of 30 grams, the number of crackers in each serving, and the kcalories per serving. On food labels, the term "Calorie" is used to refer to kcalories.

What Must Be Labeled   Food labeling laws regulate about 75% of all food consumed in the United States.[14] The FDA regulates the labeling of all foods except meat and poultry products, which are regulated by the USDA. All packaged foods except those produced by small businesses and those in packages too small to fit the labeling information must be labeled. Restaurant food and ready-to-eat food, such as that in bakeries and delicatessens, are also exempt. Raw fruits, vegetables, fish, meat, and poultry are not required to carry individual labels. The

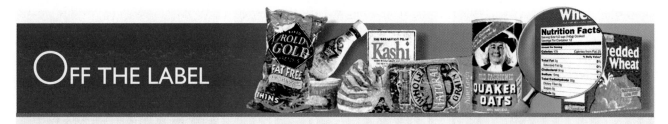

OFF THE LABEL

Food Labels: An International Perspective

Importing foods from other countries allows cuisines from around the world to be part of our diet. However, for a food to be sold in the United States it must meet U.S. standards, including those for food labeling. Likewise, foods we export to other countries must meet the labeling guidelines from those nations. Over the last decade an increase in the international trade of both raw agricultural commodities and processed foods has made food labeling an international issue.[1]

Food labels appear to be simply a source of nutrition information. So why are they an issue? The information on the label is actually of interest at the national, political, cultural, economic, as well as consumer levels.[2] Governments want labeling information to be compatible with national nutrition guidelines and food safety practices such as regulations for food additives, standards for composition of common products, and limits or thresholds of ingredients. Many countries oppose health claims that link any food with a specific disease, and some are ambivalent about nutrient content claims. Businesses want labels to emphasize features that give the product a competitive advantage. Consumers want labels to tell them how foods fit into their diets.

Achieving all of these goals among countries is a difficult task. Despite the high priority of setting international standards for trade, a standard food label is unlikely to be agreed upon.

Without standardized food labels, food for export must be specially labeled. This is expensive even when the labeling guidelines are not too different between countries. For example, if a Canadian food manufacturer wants to export cookies to the United States, they must relabel their product to meet all of the specifications of the Nutrition Labeling and Education Act. The amount of each nutrient must be adjusted to U.S. serving sizes, and the percent Daily Values must be added. For countries with no labeling guidelines, even getting the information about product composition may be costly.

Currently there are some minimum standards for international labeling of prepackaged foods. They are determined by The Codex Alimentarius Commission (Latin for "code concerned with nourishment") and state simply that "prepackaged foods should not be described or presented on any label or in any labelling material in a manner that is false, misleading, or deceptive or is likely to create an erroneous impression regarding its

character in any respect." Guidelines also state that when a nutrition claim or representation is made on the label, the declaration of a standardized list of nutrients becomes mandatory. Canadian and European nutrition labeling systems are similar to Codex guidelines. Labeling regulations in the United States are not contradictory to these but are much more stringent. In Canada, a proposal to adopt the American labeling approach was rejected in favor of a voluntary approach that offers the flexibility to accommodate bilingual labeling and ensures Canada's autonomy to establish its own nutrition policies.

Harmonization of food labels, composition requirements, formulations, and allowable additives would permit manufacturers to produce identical foods for sale in any country. Without some standardization of labeling, the burden of specially labeling foods for export will limit what foods are sold in the United States and therefore limit consumer choices, corporate choices, and government choices.

[1]Potter, N.N. and Hotchkiss, J.H. *Food Science*, 5th ed. New York: Chapman & Hall, 1995.

[2]Food labeling: a Canadian and international perspective. Nutr. Rev. 53:103–105, 1995.

FDA has asked grocery stores to voluntarily provide information for the raw fruits, vegetables, and fish most frequently eaten in the United States,[15] and the USDA encourages voluntary nutrition labeling of raw meat and poultry. The information can appear on large placards or in consumer pamphlets or brochures (Figure 2-11). In Canada, nutrition labeling is voluntary but standardized and provides information similar to that on labels in the United States.[16] (See Appendix E.)

What Must Be Listed   All labels contain basic product information such as the name of the product; the net contents or weight; the date by which the product should be sold; and the name and place of business of the manufacturer, packager, or distributor. In addition, most food labels contain a list of the food's ingredients and information about the nutrient content of the product and its contribution to a healthy diet.

List of Ingredients   The ingredients section of the label lists the contents of the product in order of their prominence by weight. An ingredients list is required on all products containing more than one ingredient. Food additives, including food colors and flavorings, must be listed among the ingredients.

Nutrition Facts   The nutrition information section of the label is entitled "Nutrition Facts" (Figure 2-12). In this section, the serving size is listed in common household and metric measures, and is based on a standard list of serving sizes. The serving size is followed by the number of servings per container. The label must then list the total kcalories, kcalories from fat, total fat, saturated fat, cholesterol, sodium, total carbohydrate, dietary fiber, sugars, and protein. The amounts of these nutrients are given per serving and listed as a percentage of a standard called the **Daily Value**, which helps consumers see how the food fits into an overall daily diet. For example, the number of grams of fat in a food may be of little help in deciding whether to select that food unless consumers know how many grams of fat they should eat in a day. The Daily Values provide this information. They are based on two sets of standards, the **Reference Daily Intakes (RDIs)** and the **Daily Reference Values (DRVs)**. To avoid confusion, only the term "Daily Value" appears on food labels.

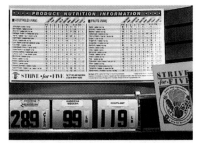

FIGURE 2-11
Fresh produce is not required to carry individual labels, but the information should be displayed voluntarily in the produce section of the store. (Dennis Drenner)

Daily Values–Nutrient reference value used on food labels to help consumers see how foods fit into their overall diets.

Reference Daily Intakes (RDIs)–Reference values established for vitamins and minerals that are based on the highest amount of each nutrient recommended for any adult age group by the 1968 RDAs.

Daily Reference Values (DRVs)–Reference values established for protein and seven nutrients for which no RDA has been established. The values are based on dietary recommendations for reducing the risk of chronic disease.

Standardized serving sizes simplify comparison of the nutrient content of similar products

Nutrition Facts

Serving Size ¹/₂ cup (95g)
Servings Per Container 4

Amount Per Serving

Calories 90   Calories from Fat 0

	% Daily Value*
Total Fat 0g	**0%**
Saturated Fat 0g	**0%**
Cholesterol 0mg	**0%**
Sodium 55mg	**2%**
Total Carbohydrate 21g	**7%**
Dietary Fiber 2g	**8%**
Sugars 5g	
Protein 2g	

Vitamin A 160% (100% as Beta Carotene)

Vitamin C 40% • Calcium 2% • Iron 4%

* Percent Daily Values are based on a 2,000 calorie diet. Your daily values may be higher or lower depending on your calorie needs:

		Calories:	2,000	2,500
Total Fat	Less than		65g	80g
Sat. Fat	Less than		20g	25g
Cholesterol	Less than		300mg	300mg
Sodium	Less than		2,400mg	2,400mg
Total Carbohydrate			300g	375g
Dietary Fiber			25g	30g

Calories per gram
Fat 9 • Carbohydrate 4 • Protein 4

The list of nutrients includes those most important to the health of today's consumer

Listing the calories from fat helps consumers follow dietary guidelines that recommend no more than 30% of calories from fat

% Daily Value shows how a food fits into the overall daily diet

Some Daily Values are maximums, such as for fat (less than 65 g), whereas others are minimums, such as for carbohydrate (300 g or more)

FIGURE 2-12
The Nutrition Labeling Act of 1990 required standardization of the information on food labels. (Federal Register 58(3), 1993, Jan 6. U.S. Government Printing Office, Superintendent of Documents, Washington, DC)

TABLE 2-3	Reference Daily Intakes*				
Nutrient	**Amount**	**Nutrient**	**Amount**	**Nutrient**	**Amount**
Vitamin A	5000 IU (1000 μg)†	Vitamin E	30 IU (10 mg)	Biotin	300 μg
Vitamin C	60 mg	Vitamin B$_6$	2.0 mg	Pantothenic acid	10 mg
Thiamin	1.5 mg	Folic acid	400 μg	Vitamin K	80 μg
Riboflavin	1.7 mg	Vitamin B$_{12}$	6 μg	Chromium	120 μg
Niacin	20 mg	Phosphorus	1000 mg	Selenium	70 μg
Calcium	1000 mg	Iodine	150 μg	Molybdenum	75 μg
Iron	18 mg	Magnesium	400 mg	Manganese	2 mg
Vitamin D	400 IU (10 μg)	Zinc	15 mg	Chloride	3400 mg
		Copper	2 mg		

*Based on National Academy of Sciences' 1968 Recommended Dietary Allowances.
†The RDIs for fat soluble vitamins are expressed in International Units (IU). The current RDAs use a newer system of measurement. Values that are approximately equivalent are given in parentheses.

The Reference Daily Intakes (Table 2-3) are used to determine Daily Values for vitamins and minerals for which RDAs have been established. Although the name has changed, most of the current RDI values are the same as the old U.S. RDAs (U.S. Recommended Daily Allowances). They are based on the highest amount of each nutrient recommended for any adult age group by the 1968 RDAs. These may overestimate the amount of a nutrient needed for some groups, but they do not underestimate the requirement for any group (except pregnant and lactating women). Label regulations require that percent Daily Values, based on RDIs, be listed for vitamin A, vitamin C, calcium, and iron. In addition to these mandatory listings, a manufacturer may voluntarily include information about other nutrients.

Daily Reference Values are designed as standards to help consumers follow recommendations for health and disease prevention. They have been established for fat, saturated fat, carbohydrate, fiber, cholesterol, sodium, potassium, and protein. The DRV for fat, for example, is based on the recommendation that dietary fat should account for less than 30% of energy, or less than 65 grams for a 2000-kcalorie diet (see Table 2-4). The DRVs are used on food labels to calculate the percent Daily Values for nutrients based on a diet containing 2000 kcalories. To illustrate that the recommended intake of some nutrients depends on energy needs, Daily Values based on DRVs are listed on food labels for both a 2000- and a 2500-kcalorie diet.

TABLE 2-4	Daily Reference Values
Food Component	**Daily Reference Value (2000 kcal)**
Total fat	Less than 65 g (30% of energy)
Saturated fat	Less than 20 g (10% of energy)
Cholesterol	Less than 300 mg
Total carbohydrate	300 g (60% of energy)
Dietary fiber	25 g (11.5 g/1000 kcal)
Sodium	Less than 2400 mg
Potassium	3500 mg
Protein	50 g (10% of energy)

Labeling Terminology and Health Claims   In addition to the required nutrition information, food labels often highlight specific characteristics of a product that might be of interest to the consumer, such as "low in Calories" or "high in fiber." Definitions for descriptors such as "free," "low," and "light" have been made based on how these terms relate to nutrient content. The specific definition of each of these descriptors is given in Table 2-5, and their use in relation to specific nutrients is discussed in *Off the Label* boxes throughout this text.

TABLE 2-5	Nutrient Content Descriptors Commonly Used on Food Labels
Free	Means that a product contains no amount of, or a trivial amount of, fat, saturated fat, cholesterol, sodium, sugars, or kcalories. For example, "sugar-free" and "fat-free" both mean less than 0.5 g per serving. Synonyms for "free" include "without," "no," and "zero."
Low	Used for foods that can be eaten frequently without exceeding the Daily Value for fat, saturated fat, cholesterol, sodium, or kcalories. Specific definitions have been established for each of these nutrients. For example, "low fat" means that the food contains 3 g or less per serving, and "low cholesterol" means that the food contains less than 20 mg of cholesterol per serving. Synonyms for "low" include "little," "few," and "low source of."
Lean and extra lean	Used to describe the fat content of meat, poultry, seafood, and game meats. "Lean" means that the food contains less than 10 g fat, less than 4.5 g saturated fat, and less than 95 mg of cholesterol per serving and per 100 g. "Extra lean" means that the food contains less than 5 g fat, less than 2 g saturated fat, and less than 95 mg of cholesterol per serving and per 100 g.
High	Can be used if a food contains 20% or more of the Daily Value for a particular nutrient. Synonyms for "high" include "rich in" and "excellent source of."
Good source	Means that a food contains 10 to 19% of the Daily Value for a particular nutrient per serving.
Reduced	Means that a nutritionally altered product contains 25% less of a nutrient or of energy than the regular or reference product.
Less	Means that a food, whether altered or not, contains 25% less of a nutrient or of energy than the reference food. For example, pretzels may claim to have "less fat" than potato chips. "Fewer" may be used as a synonym for "less."
Light	May be used in different ways. First, it can be used on a nutritionally altered product that contains one-third fewer kcalories or half the fat of a reference food. Second, it can be used when the sodium content of a low-calorie, lowfat food has been reduced by 50%. The term "light" can be used to describe properties such as texture and color as long as the label explains the intent, for example, "light and fluffy."
More	Means that a serving of food, whether altered or not, contains a nutrient that is at least 10% of the Daily Value more than the reference food. This definition also applies to foods using the terms "fortified," "enriched," or "added."
Healthy	May be used to describe foods that are low in fat and saturated fat and contain no more than 480 mg of sodium and no more than 60 mg of cholesterol per serving and provide at least 10% of the Daily Value for vitamins A or C, or iron, calcium, protein, or fiber.
Fresh	May be used on foods that are raw and have never been frozen or heated and contain no preservatives.

Federal Register 58, 1993, Jan. 6. U.S. Government Printing Office, Superintendent of Documents, Washington, DC.

TABLE 2-6	Health Claims Allowed on Food Labels
Calcium and osteoporosis	Adequate calcium intake throughout life helps maintain bone health and reduce the risk of osteoporosis.
Sodium and hypertension (high blood pressure)	Diets high in sodium may increase the risk of high blood pressure.
Dietary fat and cancer	Diets high in fat increase the risk of some types of cancer.
Saturated fat and cholesterol and cardiovascular disease	Diets high in saturated fat and cholesterol increase blood cholesterol and, thus, the risk of heart disease.
Foods high in fiber and cancer	Diets low in fat and rich in fiber-containing grain products, fruits, and vegetables may reduce the risk of some types of cancer.
Foods high in fiber and risk of cardiovascular disease	Diets low in saturated fat and cholesterol and rich in fruits, vegetables, and grain products that contain fiber, particularly soluble fiber, may reduce the risk of coronary heart disease.
Fruits and vegetables and cancer	Diets low in fat and rich in fruits and vegetables may reduce the risk of some types of cancer.
Folic acid and neural tube defect–affected pregnancy	Adequate folic acid intake by the mother reduces the risk of birth defects of the brain or spinal cord in their babies.

Food labels are also permitted to include a number of health claims if they are relevant to the product. Health claims refer to a relationship between a nutrient or a food and the risk of a disease or health-related condition. For example, milk, a good source of calcium, might include on the label a statement indicating that a diet high in calcium will reduce the risk of developing osteoporosis. Only the claims listed in Table 2-6 are currently allowed.[17]

Despite the wealth of information available on food labels, today's consumer must be educated about the benefits and pitfalls of foods that are not labeled, and about food and nutrition issues that are not addressed by food labels, such as the advantages and disadvantages of fresh, frozen, and canned produce and the safe selection, storage, and preparation of food. Food labels can't tell you what you should eat, or how you should prepare it, but they are an important source of information about what you are eating.

CRITICAL THINKING
How to Apply the Food Guide Pyramid to Your Diet

A few months ago, Naomi moved out of her parents' home and into her own apartment. For the first time in her life all her food decisions are her own. She has gained a few pounds and is beginning to realize that she needs to pay more attention to the kinds of foods she eats. To evaluate her nutrient intake, Naomi records everything she consumes for one day and compares it with the number of servings recommended by the Food Guide Pyramid.

APPLICATIONS

1. Make a form like the example shown below or use one provided to list the foods from one day of the food record you kept in Chapter 1. Next to each food, list the Food Guide Pyramid food group to which it belongs. In the next column list the number of Food Guide Pyramid servings it provides. For mixed foods, list all ingredients separately and identify the food groups that apply.

Food	Food Guide Pyramid Group	Number of Servings
2 Egg Rolls:		
Wrappers	Grain	1
Carrots ½ cup	Vegetable	1
Pork 1 oz	Meat	½
Peanut oil	Fats and sweets	1
Rice ½ cup	Grain	1

a. How many servings from each food group did you consume?
b. Does your diet meet the guidelines of the Food Guide Pyramid? If not, what types of food(s) do you need to add to or eliminate from your diet?
c. Are your food choices consistent with the selection tips described in Table 2-2? How might you modify your food choices to more closely follow these suggestions?

2. Using your food record, your kitchen cupboard, or the grocery store, select three packaged foods with food labels.
a. How does each of these foods fit into your overall daily diet with regard to total carbohydrate? Total fat? Dietary fiber?
b. If you consumed a serving of each of these three foods, how much more fat could you consume without exceeding the recommendations? How much more total carbohydrate and fiber should you consume that day to meet recommendations for a 2000-kcalorie diet?

REFERENCES

1. Wolf, G. The molecular basis of the inhibition of collagenase by vitamin A. Nutr. Rev. 50:292–294, 1992.
2. National Research Council, Food and Nutrition Board. *Recommended Dietary Allowances*, 10th ed. Washington, DC: National Academy Press, 1989.
3. United States Department of Agriculture. *The Food Guide Pyramid.* Home and Garden Bulletin No. 252. Hyattsville, MD: Human Nutrition Information Service, 1992.
4. Health and Welfare Canada. *Nutrition Recommendations. The Report of the Scientific Review Committee*. Ottawa: Minister of Supply and Services Canada, 1990.
5. FAO/WHO/UNU. Energy and Protein Requirements. WHO Technical Report Series No. 724. Geneva: World Health Organization, 1985.
6. Report of the Select Committee on Nutrition and Human Needs, U.S. Senate. *Eating in America: Dietary Goals for the United States*. Cambridge, MA: MIT Press, 1977.
7. U.S. Department of Agriculture, U.S. Department of Health and Human Services. *Nutrition and Your Health: Dietary Guidelines for Americans*, 4th ed. Home and Garden Bulletin No. 232. Hyattsville, MD: U.S. Goverment Printing Office, 1995.
8. Health and Welfare Canada. Report of the Communications/Implementations Committee. Ottawa: Minister of Supply and Services Canada, 1992.
9. U.S. Department of Health and Human Services. The Surgeon General's Report on Nutrition and Health. DHHS (PHS) Publication No. 88-50210. Washington, DC: U.S. Government Printing Office, 1988.
10. National Research Council. *Diet and Health: Implications for Reducing Chronic Disease Risk*. Washington, DC: National Academy Press, 1989.
11. *Healthy People 2000: National Health Promotion and Disease Prevention Objectives*. Washington, DC: U.S. Department of Health and Human Services, 1990.
12. The American Diabetes Association, Inc., and the American Dietetic Association. Exchange Lists for Meal Planning, 1995.
13. Federal Register 58, 1993, Jan. 6. Washington, DC: U.S. Government Printing Office, Superintendent of Documents.
14. United States Nutrition Labeling and Education Act of 1990. Nutr. Rev. 49:273–276, 1991.
15. Kurtzweil, P. Nutrition information available for raw fruits, vegetables and fish. FDA Consumer 27:6–9, Jan/Feb 1993.
16. Health and Welfare Canada. Nutrition Labels—The Inside Story. Ottawa: Minister of Supply and Services Canada, 1989.
17. Kurtzweil, P. The new food label: better information for special diets. FDA Consumer 29:19–25, Jan/Feb 1995.

The Human Body: From Meals to Molecules

CHAPTER CONCEPTS

1. All plant and animal life is made up of atoms bound together to form molecules that are organized into cells. Cells form tissues that compose the organs and organ systems of a living organism.

2. The gastrointestinal tract is a hollow tube, beginning at the mouth and ending at the anus, in which the digestion of food and absorption of nutrients take place.

3. Enzymes that act specifically on carbohydrate, lipid, or protein help digest food. Hormones help regulate digestive processes.

4. The primary site of absorption is the small intestine.

5. Water soluble materials are absorbed into the blood and most fat soluble materials are absorbed into the lymph.

6. Nutrients delivered to the cells can be used to produce energy in the form of ATP, to synthesize molecules needed for immediate use, or to synthesize molecules for storage.

7. Materials not absorbed from the gastrointestinal tract are excreted in feces. The waste products generated by metabolism are eliminated from the body via the lungs, skin, and kidneys.

JUST A TASTE

Can carbohydrate, fat, and protein be digested simultaneously?

Why are you hungry very soon after eating some meals while others stick with you longer?

Is it healthy to have bacteria living in your gastrointestinal tract?

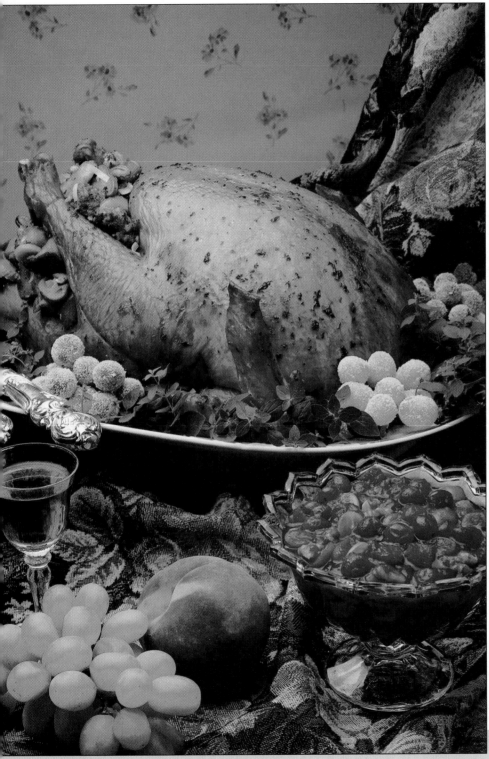

(© Victor Scocozza/FPG International)

CHAPTER OUTLINE

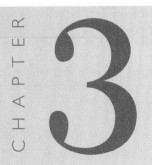

CHAPTER 3

No matter what food choices you make, the processes by which your body uses the nutrients in food are the same. After being consumed, food must be broken into smaller components, absorbed into the body, and then converted into forms that the body can use. Converting the meals we eat into energy or a part of our body involves the integration of a number of processes and interaction among almost all the systems of the body. Digestion breaks food into its component parts. Absorption takes these components into the body; and metabolism uses the nutrients for energy production, building new tissues, maintaining and repairing existing tissues, and regulating these processes. Whether you choose to eat a burrito, rice, and arroz con leche (rice milk), or a turkey sandwich, an apple, and a glass of milk—if the food cannot be properly digested, absorbed, and metabolized by the body, it is of little benefit.

An understanding of nutrition requires an understanding of the processes by which food provides fuel and function to the human body. The unique features of the digestion, absorption, and metabolism of specific nutrients will be more thoroughly discussed in subsequent chapters. In this chapter, we will discuss:

- What is the path of a meal—in this case, a turkey sandwich, apple, and glass of lowfat milk—through digestion?
- Through absorption?
- Through transport and delivery within the body?
- Through metabolism?
- And finally through the excretion of waste products?

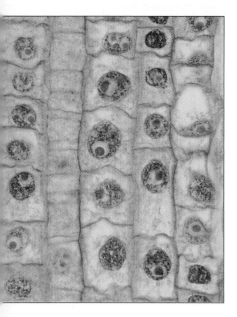

F I G U R E   3 - I
Living things are made up of cells.
(James Mauseth)

Atoms—The smallest units of an element that still retain the properties of that element.

Elements—Substances that cannot be broken down into products with different properties.

Chemical bonds—Forces that hold atoms together.

Molecules—Units of two or more atoms of the same or different elements bonded together.

Organic molecules—Substances that contain carbon atoms.

Inorganic—Substances that contain no carbon atoms.

Cells—The basic structural and functional units of plant and animal life.

Organ—A discrete structure composed of more than one tissue that performs a specialized function.

THE CHEMISTRY OF LIFE

The organization of life, as with all matter, begins with **atoms**. Atoms of different **elements** have different characteristics. Carbon, hydrogen, oxygen, and nitrogen are the most abundant elements in our bodies and in the foods we eat. These atoms can be linked by forces called **chemical bonds** to form **molecules**. The chemistry of all life on earth is based on **organic molecules**, those that contain carbon. Substances not containing carbon, such as the minerals iron and copper, are called **inorganic**.

In any living system, whether a broccoli plant, a cow, or a human being, molecules are organized into structures that form **cells**, the smallest unit of life (Figure 3-1). Cells of similar structure and function are organized into tissues. The human body contains four types of tissues: muscle, nerve, epithelial, and connective. These tissues are organized in varying combinations into **organs**, which are discrete structures that perform specialized functions in the body (Figure 3-2). The stomach, for example, is an organ that contains all four types of tissue. Most organs do not function alone but are part of a group of cooperative organs called an organ system. The organ systems in humans include the nervous system, respiratory system (lungs), urinary system (kidneys and bladder), reproductive system, cardiovascular system (heart and blood vessels), lymphatic system, muscular system, skeletal system, endocrine system (hormones), integumentary system (skin and body linings), and digestive system (Table 3-1). An organ may be part of more than one organ system. For example, the pancreas is part of the endocrine system as well as the digestive system.

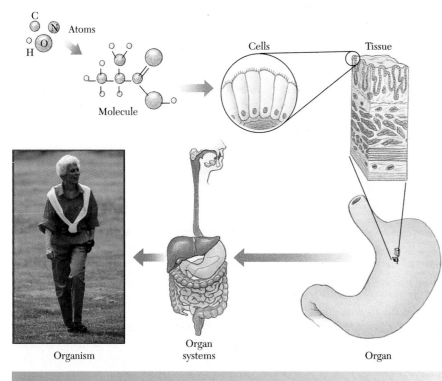

Atoms

C
N
O
H

Molecule

Cells

Tissue

FIGURE 3-2

The organization of life begins with atoms that form molecules that are organized into cells to form tissues, organs, and organisms. (Photograph, Walter Bibikow/The Image Bank)

Organism

Organ systems

Organ

TABLE 3-1	The Role of Body Organ Systems	
Organ System	**Components**	**Functions**
Nervous	Nerves, sense organs, brain, and spinal cord	Responds to stimuli from the external and internal environment; conducts impulses to activate muscles and glands; integrates activities of other systems.
Respiratory	Lungs, trachea, and air passageways	Keeps blood supplied with oxygen and removes carbon dioxide.
Urinary	Kidney and bladder	Eliminates wastes and regulates water, electrolyte, and acid-base balance of the blood.
Reproductive	Testes, ovaries, and associated structures	Produces offspring.
Cardiovascular	Heart and blood vessels	Transports blood, which carries oxygen, nutrients, and wastes.
Lymphatic	Lymph and lymph structures	Defends against foreign invaders; picks up fluid leaked from blood vessels; and transports fat soluble nutrients.
Muscular	Skeletal muscles	Provides movement and structure.
Skeletal	Bones and joints	Protects and supports the body and provides a framework for the muscles to use for movement.
Endocrine	Pituitary, adrenals, thyroid, and other ductless glands	Secretes hormones that regulate processes such as growth, reproduction, and nutrient use.
Integumentary	Skin, hair, nails, and sweat glands	Covers and protects the body, helps control body temperature.
Digestive	Mouth, esophagus, stomach, intestines, pancreas, liver, and gallbladder	Ingests and digests food; absorbs nutrients into the blood; and eliminates nonabsorbed food residues.

Marieb, E.N. *Human Anatomy and Physiology*, 3rd ed. Redwood City, CA: Benjamin/Cummings Publishing Company, 1995.

The digestive system is the organ system primarily responsible for the movement of nutrients into the body; however, several other organ systems are also important in the process of using these nutrients. The endocrine system secretes chemical messengers that help regulate food intake and absorption. The nervous system aids in digestion by sending nerve signals that help control the passage of food through the digestive tract. Once absorbed, nutrients are transported to individual cells by the cardiovascular system. The body's urinary, respiratory, and integumentary systems allow for the elimination of metabolic waste products.

THE DIGESTIVE SYSTEM: AN OVERVIEW

Digestion—The process of breaking food into components small enough to be absorbed into the body.
Absorption—The process of taking substances into the interior of the body.
Feces—Body waste, including unabsorbed food residue, bacteria, mucus, and dead cells, which is excreted from the gastrointestinal tract by way of the anus.
Gastrointestinal tract—A hollow tube consisting of the mouth, pharynx, esophagus, stomach, small intestine, large intestine, and anus, in which digestion and absorption of nutrients occur.

The digestive system provides two major functions: **digestion** and **absorption**. Carbohydrate, fat, and protein are digested and absorbed as sugars, fatty acids, and amino acids, respectively. Some substances, such as water, can be absorbed without digestion, and others, such as dietary fiber, cannot be digested by humans and so are excreted without being absorbed. These unabsorbed substances pass through the digestive tract and are excreted in the **feces**.

The main part of the digestive system is the **gastrointestinal tract**. It is also referred to as the GI tract, gut, digestive tract, intestinal tract, or alimentary canal. It can be thought of as a hollow tube that runs from the mouth to the anus. The organs of the gastrointestinal tract include the mouth, pharynx, esophagus, stomach, small intestine, large intestine, and anus (Figure 3-3). The inside of the tube

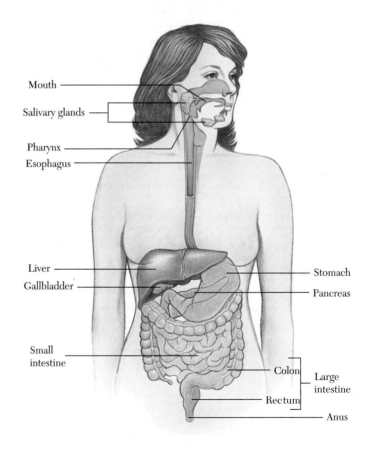

F I G U R E 3 - 3
The digestive system consists of the organs of the gastrointestinal tract: the mouth, pharynx, esophagus, stomach, small intestine, large intestine, and anus, as well as a number of accessory organs: the salivary glands, liver, gallbladder, and pancreas.

that these organs form is called the **lumen**. Food within the lumen of the gastrointestinal tract has not been absorbed and is therefore technically still outside the body. Only after food is transferred into the cells of the intestine by the process of absorption is food actually "inside" the body. The amount of time it takes for food to pass from mouth to anus is referred to as **transit time**. In a healthy adult, transit time is about 24 to 72 hours. It is affected by the composition of the diet, physical activity, emotions, medications, and illnesses. To measure transit time, researchers add a dye, which is not absorbed, to a meal and measure the time between ingestion of the dye and its appearance in the feces. The shorter the transit time, the more rapid the passage through the digestive tract.

The digestive system also includes a number of accessory organs that secrete fluids into the digestive tract. These secretions along with secretions produced by cells in the gastrointestinal tract contain substances that aid the digestive process. One of these substances is **mucus**, a viscous material produced by mucosal cells that line the gut. Mucus moistens, lubricates, and protects the digestive tract. Another important component of digestive system secretions is **enzymes**, protein molecules that speed up chemical reactions without themselves being consumed or changed by the reactions (Figure 3-4). In digestion, enzymes help the breakdown of food proceed at a rapid rate. Different enzymes are needed for the breakdown of different food components. For example, an enzyme that digests carbohydrate would have no effect on fat and one that digests fat would have no effect on carbohydrate.

In addition to secreting substances like mucus and enzymes into the lumen of the digestive tract, the digestive system secretes **hormones** into the bloodstream. Hormones are chemical messengers that are released into the blood by one organ to regulate body functions elsewhere. In the gastrointestinal tract, hormones send signals that help prepare different parts of the gut for the arrival of food and thus regulate the rate that food moves through the system.

The wall of the gastrointestinal tract contains four layers of tissue (Figure 3-5). Lining the lumen is the **mucosa**, a layer of mucosal cells that secrete mucus into the lumen. The cells of the mucosa are in direct contact with churning food and harsh digestive secretions. Therefore, these cells have a short lifespan—only about

Lumen—The inside cavity of a tube, such as the gastrointestinal tract.

Transit time—The time between the ingestion of food and the elimination of the solid waste from that food.

Mucus—A thick fluid secreted by glands in the gastrointestinal tract and other parts of the body. It acts to lubricate, moisten, and protect cells from harsh environments.

Enzymes—Protein molecules that accelerate the rate of specific chemical reactions without being changed themselves.

Hormones—Chemical messengers that are produced in one location, released into the blood, and elicit responses at other locations in the body.

Mucosa—The layer of tissue lining the gastrointestinal tract and other body cavities.

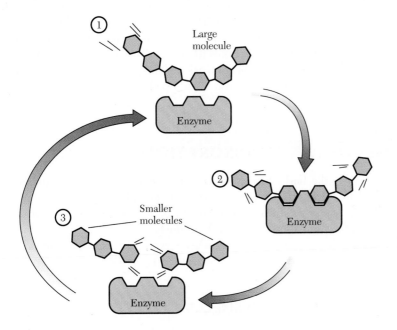

FIGURE 3-4
Enzymes speed up chemical reactions without themselves being altered by the reaction. In this example, an enzyme breaks a large molecule into smaller ones.

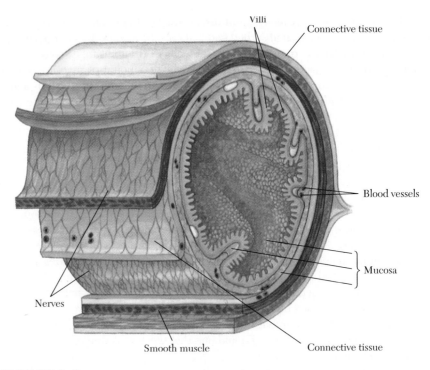

FIGURE 3-5
This cross section through the wall of the small intestine shows the four tissue layers: mucosa, connective tissue, muscle layers, and outer connective tissue layer. (Adapted from Solomon, E.P., Schmidt, R.R., and Adragna, P.J. *Human Anatomy and Physiology*, 2nd ed. Philadelphia: Saunders College Publishing, 1990.)

two to five days. When these cells die, they are sloughed off into the lumen, where some components are digested and absorbed and the remainder are excreted in the feces. Because mucosal cells reproduce rapidly, the mucosa has high nutrient requirements and is therefore one of the first areas to be affected by nutrient deficiencies. Surrounding the mucosa is a layer of connective tissue containing nerves and blood vessels. This layer provides support, delivers nutrients to the mucosa, and provides the nerve signals that control secretions and muscle contractions. Layers of smooth muscle, the type of muscle over which we do not have voluntary control, surround the connective tissue. The contraction of smooth muscles mixes food, breaks it into smaller particles, and propels it through the digestive tract. The final, external layer is also made up of connective tissue and provides support and protection.

DIGESTION AND ABSORPTION

To be used by the body, food must be eaten, digested, the nutrients absorbed, and then transported to the cells in various parts of the body. The following sections of this chapter will trace a meal through all these processes, from preparation of the meal to elimination of the waste products.

Imagine slices of oven-roasted turkey served on fresh baked bread accompanied by an apple and a glass of lowfat milk (Figure 3-6).

SIGHTS, SOUNDS, AND SMELLS

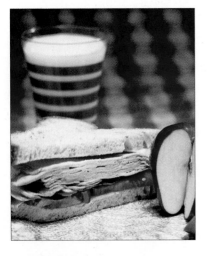

FIGURE 3-6
The sight, smell, and sounds of food preparation can initiate activity in the digestive tract. (Charles D. Winters)

Activity in the digestive tract begins before food even enters the mouth. As the meal is being prepared, sensory input such as the sight of a turkey being lifted out of the oven, the clatter of the table being set, and the smell of fresh baked bread may make your mouth become moist with **saliva** and your stomach begin to secrete digestive substances. This response occurs when the nervous system interprets sensory input and signals the digestive system to ready itself for a meal. This cephalic (which means pertaining to the head) response occurs as a result of external cues such as sight and smell even when the body is not in need of food.

Saliva—A watery fluid produced and secreted into the mouth by the salivary glands. It contains lubricants, enzymes, and other substances.

THE MOUTH

The mouth is the entry point for food into the digestive tract. In the mouth, the taste of food continues the processes begun by the smells, sights, and sounds of food preparation. The presence of food in the mouth stimulates the flow of saliva from the salivary glands located internally at the sides of the face and immediately below and in front of the ears (see Figure 3-3). Saliva contains the enzyme **salivary amylase**, which begins the digestion of carbohydrate. Salivary amylase can break the long sugar chains of starch in the bread of the turkey sandwich into shorter chains of sugars. Saliva also lubricates the upper gastrointestinal tract and moistens the food so that it can easily be tasted and swallowed.

Salivary amylase—An enzyme secreted by the salivary glands that breaks down starch.

Digestive enzymes can act only on the surface of food particles; therefore chewing is important because it breaks food into small pieces, increasing the surface area in contact with digestive enzymes. Adult humans have 32 teeth, specialized for biting, tearing, grinding, and crushing foods. Chewing also breaks apart fiber that traps nutrients in some foods. If the fiber is not broken, some nutrients cannot be absorbed. For example, the skin of the apple in the sample meal is a source of B vitamins; however, these vitamins cannot be absorbed without first being released from the fiber in the skin. Missing or decayed teeth can interfere with the proper digestion of food. Tooth decay, or caries, commonly called cavities, are caused by acid produced when bacteria break down sugars (see Chapter 4).

THE PHARYNX

The meal that entered the mouth as a turkey sandwich, apple, and milk has now been formed into a bolus, a ball of chewed food mixed with saliva. From the mouth, the bolus moves into the **pharynx**, the part of the gastrointestinal tract responsible for swallowing. It is shared by the digestive tract and the respiratory tract. Food passes through the pharynx on its way to the esophagus, and air passes here on its way to and from the lungs. During swallowing, the air passages are blocked by a valve-like flap of tissue called the epiglottis, so food passes to the esophagus, not the lungs. Sometimes food can pass into an upper air passageway and become lodged there, blocking the flow of air and causing choking. A quick reaction is required to save the life of a person whose airway is completely blocked. The Heimlich maneuver, which forces air out of the lungs by using a sudden application of pressure to the abdomen, can blow an object out of the blocked air passage (Figure 3-7).

Pharynx—An opening at the back of the throat that is responsible for swallowing.

THE ESOPHAGUS

The **esophagus** passes through the diaphragm, a muscular wall separating the abdomen from the cavity where the lungs are located, to connect the pharynx and stomach. Once the bolus of food is in the esophagus, it is moved along by rhythmic contractions of the smooth muscles. This contractile movement, called **peristalsis**, is controlled automatically by the nervous system. Peristaltic contractions, or waves, occur throughout the gastrointestinal tract from the pharynx to the large intestine (Figure 3–8).

Esophagus—A portion of the gastrointestinal tract that extends from the pharynx to the stomach.

Peristalsis—Coordinated muscular contraction that moves food through the gastrointestinal tract.

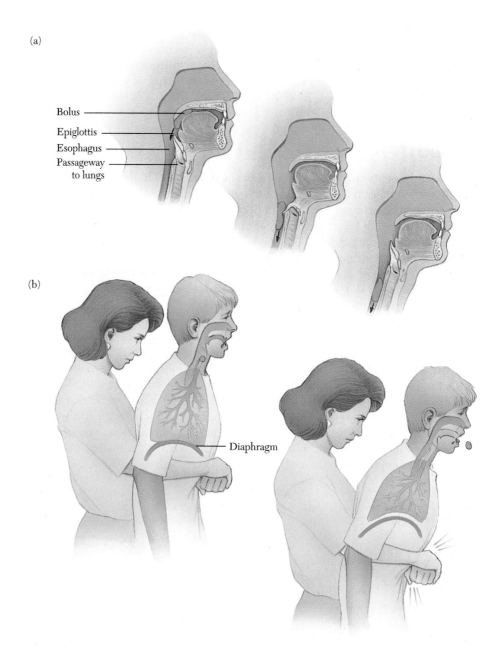

FIGURE 3-7

(a) When a bolus of food is swallowed, it pushes the epiglottis down over the opening to the air passageways. (b) If food does become lodged in the air passageways, it can be dislodged by the Heimlich maneuver, illustrated here.

THE STOMACH

Sphincter–A muscular valve that helps control the flow of materials in the gastrointestinal tract.

To move from the esophagus into the stomach, food must pass through a **sphincter**, a muscle that encircles the tube of the digestive tract and acts as a valve (See Figure 3-8). When the muscle contracts, the valve is closed. The gastroesophageal sphincter, located between the esophagus and the stomach, normally prevents foods from moving back out of the stomach. Occasionally, some of the acidic stomach contents leak up and out of the stomach into the esophagus, causing a burning sensation referred to as heartburn. Vomiting is the result of a reverse peristaltic wave that causes the sphincter to relax and allow the food to pass upward out of the stomach toward the mouth.

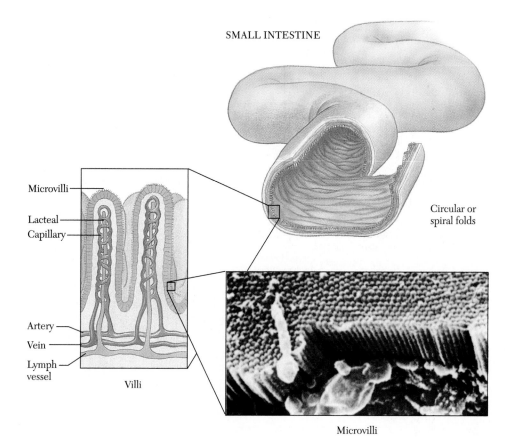

SMALL INTESTINE

Microvilli

Lacteal

Capillary

Artery

Vein

Lymph vessel

Villi

Circular or spiral folds

Microvilli

FIGURE 3-12
The small intestine contains folds, villi, and microvilli, which increase the absorptive surface area. (Courtesy of Hoskins, J.D., Henk, W.G., and Abdelbaki, Y.Z., from Am. J. Vet. Res. Vol. 43, no. 10, 1982.)

THE LARGE INTESTINE

Components of chyme that are not absorbed in the small intestine pass through the ileocecal valve to the large intestine, which includes the **colon** and **rectum**. Though most absorption occurs in the small intestine, water and some vitamins and minerals are also absorbed in the colon. Peristalsis here is slower than in the small intestine. Water, nutrients, and fecal matter may spend 24 hours in the large intestine, in contrast to the 3 to 5 hours it takes for chyme to move through the small intestine. This slow movement favors the growth of bacteria, referred to as **intestinal microflora**, which are permanent beneficial residents of this part of the gastrointestinal tract (see *Off the Shelf*: Feeding Your Flora). The microflora act on unabsorbed portions of food, such as the fiber contained in the apple and whole grain bread, producing nutrients that they can use or, in some cases, that can be absorbed into the body.[2] The microflora also synthesize small amounts of B vitamins and vitamin K, some of which can be absorbed. One additional by-product of bacterial metabolism is gas, which causes flatulence.

Materials not absorbed are excreted as waste products in the feces. The amount of water in the feces is affected by fiber and fluid intake. Fiber retains water, so when adequate fiber and fluid are consumed, feces have a high water content and are easily excreted. When inadequate fiber or fluid is consumed, feces are hard and dry, and constipation can result.

The end of the colon is connected to the rectum, where feces are stored prior to defecation. The rectum is connected to the **anus**. The rectum and anus work

Colon–The largest portion of the large intestine.
Rectum–The portion of the large intestine that connects the colon and anus.

Intestinal microflora–Microorganisms that inhabit the large intestine.

Anus–The outlet of the rectum.

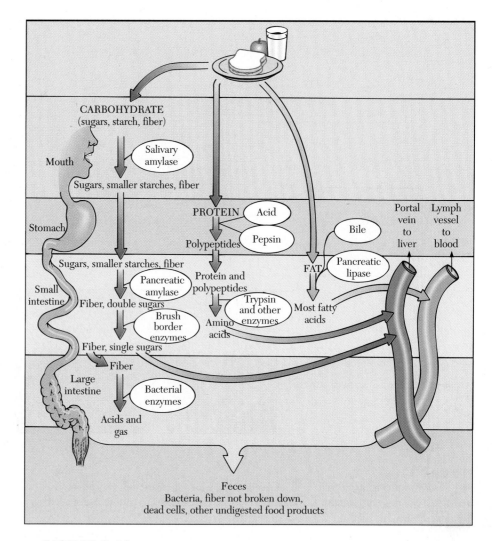

FIGURE 3-13
An overview of the digestion and absorption of a meal.

with the colon to prepare the feces for elimination. Defecation is regulated by a sphincter that is under voluntary control. It allows the contents of the colon to be eliminated at convenient and appropriate times. The digestion and absorption of carbohydrate, fat, and protein are summarized in Figure 3-13.

DIGESTIVE PROBLEMS AND SOLUTIONS

Each of the organs and processes of the digestive system is necessary for the proper digestion and absorption of food. Problems with any step along the way can inhibit the ability to obtain nutrients from food.

The inability to chew food because of dental caries or loss of teeth can limit the types of food consumed or prevent digestive enzymes from coming in contact with the nutrients in food. A delay in stomach emptying or problem in the closure of the gastroesophageal sphincter can result in heartburn. Excess acid secretion in the stomach can contribute to the formation of an ulcer of the stomach wall or the duodenum. Pancreatic problems can limit the availability of enzymes needed to digest food. Gallbladder problems can interfere with fat absorption. Abnormalities in the small intestine can reduce nutrient absorption. Some of these prob-

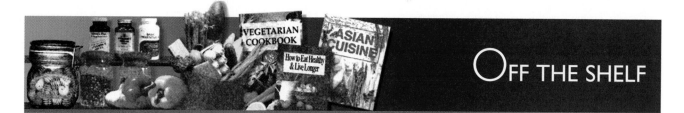

Feeding Your Flora

Bacteria growing in your gut? Sounds bad, but the large intestine of a healthy adult is home to several hundred species of bacteria. Some of these are beneficial and some are harmful.[1] Most of the time the microflora in our gastrointestinal tract have beneficial effects, but when the wrong bacteria take over the result could be diarrhea, infections, and perhaps liver disease and cancer. Should we be eating certain foods or even bacteria to promote the growth of beneficial bacteria?

The type and amount of bacteria in the gastrointestinal tract are determined by factors that affect the environment in the colon, such as diet and health. In turn, the type and amount of bacteria affect the health of the host. The beneficial bacteria improve the digestion and absorption of essential nutrients, synthesize vitamins, some of which can be absorbed, and can metabolize harmful byproducts of metabolism, such as ammonia, and thus reduce levels in the blood. They have also been hypothesized to stimulate the immune system, reduce blood cholesterol,[2,3] and prevent the formation and progression of cancerous cells.[4] A strong population of healthful bacteria can also inhibit the growth of harmful bacteria.[5,6]

It would obviously be beneficial if we could encourage the growth of the good bacteria and not the bad. One way to increase the population of healthful bacteria is to eat the bacteria themselves. Two bacterial groups that are believed to have health-promoting properties are *Bifidobacterium* and *Lactobacillus*. A number of products that contain these bacteria are available. They include yogurt with live cultures, milk with added bacterial culture (*acidophilus* milk), bottled suspensions of bacteria, and bacteria that have been pressed into tablets. When eaten alive, some of these organisms survive passage through the upper GI tract. They live temporarily in the colon but it is not known whether they actually colonize there or if they just stay for a while without proliferating and are then excreted in the feces.[7] The consumption of live bacteria, referred to as probiotics, has been hypothesized to have positive effects on diarrhea, constipation, colitis, flatulence, gastric acidity, immunity, high blood cholesterol, liver disease, and cancer. However, when the probiotic containing the bacteria is no longer consumed, the added bacteria are rapidly washed out of the colon.

A more recent approach to altering the intestinal microflora is to consume foods or other substances that encourage the growth of particular types of bacteria. These foods for bacteria, called "prebiotics," are not digested or absorbed before reaching the colon. The type of food can selectively stimulate the growth of one of a limited number of bacteria and promote host health. In order to improve some aspect of health that is affected by intestinal microflora, we may soon be consuming specially formulated bacteria food to stimulate the growth of desirable bacteria. Instead of taking antibiotics to kill the hazardous bacteria in the gut, "prebiotics" will be given to promote the growth of healthful bacteria and treat or prevent gastrointestinal problems, high blood cholesterol, liver disease, and cancer.

[1] Gibson, G.R. and Roberfroid, M.B. Dietary modulation of the human colonic microbiota: introducing the concept of prebiotics. J. Nutr. 125:1401–1412, 1995.

[2] Fukushima, M. and Nakano, M. The effect of a probiotic on fecal and liver lipid classes in arts. Br. J. Nutr. 73:701–710, 1995.

[3] Gilliland, S.E., Nelson, C.R., and Maxwell, C. Assimilation of cholesterol by *Lactobacillus acidophilus*. Appl. Environ. Microbiol. 49:377, 1985.

[4] Van Munster, I.P., Tangerman, A., and Nagengast, F.M. The effect of resistant starch on colonic fermentation, bile acid metabolism and mucosal proliferation. Dig. Dis. Sci. 39:834–842, 1994.

[5] Gibson, G.R. and Wang, X. Inhibitory effects of bifidobacteria on other colonic bacteria. J. Appl. Bacteriol. 77:412–420, 1994.

[6] Gilliland, S.E. Acidophilus milk products: a review of potential benefits to consumers. J. Dairy Sci. 72:2483–2494, 1989.

[7] Marteau, P., Pochart, P., Bouhnik, Y., and Rambaud, J.C. The fate and effects of transiting nonpathogenic microorganisms in the human intestine. World Rev. Nutr. Diet 74:1–21, 1993.

lems require adaptations in the way we obtain nutrients, whereas others are minor and can be treated with over-the-counter medications (see *Off the Shelf*: Over-the-Counter Remedies—Do They Really Cure What Ails You?).

For individuals who are unable to consume food or digest and absorb the nutrients needed to meet their requirements, several alternative feeding methods have been developed. People who are unable to chew and swallow can be fed a liquid diet through a tube inserted into the stomach or intestine. Tube feeding with either commercially prepared formula or blenderized food can provide a balanced diet containing all the essential nutrients. Tube feeding can be used for short periods following injury to the face or throat. Long-term tube feeding is often used in coma patients who cannot chew or swallow or in other individuals who cannot get food into the gastrointestinal tract. For individuals whose gastrointestinal tract is not functional, nutrients can be provided directly into the bloodstream. This is referred to as total parenteral nutrition (TPN). Carefully planned TPN can provide all the nutrients essential to life. When all nutrients are not provided in a TPN solution, nutrient deficiencies develop quickly. Inadvertently feeding patients incomplete TPN solutions has helped demonstrate the essentiality of several nutrients.

CHANGES IN THE DIGESTIVE SYSTEM THROUGHOUT LIFE

Pregnancy   Gastrointestinal problems may affect nutrition during pregnancy. During the first three months, many women experience nausea, referred to as morning sickness. This term is a misnomer, since it can occur at any time of the day. Morning sickness is believed to be due to the presence of pregnancy-related hormones in the blood. In most cases, it can be dealt with by eating frequent small meals and avoiding foods and smells that cause nausea. Eating dry crackers or cereal may also help. In severe cases, frequent vomiting occurs and requires medical intervention to obtain adequate nutrition.

Later in pregnancy, the enlarged uterus puts pressure on the stomach and intestines, making consumption of large meals uncomfortable. In addition, the placenta produces the hormone progesterone, which causes the smooth muscles of the digestive tract to relax. The muscle-relaxing effects of progesterone may relax the gastroesophageal sphincter allowing food to move back into the esophagus, causing heartburn. Symptoms of heartburn can be reduced by avoiding spicy foods; avoiding fatty foods, which slow the rate of stomach emptying; and remaining upright after eating. In the large intestine, relaxed muscles and the pressure of the uterus cause less efficient peristaltic movements, which may result in constipation. Increasing water intake, eating a diet high in fiber, and regular exercise can help relieve constipation.

Infancy   The obvious difference between the infant and adult digestive tracts is that newborns are not able to chew and swallow solid food. They are born with a suckling reflex that allows them to consume liquids from a nipple placed toward the back of the mouth. A protrusion reflex causes anything placed in the front of the mouth to be pushed out by the tongue. As head control increases, this reflex disappears, making spoon feeding possible.

Digestion and absorption also differ between infants and adults. In infants, the digestion of milk protein is aided by rennin, an enzyme produced in the infant stomach but not found in adults.[3] Low levels of pancreatic enzymes in infants limit starch digestion; however, enzymes at the brush border of the small intestine allow the milk sugar, lactose, to be digested and absorbed. The absorption of fat from the infant's small intestine is not very efficient. However, the ability to absorb intact protein is greater than in adults. The absorption of whole protein can cause food allergies (see Chapter 13), but it also allows infants to absorb immune factors from their mother's milk. These proteins provide temporary immunity to certain diseases. The bacteria in the large intestine of infants are also different from those in adults because of the all-milk diet infants consume. This is the reason that the feces of breast-fed babies are almost odorless. Another feature of the infant digestive tract is the lack of voluntary control of elimination. Between the ages of two and three, this ability develops, and toilet training is possible.

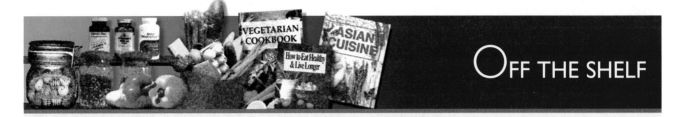

O FF THE SHELF

Over-the-Counter Remedies—Do They Really Cure What Ails You?

In the United States we spend over a billion dollars a year on nonprescription digestive remedies.[1] Formulations are available for controlling heartburn and curing constipation. Do they really do what they claim?

A variety of antacid formulations are marketed for the purpose of neutralizing stomach acid. Stomach acid is produced to help digest food, but an excess can lead to heartburn and contribute to ulcer formation. Heartburn results most commonly from overeating and tends to occur about an hour after a large meal. Anxiety and stress may also cause heartburn by stimulating stomach acid production. Although no well-controlled human studies have been done to determine whether antacids reduce heartburn, informal clinical observations suggest that antacids are effective. Self-medication with antacids to treat heartburn, however, should be limited, because repeated use may stimulate the stomach to produce more acid and aggravate some gastrointestinal problems. The sale of antacid tablets at the candy counter right next to Lifesavers

and Tic Tacs contributes to antacid overuse.

Laxatives are another bestseller. Although they may relieve constipation, they may also be the cause of constipation if used too frequently. Constipation is usually the result of behavioral factors, a poor diet, or a medical problem. Behavior can cause constipation because consistently disregarding the urge to defecate may eventually cause the rectum to fail to signal the need. Diet can cause constipation because a diet low in fiber or fluid may not provide sufficient bulk for proper bowel function. Different laxatives work in different ways. Some stimulate peristalsis, some work by softening the stools, and others add bulk. Overuse of laxatives that stimulate peristalsis can actually worsen constipation. Repeated use may irritate the mucosal lining and decrease muscle tone. Stronger and stronger stimuli are then needed to produce the muscular activity needed for defecation. According to the FDA, the safest laxatives are the bulk-producing laxatives. These contain fibers that

pass into the colon undigested and, when consumed with sufficient fluids, increase the volume of the feces and stimulate peristalsis. The same effect can be achieved by consuming fluids along with foods high in fiber such as fruits, vegetables, and whole grain products; and these have the added benefit of providing other nutrients.

[1]The editors of Consumer Reports Books. *The New Medicine Show*, 6th ed. Mount Vernon, NY: Consumers Union, 1989.

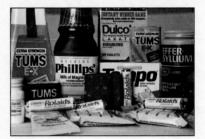

(Gregory Smolin)

Old Age   Although there are few dramatic changes in the nutrient requirements of humans as they age, changes in the digestive tract and other systems may alter the palatability of food and the ability to obtain proper nutrition. The senses of smell and taste are often diminished or even lost with age, reducing the appeal of food. Loss of teeth and improperly fitting dentures may limit food choices to soft and liquid foods or cause solid foods to be poorly chewed. The levels of intestinal secretions may also be reduced, but this rarely impairs absorption because the levels secreted in the healthy elderly are sufficient to break down food into forms that can be absorbed. A condition that is common in the elderly causes a decrease in the secretion of acid by the stomach. This may decrease the absorption of several vitamins and minerals and may permit an increase in bacterial growth (see Chapter 15).

CRITICAL THINKING

Gastrointestinal Problems Can Affect Nutrition

This chapter has followed the path of a turkey sandwich, an apple, and a glass of milk through the processes of digestion and absorption. During the journey from mouth to anus, many factors can affect how well these processes work. For each situation described below, think about how digestion and absorption might be altered.

Mouth

An individual has just had some dental work done, and chewing is difficult and painful.

What nutrients might not be absorbed if this person decided to eat the apple?

If food is not well chewed, digestive enzymes cannot come in contact with all components of the food. If the fiber in the apple skin is not chewed, the B vitamins it contains may not be available for absorption.

Stomach

After consuming the turkey sandwich, apple, and glass of milk, a large slice of high-fat cheesecake is added for dessert.

How would this affect transit time?

Transit time would increase because the cheesecake would increase the fat content of the meal. High-fat meals stay in the stomach longer, so the meal would take more time to pass from mouth to anus.

Pancreas

An individual has a disease of the pancreas that causes a deficiency of pancreatic enzymes.

What effect would this have on the digestion and absorption of the carbohydrate, fat, and protein in the sample meal?

Pancreatic enzymes are needed to digest carbohydrate, fat, and protein. If these enzymes are lacking, digestion will be incomplete, and nutrient absorption will be compromised. Carbohydrate-digesting enzymes in the mouth and intestinal brush border, as well as protein-digesting enzymes in the stomach and mucosal cells, can partially compensate for a lack of pancreatic enzymes.

Small intestine

An individual has been malnourished. The malnutrition causes the intestinal villi to become flattened.

If this individual consumed the sample meal, how would nutrient absorption be affected?

The absorption of all nutrients depends on the health of the small intestine. If the villi are flattened, the absorptive area will be decreased, so fewer nutrients will be absorbed. Malnutrition will also affect the function of the mucosal cells, so digestion and absorption that depend on these cells will also decrease.

Large intestine

An individual eats several turkey sandwiches but chooses not to drink the milk, eat the apple, or consume any other fluid.

How might this affect the feces?

A diet low in fluid might result in hard feces and constipation. This is more likely to be a problem if the diet is low in fluid and high in fiber.

Gallbladder

An individual has gallstones, which cause pain when the gallbladder contracts.

What nutrient should this person avoid?

Answer:

THE PATH OF ABSORBED NUTRIENTS

Absorbed materials are delivered to body cells by the cardiovascular system, which consists of the heart and blood vessels. The path by which nutrients enter the bloodstream varies with the nutrient. Amino acids from protein, simple sugars from carbohydrate, and the water soluble products of fat digestion are absorbed directly into the bloodstream. The products of fat digestion that are not water soluble are taken into the lymphatic system before entering the blood.

THE CARDIOVASCULAR SYSTEM

The cardiovascular system is a closed network of tubules through which blood is pumped. Blood carries nutrients and oxygen to the cells of all the organs and tissues of the body and removes waste products from these same cells. Blood also carries other substances, such as hormones, from one part of the body to another (Figure 3-14).

The heart is the workhorse of the cardiovascular system. It is a muscular pump with two circulatory loops—one that delivers blood to the lungs and one that delivers blood to the body. The blood vessels that transport blood and dissolved substances toward the heart are called **veins**, and those that transport blood and dissolved substances away from the heart are called **arteries**. As arteries carry

Veins–Vessels that carry blood toward the heart.
Arteries–Vessels that carry blood away from the heart.

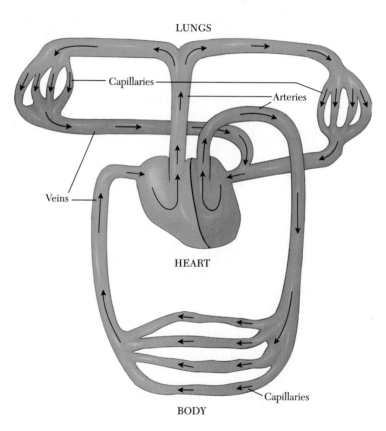

FIGURE 3-14
Blood is pumped from the heart through the arteries to the capillaries of the lungs, where it picks up oxygen. It then returns to the heart via the veins and is pumped out again into the arteries that lead to the rest of the body. In the capillaries of the body, blood delivers oxygen and nutrients and picks up wastes before returning to the heart via the veins. In this figure, red indicates blood that is rich in oxygen, and blue represents blood that is oxygen poor and carrying more carbon dioxide.

blood away from the heart, they branch many times to form smaller and smaller blood vessels. The smallest arteries are called arterioles. Arterioles then branch to form **capillaries**. Capillaries are thin-walled vessels that are just large enough to allow one red blood cell to pass at a time. In the capillaries, oxygen and nutrients carried by the blood pass out through the capillary wall into the cells, and waste products pass from the cells into the capillaries. In the capillaries of the lungs, blood releases carbon dioxide to be exhaled and picks up oxygen to be delivered to the cells. In the capillaries of the GI tract, blood picks up water soluble nutrients absorbed from the diet. Blood from capillaries then flows into the smallest veins, the venules, which converge to form larger and larger veins for return to the heart. Therefore, blood starting in the heart is pumped through the arteries to the capillaries of the lungs where it picks up oxygen. It then returns to the heart via the veins and is pumped out again into the arteries that lead to the rest of the body. In the capillaries of the body, blood delivers oxygen and nutrients and removes wastes before returning to the heart via the veins.

The blood flow and hence the amounts of nutrients and oxygen that are delivered to an organ or tissue depend on the need. When a person is resting, about 25% of the blood goes to the digestive system; 20% to the skeletal muscles; and the rest to the heart, kidneys, brain, skin, and other organs.[4] After a large meal, a greater proportion will go to the intestines to support its activity and to transport nutrients. When a person engages in strenuous exercise, large amounts of blood will be directed to the skeletal muscles to deliver nutrients and oxygen and remove carbon dioxide and waste products. Attempting to exercise after a large meal creates a conflict. The body cannot direct blood to the intestines and the muscles at the same time. The muscles win, and food remains in the intestines, often resulting in cramps.

> **Capillaries**—Small, thin-walled blood vessels where the exchange of gases and nutrients between blood and cells occurs.

HEPATIC PORTAL AND LYMPHATIC CIRCULATION

Nutrients enter the blood circulation by either the **hepatic portal circulation** or the **lymphatic system**. The villi of the intestine contain both capillaries, which form part of the portal circulation, and lacteals, small vessels of the lymphatic system.

> **Hepatic portal circulation**—The system of blood vessels that collect nutrient-laden blood from the digestive organs and deliver it to the liver.
> **Lymphatic system**—The system of lymph vessels and other lymph organs and tissues that drains excess fluid from the space between cells and provides immune function.

The Hepatic Portal Circulation

In the small intestine, water soluble products of digestion, including amino acids, sugars, and some water soluble products of fat digestion, cross the mucosal cells of the villi and enter capillaries. These capillaries merge to form venules at the base of the villi. The venules then merge to form larger and larger veins, which eventually form the **hepatic portal vein**. The hepatic portal vein transports blood directly to the liver, where absorbed nutrients are processed before they enter the general circulation (Figure 3-15).

The liver acts as a gatekeeper between substances absorbed from the intestine and the rest of the body. Some nutrients are stored in the liver, some are changed into different forms, and others are allowed to pass through unchanged. Based on the immediate needs of the body, the liver decides whether individual nutrients will be packaged for storage or delivered directly to the cells. For example, the liver, with the help of hormones from the pancreas, keeps the concentration of sugar in the blood constant by removing glucose from the portal blood and storing it, by sending absorbed glucose on to the tissues of the body, or by releasing glucose stored or synthesized in the liver to the blood. The liver is also important for the synthesis and breakdown of amino acids, proteins, and lipids. It modifies the products of protein breakdown to form molecules that can be safely transported to the kidney for excretion. The liver also contains enzyme systems that protect the body from toxins that are absorbed by the gastrointestinal tract.

> **Hepatic portal vein**—The vein that transports blood from the gastrointestinal tract to the liver.

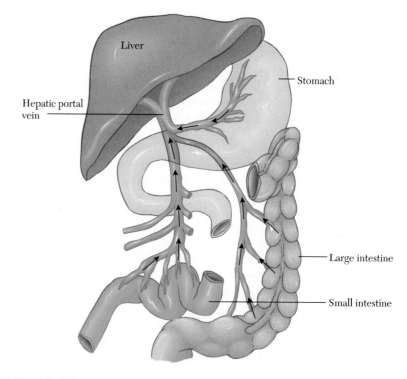

FIGURE 3-15
The hepatic portal circulation carries blood from the stomach and intestines to the hepatic portal vein and then to the liver.

The Lymphatic System The lymphatic system consists of a network of vessels that drain excess tissue fluid from the space between cells, called interstitial space, and return it to the bloodstream. Unlike the blood vessels, which carry substances to and from tissues, the lymphatic system only carries fluid away from the tissues. Fluid that is pushed out of capillaries by the force of the blood moves into the interstitial space, and is then collected by the lymph vessels. The lymphatic system prevents fluid from accumulating and causing the tissues to swell. Fat soluble substances—such as triglycerides, cholesterol, and fat soluble vitamins—and other absorbed materials too large to enter the intestinal capillaries are transported from the villi by the lymphatic system. (See Chapter 5.) Lymph vessels from the intestine and most other organs of the body drain into the thoracic duct, which empties into the bloodstream near the neck. Therefore substances that are absorbed into the lymph do not pass through the liver before entering the blood circulation.

In addition to its role in nutrient absorption and fluid balance, the lymphatic system is an extremely important part of the immune system. The role of nutrition in immune function is discussed in Chapters 6 and 15.

DESTINATION: THE CELL

Cell membrane—The membrane that encloses the cell contents.

Selectively permeable—Describes a membrane or barrier that will allow some substances to pass freely but will restrict the passage of others.

For nutrients to enter a cell, they must first cross the **cell membrane**. The cell membrane maintains homeostasis in the cell by controlling what enters and what exits. It is **selectively permeable** because some substances, such as water, can pass freely back and forth, whereas others require special transport systems or pumps to move across cell membranes. The processes that move nutrients and other substances from the bloodstream into cells are similar to those that transport nutrients from the intestinal lumen into the mucosal cells, such as diffusion and

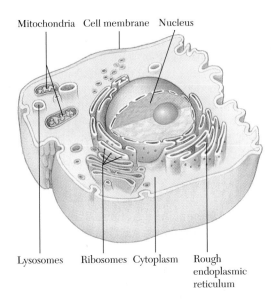

Mitochondria Cell membrane Nucleus

Lysosomes   Ribosomes Cytoplasm   Rough
endoplasmic
reticulum

FIGURE 3-16
Structure of a general animal cell. Almost all human cells contain the organelles illustrated here.

active transport. Inside the cell membrane is the **cytoplasm**, or cell fluid that contains the cell **organelles** that perform functions necessary for cell survival. Organelles are also surrounded by membranes. The largest organelle is the nucleus, which contains the cell's genetic material (Figure 3-16).

Once the nutrients have crossed the cell membrane and entered the cell, they can be broken down and used for energy, or they can be used to build the types of carbohydrates, lipids, and proteins that are needed by the human body. The sum of the reactions that convert nutrients into energy and build new molecules is called metabolism.

Cytoplasm–The cellular material outside the nucleus that is contained by the cell membrane.
Organelles–Cellular organs that carry out specific metabolic functions.

METABOLISM

A basic comprehension of how individual nutrients are used in metabolism is vital to understanding the nutritional needs of the body. The following discussion provides only a brief overview. Details about the metabolism of each nutrient will be discussed in later chapters.

Many of the reactions of metabolism occur in series known as metabolic pathways. Molecules that enter these pathways are modified at each step of the pathway with the help of enzymes. Some of the pathways are **anabolic**, using energy to build body structures, whereas others are **catabolic**, breaking large molecules into smaller ones and releasing energy.

Anabolic and catabolic processes occur in different cellular organelles. An example of an anabolic organelle is the endoplasmic reticulum, which is a maze of internal membranes. One type of endoplasmic reticulum specializes in lipid synthesis. Another type is covered with organelles called ribosomes, which are the site of protein synthesis. An example of a catabolic organelle is the lysosome, which acts as a kind of digestive system for the cell. Lysosomes contain enzymes capable of breaking down carbohydrates, fats, proteins, and other types of molecules that originate both inside and outside the cell.

The **mitochondrion** is a catabolic organelle that obtains energy from carbohydrates, fats, and proteins by **cellular respiration**. This process completely metabolizes these macronutrients in the presence of oxygen to produce carbon dioxide, water, and a form of energy that can be used by cells called **ATP (adenosine triphosphate)**. The chemical bonds of ATP are very high in energy, and when they break, the energy is released. The energy contained in ATP can be used to do work or to synthesize new molecules.

Anabolic–Refers to energy-requiring processes in which simpler molecules are combined to form more complex substances.
Catabolic–Refers to the processes by which substances are broken down into simpler molecules.

Mitochondrion–The cellular organelle responsible for generating energy in the form of ATP for cellular activities.
Cellular respiration–The reactions that break down carbohydrates, fats, and proteins in the presence of oxygen to produce energy in the form of ATP.
ATP (adenosine triphosphate)–The high-energy molecule used by the body to perform energy-requiring activities.

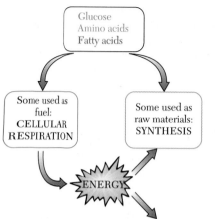

FIGURE 3-17

Nutrients delivered to cells can be used to produce energy or as raw materials for the synthesis of carbohydrates, fats, and proteins in the body.

The meal consumed at the beginning of this chapter has now been delivered to the cells. The carbohydrate in the bread has been converted to glucose. The cells can then use it to produce ATP or store it for later use. The protein in the turkey, milk, and bread has been broken down into amino acids that can be used by the cell to synthesize needed protein, to make glucose, if it is in short supply, or to produce ATP (Figure 3-17). The fat in the milk, turkey, and mayonnaise has been broken down into fatty acids. These can be used to make ATP, to produce lipids needed for body function, or they can be stored as body fat for later use.

ELIMINATION OF WASTES

The waste products left over from the digestion and metabolism of the meal must be removed from the body. Substances, such as fiber, that are not absorbed from the intestine are eliminated from the gastrointestinal tract in the feces. Waste products of cellular metabolism, such as carbon dioxide, water, and nitrogen, are eliminated by the lungs, the skin, and the kidneys.

The carbon dioxide produced by cellular respiration leaves the cells and is transported to the lungs by red blood cells. At the lungs, red blood cells release their load of carbon dioxide, which is then exhaled into the environment. In addition to carbon dioxide, the lungs lose a significant amount of water by evaporation.

Another site for the excretion of wastes is the skin. Here, some water, protein breakdown products, and minerals are lost in perspiration or sweat.

The kidney is the primary site for the excretion of water, nitrogen, and other dissolved metabolic waste products. These are excreted in the urine. The amounts of water and other substances excreted in the urine are regulated so that homeostasis is maintained. Water balance will be discussed in more detail in Chapters 10 and 12.

SUMMARY

1. The organization of all matter begins with the same basic structure—the atom. Atoms are linked by chemical bonds to form molecules. The cell is the smallest unit of life. Cells of similar structure and function are organized into tissues, and tissues into organs and organ systems.

2. The digestive system is the organ system primarily responsible for the movement of nutrients into the body. The digestive system provides two major functions: digestion and absorption. Digestion is the process by which food is broken down into units that are small enough to be absorbed. Absorption is the process by which nutrients are transported into the body.

3. The gastrointestinal tract consists of a hollow tube that begins at the mouth and continues through the pharynx, esophagus, stomach, small intestine, large intestine, and anus. The passage, digestion, and absorption of food in the lumen are aided by the secretion of mucus, enzymes, and hormones.

4. The processes involved in digestion begin in response to the smell or sight of food and continue as food enters the digestive tract at the mouth, where it is broken into smaller pieces by the teeth and mixed with saliva. Carbohydrate digestion is begun in the mouth by salivary amylase. From the mouth, food passes through the pharynx and into the esophagus. The rhythmic contractions of peristalsis propel it down the esophagus to the stomach.

5. The stomach acts as a temporary storage site for food. The muscles of the stomach mix the food into a semiliquid mass called chyme, and gastric juice containing hydrochloric acid and pepsin begins protein digestion. Stomach emptying is regulated by the amount and composition of food consumed and by signals from the small intestine.

6. The small intestine is the primary site of nutrient digestion and absorption. In the small intestine, bicarbonate from the pancreas neutralizes stomach acid, and pancreatic enzymes digest carbohydrate, fat, and protein. The digestion of fat in the small intestine is aided by bile from the gallbladder. Bile helps break fat into small droplets accessible to fat-digesting enzymes. All these secretions are regulated by the hormones secretin and cholecystokinin, produced by the duodenum.

7. The absorption of food across the intestinal mucosa occurs

by several different processes. Simple and facilitated diffusion require no energy but depend on a concentration gradient. Active transport requires energy but can transport substances against a concentration gradient. The absorptive surface of the small intestine is increased by folds and finger-like projections called villi, which are covered with tiny projections called microvilli.

8. Components of chyme that are not absorbed in the small intestine pass on to the large intestine, where some water and nutrients are absorbed. The large intestine is populated by bacteria that digest some unabsorbed materials, such as fiber, producing small amounts of nutrients and gas. The remaining unabsorbed materials are excreted in feces.

9. Absorbed nutrients are delivered to the cells of the body by the cardiovascular system. The heart pumps blood to the lungs to acquire oxygen and eliminate carbon dioxide. From the lungs, blood returns to the heart and is pumped to the rest of the body to deliver oxygen and nutrients and remove carbon dioxide and other wastes before returning to the heart. Blood is pumped away from the heart in arteries and returned to the heart in veins. Exchange of nutrients and gases occurs at the smallest blood vessels, the capillaries.

10. The products of carbohydrate and protein digestion and the water soluble products of fat digestion enter capillaries in the intestinal villi and are transported to the liver. The liver serves as a processing center, removing the absorbed substances for storage, converting them into other forms, or allowing them to pass unaltered. The liver also protects the body from toxic substances that may have been absorbed.

11. The fat soluble products of digestion and other large materials enter lacteals in the intestinal villi. The nutrients absorbed via the lymphatic system enter the blood circulation without first passing through the liver.

12. The final destination of absorbed nutrients is cells. To enter the cells, nutrients must be transported across membranes. Within the cells, some organelles are catabolic, specializing in the breakdown of nutrients to produce energy. Others are anabolic, specializing in the synthesis of molecules needed by the body. The sum of all the chemical reactions of the body is called metabolism. The reactions that completely break down macronutrients in the presence of oxygen to produce water, carbon dioxide, and energy are referred to as cellular respiration.

13. The waste products of metabolism are removed from the body through the lungs, skin, and kidneys.

SELF-TEST

1. What is an organic molecule?
2. What is the smallest unit of plant and animal life?
3. List three organ systems involved in the digestion and absorption of food.
4. How do teeth function in digestion?
5. What is peristalsis?
6. List two functions of the stomach.
7. List three mechanisms by which nutrients are absorbed.
8. Where does most digestion and absorption occur?
9. How does the structure of the small intestine aid in absorption?
10. What products of digestion are transported by the lymphatic system?
11. How does the path of an amino acid from absorption to delivery to the cell differ from the absorption and delivery path of a large fatty acid?
12. What is the form of energy used by cells?
13. List four ways that waste products are eliminated from the body.

APPLICATIONS

These exercises are designed to help you apply your critical thinking skills to your own nutrition choices.

1. Imagine you wake up on a Sunday morning and join some friends for a large breakfast consisting of a cheese omelet and sausage, foods high in fat and protein; a croissant with butter, which contains carbohydrate but is also very high in fat; and a small glass of orange juice. After the meal, you remember that you have plans to play basketball with a friend in just an hour.
   a. If you keep your plans and play basketball, what problems might you experience while exercising?
   b. Had you remembered your plans for strenuous exercise before you had breakfast, what type of meal might you have selected to ensure that your stomach would empty more quickly?
2. Most foods contain some carbohydrate, fat, and protein.
   a. Discuss where in the digestive tract the digestion of each of these nutrients begins.
   b. Does the presence of a high-protein food in the digestive tract inhibit the digestion and absorption of foods high in carbohydrate? Why or why not?

REFERENCES

1. Kang, J.Y. Peptic ulcer—a new look. Ann. Acad. Med. Singapore 24:218–223, 1995.
2. Roberfroid, M.B., Bornet, F., Bouley, C., and Cummings, J.H. Colonic microflora: nutrition and health. Summary and Conclusions of an International Life Sciences Institute (ILSI) [Europe] Workshop held in Barcelona, Spain. Nutr. Rev. 53:127–130, 1995.
3. Marieb, E.N. *Human Anatomy and Physiology*, 3rd ed. Redwood City, CA: The Benjamin/Cummings Publishing Company, 1995.
4. Solomon, E.P., Schmidt, R.R., and Adragna, P.J. *Human Anatomy and Physiology*, 2nd ed. Philadelphia: Saunders College Publishing, 1990.

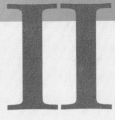

ENERGY-CONTAINING NUTRIENTS

II

LIFE CYCLE

Carbohydrates: Sugars, Starches, and Fiber

CHAPTER CONCEPTS

1. Carbohydrates from grains such as rice and wheat are the basis of the diet for most of the world.

2. There are many types of carbohydrates, including simple carbohydrates, such as that in table sugar and fruit, and complex carbohydrates, such as starch and fiber found in legumes and grains.

3. Carbohydrates provide a readily available source of energy and are central to energy production in the human body.

4. Dietary fiber cannot be digested by the human stomach or small intestine and is therefore not absorbed into the body.

5. Foods high in refined sugar are low in nutrient density; foods high in complex carbohydrates are rich sources of other nutrients.

6. Diets high in sugar and starch may promote tooth decay. Diets high in fiber may protect against chronic diseases such as diverticulosis, heart disease, and cancer.

7. The typical carbohydrate intake in the North American diet is below the recommended level of 55 to 60% of total energy.

8. Carbohydrates are added in processing to sweeten, preserve, stabilize, or thicken foods.

9. Sugar substitutes, many of which are not carbohydrates, are used to replace sugars in foods.

JUST A TASTE

Are starchy foods fattening?

Do Americans eat too much carbohydrate?

Do artificial sweeteners help you to lose weight?

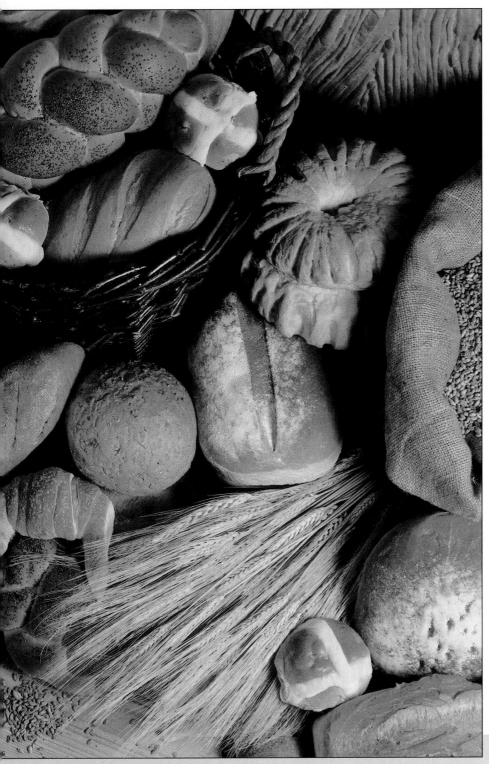

(Simon Yeo/Tony Stone Images.)

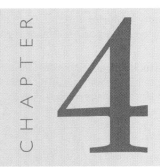

CHAPTER 4

C Carbohydrate-rich foods provide the basis of the diet for most of the world. Rice is the dietary staple in Southeast Asia, corn in South America, and cassava in parts of Africa. Although every culture eats carbohydrate, the amount and type consumed often depend on the wealth and prosperity of the society. As countries become more affluent, the intake of carbohydrate typically decreases while the intake of fat and protein increases. For example, in developing countries today, two thirds of the energy in the diet comes from carbohydrate, whereas in more economically developed Western societies, the typical intake of carbohydrate accounts for only about 40 to 50% of the energy intake. The affluence of the society also influences the form of carbohydrate consumed. Throughout history peasants have eaten brown bread and brown rice while the aristocracy has consumed refined white flour, sugar, and rice. The trend toward a diet lower in total carbohydrate and higher in sugar and refined grains may be the tide that moves a society's diet toward nutritional decline. Recommendations for a healthy diet promote diets high in whole grains, vegetables, and fruits and limited in refined and added carbohydrates.

In this chapter, we will discuss:
- What are carbohydrates?
- What role do they play in our diet and our health?
- How can you meet the recommendations for the types and amounts of carbohydrates in your diet?

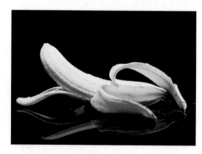

FIGURE 4-1
Bananas are a source of dietary carbohydrates. (Charles D. Winters)

Carbohydrates–Compounds containing carbon and hydrogen and oxygen in the same proportions as in water. They include sugar, starch, and fiber.

Simple carbohydrates–Carbohydrates known as sugars that include monosaccharides and disaccharides.

Refined–Refers to the process whereby the coarse parts of foods are removed, leaving behind a product of more uniform composition.

Empty kcalories–Refers to foods that contribute energy but few other nutrients.

Phytochemicals–Chemicals found in plants that are not essential nutrients but play a role in preventing chronic disease.

WHAT ARE CARBOHYDRATES?

Chemically, **carbohydrates** are compounds that contain carbon (carbo), as well as hydrogen and oxygen in the same proportion as in water (hydrate). They are found in grains, breads, fruits, vegetables, and milk, and they are the primary source of energy used to fuel the body (Figure 4-1). Carbohydrates provide 4 kcalories per gram. Most high-carbohydrate foods like bread and rice also contain protein and fat (Figure 4-2).

Carbohydrates provide 40 to 50% of the energy in the American diet. **Simple carbohydrates**, or sugars, provide about 21% of the energy. Half of this is from sugars naturally present in whole foods such as milk or fresh fruit.[1] The rest is from sugars added to foods. Added sugars are **refined** to separate them from their plant sources, such as sugar cane and sugar beets. Refined sugars are not nutritionally or chemically different from sugars occurring naturally in foods. The only difference is that they have been separated from other nutrients. Foods high in refined sugars are therefore considered **empty kcalories** because they contain energy but few other nutrients. When a whole food containing natural sources of sugar is consumed, the sugar is usually accompanied by vitamins, minerals, fiber, and other nonnutrients with health-promoting properties such as **phytochemicals**. Foods that are natural sources of sugar, therefore, have a higher nutrient density—that is, they contain more nutrients per kcalorie than do foods with added refined sugar. For example, four marshmallows contain 100 kcalories but almost no nutrients other than sugar. A large orange also has about 100 kcalories but contributes vitamin C, potassium, fiber, and some calcium.

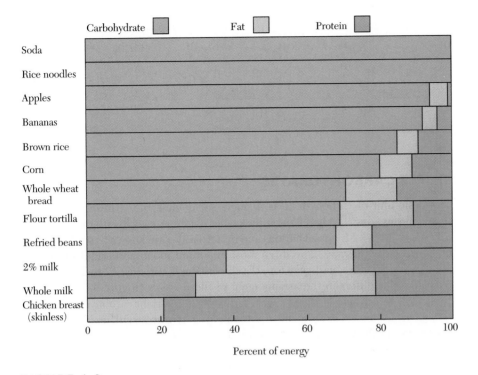

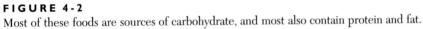

FIGURE 4-2
Most of these foods are sources of carbohydrate, and most also contain protein and fat.

Complex carbohydrates include starch and fiber. Starch is made of many sugar molecules linked together. Fiber is a mixture of substances, most of which are carbohydrate, that cannot be digested by enzymes in the human stomach and small intestine. Grains are the major source of complex carbohydrate in the North American diet. Kernels of grain provide a mixture of starch and fiber along with vitamins, minerals, and oils. The outermost part, the **bran**, is really six layers of protective fiber (Figure 4-3). The bran contains most of the fiber in the grain and is a good source of B vitamins. The **germ**, which lies at the base of the kernel, is the plant embryo where sprouting will occur. It is the source of vegetable oils such as corn or safflower oil, and it is rich in vitamin E. Together the bran layers and germ contain most of the fiber, vitamins, and minerals in the grain. The remainder of the kernel is the **endosperm**, which is the starchy food supply for the sprouting embryo. The endosperm is primarily starch but also contains most of the protein and some vitamins and minerals. During the milling of grain into flour, the grinding detaches the germ and bran from the endosperm. Whole grain flours such as whole wheat flour include the bran, germ, and endosperm. When flours are refined, these components are separated; white flour is produced from just the endosperm. Fiber and some vitamins and minerals naturally found in the whole grain are lost. For this reason, white flour and other refined grains are enriched, a process that adds back some of the nutrients lost in processing. Fiber is not added back.

Other plant foods such as vegetables and legumes are also sources of both fiber and starch. The pulp of starchy vegetables such as potatoes provides starch, whereas the skins are a source of fiber and many of the vitamins. Dried legumes, such as pinto and kidney beans, are excellent sources of starch and fiber and are a good source of protein. Other vegetables like green beans and broccoli are lower in starch and also high in fiber, making them lower in energy than the starchy vegetables.

Complex carbohydrates–Carbohydrates composed of sugar molecules linked together in straight or branching chains.

Bran–The protective outer layers of whole grains. It is a concentrated source of dietary fiber.
Germ–The embryo or sprouting portion of a kernel of grain. It contains vegetable oil and vitamins.

Endosperm–The largest portion of a kernel of grain. It is primarily starch and serves as a food supply for the sprouting seed.

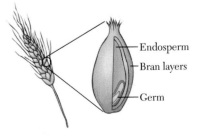

FIGURE 4-3
A grain of wheat contains outer layers of bran, the plant embryo or germ, and a carbohydrate-rich endosperm.

FIGURE 4-4

FIGURE 4-4
Common monosaccharides.

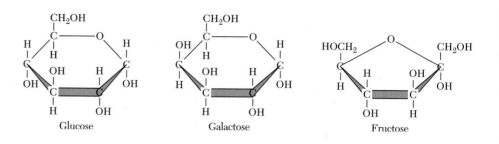

Glucose   Galactose   Fructose

SIMPLE CARBOHYDRATES

Monosaccharide–A single sugar molecule, such as glucose.
Disaccharide–A sugar formed by linking two monosaccharides.

Glucose–A monosaccharide that is the primary form of carbohydrate used to produce energy in the body. It is the sugar referred to as blood sugar.
Photosynthesis–The metabolic process by which plants trap energy from the sun and use it to make sugars from carbon dioxide and water.

The basic unit of carbohydrate is a single sugar molecule, a **monosaccharide** (*mono* means "one"). When 2 sugar molecules combine, they form a **disaccharide** (*di* means "two"). Monosaccharides and disaccharides are known as simple sugars, or simple carbohydrates. The three most important monosaccharides in the diet are glucose, fructose, and galactose. Each contains 6 carbons, 12 hydrogens, and 6 oxygens but differs in the arrangement of these atoms (Figure 4-4). **Glucose**, commonly referred to as blood sugar, is the most important carbohydrate fuel for the body. It is produced in plants by the process of **photosynthesis**, which uses energy from the sun to combine carbon dioxide and water (Figure 4-5). Glucose rarely occurs as a monosaccharide in food. It is most often found as part of a disaccharide or starch. Fructose is a monosaccharide that tastes sweeter than glucose. It is found in fruits and vegetables and makes up more than half the sugar in honey. Galactose occurs most often as a part of lactose, the disaccharide in milk, and is rarely present as a monosaccharide in the food supply.

Disaccharides are simple carbohydrates made up of 2 monosaccharides linked together (Figure 4-6). Maltose is the disaccharide formed when 2 molecules of glucose are joined. This sugar is made whenever starch is broken down. For example, it is responsible for the slightly sweet taste experienced when bread is held in the mouth for a few minutes. As salivary amylase begins digesting the starch, some sweeter tasting maltose is formed. Sucrose, or common white table sugar, is the disaccharide formed by linking glucose to fructose. It is found in sugar cane,

FIGURE 4-5
The process of photosynthesis uses energy from the sun to synthesize glucose from carbon dioxide and water.

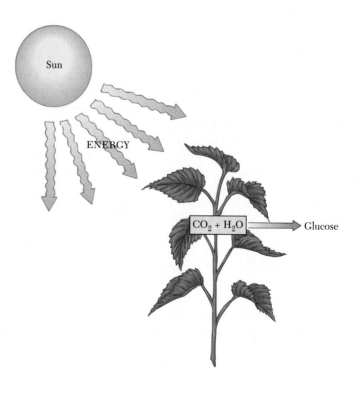

Sun

ENERGY

$CO_2 + H_2O$ → Glucose

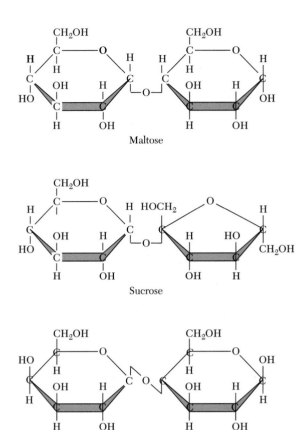

FIGURE 4-6
Common disaccharides.

Maltose

Sucrose

Lactose

sugar beets, honey, and maple syrup. Sucrose is the only sweetener that can be called sugar in the ingredients list on food labels in the United States. Lactose, or milk sugar, is glucose linked to galactose. Lactose is the only sugar found naturally in animal foods. It contributes about 30% of the energy in whole cow's milk and about 40% of the energy in human milk.

COMPLEX CARBOHYDRATES

Complex carbohydrates are made up of many monosaccharides linked together in chains. They are generally not sweet to the taste like simple carbohydrates. Short chains of three to ten monosaccharides are called **oligosaccharides** and longer chains are called **polysaccharides** (*poly* means "many"). The polysaccharides include glycogen in animals and starch and fiber in plants (Figure 4-7).

Oligosaccharides—Short chain carbohydrates containing 3 to 10 sugar units.
Polysaccharides—Carbohydrates containing many sugar units linked together.

Oligosaccharides   Two oligosaccharides found in beans and other legumes are raffinose and starchyose. These cannot be digested by enzymes in the human stomach and small intestine, so they pass undigested into the large intestine. Here bacteria digest them, producing gas and other byproducts. Plant breeders and genetic engineers are trying to develop varieties of legumes with lower amounts of these oligosaccharides to reduce the amount of intestinal gas produced when they are consumed.

Glycogen   **Glycogen** is the storage form of carbohydrate in animals. It is made up of highly branched chains of glucose molecules. The branched structure allows it to be broken down quickly when glucose is needed. In humans, glycogen is stored in the muscles and in the liver. Muscle glycogen provides glucose as a source

Glycogen—A carbohydrate made of many glucose molecules linked together in a highly branched structure. It is the storage form of carbohydrate in animals.

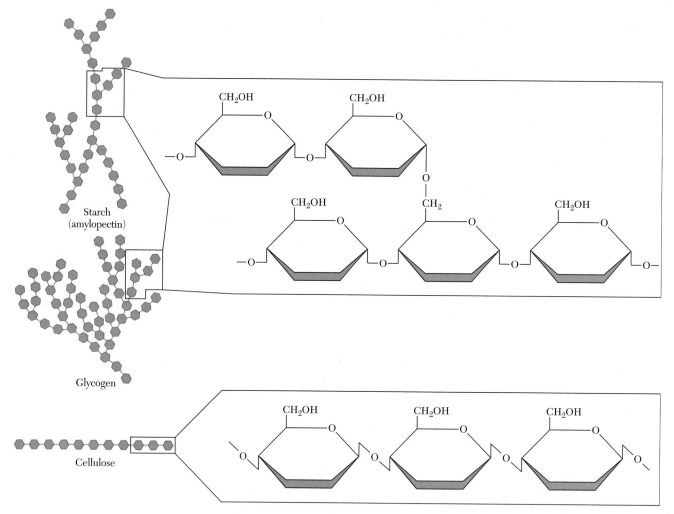

FIGURE 4-7
Complex carbohydrates are made up of straight or branching chains of monosaccharides.

Carbohydrate loading–A regimen of diet and exercise, followed in preparation for endurance activities, that is designed to load muscle glycogen stores beyond their normal capacity.

Starch–A carbohydrate made of many glucose molecules linked in straight or branching chains. The bonds that hold the glucose molecules together can be broken by the human digestive enzymes.

of energy for the muscle during activity, whereas liver glycogen supplies glucose when blood levels drop.

The amount of glycogen in the body is relatively small—about 200 to 500 grams.[2] The amount stored in muscle can be temporarily increased by **carbohydrate loading**, a diet and exercise regimen followed by endurance athletes to build up glycogen stores before an event. Extra glycogen can mean the difference between running only 20 miles or finishing a 26-mile marathon before exhaustion takes over. Carbohydrate loading is discussed in more detail in Chapter 12.

Starches   **Starch** is a storage form of carbohydrate in plants. It is found in two forms: amylose, which consists of long straight chains of glucose molecules, and amylopectin, which consists of branched chains of glucose molecules. Starch accumulates in seeds, where it provides an energy source for the developing plant embryo, and in roots and tubers, where it provides stored energy for the growth and reproduction of the plant. In our diet, we take advantage of these plant energy stores. When we eat products made from corn, rice, wheat, or oats, we are eating the starch from a seed. When we eat legumes such as peas, lentils, soybeans, and kidney beans, we are also eating a starchy seed but from a plant that produces

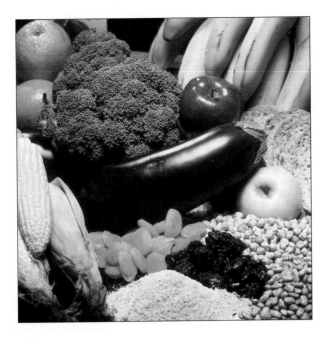

FIGURE 4-8
These foods are good sources of dietary fiber. (Charles D. Winters)

seeds in a pod. When we eat potatoes and yams, we are eating the underground energy storage organ of plants called tubers; and when we eat cassava, a starchy root is being used as a food source.

Dietary Fiber **Dietary fiber** consists of substances that cannot be digested in the stomach and small intestine because humans lack the enzymes necessary to break the bonds that connect the monosaccharide units. Since fiber cannot be digested, it cannot be absorbed into the body and used for energy. Some fiber is digested by microflora in the large intestine, producing gas and short chain fatty acids, small quantities of which can be absorbed.

Fibers are categorized by their ability to dissolve in water. **Insoluble fibers** are primarily those that are derived from the structural parts of plants such as the cell walls. These substances include cellulose and some hemicelluloses, which are carbohydrates, and lignins, which technically are not carbohydrates but are classified as insoluble dietary fiber. Food sources of insoluble fiber include wheat bran and rye bran, which are mostly hemicellulose and cellulose, and vegetables such as broccoli, which contain woody fibers composed partly of lignins. **Soluble fibers** are found around and inside plant cells. These carbohydrates either absorb water or dissolve in water. They include pectins, gums, and some hemicelluloses. Food sources of soluble fibers include oat bran, apples, beans, and seaweed. Pectins from fruit are used to gel jams and jellies. Gums found in seaweed are often added to processed foods as thickeners; for example, gums are used to thicken fat-free salad dressings. Most foods of plant origin contain mixtures of soluble and insoluble fibers (Figure 4-8).

Dietary fiber—Substances in food that are not broken down by the digestive processes in the human stomach and small intestine.

Insoluble fibers—Fiber that, for the most part, does not dissolve in water. It includes cellulose, hemicellulose, and lignin.

Soluble fibers—Fiber that either dissolves when placed in water or absorbs water. It includes pectins, gums and some hemicelluloses.

CARBOHYDRATES IN THE BODY

The major function of carbohydrate in the body is to provide energy to the cells. The main source of this energy is glucose. After absorption, monosaccharides travel via the hepatic portal vein to the liver where much of the fructose and

OFF THE SHELF

Honey and Molasses: Are "Natural" Sugars Better?

Some people think honey is healthy. Honey, blackstrap molasses, and other less refined sugars have been promoted as healthier alternatives to table sugar, since they contain some nutrients that have been processed out of pure white table sugar. Candy and baked products made with these sweeteners are marketed as more nutritious. Although these sweeteners do have more micronutrients than table sugar, the amounts are too small to add much to the diet.

Honey is derived from the nectar of flowering plants, which contains sucrose. Bees collect honey and convert the sucrose into fructose and glucose. The color, flavor, and proportions of the sugars in honey vary with the source of the nectar. Honey supplies a concentrated source of energy but only traces of vitamins and minerals, so it cannot be considered a nutrient-dense food. Since sucrose from any source is broken into glucose and fructose before it is absorbed in the small intestine, the body cannot distinguish whether the glucose and fructose it absorbs come from honey or from refined white table sugar. The benefit of honey as a home remedy

for a cough when mixed with lemon juice is only anecdotal. Honey is somewhat sweeter than sucrose, so smaller amounts may be used for the same level of sweetness. Because honey may contain spores of the bacteria *Clostridium bolulinum* (see Chapters 13 and 16), it should not be fed to infants.

Blackstrap molasses is a byproduct of the refining of sucrose from sugar cane or sugar beets. It is a thick brown syrup that remains after the sucrose has crystallized. Refining of blackstrap molasses produces light and medium molasses. Curative properties for cancer and other disorders have often been attributed to molasses, but there is no scientific support for these claims. Unlike any other concentrated nutritive sweetener, it does contain significant amounts of some minerals. When it is made in old-fashioned iron vats with iron pipes, it is rich in this nutrient.

Other sweeteners such as brown sugar and maple syrup are also believed by some to be healthier than sucrose. In fact, most are not significantly different from sucrose. Most brown sugar is simply refined white

sugar containing some molasses to color it brown. Maple syrup is formed by boiling down the sap of maple trees. It is composed primarily of sucrose, which has been browned by the heat involved in processing.

Sweeteners promoted as natural, such as honey, molasses, brown sugar, and maple syrup, are all processed in some way, either by humans or, in the case of honey, by bees. Though these sweeteners contribute distinctive flavors to the foods to which they are added, their nutritional contribution is not significantly different from that of refined white sugar.

Foods that are high in added refined sugars provide energy but few nutrients. So, guidelines for a healthy diet recommend that refined sugars be consumed in moderation. There are some easy ways to do this—use less sugar in coffee or on cereal and reduce sweetened soft drink consumption. But finding and eliminating other sources of refined sugar in the diet isn't always easy. Consumers need to understand the information provided on food labels before they can sort out their sugar intake.

galactose is converted into glucose. Glucose circulates in the blood, reaching cells throughout the body.

In addition to its role in energy production, there are several other functions of carbohydrates in the body. The monosaccharide galactose is an important molecule in nervous tissue. It also combines with glucose to make lactose in women who are producing breast milk. Two other monosaccharides that are of great importance to the body are deoxyribose and ribose. These sugars are components of DNA and RNA (ribonucleic acid), which contain the genetic information for the synthesis of proteins. Deoxyribose and ribose can be synthesized by the body and are not found in significant amounts in the diet. Ribose is also a component of the vitamin riboflavin. Oligosaccharides are also important in our bodies. They are found attached to proteins or lipids on the surface of cells where they help to signal information about cells.

Fiber cannot be digested by human enzymes, so it cannot be absorbed. However, it is important for the health of the gastrointestinal tract.

Nutritional Value of Various Sweeteners
(Nutrients per tablespoon of sweetener)

	Light Molasses	Medium Molasses	Blackstrap Molasses	Honey	Brown Sugar	Table Sugar
Energy (kcal)	40	38	35	61	52	46
Protein (g)	0.4	0.4	0.4	0.1	0	0
Carbohydrate (g)	10	9	8	16.5	13.4	11.9
Calcium (mg)	25	44	103	1	11	0.7
Phosphorus (mg)	7	10	13	1	5	0
Sodium (mg)	2	6	14	1	3	0
Magnesium (mg)	31	31	31	1	9	0
Potassium (mg)	138	159	439	10	32	0.7
Iron (mg)	0.6	0.9	2.4	0.1	0.4	0
Zinc (mg)	0.1	0.1	0.1	0.1	0.1	0
Copper (mg)	0.1	0.1	0.1	0	0	0
Thiamin (mg)	0.02	0.02	0.02	0	0	0
Riboflavin (mg)	0.02	0.02	0.03	0	0	0
Niacin (mg)	0.03	0.2	0.3	0	0	0
Pantothenic acid (mg)	0.1	0.1	0.1	0.2	0.01	0
Vitamin B_6 (mg)	0.03	0.03	0.03	0.1	0	0
Folic acid (μg)	2.0	1.4	1.4	0.24	0.09	0
Biotin (μg)	1.4	1.4	1.4	0	0	0

CARBOHYDRATES IN THE DIGESTIVE TRACT

The digestion of carbohydrate begins in the mouth, where salivary amylase starts breaking starch into shorter polysaccharides and maltose (see Figure 4-9). The majority of starch digestion occurs in the small intestine, where pancreatic amylases complete the job of breaking starch into maltose. The digestion of carbohydrate is completed by enzymes attached to the brush border of the villi in the small intestine. Here sucrose from table sugar is broken down by the enzyme sucrase to glucose and fructose; lactose from milk is broken down by lactase to form glucose and galactose; and maltose from starch is broken down into two glucose molecules by maltase. The resulting monosaccharides are then absorbed and transported to the liver via the hepatic portal circulation.

Lactose Intolerance   When lactose, the carbohydrate found in dairy products, is not completely digested, it passes into the large intestine, where it is me-

FIGURE 4-9
An overview of carbohydrate digestion and absorption.

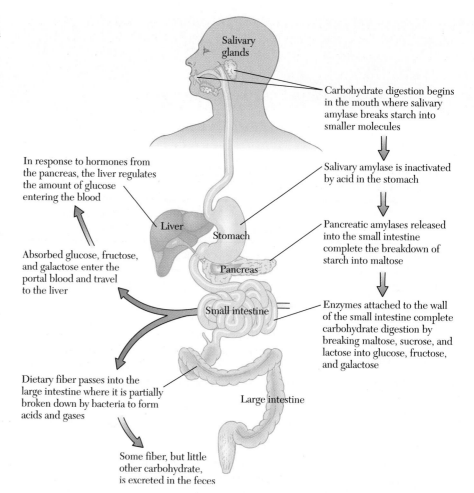

Carbohydrate digestion begins in the mouth where salivary amylase breaks starch into smaller molecules

Salivary amylase is inactivated by acid in the stomach

Pancreatic amylases released into the small intestine complete the breakdown of starch into maltose

Enzymes attached to the wall of the small intestine complete carbohydrate digestion by breaking maltose, sucrose, and lactose into glucose, fructose, and galactose

In response to hormones from the pancreas, the liver regulates the amount of glucose entering the blood

Absorbed glucose, fructose, and galactose enter the portal blood and travel to the liver

Dietary fiber passes into the large intestine where it is partially broken down by bacteria to form acids and gases

Some fiber, but little other carbohydrate, is excreted in the feces

Salivary glands

Liver

Stomach

Pancreas

Small intestine

Large intestine

Lactose intolerance—The inability to digest lactose because of a deficiency of the enzyme lactase. It causes symptoms such as gas and bloating after dairy products are consumed.

tabolized by bacteria. Acids and gas produced by the bacteria can draw in water, cause abdominal distension, flatulence, cramping, and diarrhea. This inability to digest lactose is called **lactose intolerance**. Although frequently called a milk allergy, lactose intolerance is not an allergy but rather a reduction in lactase, the enzyme needed to break lactose into glucose and galactose. Lactase is produced by almost everyone at birth, so milk digestion is rarely a problem in infants and children. However, in most ethnic groups, lactase levels decrease with age. This decrease occurs in 5% of Northern Europeans and in almost 100% of individuals in Far Eastern cultures.[3] In the United States, it is common in Asians and African Americans. Lactose intolerance may also occur as a result of an intestinal infection or other disease. It is then referred to as secondary lactase deficiency and may disappear when the other condition is resolved.

In cultures where lactose intolerance is common, traditional diets provide sources of calcium other than milk. For example, in Asia, tofu and fish consumed with bones supply calcium, and in the Near East fermented cheese and yogurt provide much of the calcium. In the United States milk is the most important source of calcium. The Food Guide Pyramid recommends 2 to 3 servings from the milk group each day. Individuals who are lactose intolerant must select diets that contain calcium-rich foods other than milk. Those who can tolerate lactose in small doses, can divide the 2 to 3 servings into many smaller portions or try yogurt, since the bacteria used to make yogurt digest some of the lactose. Cheese may also be tolerable, since much of the lactose is lost in processing. Those who cannot tolerate any lactose can meet their calcium needs with tofu, fish, calcium-rich vegetables, and milk treated with the enzyme lactase. Lactase breaks the lactose into glucose and galactose, producing a somewhat sweeter-tasting but lactose-free milk. Lactase tablets, which can be consumed with or before milk products, are also available. The enzymes in these tablets digest the lactose before it passes into the large intestine (Figure 4-10).

Fiber: Indigestible but Indispensable

Even though dietary fiber cannot be digested by the enzymes of the human digestive tract, fiber does have important properties that affect the digestive tract and maintain healthy bowel function. Soluble fibers, such as pectins and gums, absorb water. For example, the soluble fiber in a carrot can hold 20 to 30 times its weight in water. In the gastrointestinal tract, soluble fibers absorb water, forming viscous solutions that slow the rate at which nutrients are absorbed. The delay in glucose absorption caused by fiber is beneficial for individuals with diseases that affect the regulation of blood glucose levels (diabetes and hypoglycemia) because it slows the rate at which glucose reaches the bloodstream. Insoluble fibers, such as wheat bran, increase the amount of material in the intestine. Together the increased bulk of insoluble fibers and the fluid drawn in by soluble fibers result in an increased volume of material in the intestine. This promotes healthy bowel function because it stimulates peristalsis, causing the muscles of the colon to work more, become stronger, and function better. The increase in peristalsis also reduces transit time, the time it takes food and fecal matter to move through the intestine. In African countries, where the diet contains 40 to 150 grams of fiber per day, the transit time is 36 hours or less. In the United States, where fiber intake is less than 20 grams per day, it is not uncommon for transit time to be as long as 96 hours.

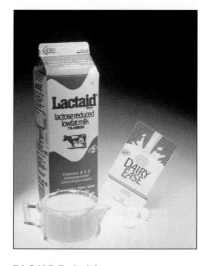

FIGURE 4-10
These products can allow individuals with lactose intolerance to consume milk. (Charles D. Winters)

CARBOHYDRATE METABOLISM

Body cells receive a constant supply of glucose via the bloodstream. This supply is regulated by the liver and by hormones secreted from the pancreas. Once glucose reaches the cells, it is metabolized to produce energy.

Delivery of Glucose to Cells

After a meal, glucose is absorbed and enters the bloodstream, causing blood levels to rise. How quickly blood glucose levels rise after a meal, referred to as **glycemic response**, or **glycemic index**, is affected by the composition of the diet. Foods that leave the stomach quickly and are readily absorbed raise blood glucose levels most rapidly and so have the highest glycemic index. For example, when a food that is mostly sucrose, such as a gumdrop, is consumed alone, blood glucose levels rise within minutes. Fat and protein consumed with carbohydrate cause the stomach to empty more slowly and therefore delay the rate at which glucose enters the small intestine, where it is absorbed. This causes a longer, slower rise in blood glucose. Foods high in fiber also take longer to leave the stomach and may slow the rise in blood glucose. After a mixed meal of chicken, rice, and green beans, for example, it will take 30 to 60 minutes before blood glucose begins to rise.

Glucose is transported in the blood to the liver and other body cells. The amount of glucose in the blood is regulated at about 60 to 100 mg per 100 ml of blood (70 to 120 mg/100 ml serum). This ensures adequate glucose delivery to body cells, which is particularly important for brain and red blood cells that rely almost exclusively on glucose as an energy source. If blood glucose levels rise too high or drop too low, hormonal signals from the pancreas act to decrease or increase levels, respectively.

A rise in blood glucose triggers the pancreas to release the hormone **insulin**, which allows glucose to be taken into the cells of the body. In the liver, insulin promotes the storage of glucose as glycogen and, to a lesser extent, fat.[4] In muscle, insulin stimulates the uptake of glucose for energy production and the synthesis

Glycemic response or **glycemic index**—A measure of how quickly blood glucose levels increase after a food or a meal is consumed.

Insulin—A hormone made in the pancreas that allows the uptake of glucose by body cells and stimulates the synthesis of glycogen in liver and muscle.

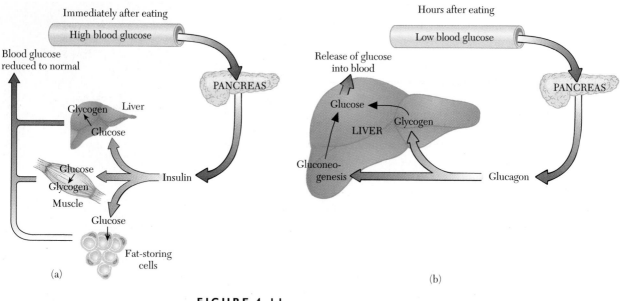

FIGURE 4-11

Blood glucose is regulated by hormones secreted by the pancreas. (a) Immediately after a meal, when blood glucose is high, insulin stimulates the uptake and storage of glucose. (b) Several hours after a meal, when blood glucose levels begin to decrease, glucagon stimulates the breakdown of glycogen into glucose and glucose production via gluconeogenesis.

of muscle glycogen for energy storage. In fat-storing cells, insulin increases glucose uptake from the blood and stimulates lipid synthesis. All of these actions remove glucose from the blood, causing blood glucose levels to decrease to the normal range (Figure 4-11a).

Glucose Metabolism   Once glucose has left the bloodstream and been taken up by a cell, it can be metabolized through cellular respiration to produce carbon dioxide, water, and energy in the form of ATP. Providing energy through cellular respiration involves four interconnected phases. The first takes place in the cytoplasm of the cell and is called **glycolysis** (meaning "glucose breakdown"). In this process, the 6-carbon sugar, glucose, is broken into two 3-carbon pyruvate molecules and produces 2 molecules of ATP (Figure 4-12).

In the next phase of cellular respiration, which occurs in the mitochondria, 1 carbon is removed from pyruvate to form acetyl-CoA. Acetyl-CoA then enters the third stage of breakdown, the **citric acid cycle**. To begin the cycle, acetyl-CoA combines with a 4-carbon compound to form a 6-carbon molecule. The citric acid cycle then removes 1 carbon at a time, as carbon dioxide, from this molecule until the 4-carbon molecule is reformed. These chemical reactions produce 2 ATP molecules per glucose but also remove **electrons**, which are passed to shuttling molecules for transport to the last stage of respiration, the **electron transport chain**. The electron transport chain is a series of molecules, most of which are proteins, in the inner membrane of the mitochondria. These molecules accept the electrons from the shuttle molecules and pass them from one to another down the chain until they are finally given to oxygen to form water. As the electrons are passed along, their energy is trapped and used to make ATP. These reactions, which convert glucose into carbon dioxide, water, and energy in the form of ATP, are central to all energy-producing processes in the body.

Using Protein to Make Glucose   When no carbohydrate has been eaten for a few hours, the glucose level in the blood—and consequently glucose available to

Glycolysis–A metabolic pathway in the cytoplasm of the cell that splits glucose into two 3-carbon pyruvate molecules. The energy released is used to make 2 ATP molecules.

Citric acid cycle–Also known as the *Krebs cycle* or the *tricarboxylic acid cycle,* this is the stage of respiration in which a 2-carbon compound is completely broken down to carbon dioxide and water.
Electrons–High-energy particles carrying a negative charge that orbit the nucleus of an atom.
Electron transport chain–The final stage of cellular respiration in which electrons are passed down a chain of molecules to oxygen and ATP is formed.

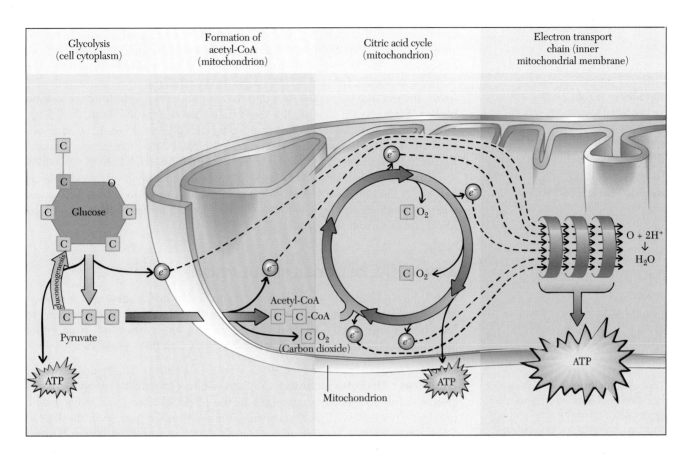

FIGURE 4-12

An overview of glucose metabolism. In the cytoplasm, glycolysis breaks glucose into two 3-carbon pyruvate molecules that enter the mitochondria, where they are converted into acetyl-CoA, which enters the citric acid cycle. High-energy electrons are released and transferred to the electron transport chain, where their energy is trapped to produce ATP.

the cells—begins to decrease. This triggers the pancreas to secrete **glucagon** (Figure 4-11b). Glucagon signals liver cells to break down glycogen into glucose, which is released into the bloodstream. Glucagon also stimulates the synthesis of new glucose, using a pathway called **gluconeogenesis** (meaning "production of new glucose"). Gluconeogenesis occurs in the liver and kidneys and requires energy in the form of ATP. This pathway makes glucose from 3-carbon molecules. Since 3-carbon molecules are not generated by the breakdown of fatty acids, amino acids from protein are the primary source of carbons. Newly synthesized glucose is released into the blood to prevent blood glucose from going below the normal range. Gluconeogenesis is also stimulated by another hormone, epinephrine. This hormone, also known as adrenaline, enables the body to respond to emergencies. For example, epinephrine is released in response to dangerous or stressful situations. It causes a rapid release of glucose into the blood to supply the energy needed for action.

Though gluconeogenesis is essential for meeting the body's immediate need for glucose, particularly when carbohydrate intake is very low, it takes protein from other essential functions such as growth and maintenance of muscle tissue. When carbohydrate is plentiful in the diet, protein is not needed to synthesize glucose. Therefore, carbohydrate is said to spare protein.

Carbohydrate Is Needed to Produce Energy from Fat Even tissues that can use fat as an energy source must have a small amount of carbohydrate available to completely metabolize the fat. When fat is used to produce energy, it is broken

Glucagon—A hormone made in the pancreas that stimulates the breakdown of liver glycogen and the synthesis of glucose to increase blood sugar.

Gluconeogenesis—The synthesis of glucose from simple noncarbohydrate molecules. Amino acids from protein are the primary source of carbons for glucose synthesis.

Ketones or **ketone bodies**–Molecules formed when there is not sufficient carbohydrate to completely metabolize the acetyl-CoA produced from fat breakdown.

Ketosis–High levels of ketones in the blood.

into molecules of acetyl-CoA. Acetyl-CoA can be used to produce energy via the citric acid cycle only if it can combine with a 4-carbon molecule derived from carbohydrate metabolism. When carbohydrate is not available to provide the 4-carbon molecule, the acetyl-CoA cannot be metabolized to carbon dioxide and water. Instead, the liver converts it into compounds known as **ketones** or **ketone bodies** (Figure 4-13). The ketones travel in the blood and can be used for energy by cells, such as those in the heart, muscles, and kidneys. Eventually, as an adaptation to starvation, even the brain can obtain some of its energy from ketones. Excess ketones are excreted by the kidney in urine. Although ketone production is a normal response, ketones not used for fuel can build up in the blood, causing **ketosis**. If fluid intake is too low to produce enough urine to excrete ketones or if ketone production is high, ketosis will result. Ketosis increases the acidity of the blood and can result in coma and death.

ABNORMAL GLUCOSE REGULATION

Blood glucose levels are normally tightly controlled by insulin, glucagon, and other hormones. Levels of glucose above or below this range can be detrimental to homeostasis and health. Abnormal blood glucose levels can result from either abnormal levels of hormones or abnormal responses to these hormones.

Diabetes mellitus–A disease caused by either insufficient insulin production or decreased sensitivity of cells to insulin. It results in elevated blood glucose levels.

Diabetes   **Diabetes mellitus** is a disease involving an inability to regulate blood glucose levels so glucose accumulates in the blood. Diabetes is a major health problem. It is estimated that between 6.5 and 14 million people in the United States have diabetes. The prevalence is highest among minorities such as Hispanics, African Americans, and Native Americans.[5] Diabetes increases the risks of hypertension, heart disease, and kidney failure.[6] The high level of glucose in the blood is believed to bind proteins, alter their functions, and damage body tissues. The eyes, kidneys, and blood vessels are particularly susceptible to damage. Dia-

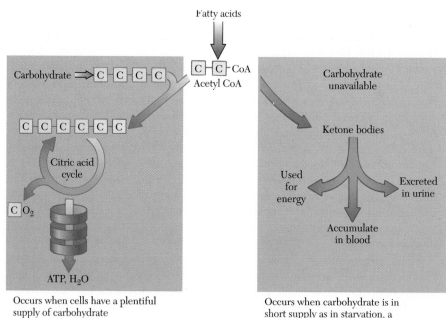

FIGURE 4-13

If carbohydrate is in short supply, the acetyl-CoA from fatty acid breakdown is unable to enter the citric acid cycle and instead is used to make ketone bodies.

betes accounts for 30% of all cases of kidney failure, half of all cases of blindness in adults, and half of all amputations not due to trauma.[7] There are two major types of diabetes: insulin-dependent and noninsulin-dependent.

Insulin-Dependent Diabetes   About 10% of diabetics are diagnosed with insulin-dependent diabetes (Type I or juvenile onset).[8] This form of diabetes is usually diagnosed before the age of 30. It involves a reduction or cessation of insulin secretion by the pancreas. Insulin-dependent diabetes is believed to be an **autoimmune disease** in which the immune system destroys the insulin-secreting cells of the pancreas. In this disease blood levels of glucose rise, but since insulin is unavailable, the glucose cannot enter cells to be used or stored as an energy source (Figure 4-14). The body responds as it does in starvation, and fat is used for energy. Since glucose cannot enter cells, fat cannot be completely broken down and large quantities of ketones are produced, causing ketosis.

Autoimmune disease—A disease that results from immune reactions that destroy normal body cells.

The goal in treating insulin-dependent diabetes is to maintain blood glucose levels within the normal range to prevent the damage caused by elevated glucose levels. This requires insulin injections, a modified diet, and adequate exercise. Insulin must be injected because it is a protein that would be broken down in the gastrointestinal tract if taken orally. Treatment also requires dietary modification to regulate the rate at which glucose enters the bloodstream.[9] The amount of carbohydrate consumed must be coordinated with the schedule of insulin injections so that glucose and insulin are available in the proper proportions at the same time. The diet must be adequate in energy, protein, and micronutrients, and be limited in fat because heart disease is more common in diabetics.[10] Diet planning can be based on the exchange system or on a system of carbohydrate counting with the goal of limiting the amount of carbohydrate entering the bloodstream at any given time. Exercise can also reduce blood glucose levels, so individuals with diabetes are encouraged to maintain regular exercise patterns. A change in exercise may affect the amount of insulin required.

Noninsulin-Dependent Diabetes   The other 90% of diabetics have noninsulin-dependent diabetes (Type II or maturity onset). This form usually appears in overweight persons over the age of 40.[7] In this disease, insulin secretion may be normal but body cells are resistant to the effects of insulin. Large amounts of insulin are therefore required for cells to take up enough glucose to meet their

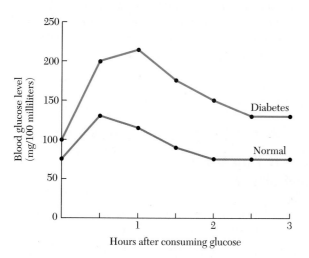

FIGURE 4-14
These glucose tolerance curves compare normal blood sugar patterns with those commonly seen in individuals with diabetes. The values are measured in blood drawn every 30 minutes for 3 hours after an individual consumes 75 grams of glucose.

energy needs. Since some glucose does enter the cells, ketosis rarely occurs in this form of diabetes.

Noninsulin-dependent diabetes can be controlled with diet and exercise. Because excess body fat increases insulin resistance, dietary modification to reduce body fat is ideal. But since the long-term maintenance of weight loss is usually poor, the current emphasis of dietary treatment is to promote a diet and exercise pattern that will maintain normal blood glucose and blood lipid levels and control blood pressure.[8] When these fail to normalize blood sugar, medications that increase pancreatic insulin production, and in some cases insulin itself, are prescribed.

Many foods on the market are targeted for diabetics. In general, these products are low in sugar, so they do not raise blood glucose levels rapidly. Fructose-containing foods are promoted because fructose causes smaller increases in blood sugar than sucrose. However, since fructose causes a rise in blood lipid levels, it may offer no long-term benefit over other sweeteners.[8]

Gestational Diabetes   A third form of diabetes, called gestational diabetes, sometimes occurs in women during pregnancy. This form of diabetes may be caused by the hormonal changes that occur during pregnancy. The high levels of glucose in the mother's blood increase the risk of complications for the unborn child (see Chapter 13). Women with gestational diabetes are treated with diet to regulate blood glucose levels, as are other diabetics. Gestational diabetes usually disappears once the pregnancy is complete and hormones return to nonpregnant levels. However, individuals who have had gestational diabetes are at risk for developing other forms of the disease.[11]

Hypoglycemia–A low blood glucose level, usually below 40 to 50 mg of glucose per 100 ml of blood.

Hypoglycemia   **Hypoglycemia**, or low blood glucose, results from an overproduction of insulin. The symptoms of hypoglycemia include irritability, nervousness, sweating, shakiness, anxiety, rapid heartbeat, headache, hunger, weakness, and sometimes seizure and coma. There are two forms of hypoglycemia. Reactive hypoglycemia occurs an hour or so after consumption of high-carbohydrate foods. The rise in blood glucose from the carbohydrate stimulates insulin release. However, too much insulin is secreted, resulting in a rapid fall in blood glucose to an abnormally low level. The treatment for reactive hypoglycemia is a diet that prevents rapid changes in blood glucose. Small, frequent meals low in simple carbohydrates and high in protein and fiber are recommended. The second form of hypoglycemia, fasting hypoglycemia, is not related to food intake. In this disorder, abnormal insulin secretion results in episodes of low blood glucose levels. This condition is often caused by pancreatic tumors.

CRITICAL THINKING

What Happens if You Consume Too Little Carbohydrate?

Bob weighed about 30 pounds more than he wanted to weigh, so he decided to try to shed pounds quickly with a low-carbohydrate weight-loss diet. The diet allowed an unlimited amount of beef, chicken, and fish as well as limited fruits and vegetables; breads and cereals were forbidden. Bob was overjoyed with his initial rapid weight loss, but after about a week his weight loss slowed down and he began to feel tired and light-headed. He was having headaches and noticed a funny smell on his breath.

Nutritional assessment

A nutritional assessment suggested that Bob needed about 2500 kcalories a day to maintain his weight. His weight-loss diet provided about 1000 kcalories, 25 grams of carbohydrate, 125 grams of protein, and 44 grams of fat per day. He consumed only about 3 cups of fluid daily.

What's wrong with Bob's diet plan?

Bob's diet is very low in energy and carbohydrate. This low energy intake caused Bob to use stored fat to meet his energy needs. Because his diet didn't contain enough carbohydrate to allow fat to be burned completely, ketones were produced and began to accumulate in his blood. Some of the ketones were used by cells for energy; some were excreted in the urine. However, since Bob was not consuming much fluid, the rate of ketone production exceeded the ability of his kidneys to excrete them, and they began to accumulate in his blood.

Ketone accumulation caused Bob's symptoms.

High blood ketone levels probably caused the headaches and light-headedness Bob was experiencing. Some blood ketones were lost through the lungs, giving him funny-smelling breath.

What would happen if Bob switched to a diet high in carbohydrate and fluids but still low in energy?

A 1000-kcalorie diet, including 150 grams of carbohydrate, would allow his body to burn fat more completely and therefore produce fewer ketones. Also, a high fluid intake would increase his urine production and lower his blood ketone level. However, it is unlikely that he will be able to meet his micronutrient needs on this restrictive diet.

Why can insulin-dependent diabetics develop ketosis even when consuming plenty of carbohydrate?

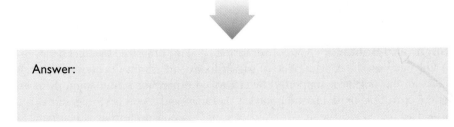

Answer:

CARBOHYDRATES AND HEALTH

Carbohydrates have been accused of either causing or curing most of the major health problems of the 20th century. It is hard to find a nutrient that has been craved and criticized more than the simplest carbohydrate, sugar. The consumption of sugary foods has been blamed for a myriad of chronic health problems from hyperactivity to obesity and heart disease.[12–14] While sugar is being condemned, nutritional respect for complex carbohydrates in the diet has increased. This dichotomy is reflected in nutrition messages from the *Dietary Guidelines*, food labels, and the Food Guide Pyramid, all of which recommend that we increase our intake of complex carbohydrates, but limit our sugar intake.

IS SUGAR REALLY THAT BAD?

Despite the negative press that has hounded sugar, very few diseases are directly related to a high sugar intake. Studies by both the FDA and the National Academy of Sciences concluded that other than its contribution to dental caries, sugar poses no proven health risk in the amounts currently consumed.[15] The problem with sugar is that it is a source of empty kcalories, and when it replaces more nutrient-dense foods, it reduces the nutritional value of the diet as a whole. There is nothing wrong with an occasional sweet treat. However, nutritional deficiencies may result when a large percentage of the energy in the diet is from low-nutrient-density foods (Figure 4-15).

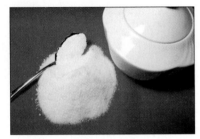

FIGURE 4-15
Refined table sugar is a source of empty kcalories. (Gregory Smolin)

Dental caries or **tooth cavities**—The decay and deterioration of teeth caused by acid produced when bacteria on the teeth metabolize carbohydrate.

Sugar Intake and Disease   Sugar has been accused of increasing the risks of heart disease and diabetes.[16] These accusations were probably based on observations of the body's metabolic responses to sugar consumption. For example, a diet high in sugar causes an increase in blood lipids, and the risk of heart disease is increased by high blood lipid levels; a high-sugar meal causes blood glucose to rise, and diabetes is characterized by high blood glucose levels. However, a cause and effect relationship between sugar consumption and these diseases has not been supported by scientific experimentation.[12]

The most significant health problem associated with a diet high in sugar is **dental caries**, or **tooth cavities**. Dental caries are formed when bacteria that live in the mouth metabolize sugar from the diet and produce acids. The acid can then dissolve the enamel and underlying structure of the teeth. Simple carbohydrate, particularly sucrose, is the most rapidly utilized food source for these microbes; however, any carbohydrate-containing foods that stick to the teeth can also cause cavities. The length of time that carbohydrate-containing food is in contact with the teeth determines the likelihood that a cavity will develop. Certain foods, such as sticky candies, cereals, crackers, and cookies, tend to remain on people's teeth longer, providing a continuous supply of nutrients to decay-causing bacteria. Other foods, such as chocolate, ice cream, and bananas, are rapidly washed away from the teeth. Frequent snacking also increases contact time by providing a continuous food supply for the bacteria. Limiting sugar can help prevent dental caries, but since starch is also eventually metabolized into acid, proper dental hygiene is important even if the diet is low in sugar.[17]

Sugar and Behavior   Carbohydrate has been hypothesized to affect behavior. A link between the consumption of sugary foods and criminality and hyperactive behavior has not been supported by controlled experiments. But support for an effect of carbohydrate consumption on the brain and mood is strong and is believed to play a role in the drive to consume carbohydrate that is common in disorders ranging from obesity to several types of depression.

Sugar and Criminal Behavior   In 1978, Dan White blamed overconsumption of Hostess Twinkies for the mental state that led him to gun down the mayor and city supervisor of San Francisco. This became known as the "Twinkie Defense." In response to the idea that high sugar consumption leads to criminal behavior, some correctional facilities removed candy machines and reduced the sugar in their menus. However, controlled studies of sugar intake and aggressive behavior have found no relationship.[14]

Sugar and Hyperactivity   The consumption of sugary foods has also been suggested as a cause of hyperactivity in children (see Chapter 14). The increase in blood glucose after a meal high in simple carbohydrates is hypothesized to provide the energy for the excessive activities of a hyperactive child. However, no clinical evidence exists to support a connection between sugar intake and hyperactivity.[14,18]

Carbohydrate Craving   An abnormal craving for carbohydrate-rich foods has been identified in individuals with a variety of disorders including obesity, premenstrual syndrome, bulimia, depression, and seasonal affective disorder.[19–21] The reason these individuals crave carbohydrates is believed to be an abnormality in the regulation of brain levels of the **neurotransmitter** serotonin, which functions in the sleep center of the brain.[14] In most people, a high-carbohydrate meal causes the amount of serotonin in the brain to increase, which results in sleepiness and the inability to concentrate. In carbohydrate cravers, the effect of carbohydrate consumption is different. It alleviates tension, anxiety, and mental fatigue, causing them to feel calm and clearheaded after their carbohydrate "fix."

Neurotransmitter–A chemical substance produced by a nerve cell that can stimulate or inhibit another cell.

WHAT'S SO GOOD ABOUT COMPLEX CARBOHYDRATES?

Sugar's bad reputation is balanced by the good reputation of complex carbohydrate, particularly fiber. Foods that are high in complex carbohydrates are generally also good sources of other nutrients such as vitamins and minerals. Despite the lingering belief that starchy foods are fattening, a gram of starch has less than half the energy of a gram of fat. It is the fat that is added to or baked into starches that increases the kcalorie tally. A medium baked potato provides about 110 kcalories, but the 2 tablespoons of sour cream you add brings the total to 175 kcalories (Figure 4-16). A plate of plain pasta has about 200 kcalories, but with a high-fat sauce, the kcalories rise to 300—add sausage and the meal is now 450 kcalories. A healthy-looking bran muffin may contain 50 kcalories from complex carbohydrates and another 65 from fat.

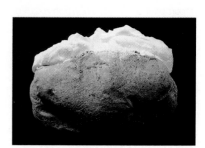

FIGURE 4-16
High-carbohydrate foods are not high in kcalories, but the toppings used on them often are. (Dennis Drenner)

This is not to say that starch consumed in excess of energy needs will not add pounds. Any energy source consumed in excess of requirements can cause weight gain. But carbohydrate is no more fattening than any other energy source. In fact, excess carbohydrate in the diet is less efficient at producing body fat than excess fat in the diet (see Chapter 7).

The dietary fiber that is plentiful in many foods high in complex carbohydrate is also important in health maintenance. Epidemiological research comparing the incidence of certain chronic diseases in populations with different fiber intakes found high-fiber diets to be associated with a lower incidence of certain bowel disorders, heart disease, and colon cancer.[22]

Dietary Fiber and Chronic Bowel Disorders   A diet high in fiber can relieve or prevent some chronic bowel disorders. Fiber adds bulk and absorbs water, making the feces larger and softer and reducing the amount of pressure needed for defecation. This helps to reduce the incidence of constipation and **hemorrhoids**, the swelling of veins in the rectal or anal area. Reducing the pres-

Hemorrhoids–Swollen veins in the anal or rectal area.

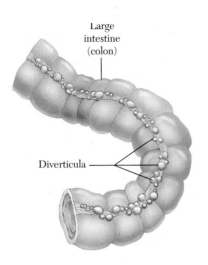

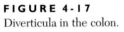

FIGURE 4-17
Diverticula in the colon.

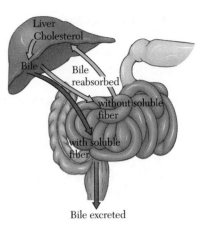

FIGURE 4-18
When the diet is low in soluble fiber, bile, which contains cholesterol and bile acids made from cholesterol, is reabsorbed and returned to the liver. When soluble fiber is present, it binds cholesterol and bile acids so they are excreted rather than absorbed.

Diverticula—Sacs or pouches that protrude from the wall of the large intestine in the disease diverticulosis. When these become inflamed, the condition is called diverticulitis.

sure in the lumen of the colon can also reduce the possibility of developing **diverticula**, outpouchings in the intestinal wall (Figure 4-17). In the United States, about 50% of elderly people have diverticulosis. Fecal matter may occasionally accumulate in these outpouchings, causing irritation, pain, inflammation, and infection. This condition is known as diverticulitis. Treatment of diverticulitis usually includes antibiotics to reduce bacterial growth and a decrease in fiber intake to prevent irritation of the inflamed tissues. Once the inflammation is resolved, however, a high-fiber intake is recommended to increase fecal bulk, decrease transit time, ease stool elimination, and reduce future attacks.[23]

Dietary Fiber and Blood Cholesterol and Heart Disease Blood cholesterol levels can be reduced by increasing the consumption of fiber-rich foods.[24] High blood cholesterol levels are a risk factor for the development of heart disease (see Chapter 5). By reducing blood cholesterol levels, the risk of heart disease is reduced. Not all dietary fiber, however, has a cholesterol-lowering effect. Studies in humans indicate that soluble fiber such as that in legumes, rice and oat bran, guar gum, pectin, and psyllium, a grain used in over-the-counter bulk-forming laxatives such as Metamucil, are more effective at lowering blood cholesterol levels than insoluble fibers such as wheat bran or cellulose.[25] This may be due to the ability of soluble fibers to bind cholesterol and **bile acids**, which are made from cholesterol, in the digestive tract. Normally, cholesterol and bile acids are absorbed and reused. When bound to fiber, cholesterol and bile acids are excreted in the feces rather than being absorbed. The liver must then use cholesterol from the blood to synthesize new bile acids. This provides a mechanism for eliminating cholesterol from the body and reducing blood cholesterol (Figure 4-18). Another theory suggests that the short chain fatty acids produced by the microbial digestion of fiber enter the circulation and travel to the liver where they inhibit cholesterol synthesis.[26] Regardless of the mechanism, diets high in soluble fiber help to reduce blood cholesterol levels.

Bile acids—Emulsifiers present in bile that are synthesized by the liver from cholesterol.

Dietary Fiber and Colon Cancer Epidemiological studies have shown that the incidence of colon cancer is lower in populations consuming diets high in fiber.[22] The role of fiber in preventing the development of colon cancer may be related to its ability to decrease contact between the mucosal cells of the large intestine and the fecal contents. Cancer cells develop as a result of **mutations**, or changes in their genetic material. Mutations occur most frequently in cells that divide rapidly, such as mucosal cells. Mutations can be caused by many factors, including contact with chemical substances in the environment. In the case of the colon, mutations may be caused by substances consumed in the diet or produced in the gastrointestinal tract. Fiber increases fecal bulk, dilutes the colon contents, and speeds transit, thereby decreasing contact time between the mucosal cells and potentially cancer-causing substances. In addition, the metabolism of fiber by microflora may produce chemicals that affect the promotion and progression of cancer in the colon.[27]

Mutations–Changes in DNA caused by chemical or physical agents.

Problems with High-Fiber Diets   Although a high-fiber diet has many benefits, a very high fiber intake can cause problems. The more fiber there is in the diet, the more water is needed to prevent the stool from becoming hard and difficult to eliminate. If not enough water is consumed, intestinal blockage can occur when large amounts of fiber are consumed.[28] A sudden increase in fiber intake may also cause discomfort due to the production of intestinal gas from the bacterial breakdown of fiber. Another problem with a high-fiber diet is that fiber may decrease nutrient absorption. This occurs for two reasons. First, the increased volume of intestinal contents that occurs with a high-fiber diet may prevent enzymes from coming in contact with food. If a food cannot be broken down, nutrients may not be absorbed. Second, fiber may bind some micronutrients, preventing their absorption. For instance, wheat bran fiber binds the minerals zinc, calcium, magnesium, and iron, reducing their absorption.

A high-fiber diet also increases the volume of food needed to meet energy requirements. For example, consuming 200 kcalories of broccoli, a high-fiber food, requires eating a large volume of food—about 4 cups. A diet that is very high in fiber may satisfy hunger before nutrient requirements are met. Generally this is a problem only when the diet is low in micronutrients or when high-fiber diets are consumed by young children whose small stomachs limit the amount of food they can eat.

HOW MUCH CARBOHYDRATE SHOULD WE EAT?

The typical carbohydrate content of the North American diet today is about 40 to 50% of energy. Much of this comes from baked goods, sugared soft drinks, fruit drinks, and table sugar.[1] Public health guidelines such as the *Dietary Guidelines* recommend that the complex carbohydrate content of the diet be increased while sugar be limited (Figure 4-19).

RECOMMENDATIONS FOR CARBOHYDRATE INTAKE

An RDA for carbohydrate has not been established. In a diet that meets energy needs, a minimum of about 50 to 100 grams of carbohydrate is needed to meet glucose needs and to prevent ketosis. This amount of carbohydrate is easy to obtain. For example, two slices of toast and a cup (240 ml) of juice provide about 60 grams. If, however, only this small amount of carbohydrate were consumed, the total diet would be higher in fat and protein than is desirable.

Recommendations for a healthy diet suggest that the carbohydrate content of the diet be increased to 55 to 60% of the total energy intake. This can be accomplished by increasing consumption of grains, vegetables, and fruits, as is recommended by the *Dietary Guidelines*, Healthy People 2000, food labels, and the

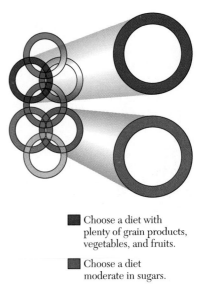

■ Choose a diet with plenty of grain products, vegetables, and fruits.

■ Choose a diet moderate in sugars.

FIGURE 4-19
The *Dietary Guidelines for Americans* recommend a diet high in complex carbohydrates with moderate amounts of refined sugars. (USDA, DHHS, 1995)

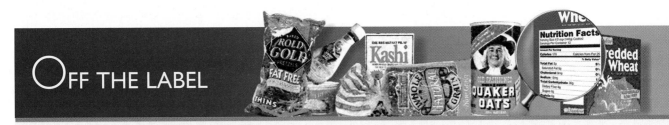

OFF THE LABEL

Identifying High-Fiber Products

Consumers flock to brown breads and bran cereals in an effort to increase dietary fiber. The color and name of a product, however, often reveal little about the fiber content. Better places to look are the list of ingredients and the Nutrition Facts section of the food label.

On the Ingredients List of breads, cereals, pastas, crackers, and other grain products, the term "whole" before the name of the grain indicates that the bran layer is still present in the food. Wheat flour, used to describe refined white flour made from wheat, is often confused with whole wheat flour. Only when whole wheat flour is the first ingredient, as it is in the label shown here from whole wheat bread, is the product made with mostly wheat flour containing the bran layer. The first ingredient on the "wheat" bread label shown in the figure is enriched wheat flour,

rather than whole wheat flour. For products containing oats, the term "rolled" indicates that the whole oat grain has been used. Fiber added to processed foods can also be identified from the list of ingredients. Insoluble fibers, such as the wheat bran added to the wheat bread shown here, are usually added to decrease the energy content of a product or to meet consumer demands for a high-fiber product. Except for oat bran, most added soluble fibers, such as pectins and gums, are used to thicken and stabilize foods and rarely contribute a significant amount of fiber.

The Nutrition Facts section of a food label provides information about how much dietary fiber is in a product and how it fits into the recommendations for an overall diet. It lists the total dietary fiber contained in a serving of the product; the amounts of soluble and insoluble fiber are not mandatory,

but some manufacturers choose to include them. The percent Daily Value, based on the Daily Value for fiber of 25 grams for a 2000-kcalorie diet, is also listed. For example, the whole wheat bread shown here contains 2 grams of fiber, which is 8% of the recommended 25 grams. Foods that contain 20% or more of the Daily Value for fiber per serving can state on the label that they are "high in dietary fiber." Products containing 10 to 19% of the Daily Value can state that they are "a good source of dietary fiber."

Food labels may also carry health claims related to fiber and chronic disease risk. Foods that contain at least 2.5 grams of fiber per serving and are low in fat may claim to reduce the risk of cancer. Foods that contain at least 0.6 gram of fiber per serving and are low in total fat, saturated fat, and cholesterol may claim to reduce the risk of heart disease.

Food Guide Pyramid. An increase in dietary fiber above the current intake[29] is also recommended. Expert panels in both Canada and the United States recommend 10 to 13 grams of fiber per 1000 kcalories, or about 20 to 35 grams of fiber per day.

DETERMINING YOUR CARBOHYDRATE INTAKE

The amount of carbohydrate in your diet can be calculated using values from food composition tables, computer databases, food labels, or the exchange system. Food composition tables and databases generally give information on the carbohydrate and fiber content of foods. Occasionally, they give **crude fiber** values. Crude fiber is an outdated method for measuring the fiber content of foods. Crude fiber is determined using what remains after food has been treated in the laboratory with strong acids and bases. This treatment destroys all the soluble fiber as well as some of the insoluble fiber in food and so gives little information about what acts as fiber in the body. The current methods of measuring fiber, as dietary fiber, are more similar to the digestive processes that occur in the human body; however, even these are not ideal, and results are often inconsistent.

Food labels list the grams of total carbohydrate, fiber, and sugars. Total carbohydrate and fiber are listed also as a percent of the Daily Value. The Daily Value

Crude fiber–Fiber that remains after a food has been treated in the laboratory with acid and base. It consists primarily of cellulose and lignin.

Whole Wheat Bread

Nutrition Facts	Amount/Serving	%DV*	Amount/Serving	%DV*
Serving Size 1 Slice (27g)	**Total Fat** 1g	**2%**	**Total Carb.** 12g	**4%**
Servings Per Container 17	Sat. Fat 0g	**0%**	Dietary Fiber 2g	**8%**
Calories 70	**Cholesterol** 0mg	**0%**	Sugars 2g	
Calories from Fat 10	**Sodium** 10mg	**0%**	**Protein** 2g	

Vitamin A 0% • Vitamin C 0% • Calcium 4% • Iron 4%

Thiamin 4% • Riboflavin 2% • Niacin 4%

*Percent Daily Values (DV) are based on a 2,000 calorie diet. Your daily values may be higher or lower depending on your calorie needs:

	Calories:	2,000	2,500
Total Fat	Less than	65g	80g
Sat Fat	Less than	20g	25g
Cholesterol	Less than	300mg	300mg
Sodium	Less than	2,400mg	2,400mg
Total Carbohydrate		300g	375g
Dietary Fiber		25g	30g

NOT A SODIUM FREE FOOD

INGREDIENTS: WHOLE WHEAT FLOUR, WATER, SWEETENERS (HIGH FRUCTOSE CORN SYRUP, MOLASSES), WHEAT GLUTEN, SOYBEAN OIL, CONTAINS 2% OR LESS OF THE FOLLOWING: YEAST, DOUGH CONDITIONERS (MONO & DIGLYCERIDES, ETHOXYLATED MONO & DI-GLYCERIDES, CALCIUM STEAROYL-2-LACTYLATE), YEAST NUTRIENTS (CALCIUM SULFATE, MONO- CALCIUM PHOSPHATE), CALCIUM PROPIONATE (A PRESERVATIVE).

Wheat Bread

Nutrition Facts	Amount/Serving	%DV*	Amount/Serving	%DV*
Serving Size 1 Slice (28g)	**Total Fat** 1g	**2%**	**Total Carb.** 13g	**4%**
Servings Per Container 20	Sat. Fat 0g	**0%**	Dietary Fiber 1g	**4%**
Calories 80	**Cholesterol** 0mg	**0%**	Sugars 2g	
Calories from Fat 15	**Sodium** 190mg	**8%**	**Protein** 2g	

Vitamin A 0% • Vitamin C 0% • Calcium 4% • Iron 4%

Thiamin 4% • Riboflavin 4% • Niacin 4%

*Percent Daily Values (DV) are based on a 2,000 calorie diet. Your daily values may be higher or lower depending on your calorie needs:

	Calories:	2,000	2,500
Total Fat	Less than	65g	80g
Sat Fat	Less than	20g	25g
Cholesterol	Less than	300mg	300mg
Sodium	Less than	2,400mg	2,400mg
Total Carbohydrate		300g	375g
Dietary Fiber		25g	30g

INGREDIENTS: ENRICHED WHEAT FLOUR, (WHEAT FLOUR, BARLEY MALT, NIACIN, IRON, THIAMIN MONONITRATE, RIBOFLAVIN), WATER, WHOLE WHEAT FLOUR, SWEETENERS, (HIGH FRUCTOSE CORN SYRUP, MOLASSES, HONEY), WHEAT BRAN, YEAST, SOYBEAN OIL, CONTAINS 2% OR LESS OF THE FOLLOWING: SALT, DOUGH CONDITIONERS (MONOGLYCERIDES, SODIUM STEAROYL LACTYLATE), YEAST NUTRIENTS (AMMONIUM SULFATE, CALCIUM SULFATE), CALCIUM PROPIONATE (A PRESERVATIVE).

for total carbohydrate is calculated as 60% of the energy. For a 2000-kcalorie diet this represents 300 grams of carbohydrate (2000 kcal × 60% ÷ 4 kcal/g of carbohydrate = 300 g). The Daily Value for fiber is based on a recommended intake of about 11.5 grams per 1000 kcalories, which is rounded to 25 grams in a 2000-kcalorie diet. No Daily Value has been established for sugars, but labels can help identify high-sugar products. The number of grams of sugars listed in the Nutrition Facts includes all monosaccharides and disaccharides but does not distinguish between refined and naturally occurring sugars. For example, the fructose found naturally in frozen strawberries and high-fructose corn syrup added to soft drinks are both listed as sugars. Nutrient claims provide some information about whether a food contains added refined sugar. The presence of a claim such as "no added sugar" or "without added sugar" indicates that no sugars have been added in processing. The list of ingredients also provides information about the types of sweeteners added to a food. Only added sugars are listed here and the only type of sweetener that can be called "sugar" is sucrose. Since sucrose may represent only one of many added sweeteners, consumers need to increase their carbohydrate vocabulary to recognize all the sweeteners on the label. High-fructose corn syrups, invert sugar, dextrose, lactose, honey, and mannitol are just a few.

Although the exchange system does not distinguish between complex and simple carbohydrate, it can be used to give a quick estimate of the total amount

TABLE 4-1	Using Exchange Lists to Calculate the Carbohydrate Content of a Diet

Exchange Groups/Lists	Carbohydrate Content (g)
Starch ½ cup rice, cereal, potatoes, 1 slice bread	15
Fruit ½ cup canned water-pack fruit, ½ banana, 1 small fresh pear, peach, apple	15
Milk 1 cup fluid milk or yogurt	12
Vegetables ½ cup cooked vegetables, 1 cup fresh greens	5
Meat and meat substitutes 1 oz meat or hard cheese, 1 Tbsp peanut butter, ½ cup legumes	0
Fat 1 tsp butter, margarine, mayonnaise, oil	0

of carbohydrate in a food or in the diet (Table 4-1). One serving of bread or fruit provides 15 grams of carbohydrate, 1 milk serving provides 12 grams, and vegetables provide about 5 grams. Meats and fats provide no carbohydrate. The exchange lists cannot be used for calculating fiber intake, but Table 4-2 offers a method for estimating fiber in foods.

To calculate your carbohydrate intake as a percent of energy, you need to know the grams of carbohydrate in your diet and the amount of energy you consume. For example, if you consume 2500 kcalories and 350 grams of carbohydrate, you can calculate your percent of energy as carbohydrate.

350 g of carbohydrate $\times$ 4 kcal/g = 1400 kcal of carbohydrate

1400 kcal $\div$ 2500 total kcal $\times$ 100 = 56% energy (kcal) as carbohydrate

CHOOSING A DIET TO MEET RECOMMENDATIONS

To meet the recommendations of 55 to 60% of energy from carbohydrate and a moderate intake of refined sugar, most people need to increase the total carbohydrate in their diets but limit their intake of sugar. To do this without increasing energy, complex carbohydrate should be substituted for foods high in refined sugar, fat, and protein. For example, choosing a stir-fry meal of beef and vegetables on rice or a meal of spaghetti and meatballs can provide the same energy but more carbohydrate than a dinner of steak and french fries. These carbohydrate-based meals are also lower in fat and cost less than meat-based meals. To limit refined sugars, soft drinks and candy bars should be rare treats, and fruits should be substituted for sugary desserts.

The recommendations of the Food Guide Pyramid can be used to plan a diet high in carbohydrate. Six to 11 servings should be selected from the bread, cereal, rice, and pasta group, the base of the pyramid. If whole grain products are selected, this group will also provide an excellent source of fiber. The next level of the Pyramid contains the vegetable group and fruit group, which are also good sources of complex carbohydrate, fiber, and naturally occurring simple carbohydrate. It is recommended that 3 to 5 servings from the vegetable group and 2 to 4 servings from the fruit group be consumed each day. On the next level of the Pyramid, the milk group provides carbohydrate in the form of lactose. To emphasize moderation in the consumption of refined sugar, the Food Guide Pyramid recommends that added sweets be used sparingly. The relative amounts of added sugar in each of the food groups is indicated by an upside-down triangle symbol (∇). The food groups that contain a higher proportion of foods with added sugar have more of

disease among men has been declining since the 1950s, the incidence among women has increased.[14] One of the goals of Healthy People 2000 is to reduce the incidence of heart disease by promoting healthy diets and lifestyles.[13]

How Does Atherosclerosis Develop?   An article published over 60 years ago concluded that cholesterol in the food we eat is transported into the bloodstream and deposited in the arteries.[15] This article provided a simplistic description of the connection between diet and the development of **atherosclerosis**, a type of **cardiovascular disease** in which lipids are deposited in the artery walls, reducing elasticity and eventually blocking blood flow. Since this initial description, a great deal of research has been done to determine how cholesterol deposits form in arteries, how diet affects blood cholesterol levels, and if changes in diet can decrease the risk of developing atherosclerosis.

Our current understanding of how atherosclerosis develops is based on the Nobel-Prize-winning work of Michael Brown and Joseph Goldstein, who discovered LDL receptors on cells. LDL receptors regulate the level of cholesterol in the blood by binding LDL particles and allowing them to be taken up by the cells. If the amount of cholesterol in the blood exceeds the amount that can be taken up by cells, because there is either too much cholesterol or too few LDL receptors, the result is a high level of LDL cholesterol in the blood.[16] Excess LDL cholesterol in the blood can lead to the deposition of cholesterol in the artery walls, causing atherosclerosis.

The exact events that initiate the buildup of cholesterol in arterial walls are still unknown. One theory is that atherosclerosis develops in response to an injury to the arterial wall caused by high blood pressure, high cholesterol levels, viruses, chemicals, or some other factor. Once the initial injury has occurred, LDL particles, white blood cells, and blood cell fragments involved in blood clotting, called platelets, enter the artery wall. Inside the artery wall, LDL that comes in contact with highly reactive oxygen molecules is transformed into **oxidized LDL cholesterol**. Oxidized LDL cholesterol binds to scavenger receptors located on the surface of the white blood cells.[17] As white blood cells fill with more and more oxidized LDL cholesterol, the white blood cells are transformed into cholesterol-filled foam cells. Foam cells accumulate in the artery wall and then burst, depositing cholesterol to form a fatty streak. Platelets signal muscle cells to invade the fatty streak and secrete fibrous proteins. The result is a mass of cholesterol, muscle cells, and fibrous tissue called a **plaque** (Figure 5-13). Eventually, calcium collects in the plaque and causes it to harden. Blood clots form around the plaque and it continues to enlarge, causing the artery to narrow and lose its elasticity. The plaque can become so large that it completely blocks the artery, or a clot can break loose and block an artery elsewhere. When an artery is blocked, blood can no longer move through it to supply oxygen and nutrients to the cells, and they die quickly. If blood flow to the heart muscle is interrupted, heart cells die, resulting in a heart attack or myocardial infarction. If the blood flow to the brain is interrupted, a stroke results.

Risk Factors for Heart Disease   The risk of developing heart disease is directly affected by blood cholesterol levels, blood pressure, and diabetes. Age, genetics, and lifestyle factors such as exercise and diet can also affect risk either directly or indirectly by altering blood cholesterol, blood pressure, or the risk of diabetes. Age and genetics are risks that cannot be changed, but diet and lifestyle factors can.

Elevated levels of LDL cholesterol increase the risk of heart disease, whereas high HDL levels offer a protective effect. High blood pressure increases the risk of heart disease, as does diabetes. The risk of heart disease increases with age.[18] Men are affected by heart disease generally a decade earlier than women.[19] In-

Atherosclerosis—The buildup of fatty material in the artery walls. It is a type of **cardiovascular disease**. Cardiovascular disease refers to all diseases of the heart and blood vessels.

Oxidized LDL cholesterol—A substance formed when the cholesterol in LDL particles is oxidized by reactive oxygen molecules. It is key in the development of atherosclerosis because it is taken up by scavenger receptors on white blood cells.

Plaque—The cholesterol-rich material that is deposited in the blood vessels of individuals with atherosclerosis. It consists of cholesterol, smooth muscle cells, and fibrous tissue.

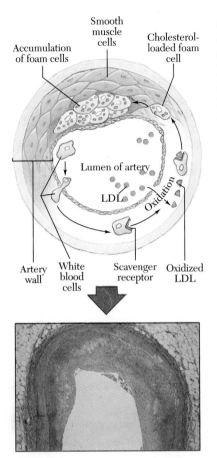

Accumulation of foam cells

Smooth muscle cells

Cholesterol-loaded foam cell

Lumen of artery

LDL

Oxidation

Artery wall

White blood cells

Scavenger receptor

Oxidized LDL

FIGURE 5-13
An atherosclerotic plaque develops when white blood cells and LDL particles penetrate the artery wall. LDLs become oxidized and enter the white blood cells by binding to scavenger receptors. The cholesterol-filled white blood cells are transformed into foam cells that burst, depositing cholesterol in the artery wall. (Photo, CNRI/Phototake NYC)

dividuals with a male family member who exhibited heart disease before the age of 55 or a female family member who exhibited heart disease before the age of 65 are considered to be at greater risk. An inactive lifestyle increases the risk of heart disease. Regular exercise improves cardiovascular fitness and increases HDL cholesterol levels.[20] Cigarette smoking and a stressful lifestyle increase the risk of heart disease. The effect of diet on the risk of heart disease has been investigated using epidemiology and studies that use dietary modification.

Diet and Heart Disease   Epidemiology has demonstrated a relationship between diet and the incidence of heart disease. In the United States the diet is high in fat and saturated fat and low in vegetables and fruits, and the risk of heart disease is high. In China, the diet is low in total fat and saturated fat and high in grains and vegetables, and the incidence of heart disease is low.[21] The diet in Mediterranean countries is high in monounsaturated fat, grains, and vegetables, and there is low mortality from heart disease.[22,23] And populations that consume a diet high in omega-3 fatty acids, such as the Inuits in Greenland, have a low incidence of heart disease.[24,25] Not only do the type and amount of fat differ among these countries, but the total diet and lifestyle differ. The higher intake of grains and vegetables and the active low-stress lifestyles in many Asian and Mediterranean populations may be as important as fat intake in reducing the risk of heart disease.

Diet can affect the risk of heart disease by altering blood cholesterol levels, blood pressure, and the risk of diabetes. Diets high in fat and energy can lead to obesity, which can affect blood cholesterol levels and increase the risk of high blood pressure and diabetes. A diet low in vegetables and fruits and high in salt can increase blood pressure. A diet high in fat, saturated fat, and energy increases blood cholesterol levels. Different amounts and types of various lipids—cholesterol, saturated fat, polyunsaturated fat, monounsaturated fat, trans fatty acids—have different effects on blood cholesterol levels. Different types and amounts of dietary fiber can also affect blood cholesterol levels.

Dietary Cholesterol   Cholesterol in the blood comes from cholesterol consumed in the diet and that made by the liver. The extent to which dietary cholesterol affects blood levels varies with the individual. Generally, about three to four times more cholesterol is made by the body than is consumed in the diet. In some individuals, as dietary cholesterol increases, liver cholesterol synthesis decreases so that blood levels do not change.[26] In others, however, increases in dietary cholesterol do not result in decreased liver synthesis, so concentrations of cholesterol increase in the blood.

Dietary Saturated Fat   Diets high in saturated fat increase blood cholesterol.[27] It is hypothesized that when saturated fat intake is high, there are fewer LDL receptors in the liver, so that LDL cholesterol cannot be removed from the blood. When saturated fat intake is low, the number of LDL receptors increases, allowing more cholesterol to be removed from the bloodstream.[28] However, not all saturated fats cause a rise in blood cholesterol. Saturated short and medium chain fatty acids and stearic acid, a long chain of saturated fatty acid found in chocolate and beef, do not increase blood cholesterol levels when compared with other saturated fatty acids. Stearic acid may, however, cause a reduction in the levels of HDL cholesterol, the type of cholesterol that offers a protective effect against heart disease.[29]

Dietary Polyunsaturated Fat   When saturated fat in the diet is replaced by polyunsaturated fat, there is a decrease in LDL cholesterol.[30] However, a high intake of polyunsaturates may decrease HDL cholesterol as well. In contrast to other polyunsaturated fatty acids, omega-3 fatty acids, such as those found in fish oils, do not lower HDL cholesterol and may even increase it.[31] In addition to these effects on blood lipids, omega-3 fatty acids have effects on blood clotting, blood pressure, and immune function that may alter the risk of cardiovascular disease. Studies of omega-3 fatty acids show that replacing some of the fat in the diet with sources of omega-3 fatty acids reduces the incidence of heart disease. The reductions are greater if the omega-3 fatty acids come from fish rather than supplements.[25]

Unsaturated fats with trans double bonds may also affect blood cholesterol levels. When partially hydrogenated vegetable oils containing trans fatty acids are substituted for animal or vegetable fats rich in saturated fatty acids, they lower total and LDL cholesterol concentrations in the blood. But when they replace unhydrogenated polyunsaturated oils in the diet, they raise total and LDL cholesterol concentrations in the blood. The effect on HDL cholesterol has not been clearly demonstrated.[32]

Dietary Monounsaturated Fat   Monounsaturated fat may also have a protective effect against heart disease. Populations with diets high in monounsaturated fats, such as those in Mediterranean countries, where olive oil is commonly used, have a mortality rate from heart disease that is half that of the United States. This is true even when total fat intake is high.[21,33] Substituting monounsaturated fat for saturated fat reduces LDL cholesterol and has little effect on HDL cholesterol.[31]

Fiber and Energy   Soluble fibers, such as those in oat bran, legumes, psyllium, pectin, and gums, have been shown to reduce blood cholesterol levels. These fibers are believed to bind cholesterol and bile acids in the small intestine and cause them to be excreted (see Figure 4-18). Excess energy intake affects blood cholesterol because it results in excess body fat or obesity, which is a separate risk factor for elevated blood cholesterol levels. A reduction in body weight to achieve desirable weight has been shown to reduce blood cholesterol levels.[34,35]

Dietary Recommendations for Reducing the Risk of Heart Disease

It is estimated that 29% of adult Americans have blood cholesterol levels that put them at risk for developing heart disease.[36] The National Cholesterol Education Program (NCEP), a nationwide program designed to evaluate and reduce the risks of heart disease, has recommended that all adults have their blood lipids measured every five years (Figure 5-14).[37]

The desirable level for total blood cholesterol in adults is below 200 mg per 100 ml. LDL levels should be below 130 mg per 100 ml (see Table 5-1). Since HDL cholesterol has a protective effect against heart disease, a high ratio of total cholesterol to HDL cholesterol is beneficial. The ratio of total blood cholesterol to HDL cholesterol should be no more than 4 to 1. For example, if your total cholesterol is 200 mg per 100 ml, your HDL cholesterol should be at least 50 mg per 100 ml.

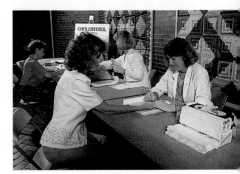

FIGURE 5-14
The National Cholesterol Education Program recommends that all adults have their blood cholesterol levels checked at least every five years. (Blair Seitz/Photo Researchers, Inc.)

TABLE 5-1	Blood Cholesterol Levels and the Risk of Cardiovascular Disease		
	Desirable	**Borderline-High**	**High**
Total cholesterol	<200 mg/100 ml	200–239 mg/100 ml	≥240 mg/100 ml
LDL cholesterol	<130 mg/100 ml	130–159 mg/100 ml	≥160 mg/100 ml
Ratio total/HDL	<4:1		

The NCEP recommends that individuals with LDL cholesterol above 160 mg per 100 ml and those with LDL cholesterol between 130 and 159 mg per 100 ml who have heart disease or two other risk factors should begin a dietary program to reduce blood cholesterol levels. This program recommends reducing fat intake to no more than 30% of energy, saturated fat to less than 10%, and cholesterol intake to less than 300 mg per day. If after six months of consuming this diet, blood cholesterol levels have not decreased, a more restrictive dietary program should be initiated. The NCEP also recommends drug therapy in addition to diet therapy for individuals with extremely high cholesterol levels or those in whom diet therapy fails. Two types of drugs are used to lower blood cholesterol levels. One type acts in the gastrointestinal tract by preventing cholesterol and bile absorption, and the other blocks cholesterol production in the liver.

Other public health recommendations, such as the *Dietary Guidelines*, also promote diets low in fat, saturated fat, and cholesterol to reduce the risk of cardiovascular disease. In addition to recommendations about fat, the *Dietary Guidelines* promote diets high in grains, vegetables, and fruits; an increase in physical activity; maintenance of a healthy body weight; and moderate alcohol consumption. Higher levels of alcohol increase heart disease risk and should be avoided. Another recommendation proposes consuming 1 to 2 servings of fish per week to decrease the incidence of heart disease.[25] The impact of any change, whether it is to reduce total fat intake, substitute monounsaturated fats for saturated fats, or increase activity level, must be considered within the context of one's total diet and lifestyle. For example, a glass of wine with dinner, as is traditional in Mediterranean diets, may be associated with a lower risk of heart disease. But if the rest of the diet is high in saturated fat and low in vegetables and fruits, the risk of heart disease may still be high.

DIETARY FAT AND CANCER

Cancer is the second leading cause of death in the United States, and it is estimated that 35% of cancers are related to diet.[13] As with cardiovascular disease, there is a body of epidemiological evidence correlating diet and lifestyle with the incidence of cancer, particularly cancers of the esophagus, breast, prostate, and colon. Diets high in fat and low in fiber and plant foods are correlated with an increased risk of cancer.[38] The mechanism whereby a high intake of dietary fat increases the incidence of various cancers is less well understood than the relationship between dietary fat and cardiovascular disease.

How Do Cancers Develop?   Different cancers originate in different parts of the body and have different causes and effects. However, cancer cells share two traits that distinguish them from other body cells. First, they reproduce without restraint. Normal body cells reproduce only to replace lost cells or during normal growth, but cancer cells divide continuously, forming enlarged cell masses known as tumors (Figure 5-15). Second, they invade and colonize areas reserved for other cells. A normal breast cell will stay in the breast, whereas a cancerous breast cell could travel to the liver, bone, or other tissue and begin dividing in the new location. Therefore, cancer cells eventually crowd out the normal cells, robbing them of nourishment and preventing them from functioning properly.

Cells become cancerous as a result of mutations in their genetic material. The type of cancer depends on the type of cell that is originally affected—for example, lung, breast, or colon—and on how the genetic material is altered by the mutations. Most mutations are thought to be caused by environmental factors, such as diet, tobacco use, and air pollution. Any substance that causes a cell to have cancerous potential is called a **tumor initiator**. Tumor initiators sow the seeds of cancer but alone do not create cancerous cells. For the affected cell to begin

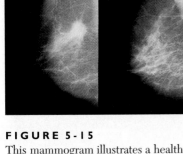

FIGURE 5-15
This mammogram illustrates a healthy breast (right) and one with a tumor (left). (Medical Illustration SBHA/ Tony Stone Images)

Tumor initiator—A substance that causes mutations and therefore may predispose a cell to becoming cancerous.

growing and dividing as a cancer cell, it must be exposed to a **tumor promoter**. Although tumor promoters allow mutated cells to begin dividing, they do not cause mutations themselves. Dietary fat has been suggested to be both a tumor initiator and a tumor promoter.

Tumor promoter–A substance that stimulates a mutated cell to begin dividing.

Dietary Fat and Breast Cancer   Breast cancer is the leading form of cancer in women worldwide. In the United States it affects 182,000 women annually. The incidence is similar among all ethnic groups, but the mortality is higher among minority women. Breast cancer is more common in older women, in women who have had no children or who had children late in life, and in women with a family history of the disease. In populations where the diet is high in fat and low in fiber, the incidence of breast cancer is high. In populations where the typical fat intake is low, the incidence is lower and the survival rate is better in people with the disease. Currently major studies are under way to determine if reducing fat intake to less than 20% of energy will reduce cancer risk or mortality.[39]

The mechanism by which diet affects breast cancer has been studied in laboratory animals. Since most laboratory animals do not get breast cancer, studies are conducted by implanting breast tumors and examining how diet affects their growth. The tumors are more likely to grow in mice fed a high-fat diet than in those fed a lowfat diet. Diets high in linoleic acid are stronger tumor promoters than diets high in saturated fatty acids or omega-3 fatty acids.[40,41] This is the rationale for the recommendation that the intake of omega-6 polyunsaturated fat in the diet not exceed 10% of energy.

Diet and Colon Cancer   Epidemiology has correlated the incidence of colon cancer with high-fat, low-fiber diets.[42] Many of these studies found a stronger correlation between diets high in animal fats and colon cancer incidence than diets with vegetable fats.[43] The connection between dietary fat and colon cancer may be related to breakdown products of fat in the large intestine. Here bacteria metabolize dietary fat and bile, producing substances that may cause mutations. These mutation-producing substances, or mutagens, may act as tumor initiators. A high intake of fiber tends to dilute these mutagens by increasing the volume of feces. High-fiber diets also decrease transit time. Both of these effects reduce the exposure of the intestinal mucosa to the hazardous substances (see Chapter 4).

Dietary Recommendations for Reducing Cancer Risk   Recommendations for reducing cancer risk include modifying the diet to decrease total fat intake[44] and increase fiber, vegetable, and fruit intake (Table 5-2). These recommendations support the goal of reducing cancer incidence in the United States by 50% by the year 2000.[13]

TABLE 5-2	Dietary Recommendations for Reducing Cancer Risk

Maintain a desirable body weight.

Eat a varied diet.

Include a variety of fruits and vegetables in the daily diet.

Eat more high-fiber foods such as whole grain cereals, legumes, vegetables, and fruits.

Cut down total fat intake.

Limit consumption of alcoholic beverages, if you drink.

Limit consumption of salt-cured, smoked, or nitrate-preserved foods.

Work Study Group on Diet, Nutrition and Cancer. American Cancer Society Guidelines on Diet, Nutrition and Cancer. Cancer 41:335–339, 1991.

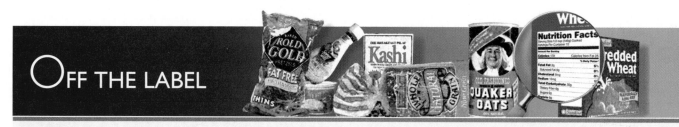

OFF THE LABEL

Using Food Labels to Trim the Fat

The information about fat on food labels is designed to make it easier to identify sources of dietary fat. Understanding how to use this information can help consumers make more informed choices.

Food labels provide a number of different types of information concerning the fat in a food. The Ingredients List includes the source of fat, such as corn oil or soybean oil, and the Nutrition Facts provides the kcalories from fat, the grams of fat and saturated fat, and the milligrams of cholesterol in a serving. These are also presented as a percent of the Daily Value. The Daily Values are calculated for a diet containing 2000 kcalories and are based on the recommendation that the diet should contain no more than 30% of energy from fat (65 g), no more than 10% from saturated fat (20 g), and no more than 300 mg of cholesterol per day. The percent Daily Value allows consumers to tell at a glance how one food will fit into the recommendations for fat intake for the day. For example, if a serving provides 50% of the Daily Value for fat, that is, half the

recommended daily intake for a 2000-kcalorie diet, the rest of the day's intake will have to be carefully selected to not exceed the recommended amount.

Food labels may also contain terms like "fat free," "low cholesterol," or "lean." These descriptors are added by manufacturers trying to capitalize on the public's interest in decreasing fat intake. To make these descriptors helpful to consumers as well as to manufacturers, food labeling regulations have developed standard definitions for these terms. For instance, a product labeled "lowfat" cannot contain more than 3 grams of fat in a serving (see table). These terms can be used only in ways that do not confuse consumers. For instance, since saturated fat in the diet raises blood cholesterol, a food that is low in cholesterol but high in saturated fat, like crackers containing coconut oil, cannot be labeled "low cholesterol," since it may actually raise blood cholesterol.

A component of food labels that may be confusing to consumers is the

claim that a product is a certain percent fat free. This refers to percent by weight, not by energy. To avoid deception, labeling laws require that a product can claim to be a certain percent fat free only if it is also a fat-free or lowfat food. For example, lowfat hot dogs that are labeled 97% fat free contain 1.5 grams of fat, which represents 10% of the total kcalories and accounts for 2% of the Daily Value.

Although packaged meats must be labeled, fresh raw meats such as steak, which are one of the greatest contributors of fat, are not required to carry standard labels. Labels on ground beef can be particularly misleading because they may mention a certain "% lean." In this case "% lean" refers to the weight of the meat that is lean. So when the label says it is 78% lean, it means that 22% of the weight of the meat is fat, or 22 grams of fat in 3.5 ounces (100 g) of raw hamburger. This calculates out to about 55% energy as fat. Only ground beef that is 90% lean or greater meets the governments definition of lean— less than 10 grams of fat per serving.

HOW MUCH FAT SHOULD WE EAT?

Whether you are trying to consume a generally healthy diet or are concerned about your risks of heart disease or cancer, the recommendation is that most people should reduce their fat intake while meeting their needs for essential fatty acids (Figure 5-16).

RECOMMENDATIONS FOR FAT INTAKE

Some fatty acids are essential nutrients. Although there is no RDA for fatty acids, the recommendation for a minimally adequate adult intake is 1 to 2% of energy or 3 to 6 grams per day of the omega-6 fatty acid, linoleic acid. This is well below the approximately 7% of the energy from linoleic acid in a typical adult diet in the United States. The RDAs do not currently make recommendations for the intake of omega-3 fatty acids, but such an allowance is being considered for the future. The Canadian RNIs recommend that at least 3% of energy come from omega-6 fatty acids and that at least 0.5% of energy come from omega-3 fatty acids, with

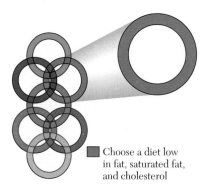

Choose a diet low in fat, saturated fat, and cholesterol

FIGURE 5-16
The *Dietary Guidelines for Americans* recommend a diet low in fat, saturated fat, and cholesterol. (USDA, DHHS, 1995)

Definitions Related to Fat and Cholesterol

Descriptor	Definition
Fat free	Contains less than 0.5 gram of fat per serving.
Saturated fat free	Contains less than 0.5 gram of saturated fat per serving and less than 0.5 gram trans fatty acids per serving.
Lowfat	Contains 3 grams or less of fat per serving.
Percent fat free	This may be used only to describe foods that meet the definition of fat free or lowfat.
Reduced or less fat	Contains at least 25% less fat per serving than the regular or reference product.
Low saturated fat	Contains 1 gram or less of saturated fat and not more than 15% of kcalories from saturated fat per serving.
Reduced or less saturated fat	Contains at least 25% less saturated fat than the regular or reference product.
Cholesterol free	Contains less than 2 mg of cholesterol and 2 grams or less of saturated fat per serving.
Low cholesterol	Contains less than 20 mg of cholesterol and 2 grams or less of saturated fat per serving.
Reduced or less cholesterol	Contains at least 25% less cholesterol than the regular or reference product and 2 grams or less of saturated fat per serving.
Lean	Contains less than 10 grams of fat, 4.5 grams or less of saturated fat, and less than 95 mg of cholesterol per serving and per 100 grams.
Extra lean	Contains less than 5 grams of fat, less than 2 grams of saturated fat, and less than 95 mg of cholesterol per serving and per 100 grams.

Kurtzweil, P. The new food label. Help in preventing heart disease. FDA Consumer 28:19–24, Dec, 1994.

the ratio of omega-6 to omega-3 in the range of 4:1 to 10:1.[45] The recommendations of the World Health Organization are similar, recommending a ratio of linoleic to alpha-linolenic acid in the diet between 5:1 and 10:1.[4]

The amounts of essential fatty acids needed are minuscule compared with the amount of fat most Americans consume. Of more concern than fatty acid deficiency is the chronic disease risk related to the typical American diet. Although the specifics of recommendations differ depending on whether they address cancer or heart disease risk, the principles are the same. Reduce dietary fat intake and increase consumption of grains, vegetables, and fruits, which are high in fiber, micronutrients, and phytochemicals, all of which may be protective against chronic disease. Total fat in the diet should be divided equally between saturated fat, polyunsaturated fat, and monounsaturated fat, and should account for no more than 30% of energy. Cholesterol intake should be no more than 300 mg per day.

Guidelines for Special Groups   The recommendations for fat intake are designed for all individuals over the age of two years. None of the recommendations to restrict fat and cholesterol intake have been suggested for children under the age of two because of their high energy needs and because lipids are needed to support the rapid brain development that occurs in young children. Children between the ages of 2 and 19 with cholesterol levels above 170 mg per 100 ml are at high risk for heart disease and should reduce their fat intake and be followed carefully by their physicians.

During pregnancy, there is an increase in blood cholesterol. This increase appears to be independent of diet, and levels return to normal about eight weeks after the baby is born. Reducing fat intake to 30% of energy intake has not been shown to be detrimental during pregnancy as long as energy, protein, and micronutrient needs are met.

In the elderly, the value of dietary fat reduction must be balanced with the risk of undernutrition. Reducing fat intake to 30% of energy causes little risk, though further reduction may increase the risk for protein or micronutrient malnutrition in this group.

DETERMINING YOUR FAT INTAKE

How much fat is in your diet? The amount of fat in a diet can be calculated using values from food composition databases and tables, food labels, or exchange lists. Databases and composition tables provide information on a wide variety of foods. Food labels provide a more accessible source of information on packaged foods. The Nutrition Facts portion of food labels lists the grams of total fat, saturated fat, and cholesterol in the product as well as the number of kcalories from fat in that food. Daily Values help determine how much fat, saturated fat, and cholesterol is in a food relative to the daily amount recommended for a 2000-kcalorie diet. Unfortunately, food labels are not available on fresh meats, which are one of the main contributors of fat in our diets. If a quick estimate of the fat content of foods is required, the exchange system can be used (Table 5-3). An exchange of fruits

TABLE 5-3	Using Exchange Lists to Calculate the Fat Content of a Diet	
Exchange Groups/Lists		**Fat Content (g)**
Starch ½ cup rice, cereal, potatoes, 1 slice bread		1 or less
Fruit ½ cup canned water-pack fruit, ½ banana, 1 small fresh pear, peach, apple		0
Milk 1 cup skim milk or yogurt		0
1 cup lowfat (1%) milk or yogurt		2.5
1 cup lowfat (2%) milk or yogurt		5
1 cup whole milk or yogurt		8
Vegetables ½ cup cooked vegetables, 1 cup fresh greens		0
Meat and Meat Substitutes Very-Lean: 1 oz chicken or turkey, white meat, no skin; tuna in water; non-fat cheese		0–1
Lean: 1 oz lean beef, pork or skinless dark poultry, or fish		3
Medium-fat: 1 oz mostly bean and pork, lamb, poultry with skin, fried fish		5
High-fat: 1 oz sausage, processed meat or hard cheese, 1 Tbsp peanut butter		8
Fat 1 tsp butter, margarine, mayonnaise, oil		5

other energy-containing nutrients, so the energy content of fat-free foods may not be significantly reduced. For instance, a brownie contains about 6.5 grams of fat and 650 kcalories. Reduced-fat brownies contain between 0.5 and 1.8 grams of fat and 590 to 550 kcalories. Fat-free products can help reduce the amount of fat in the diet, but they cannot be eaten liberally without affecting energy intake.

SUMMARY

1. Lipids are a group of organic compounds, most of which do not dissolve in water. In the body, they provide a concentrated source of energy; insulate against shock and temperature changes; are a structural component of cell membranes; and are used to synthesize hormones and other molecules. In the diet, they provide energy and contribute to the texture and flavor of food.

2. Fatty acids consist of a carbon chain with an acid group at one end. The length of the carbon chain and the number and position of double bonds determine the characteristics of the fat. Linoleic acid and alpha-linolenic acid are considered essential fatty acids because they cannot be synthesized by the body. Other omega-3 and omega-6 fatty acids may be essential when they cannot be synthesized in adequate amounts for proper physiological function. In the body and in the diet, most fatty acids are found as part of triglycerides.

3. Triglycerides, the storage form of fat, consist of a backbone of glycerol with three fatty acids attached.

4. Phosphoglycerides consist of a backbone of glycerol, two fatty acids, and a phosphate group. Phosphoglycerides are an important part of cell membranes and lipoproteins because one end is water soluble and one end is lipid soluble.

5. Sterols, of which cholesterol is the best known, are made up of multiple chemical rings. Cholesterol is made by the body and consumed in animal foods in the diet. In the body, it is a component of cell membranes and is used to synthesize vitamin D, bile acids, and a number of hormones.

6. In the small intestine, fats from the diet form micelles with bile and are digested by pancreatic lipase. The products of fat digestion pass into the cells of the small intestine.

7. In body fluids, lipids are transported as lipoproteins. Lipids absorbed from the intestine are packaged with protein to form chylomicrons, which enter the lymphatic system before entering the blood. The triglycerides in chylomicrons are broken down by lipoprotein lipase on the surface of cells lining the blood vessels. Fatty acids are released and are taken up by surrounding cells. The chylomicron remnants that remain are returned to the liver.

8. VLDLs are lipoproteins synthesized by the liver. They deliver triglycerides to the tissues. Once the triglycerides have been removed, IDLs are transformed into LDLs. LDLs deliver cholesterol to tissues by binding to LDL receptors on the cell surface. High levels are associated with cardiovascular disease. HDLs are made by the liver and small intestine. They help remove cholesterol from cells and protect against cardiovascular disease.

9. After eating, chylomicrons and VLDLs deliver triglycerides to cells for energy or storage. During fasting, triglycerides from adipose cells are broken down by hormone sensitive lipase and the fatty acids and glycerol are released into the blood.

10. Diets high in fat have been associated with the development of cardiovascular disease. This may be related to the effect of dietary fats on blood lipid levels. Saturated fat and cholesterol increase blood cholesterol; omega-6 polyunsaturated fatty acids reduce both LDL and HDL cholesterol; and omega-3 fatty acids and monounsaturated fatty acids decrease LDL but not HDL cholesterol. Since fat is only one component of the diet, the overall effect of the amounts and types of fats on blood lipids must be viewed within the context of the diet as a whole.

11. Diets high in fat correlate with an increased incidence of certain types of cancer. In general, diets very low in fat are associated with a lower risk of breast cancer, and high intakes of linoleic acid may promote tumor growth. Diets high in fat and low in fiber also increase colon cancer risk. As with heart disease, the overall diet is probably more important in cancer prevention than fat intake alone.

12. There is no RDA for fat, but a minimum of 2 to 6 grams of essential fatty acids is recommended. To reduce chronic disease risk, it is recommended that total fat in the diet be divided equally between saturated fat, polyunsaturated fat, and monounsaturated fat, and account for no more than 30% of energy and that dietary cholesterol be no more than 300 mg per day.

13. Reducing fat intake requires decreasing intake of obvious sources of fat such as butter and oils, as well as baked goods, fast foods, and processed convenience food that contain hidden fats. To reduce health risks, the total diet, including consumption of grains, fruits, and vegetables, is as important as a lowfat intake.

14. The types of fats used in processing depend on the desired characteristic. Tropical oils are used because they remain liquid at room temperature and have good storage properties. Partially hydrogenated vegetable oils are used to improve storage characteristics and increase melting point.

15. Artificial fats are used to create lowfat products with taste and texture similar to the original. Some lowfat products are made by using mixtures of carbohydrates or proteins to simulate the properties of fat, and some use artificial fats made from lipids that are not well absorbed.

SELF-TEST

1. What is a lipid?
2. Name four classes of lipids found in the body.
3. What distinguishes a saturated fat from a monounsaturated or a polyunsaturated fat?
4. Name two functions of fat in foods.
5. What are the functions of fat in the body?
6. What is the advantage of storing fat rather than carbohydrate for energy?
7. What is the function of bile in fat digestion?
8. How do chylomicrons and VLDLs differ?
9. How do HDLs differ from LDLs?
10. How are blood levels of LDLs and HDLs related to the risk of cardiovascular disease?
11. What types of foods contain cholesterol?
12. What are the recommendations for dietary fat intake?
13. What is hydrogenation and how is it related to trans fatty acids?
14. Is essential fatty acid deficiency common in developed countries? Why or why not?

APPLICATIONS

These exercises are designed to help you apply your critical thinking skills to your own nutrition choices. Many are best performed using a diet analysis software program. If you do not have access to a computer program, the exercises can be hand calculated using the information in this text and its appendices.

1. Calculate your average fat, saturated fat, and cholesterol intake using the three-day food record you kept in Chapter 1.
   a. How many grams of fat and saturated fat do you consume?
   b. What percent of your energy intake is fat? Saturated fat?
   c. How does your fat intake compare with the recommendation of no more than 30% of energy from total fat and 10% from saturated fat?
   d. If your diet contains more than 30% of energy from fat, make food substitutions or deletions that would decrease your fat intake to 30% or less of energy without changing your energy intake. If your diet already contains less than 30% of energy from fat, list foods you typically consume that are high in fat.
   e. If your diet contains more than 10% of energy from saturated fat, suggest food substitutions that would decrease the amount of saturated fat in your diet.
   f. How does your cholesterol intake compare with the suggested limit of 300 mg per day?
2. Review all three days of the food record you kept in Chapter 1. Identify two foods from your diet that are sources of each of the following lipids. If your diet does not contain any foods that are sources of these, name foods that do contain them.
   a. Cholesterol
   b. Saturated fat
   c. Polyunsaturated fat
   d. Monounsaturated fat
   e. Omega-3 fatty acids
   f. Partially hydrogenated vegetable oils

REFERENCES

1. Anonymous. Daily dietary fat and total food energy intakes. Third National Health and Nutrition Examination Survey. MMWR 43:116–126, 1995.
2. Emken, E.A. Trans fatty acids and coronary heart disease risk. Physiochemical properties, intake and metabolism. Am. J. Clin. Nutr. 62(suppl):659S–669S, 1995.
3. Connor, W.E., Neuringer, M., and Reisbick, S. Essential fatty acids: the importance of n-3 fatty acids in the retina and brain. Nutr. Rev. 50:21–29, 1992.
4. WHO and FAO Joint Consultation. Fats and oils in human nutrition. Nutr. Rev. 53:202–205, 1995.
5. Carlson, S.E., Werkman, S.H., Peeples, J.M., and Wilson, W. Long-chain fatty acids and early visual and cognitive development of preterm infants. Eur. J. Clin. Nutr. 48(suppl):27S–30S, 1994.
6. Wood, J.L. and Allison, R.G. Effects of consumption of choline and lecithin on neurological and cardiovascular systems. Fed. Proc. 41:3015, 1982.
7. Gerster, H. The use of n-3 PUFAs (fish oil) in enteral nutrition. Int. J. Vitam. Nutr. Res. 65:3–20, 1995.
8. Hamosh, M., Iverson, S.J., Kirk, C.L., and Hamosh, P. Milk lipids and neonatal fat digestion: relationship between fatty acid composition, endogenous and exogenous digestive enzymes and digestion of milk fat. World Rev. Nutr. Diet. 75:86–91, 1994.
9. Thomson, A.B., Scholler, C., Keelan, M., et al. Lipid absorption: passing through the unstirred layers, brush-border membrane and beyond. Can. J. Physiol. Pharmacol. 71:531–555, 1993.
10. Fielding, C.J. and Fielding, P.E. Molecular physiology of reverse cholesterol transport. J. Lipid Res. 36:211–228, 1995.
11. Linscheer, W.G. and Vergroesen, A.J. Lipids. In *Modern Nutrition in Health and Disease*, 8th ed. Shils, M.E., Olson, J.A., and Shike, M., eds. Philadelphia: Lea & Febiger, 1994.
12. Keys, A. *Seven Countries: A Multivariate Analysis of Diet and Coronary Heart Disease*. Cambridge, MA: Harvard University Press, 1980.
13. Healthy People 2000: National Health Promotion and Dis-

ease Prevention Objectives. Washington, DC: U.S. Department of Health and Human Services, 1990.

14. Geil, P.B., Anderson, J.W., and Gustafson, N.J. Women and men with hypercholesterolemia respond similarly to an American Heart Association Step 1 Diet. J. Am. Diet. Assoc. 95:436–441, 1995.

15. Gordon, T. The diet-heart idea. Am. J. Epidemiol. 127:220–223, 1988.

16. Brown, M.S. and Goldstein, J.L. How LDL receptors influence cholesterol and atherosclerosis. Sci. Am. 251:58–66, 1984.

17. Brown, M.S. and Goldstein, J.L. Scavenging for receptors. Nature 343:508–509, 1990.

18. Schaefer, E.J., Lichtenstein, A.H., Lamon-Fava, S., et al. Lipoproteins, nutrition, aging, and atherosclerosis. Am. J. Clin. Nutr. 61(suppl):726S–740S, 1995.

19. American and Canadian Dietetics Association. Position paper of the American Dietetic Association and the Canadian Dietetic Association on: Women's Health and Nutrition. J. Am. Diet. Assoc. 95:362–366, 1995.

20. Sagiv, M. and Goldbourt, U. Influence of physical work on high density lipoprotein cholesterol: implications for the risk of coronary heart disease. Int. J. Sports Med. 15:261–266, 1994.

21. Campbell, T.C. and Junshi, C. Diet and chronic degenerative diseases: perspectives from China. Am. J. Clin. Nutr. 59(suppl):1153S–1161S, 1994.

22. Nestle, M. Mediterranean diets: historical and research overview. Am. J. Clin. Nutr. 61(suppl):1313S–1320S, 1995.

23. Keys, A. Mediterranean diet and public health: personal reflections. Am. J. Clin. Nutr. 61(suppl):1321S–1323S, 1995.

24. Ascherio, A., Rimm, E.B., Stampfer, M.J., et al. Marine n-3 fatty acids, fish intake, and the risk of coronary disease among men. N. Engl. J. Med. 332:977–982, 1995.

25. Schoene, N.W. and Fitzgerald, G.A. Thrombogenic potential of dietary long-chain polyunsaturated fatty acids: session summary. Am. J. Clin. Nutr. 56(suppl):825S–826S, 1992.

26. Denke, M.A. Review of human studies evaluating individual dietary responsiveness in patients with hypercholesterolemia. Am. J. Clin. Nutr. 62(suppl):471S–477S, 1995.

27. Norum, K.R. Dietary fat and blood lipids. Nutr. Rev. 50:30–37, 1992.

28. Grundy, S.M. Cholesterol and coronary heart disease: future directions. JAMA 264:3053–3059, 1990.

29. Kris-Etherton, P.M., Derr, J., Mitchell, D.C., et al. The role of fatty acid saturation on plasma lipids, lipoproteins, and apolipoproteins: I. Effects of whole food diets high in cocoa butter, olive oil, soybean oil, dairy butter, and milk chocolate on plasma lipids of young men. Metabolism 42:121–129, 1993.

30. Grundy, S.M. and Denke, M.A. Dietary influences on serum lipids and lipoproteins. J. Lipid Res. 31:1149–1172, 1990.

31. Katan, M.B., Zock, P.L., and Mensink, R.P. Dietary oils, serum lipoproteins, and coronary heart disease. Am. J. Clin. Nutr. 61(suppl):1368S–1373S, 1995.

32. Trans fatty acids and coronary heart disease risk. Report of the expert panel on trans fatty acids and coronary heart disease. Am. J. Clin. Nutr. 62(suppl):655S–708S, 1995.

33. Willett, W.C., Sacks, F., Trichopouluo, A., et al. Mediterranean diet pyramid: a cultural model for healthy eating. Am. J. Clin. Nutr. 61(suppl):1402S–1406S, 1995.

34. Denke, M.A., Sempos, C.T., and Grundy, S.M. Excess body weight: an under-recognized contributor to high blood cholesterol in Caucasian American men. Arch. Intern. Med. 153:1093–1103, 1993.

35. Denke, M.A., Sempos, C.T., and Grundy, S.M. Excess body weight: an under-recognized contributor to dyslipidemia in white American women. Arch. Intern. Med. 154:401–410, 1994.

36. Van Horn, L., Bujnowski, M., Schwaba, J., et al. Dietitians' contributions to cholesterol education: A decade of progress. J. Am. Diet. Assoc. 11:1263–1267, 1995.

37. The Expert Panel. Summary of the Second Report of the National Cholesterol Education Program. Expert panel on Detection, Evaluation and Treatment of High Blood Cholesterol in Adults. JAMA 269:3015–3023, 1993.

38. Dwyer, J.T. Diet and nutritional strategies for cancer risk reduction. Cancer 72:1025–1031, 1993.

39. Chlebowski, R.T., Rose, D., Buzzard, M., et al. Adjuvant dietary fat intake reduction in postmenopausal breast cancer patient management. Breast Ca. Res. Treat. 20:73–84, 1991.

40. De Vries, C.E. and van Noorden, C.J. Effects of dietary fatty acid composition on tumor growth and metastasis. Anticancer Res. 12:1513–1522, 1992.

41. Noguchi, M., Rose, D.P., Earashi, M., and Miyazaki, I. The role of fatty acids and eicosanoid synthesis inhibitors in breast carcinoma. Oncology 52:265–271, 1995.

42. Reddy, B.S. Nutritional factors and colon cancer. Crit. Rev. Food Sci. Nutr. 35:175–190, 1995.

43. Giovannucci, E. and Willett, W.C. Dietary factors and risk of colon cancer. Ann. Med. 26:443–452, 1994.

44. Work Study Group on Diet, Nutrition and Cancer. American Cancer Society Guidelines on Diet, Nutrition and Cancer. Cancer 41:335–339, 1991.

45. Health and Welfare Canada. *Nutrition Recommendations. The Report of the Scientific Review Committee.* Ottawa: Minister of Supply and Services Canada, 1990.

46. Elson, C.E. Tropical oils: nutritional and scientific issues. Crit. Rev. Food Sci. Nutr. 31:79–102, 1992.

47. Miraglio, A.M. Nutrient substitutes and their energy values in fat substitutes and replacers. Am. J. Clin. Nutr. 62(suppl):1175S–1179S, 1995.

48. Gershoff, S.N. Nutrition evaluation of dietary fat substitutes. Nutr. Rev. 53:305–313, 1995.

Protein: The Privileged Nutrient

CHAPTER CONCEPTS

1. Most people in economically developed countries consume more than enough protein.
2. Protein is found in animal and plant foods.
3. Proteins are made up of chains of amino acids folded into three-dimensional shapes.
4. Some amino acids that cannot be made by the body are essential in the diet.
5. Amino acids can be used to synthesize body protein, to synthesize nonprotein molecules, and to provide energy.
6. Protein is necessary to maintain structure and regulate functions in the body.
7. Protein intake must be adequate to maintain body protein and, in some phases of the life cycle, allow for growth.
8. The quality of dietary protein reflects its amino acid composition and therefore how efficiently it can be used to make body proteins.
9. Protein from animal sources is generally of higher quality than plant protein, but plant protein can also meet body needs as long as it is consumed from a variety of sources.
10. Protein and amino acids are added to alter the texture, flavor, and nutritional characteristics of food products.

JUST A TASTE

Do Americans eat enough protein?

Does a high-protein diet make your muscles bigger?

Can vegetarian diets meet protein needs?

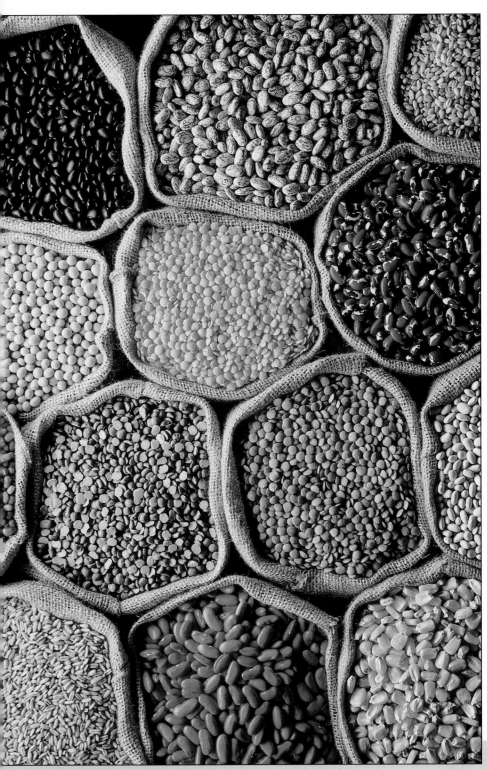

(Thomas Brase/Tony Stone Images)

CHAPTER OUTLINE

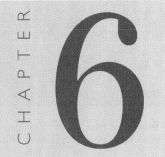

CHAPTER **6**

Protein is a nutrient that conjures up images of vitality and strength. Unlike carbohydrate and fat, protein has had the privilege of being associated with positive effects. It hasn't been accused of being fattening, causing tooth decay, or increasing the risk of heart disease. It is associated with strong muscles and good health. As a result protein is a big seller. Protein drinks, pills, and powders fill the shelves of health-food stores. Advertisers use claims about protein to sell everything from breakfast cereals to hand lotions and shampoos. Consumers often choose foods high in protein because of its association with good health. Is protein worthy of its lofty reputation? Do we need more protein in our diets?

Protein is an essential nutrient. Dietary recommendations such as the *Dietary Guidelines* don't specifically target protein, but following these recommendations will affect the amount and sources of protein in the overall diet and can have an impact on health. In the United States and other economically developed countries, the diet contains plenty of protein and most of it comes from animal foods. Although the protein in these foods easily meets the need for protein, these foods contribute to an overall diet that is too high in fat and too low in carbohydrate. This dietary pattern has been associated with heart disease and cancer. Most of the world relies on plant sources of protein such as grains and vegetables to meet the need for this essential nutrient. Such diets are associated with a lower risk of chronic disease, but when the diet does not include animal sources of protein, the possibility of protein and other nutrient deficiencies is increased, particularly in children.

In this chapter, we will discuss:
- What is protein?
- What role does it play in our diet and our health?
- Does your diet meet current recommendations for protein intake?

Protein—A group of compounds made up of one or more strands of amino acids folded into complex three-dimensional shapes. Unlike carbohydrate and lipid, protein contains nitrogen.

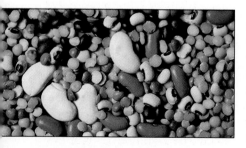

FIGURE 6-1
Legumes are an excellent plant source of protein. (Charles D. Winters)

WHAT IS PROTEIN?

Protein is distinguished from carbohydrate and lipid by the fact that it contains the element nitrogen in addition to oxygen, carbon, and hydrogen. Protein is essential in the diet in order to maintain body structure, regulate body functions, and allow for growth.

Most people in developed countries consume more than enough protein. One fast-food cheeseburger provides about 20 grams of protein, more than a third of the recommended daily intake for an average man and almost half that for a woman. In a typical day most North Americans consume 12 to 17% of their energy as protein or about 70 to 105 grams of protein.[1] Most of this comes from animal sources such as meat, milk, and eggs—the most concentrated sources of protein. One egg or an ounce of meat contains about 7 grams of protein, and a cup of milk contains 8 grams. Plants also provide protein. Although plant sources of protein are not used as efficiently as animal sources to make body proteins, a diet including a variety of sources of plant proteins can still meet body needs. The best plant sources of protein are legumes, such as lentils, soybeans, peanuts, black-eyed peas, chickpeas, red beans, pinto beans, kidney beans, and black beans (Figure 6-1).

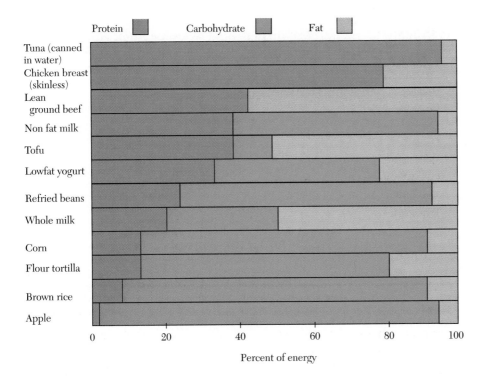

FIGURE 6-2
These foods provide varying amounts of dietary protein and also contain carbohydrate and fat.

One-half cup of any of these provides 6 to 10 grams of protein. Nuts and seeds, although high in fat, are also good sources of protein, providing about 5 to 10 grams per quarter cup. Breads and cereals are moderately good sources of protein. One serving provides 2 to 3 grams (Figure 6-2). Vegetables also contain protein, about 2 grams per half cup.

If protein is plentiful in plant and animal sources, why then do we worry about getting enough in our diets? This is probably because proteins are essential to virtually every aspect of body function. They provide structure to cells, tissues, and organs; regulate the body's ability to use other nutrients; and aid in the transport of molecules through the bloodstream and in and out of cells. Dietary protein provides the raw material to make all the various types of proteins that the body needs. Any protein consumed in excess of needs can be used for energy, providing 4 kcalories per gram, or converted into carbohydrate or fat.

PROTEINS ARE MADE OF AMINO ACIDS

A protein molecule, whether found in a steak, a kidney bean, or a part of the human body, is constructed of one or more folded chainlike strands of **amino acids**. A particular protein contains a specific number of amino acids in specific proportions and in a specific order. Variations in the number, proportions, and order of amino acids allow for an infinite number of different protein structures.

There are approximately 20 amino acids commonly found in proteins. Each amino acid consists of a carbon atom bound to four structures: a hydrogen atom; an amino group, which contains nitrogen; an acid group; and a side chain that varies in length and structure (Figure 6-3). Different side chains give specific properties to individual amino acids.

Of the 20 amino acids commonly found in protein, 9 cannot be made by the adult human body. These amino acids, called **essential or indispensable amino acids**, must be consumed in the diet (Table 6-1). If the diet is deficient in one or more these amino acids, body proteins containing them cannot be made unless

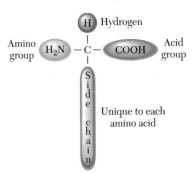

FIGURE 6-3
All amino acids have a similar structure, but each has a different side chain.

Amino acids—The building blocks of proteins. Each contains a carbon atom bound to a hydrogen atom, an amino group, an acid group, and a side chain.

Essential or indispensable amino acids—Amino acids that cannot be synthesized by the human body in sufficient amounts to meet needs and therefore must be included in the diet.

TABLE 6-1	Classification of Amino Acids for Adult Humans	
Essential Amino Acids		**Nonessential Amino Acids**
Histidine		Alanine
Isoleucine		Arginine
Leucine		Asparagine (aspartate)
Lysine		Aspartic acid
Methionine		Cysteine (cystine)°
Phenylalanine		Tyrosine°
Threonine		Glutamic acid (glutamate)
Tryptophan		Glutamine
Valine		Glycine
		Proline
		Serine

°These amino acids are also classified as semiessential. If not enough is supplied in the diet, they must be made from essential amino acids. If those essential amino acids are in short supply, the semiessential amino acids can become essential.

Nonessential or dispensable amino acids–Amino acids that can be synthesized by the human body in sufficient amounts to meet needs.

Transamination–The process by which an amino group from one amino acid is transferred to a carbon compound to form a new amino acid.

Semiessential or conditionally essential amino acids–Amino acids that are essential in the diet only under certain conditions or at certain times of life.

other body proteins are broken down to provide them. The 11 **nonessential or dispensable amino acids** that can be made by the human body are not required in the diet. When a nonessential amino acid, needed for protein synthesis, is not available from the diet, it can be made in the body. Most of the nonessential amino acids can be made by the process of **transamination** in which an amino group from one amino acid is transferred to a carbon-containing molecule to form a different amino acid (Figure 6-4).

Some amino acids are **semiessential** or **conditionally essential**. These are essential only under certain circumstances. Tyrosine and cysteine, for example, can be formed in the body from the metabolism of the essential amino acids phenylalanine and methionine, respectively. If the essential amino acid from which they are made is in short supply, the semiessential amino acids then become essential. For example, if the diet is low in cysteine, it can be made from methionine. However, if the diet is low in methionine, adequate cysteine must be consumed, since not enough methionine is available to make it. Other amino acids may be essential under certain conditions such as in premature infancy.

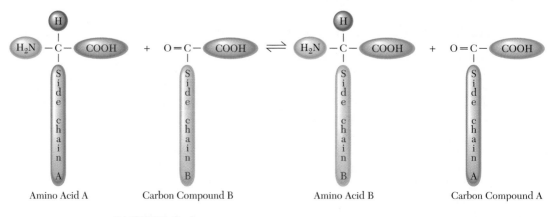

FIGURE 6-4
By the process of transamination, a carbon compound, shown as B in this figure, is combined with the amino group from a nonessential amino acid, A in this figure, to form amino acid B and carbon compound A.

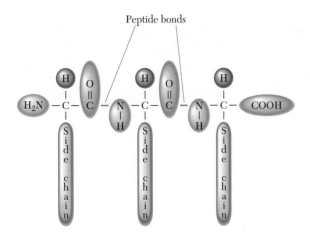

Peptide bonds

FIGURE 6-5
Amino acids in proteins are linked by peptide bonds.

PROTEIN STRUCTURE

Amino acids are linked together to form proteins by a unique type of chemical bond called a **peptide bond**. This bond is formed between the acid group of one amino acid and the nitrogen atom of the next amino acid (Figure 6-5). When two amino acids are linked with a peptide bond, they are called a **dipeptide**; when three amino acids are linked, they form a **tripeptide**. Many amino acids bonded together constitute a **polypeptide**. Proteins are polypeptide chains folded into a complex three-dimensional shape. The three-dimensional shape of the protein is determined by the order of the amino acids, and it is the shape of a protein that determines its function. If the shape changes, the function is altered. For example, the genetic disease sickle-cell anemia results from a change in only one of the amino acids in hemoglobin, the protein that carries oxygen in the blood. The altered amino acid chain causes the characteristics of the molecule to change. Sickle-cell hemoglobin molecules bind together, forming long chains, whereas normal hemoglobin molecules do not bind together. A red blood cell containing normal hemoglobin is disc shaped, whereas a cell containing chains of sickle-cell hemoglobin is crescent or sickle shaped (Figure 6-6). These distorted red blood cells can block capillaries, causing inflammation and pain, and they rupture easily, leading to anemia from a shortage of red blood cells.

Changes in protein structure can also be caused by heat or acid. This change in structure is called **denaturation** (a change from the natural). In food, cooking denatures protein, thereby changing its shape and physical properties. A raw egg

Peptide bond—The chemical linkage between the amino group of one amino acid and the acid group of another.
Dipeptide—Two amino acids linked by a peptide bond. A **tripeptide** is three amino acids linked by peptide bonds, and a **polypeptide** is a chain of three or more amino acids linked by peptide bonds.

Denaturation—The alteration of a protein's three-dimensional structure.

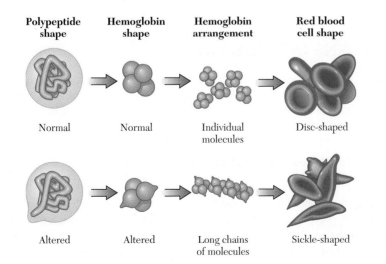

Polypeptide shape	Hemoglobin shape	Hemoglobin arrangement	Red blood cell shape
Normal	Normal	Individual molecules	Disc-shaped
Altered	Altered	Long chains of molecules	Sickle-shaped

FIGURE 6-6
In sickle-cell anemia, a change in the sequence of amino acids in hemoglobin causes a change in the shape and function of the protein molecule.

OFF THE SHELF

Are Vegetarian Diets Better for Our Environment?

Concern about the environment is one reason that people choose to adopt vegetarian diets. Modern methods of animal production waste energy and water, destroy forests and grazing lands, and pollute the air and water. Will becoming a vegetarian eliminate the need to produce animals and therefore save the planet from environmental destruction? To answer this question, one needs to look at the way animals are being raised, the numbers of animals being raised, and their roles in the ecosystem.

In developed nations, the drive to produce animals more efficiently and more profitably has moved them off the family farm and into large agribusinesses. This has had an impact on energy use, land and water use, and air quality. On a small farm animals can turn crop wastes, kitchen scraps, and cellulose grasses that people can't eat into meat, milk, and eggs that make an important contribution to the diet. This isn't true in large agribusinesses. Animals are fed grain rather than grasses and kitchen scraps. This is energetically inefficient because hu-

mans who eat the animals get back only a fraction of the energy they could have gotten from eating the grain. For every 100 kcalories of plant material a cow eats, only 10 kcalories are stored in the cow and can be consumed by humans.[1] Worldwide, 38% of the total grain produced is fed to chickens, pigs, and cows. In the United States, as much as 70% of the grain is fed to animals. Producing feed grain also uses energy and depletes topsoils. In the United States, 1 pound of pork provides 1000 to 2000 kcalories in the diet and costs 14,000 kcalories to produce. Livestock production also uses water—430 gallons to produce 1 pound of pork in the United States. For the world to adopt the American diet would require "more grain than the world can grow and more energy, water, and land than the world can supply."[2]

In addition to feeding animals, their waste materials must be managed. On small farms manure is used for fertilizer, but when thousands of animals are confined to a small area as in agribusiness, manure may pollute

nearby rivers and lakes. The excess nutrients that should have been returned to the land cause algae overgrowth that chokes out other aquatic life and causes nitrate pollution of drinking water.[3] Animal wastes also produce gases that are released into the atmosphere, contributing to acid rain.

The sheer number of domestic animals is also destructive to the environment. Pastures are overstocked; grazing lands, even in the United States, are overgrazed; and forests in the Amazon and other parts of the world are being cut down to create grazing land for cattle. Forests serve to absorb carbon dioxide. When trees are cut down, carbon dioxide produced by animals and the burning of fossil fuels accumulates in the atmosphere and contributes to global warming. The cattle also produce methane gas that contributes to global warming. If global warming continues it will cause changes in climate—probably the single most important environmental issue of today. So whether domestic animals are con-

---

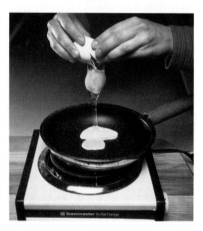

FIGURE 6-7
The protein in egg white is denatured by heat when the egg is cooked. (Charles D. Winters)

white is clear and liquid, but once it has been denatured by cooking, it becomes white and firm (Figure 6-7).

PROTEINS IN THE BODY

To be used by the body, dietary proteins must be digested and absorbed. Their amino acids then become available to synthesize the specific proteins needed by the body, to synthesize nonprotein molecules, or to provide energy.

PROTEIN DIGESTION AND ABSORPTION

The proteins that enter the digestive tract come from the diet, as well as from gastrointestinal secretions and from dead mucosal cells that are sloughed off. The digestion of protein begins in the stomach, where hydrochloric acid denatures protein, opening up its folded structure to make it more accessible to enzyme attack. The acid also activates the protein-digesting enzyme pepsin, which breaks

fined or free, the natural resources of the earth are no longer able to sustain their increasing numbers without serious ecological consequences. Is elimination of animal foods the answer?

The environmental problems caused by animal production occur both because of the way they are raised and because there are too many of them, not because of their existence per se. In parts of the developing world, small amounts of meat and milk obtained from animals may mean the difference between survival and starvation. Manure is a valuable fertilizer and a source of fuel. When integrated into farming, animal products provide extra income during good times and insurance during bad times. In the United States, we rely on animal foods to provide vitamin B_{12}, much of our calcium, and a highly absorbable source of iron and zinc. Eliminating animals entirely would result in less food and is no more ecologically sound than raising them with the methods we are using today.

If we are to both feed the world and preserve the environment, sustainable agricultural systems must be adopted. The aim of sustainable agriculture is to produce vegetable and animal foods while preserving the long-term fertility and productiveness of the planet. The natural ecosystems of the planet include both plants and animals, so it is not surprising that agricultural systems modeled after natural ecosystems would require both. For example, in a sustainable system cattle and sheep would eat from grazing lands not suitable for growing crops rather than eating grains that humans can eat. Without these animals the grazing land would go unused. This type of system uses fewer resources but also produces many fewer animals than the present system. For example, if U.S. agriculture were to eliminate feed grains, energy inputs into animal agriculture would be reduced by 60%, but milk, meat, and egg production would be cut by at least half.[4] To absorb the decrease in productivity the demand for animal products would have to decrease in developed nations. Consuming a diet that is higher in grains, vegetables, and fruits and lower in animal products is therefore a goal that is compatible not only with the recommendations of the *Dietary Guidelines* but also with the ecology of the planet. Completely eliminating animal products is neither necessary nor beneficial. Both plants and animals are essential for a diversified ecosystem, and both plant and animal foods make a valuable contribution to the diet.

[1] Raven, P.H., Berg, L.R., and Johnson, G.B. *Environment*, 1995 Version. Philadelphia: Saunders College Publishing, 1993.

[2] Durning, A.T. Fat of the land. World Watch 4:7–11, 1991.

[3] Gussow, J.D. Ecology and vegetarian considerations: does environmental responsibility demand the elimination of livestock? Am. J. Clin. Nutr. 59(suppl):1110s–1116s, 1994.

[4] Pimentel, D., Vitenzcu, P.A., Nesheim, M.C., et al. The potential for grass-fed livestock: resource constraints. Science 207:843–848, 1980.

the protein into polypeptides and amino acids. When the polypeptides enter the small intestine, they are broken into smaller peptides by the enzymes trypsin and chymotrypsin secreted by the pancreas. Small peptides are broken into single amino acids by protein-digesting enzymes from the small intestine. Single amino acids, dipeptides, and tripeptides can be absorbed by the mucosal cells of the small intestine.[2] Once inside the mucosal cells, dipeptides and tripeptides are broken into single amino acids (Figure 6-8).

Amino acids cross the mucosal cell of the small intestine using one of several active transport systems. Those with similar structures share the same transport system and therefore compete for absorption. In general, proteins in foods contain enough of all competing amino acids so that no individual one is absorbed in excessively large quantities. However, if the diet is supplemented with a large amount of one amino acid, absorption of other amino acids that share the same transport system may be impaired. This is because the supplemented amino acid will monopolize the transport system and reduce absorption of the others (Figure 6-9). For example, the amino acids leucine, isoleucine, and valine share the same transport system. If a leucine supplement is ingested, the absorption of isoleucine and valine will be slowed.

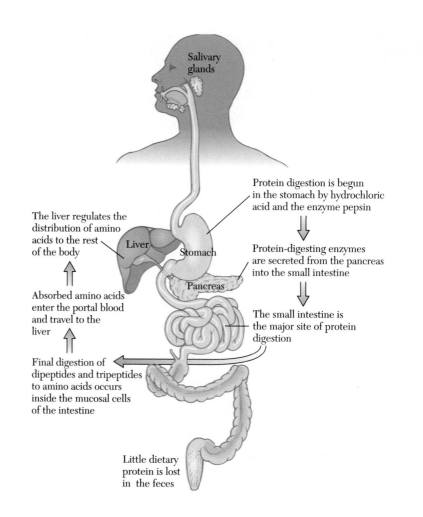

FIGURE 6-8
An overview of protein digestion and absorption.

The liver regulates the distribution of amino acids to the rest of the body

Absorbed amino acids enter the portal blood and travel to the liver

Final digestion of dipeptides and tripeptides to amino acids occurs inside the mucosal cells of the intestine

Salivary glands

Liver

Stomach

Pancreas

Protein digestion is begun in the stomach by hydrochloric acid and the enzyme pepsin

Protein-digesting enzymes are secreted from the pancreas into the small intestine

The small intestine is the major site of protein digestion

Little dietary protein is lost in the feces

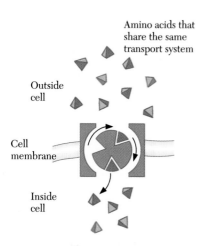

Amino acids that share the same transport system

Outside cell

Cell membrane

Inside cell

FIGURE 6-9
The amino acids in this figure share the same transport system, and since there are more of the purple ones than the green ones, more of the purple amino acids are able to cross the membrane into the cell.

In adults, whole proteins are not usually absorbed. If a protein from the diet is absorbed without being completely digested, an allergic reaction can occur (see Chapter 13). The absorbed protein is recognized as a foreign substance by the immune system, which mounts an attack. Symptoms of food allergies can include reactions of the respiratory tract (sneezing and asthma), skin (rashes or hives), nervous system (headache and dizziness), cardiovascular system (rapid heart rate), urinary tract (blood in the urine), or digestive system (vomiting and diarrhea).

Allergies are most common in people with gastrointestinal disease and infants whose gastrointestinal tract is still immature. Once an infant's intestinal mucosa matures, absorption of whole proteins is less likely and food allergies usually disappear. The absorption of whole proteins by very young infants, however, can also be of benefit because antibody proteins present in breast milk can be absorbed and provide temporary protection against certain diseases (see Chapter 13).

PROTEIN METABOLISM: AMINO ACIDS FOR SYNTHESIS AND ENERGY

Once amino acids are absorbed, they enter the hepatic portal vein and travel to the liver. The liver plays an important role in determining how amino acids will be used by the rest of the body. The liver can use the amino acids to synthesize blood or liver proteins, release them into the general circulation for use by other tissues, or degrade them for energy. Some amino acids are also used by the liver and other tissues to form nonprotein molecules of biological importance such as neurotransmitters.

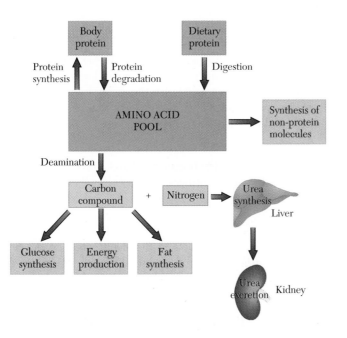

FIGURE 6-10
Amino acids enter the available pool from the diet and from the breakdown of body proteins. They are used to synthesize body proteins and non-protein molecules and to provide energy.

Recycling Amino Acids   The amino acids in body tissues and fluids are available to the body and are referred to collectively as the body **amino acid pool**. Amino acids enter this so-called pool from protein in the diet as well as from the breakdown of body proteins. Of the approximately 300 grams of protein synthesized by the body each day, only about 100 grams is made of amino acids from the diet. The other 200 grams is made from amino acids recycled from protein broken down in the body. When dietary intake of protein and energy is adequate but not excessive, most amino acids in the amino acid pool are used to synthesize body proteins and other nitrogen-containing compounds (Figure 6-10). Under some circumstances, as discussed below, amino acids are used for energy.

Amino acid pool—All of the amino acids in body tissues and fluids that are available for protein synthesis.

Protein Synthesis   Protein synthesis is precisely controlled and orchestrated by the DNA in the nucleus of each cell. DNA provides the blueprint for the structure of each of the proteins in the body. The DNA blueprint is used to synthesize RNA, which travels out of the nucleus to ribosomes in the cytoplasm of the cell where protein synthesis occurs. The RNA dictates which amino acids are used and in what order they will be bonded together (Figure 6-11). During the construction of a protein, a shortage of one needed amino acid can stop protein synthesis until the missing amino acid can be supplied. Just as on an assembly line, if one part is missing, the line stops—a different part cannot be substituted. If the missing amino acid is a nonessential amino acid, it can be synthesized in the body

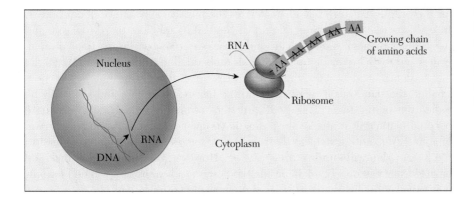

FIGURE 6-11
DNA in the nucleus of cells provides a blueprint for the sequence of amino acids in proteins. RNA transcribes the blueprint and carries it to the ribosomes where amino acids are linked together to form proteins.

Limiting amino acid–The essential amino acid that is available in the lowest concentration in relation to the body's needs.

and protein synthesis can continue. If the missing amino acid is an essential amino acid, the body can break down its own proteins to obtain the missing amino acid. If an amino acid cannot be supplied, protein synthesis will stop. The essential amino acid present in shortest supply relative to need is called the **limiting amino acid**, because lack of this amino acid limits the ability to make the protein. If all amino acids are present in adequate amounts at the time of synthesis, proteins will be completed and released for further processing by the cell.

Synthesis of Nonprotein Molecules   Some amino acids are also used to synthesize biologically important nitrogen-containing molecules. A number of neurotransmitters are made from amino acids. Neurotransmitters are chemical messengers that transmit signals from nerve cells to target cells such as muscles or other nerves. For example, the amino acid tryptophan is used to synthesize the neurotransmitter serotonin, which acts in the sleep center of the brain. Other molecules synthesized from amino acids include DNA, the skin pigment melanin, and histamine, which causes blood vessels to dilate.

Energy Production   Although carbohydrate and fat are more efficient energy sources, protein can also be used for energy. This occurs when the diet does not provide enough total energy to meet needs, as in starvation, and when protein is consumed in excess of needs. When energy is deficient, proteins, such as muscle and enzyme proteins, are broken down to amino acids that can then be used as fuel. Before amino acids can be used for energy, the nitrogen in them must be removed in a process called **deamination**. The nitrogen is then converted by the liver into the waste product **urea**, which can be excreted by the kidneys. The carbon compounds remaining after nitrogen is removed from the amino acids can enter the citric acid cycle and pass electrons to the electron transport chain to make ATP or be used to make glucose via gluconeogenesis (Figure 6-12). This provides energy in times of need, but it also robs the body of functional proteins.

Deamination–The removal of the amino group from an amino acid.
Urea–A nitrogen-containing waste product from the breakdown of proteins that is excreted in the urine.

Amino acids can also be used for energy when protein intake exceeds protein needs. The extra amino acids are not stored as protein; rather, they are deaminated and used as an energy source or converted into either glucose or fatty acids, depending on their structure.

FUNCTIONS OF PROTEINS IN THE BODY

The number of different proteins made by the human body is vast. Each protein molecule has a specific function. Some provide structure, and some help regulate body processes.

Structural Proteins   Protein provides body structure for individual cells and for the overall structure that characterizes the physical appearance of our bodies. In cells, proteins are an integral part of the cell membrane, the cytoplasm, and the cellular organelles. Skin, hair, and muscle are composed largely of protein. Bones and teeth are made up of minerals embedded in a protein base. When the diet is deficient in protein, these structures break down. The muscles become smaller, the skin loses its elasticity, and the hair becomes thin and can easily be pulled out by the roots. These outward signs of dietary protein deficiency have become marketing strategies for cosmetic companies. Shampoo and hand lotion manufacturers add protein to their products, suggesting that protein applied to the hair or skin will improve the structure. However, the proteins that make up hair and skin can only be made inside the body, so a healthy diet will do more for hair and skin quality than expensive protein shampoos or lotions.

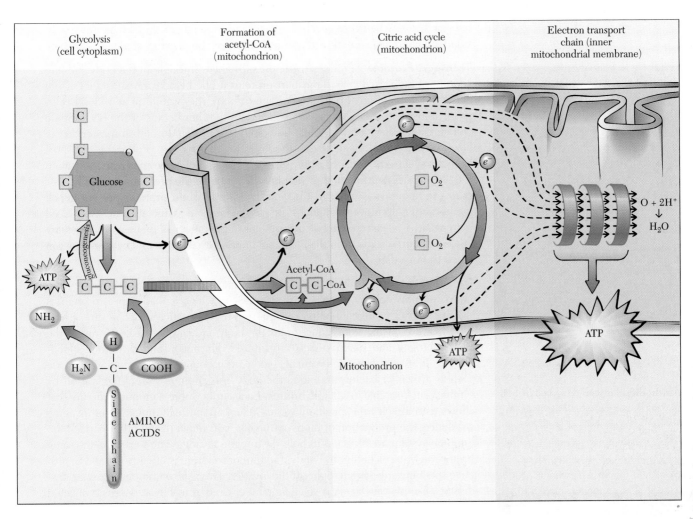

FIGURE 6-12
Deaminated amino acids can be metabolized to produce energy.

Regulatory Proteins   While some proteins provide structure, others help regulate the body's many different processes to maintain homeostasis. Regulatory proteins include enzymes; transport proteins in the blood and in cells; immune system proteins; protein hormones; and proteins that aid in muscle contraction, fluid balance, and acid balance.

Enzymes   Enzymes are protein molecules that speed up the metabolic reactions of the body but are not used up or destroyed in these reactions. All the reactions involved in the production of energy, the synthesis and breakdown of carbohydrates, lipids, proteins, and other molecules, are expedited by enzymes. Each reaction requires a specific enzyme with a specific structure. If the structure of the enzyme molecule is changed, it can no longer function in the reaction it is designed to speed up.

Enzymes that function in the body are made by the body and therefore do not need to be consumed in the diet. Enzymes contained in cooked foods are denatured by the cooking process and are no longer functional when eaten. The enzymes in raw foods, such as papain in papaya, are broken down like other proteins during digestion in the gastrointestinal tract. Purified enzymes sold as dietary supplements to enhance digestion or to protect the body from disease or old age are also broken down in the gut. Some enzyme products, such as lactase taken by individuals with lactose intolerance, are coated to protect them from the acid and digestive enzymes in the stomach. These are not digested in the stomach and become active when they reach the small intestine where they break down substances that are consumed with them. Eventually, they are digested and absorbed.

Transport Proteins   Proteins transport substances throughout the body and into and out of individual cells. Transport proteins in the blood carry substances from one organ to another. For example, hemoglobin, the protein in red blood cells, picks up oxygen in the lungs and transports it to other organs of the body. Some vitamins, such as vitamin A, must be bound to a protein to be transported in the blood. When protein is deficient, the nutrients that require protein for transport cannot travel to the cells. For this reason, a protein deficiency can cause a vitamin A deficiency. Even though the vitamin is in the body, the protein needed to transport it to tissues is lacking. At the cellular level transport proteins present in cell membranes help move substances such as glucose and amino acids across the cell membrane. For example, transport proteins in the intestinal mucosa are necessary to absorb amino acids from the intestinal lumen into the mucosal cells so they can reach the bloodstream.

Defense Proteins   Proteins play an important role in protecting the body from injury and invasion by foreign substances. Skin, which is made up of protein, is the first barrier against infection and injury. Foreign particles such as dirt or bacteria that are on the skin cannot enter the body and can be washed away. If the skin is broken and blood vessels are injured, fibrinogen and thrombin, blood-clotting proteins, prevent too much blood from being lost. If a foreign particle such as a virus or bacterium enters the body, the immune system fights it off by synthesizing proteins called **antibodies**. Each antibody has a unique structure that allows it to attach to a specific invader. When an antibody binds to an invading substance, the production of more antibodies is stimulated, and other parts of the immune system are signaled to help destroy the invader. The next time the same bacterium or virus enters the body, the immune system is already primed to produce specific antibodies to fight off the invader. This is how immunizations against diseases like measles work. A small amount of dead or inactivated virus is injected into the body (Figure 6-13). The injected material does not cause disease, but it does stimulate the immune system to produce antibodies to the virus. The next time the body comes in contact with the virus, a large-scale immune attack is mounted, and the infection is prevented. When the immune system malfunctions, because of protein deficiency or other causes such as HIV infection, the ability to protect the body from infection is decreased.

Antibodies–Proteins produced by cells of the immune system that destroy or inactivate foreign substances in the body.

Contractile or Motile Proteins   Some proteins give cells and organisms the ability to move, contract, and change shape. Actin and myosin function in the contraction of muscles. These two proteins slide past each other to shorten the muscle and cause contraction. For example, when you do a pull-up, the muscles in your arms shorten as the alternating actin and myosin proteins slide past one another. A similar process causes contraction in heart muscle and the muscles that cause constriction in the digestive tract, blood vessels, and body glands. Actin and myosin can also cause contraction in nonmuscle cells. This contraction may help individual cells such as white blood cells change shape and move. The energy for muscle contraction comes from ATP, which is derived primarily from the metabolism of carbohydrate and fat.

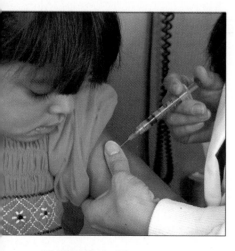

FIGURE 6-13
Immunizations stimulate the production of antibodies against disease-causing organisms. (© Matt Meadows/Peter Arnold, Inc.)

Protein Hormones   Hormones are chemical messengers that are secreted into the blood by one tissue and act on target cells in another part of the body. Some hormones are made of lipid; others are made of amino acids and so are classified as peptides or proteins. For instance, insulin is a protein hormone. A deficiency of insulin causes diabetes and must be treated with injections. The disease cannot be treated by consuming insulin in the diet because the hormone would be broken down in the gastrointestinal tract and therefore have no physiological effect on the body.

Proteins in Fluid Balance The distribution of fluid in body cells, in the bloodstream, and in the interstitial space between cells is important for homeostasis. Fluid moves back and forth across membranes to maintain appropriate concentrations of particles and fluids inside and outside cells and tissues (see Chapter 10). Proteins help regulate this fluid balance in two ways. First, protein pumps located in cell membranes transport particles from one side of a membrane to another. Second, large protein molecules present in the blood keep fluid in the blood both by preventing it from being forced into tissues and by attracting fluid in tissues back into blood vessels. In cases of malnutrition, the concentration of these large proteins in the blood decreases, fluid is no longer held in the blood, and it accumulates in the tissues.

Proteins in Acid Balance The chemical reactions of metabolism require a specific level of acidity or **pH** to function properly. In the gastrointestinal tract, acidity varies widely. The digestive enzyme pepsin works best in the acid environment of the stomach, whereas the pancreatic enzymes operate best in the more neutral environment of the small intestine. Inside the body, large fluctuations in pH can prevent metabolic reactions from proceeding. Proteins in the blood help prevent large changes in the acidity of the blood. For instance, the negative effects of ketosis occur because ketones are acids. Proteins in the blood neutralize some of the ketones, preventing changes in pH. Ketones cause damage only when the capacity of the blood to neutralize them is exceeded.

pH–A measure of acidity.

PROTEIN AND HEALTH

A diet adequate in protein is essential to health. Dietary protein is needed for growth and to replace protein that is broken down and lost each day. Adequate dietary protein allows the body to maintain all of the functions that depend on protein. If too little protein is consumed, the consequences are dramatic and devastating, but too much protein, particularly if it is derived primarily from animal sources, may also have health implications.

PROTEIN DEFICIENCY

Because of the availability and variety of foods in industrialized countries, protein deficiency is uncommon. However, in developing nations, concerns about inadequate protein are very real. A deficiency of protein in the absence of an energy deficiency is rare. This situation can result when food choices are extremely limited and the staple food of a population is very low in protein. The term **protein-energy malnutrition (PEM)** is used to refer to the continuum of conditions ranging from pure protein deficiency, called **kwashiorkor**, to energy deficiency, called **marasmus** (Figure 6-14).

Kwashiorkor Kwashiorkor is typically a disease of children. Since children are growing, their protein needs per unit of body weight are higher than those of adults, and the effects of a deficiency become obvious much more quickly. The word "kwashiorkor" literally means the disease that the first child gets when a second child is born. When the new baby is born, the older child is no longer breast fed. Rather than protein-rich breast milk, the young child is fed a watered-down version of the diet eaten by the rest of the family. This diet is low in protein and is often high in fiber and difficult to digest. The child, even if able to get adequate energy, is not able to eat a large enough quantity to get adequate protein. The symptoms of kwashiorkor can be predicted from the roles that proteins play in the body. Since protein is needed for the synthesis of new tissue, growth in

Protein-energy malnutrition–A condition characterized by wasting and an increased susceptibility to infection that results from the long-term consumption of insufficient energy and protein to meet needs.

Kwashiorkor–A form of protein-energy malnutrition in which only protein is deficient. It is most common in young children who are unable to meet their high protein needs with the available diet.

Marasmus–A form of protein-energy malnutrition in which a deficiency of energy in the diet causes severe body wasting.

FIGURE 6-14
Kwashiorkor (a) is characterized by a bloated belly, whereas marasmus (b) presents as severe wasting. Most protein-energy malnutrition is a combination of the two. a, Dourdin, Rapho Division/Photo Researchers, Inc.; b, Scott Dani Peterson/Gamma Liaison, Inc.)

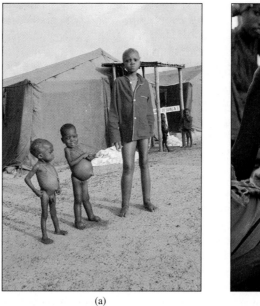
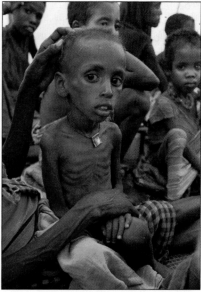

(a)   (b)

terms of both height and weight is hampered. Since proteins are important in immune function, there is an increased susceptibility to infection. There are changes in hair color because the skin pigment melanin is not made; the skin flakes because structural proteins are not available to provide elasticity and support. The cells lining the digestive tract die and cannot be replaced, so nutrient absorption is impaired. The bloated belly typical of this condition is a result of both fat accumulating in the liver because there is no protein to transport it and fluid accumulating in the abdomen because there is not enough protein in the blood to draw fluids out of the tissues. Kwashiorkor is commonly found in Africa, South and Central America, the Near East, and the Far East. It has also been reported in poverty-stricken areas in the United States. Although kwashiorkor is often thought of as a disease of children, it is seen in hospitalized adults who have high protein needs due to infection or trauma and a low protein intake because they are unable to eat.

Marasmus   At the other end of the continuum of protein-energy malnutrition is marasmus, meaning to waste away. Marasmus is primarily due to a deficiency of energy, but protein and other nutrients are usually also insufficient to meet needs. Marasmus may have some of the same symptoms as kwashiorkor, but there are also differences. In kwashiorkor, some fat stores are retained, since energy intake is adequate. Marasmic individuals have used their body fat stores to provide energy. Since fat is a major energy source and carbohydrate is limited, ketosis may occur in marasmus. This is not so in kwashiorkor because carbohydrate intake is adequate—only protein is deficient.

Marasmus occurs in infants and children 6 to 18 months of age in impoverished neighborhoods all over the world. Since most brain growth takes place in the first year of life, poor nutrition early in life can result in permanent loss of function, such as decreased intelligence and ongoing learning disability. Marasmus often occurs in children who are fed improperly mixed formulas that do not provide sufficient energy. This occurs when caregivers dilute formula to stretch limited supplies. Marasmus occurs less often in breast-fed infants. It can also occur in individuals of all ages during famine and is the form of malnutrition that occurs with eating disorders (see Chapter 7).

kilogram is recommended. As the growth rate slows, requirements per unit of body weight decrease but continue to be greater than adult requirements until about 18 years of age.

Pregnancy   Pregnancy increases protein needs to provide for the growth of both the mother and the unborn child (Figure 6-16). Protein in the mother's diet is needed for the expansion of her blood volume, enlargement of her uterus and breasts, development of the placenta, and growth and development of the fetus. An allowance of an additional 10 grams per day is recommended. Pregnant adolescents should consume enough protein to meet both the protein needs for their own growing body and needs of pregnancy.

Lactation   The quantity of milk produced and the protein content of the milk determine the additional protein needs of lactation. An additional 15 to 20 grams per day of dietary protein is recommended for lactation.

Physical Stress   Extreme stresses on the body such as infections, fevers, burns, or surgery increase protein breakdown. These losses must be replaced by dietary protein. Requirements for these types of stresses must be assessed on an individual basis, depending on the extent of the losses. For example, a severe infection increases requirements by about one third. Burns can increase requirements to two to four times above normal.

Exercise   The marketing of protein powders and amino acid supplements to athletes might lead people to believe that protein is in short supply in the athlete's diet. Most athletes get plenty of protein in their diets without supplements. Endurance athletes and those building muscle may benefit from 1 to 1.5 grams of protein per kilogram of body weight, which is slightly more than the RDA.[8] Weight lifters and body builders require this extra protein to supply amino acids to build muscle protein; dietary protein in excess of this does not increase muscle growth. Muscle growth occurs in response to exercise, which is fueled primarily by glycogen stored in the muscles. For example, a 200-pound man who is lifting weights to build muscle would need about 91 grams of protein in his diet. This is approximately the amount contained in a typical North American diet without protein supplements. Endurance athletes who engage in events such as triathlon competitions may have slightly increased protein requirements because protein may contribute some energy during prolonged exercise. The protein needs of athletes are discussed more extensively in Chapter 12.

DETERMINING YOUR PROTEIN INTAKE

To determine if your protein intake meets recommendations, the protein content of your diet can be calculated using food composition tables or databases, the information on food labels, or exchange lists. Food composition tables and databases contain information on all types of foods and supplements. Food labels provide a more readily available source of information; however, since the labeling of raw meats and fish is voluntary, many of the greatest sources of protein in the diet do not carry food labels. Another way to estimate protein in the diet is to use the exchanges shown in Table 6-2. According to the exchange lists, a 1-ounce serving of meat (28 g) provides 7 grams of protein. A cup of milk provides 8 grams, and grains and vegetables provide 2 to 3 grams per serving. For diets consisting of only plant proteins, protein quality must also be considered.

Protein Quality   The recommendations for protein intake assume that the diet contains proteins of various quality. **Protein quality** is a measure of how useful a protein in the diet is for building body protein. This depends on the proportion of amino acids present in the protein. Animal proteins usually contain

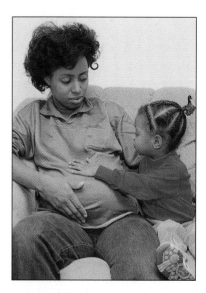

FIGURE 6-16
Protein needs are affected by the stages of life (Photo Edit/Robert Brenner).

Protein quality—A measure of how efficiently a protein in the diet can be used to make body proteins.

TABLE 6-2   Using Exchanges to Calculate the Protein Content of a Diet

Exchange Groups/Lists	Protein Content (g)
Starch ½ cup rice, cereal, potatoes, 1 slice bread	3
Fruit ½ cup canned water-pack fruit, ½ banana, 1 small fresh pear, peach, apple	0
Milk 1 cup fluid milk or yogurt	8
Vegetables ½ cup cooked vegetables, 1 cup fresh greens	2
Meat and meat substitutes 1 oz meat or hard cheese, 1 Tbsp peanut butter, ½ cup cooked legumes	7
Fat 1 tsp butter, margarine, mayonnaise, oil	0

a ratio of amino acids closer to that needed by the body than do plant proteins. Therefore, they are said to be of higher quality. Plant proteins are limiting in one or more amino acids and are therefore said to be of lower quality. Since foods with high-quality protein provide more of the essential amino acids in the proportions needed by the body than do foods with low-quality protein, less total protein is needed when the diet contains high-quality protein.

Measuring Protein Quality   Protein quality is evaluated experimentally in a number of ways. One way is to compare the amino acid pattern of the food being evaluated with that found in a reference protein known to be of high quality, such as egg protein. A **chemical score** is calculated by comparing the amount of the limiting amino acid in the test protein with the amount of that amino acid in egg protein. In this system, proteins with the most desirable proportions of amino acids will have the highest scores. For example, if a test protein has a limiting amino acid that is present at 75% of the level found in egg, it will be assigned a chemical score of 75.

Chemical score–A measure of protein quality determined by comparing the amount of the limiting amino acid in a food with that in a reference protein.

$$\text{Chemical score} = \frac{\text{mg of limiting amino acid per g of test protein}}{\text{mg of amino acid per g of egg protein}} \times 100$$

Chemical score is an easy way to estimate protein quality in theory but does not take into account how well the body can use the protein that is being evaluated. The simplest estimate of protein quality that takes into account usage by the body is the **protein efficiency ratio**. This is calculated by comparing the weight gain of growing animals fed a test protein with the weight gain of those fed a reference protein. Other methods use balance studies with humans or animals to measure not just weight gain but also how well a protein is used for growth and maintenance. **Net protein utilization** measures how much of the protein eaten in the diet is retained for use by the body. Since not all the protein eaten in the diet is absorbed, another measure, **biological value**, compares the amount of nitrogen retained in the body for maintenance and growth with the amount absorbed from the diet. The high-quality protein in egg has a biological value of 100, meaning that 100% of the egg protein that is absorbed is retained by the body. The protein in corn has a biological value of only 60, meaning that only 60% of that which is absorbed is retained for use by the body.

Protein efficiency ratio–A measure of protein quality determined by comparing the weight gain of a laboratory animal fed a test protein with the weight gain of an animal fed a reference protein.

Net protein utilization–A measure of protein quality determined by comparing the amount of nitrogen retained in the body with the amount eaten in the diet.

Biological value–A measure of protein quality determined by comparing the amount of nitrogen retained in the body with the amount absorbed from the diet.

$$\text{Net protein utilization} = \frac{\text{nitrogen retained}}{\text{nitrogen intake}} \times 100$$

$$\text{Biological value} = \frac{\text{nitrogen retained}}{\text{nitrogen absorbed}} \times 100$$

APPLICATIONS

These exercises are designed to help you apply your critical thinking skills to your own nutrition choices. Many are best performed using a diet analysis software program. If you do not have access to a computer program, the exercises can be hand calculated using the information in this text and its appendices.

1. Calculate your average protein intake using the three-day food record you kept in Chapter 1.
   a. What is your average daily protein intake?
   b. Is your intake higher or lower than the RDA for protein for someone of your weight and age?
   c. If you consumed more than the RDA for protein, do you think you should decrease your protein intake? Why or why not?
   d. If you consumed less than the RDA for protein, modify one day of your diet to meet your protein needs. How did these changes affect the amount of fat in your diet?
   e. List two good sources of plant protein in your diet.

   f. The Canadian RNI for protein is 0.86 g per kilogram. The American RDA is 0.8 g per kilogram. Do Canadians need more protein than Americans?
2. Imagine that you have decided to become a lacto vegetarian. Make a list of the nondairy animal foods in your diet and then list plant foods you could substitute. Use protein complementation (Figure 6-17) to be sure that you meet your need for essential amino acids.
   a. Does your diet meet the serving recommendations of the vegetarian Food Guide Pyramid in Figure 6-19? If not, what changes would you suggest?
   b. How much protein is in your lacto vegetarian diet? Does it meet your RDA for protein?
   c. If you already consume a lacto vegetarian diet, design a vegan diet by substituting plant sources of protein for dairy products. Make sure the diet includes at least 2 servings of calcium-rich foods.

REFERENCES

1. Crane, N.T., Lewis, C.J., and Yetley, E.A. Do trends in food supply levels of macronutrients reflect survey estimates of macronutrients intake? Am. J. Public Health 82:862–866, 1992.
2. Crim, M.C. and Munro, H.N. Proteins and amino acids. In *Modern Nutrition in Health and Disease*, 8th ed. Shils, M.E., Olson, J.A., and Shike, M., eds. Philadelphia: Lea & Febiger, 1994, pp. 3–35.
3. National Research Council. *Diet and Health: Implications for Reducing Chronic Disease Risk*. Washington, DC: National Academy Press, 1989.
4. Buckalew, V.M., Jr. End-stage renal disease: can dietary protein restriction prevent it? South. Med. J. 87:1034–1037, 1994.
5. Barger-Lux, M.J. and Heaney, R.P. The role of calcium intake in preventing bone fragility, hypertension, and certain cancers. J. Nutr. 124:1406S–1411S, 1994.
6. Campbell, T.C. and Junshi, C. Diet and chronic degenerative disease: perspectives from China. Am. J. Clin. Nutr. 59(suppl):1153S–1161S, 1994.
7. Willett, W.C. Micronutrients and cancer risk. Am. J. Clin. Nutr. 59(suppl):1162S–1165S, 1994.
8. Clark, N., Tobin, J., and Ellis, C. Feeding the ultraendurance athlete: practical tips and a case study. Am. J. Clin. Nutr. 92:1258–1262, 1992.
9. Young, V.R. and Pellett, P.L. Plant proteins in relation to human protein and amino acid nutrition. Am. J. Clin. Nutr. 59(suppl):1203S–1212S, 1994.
10. Beilin, L.J. Vegetarian and other complex diets, fats, fiber, and hypertension. Am. J. Clin. Nutr. 59(suppl):1120S–1135S, 1994.
11. Mills, P.K., Beeson, W.L., Phillips, R.L., and Fraser, G. Cancer incidence among California Seventh Day Adventists. Am. J. Clin. Nutr. 59(suppl):1136S–1142S, 1994.
12. Fonnebo, V. The healthy Seventh Day Adventist. Am. J. Clin. Nutr. 59(suppl):1124S–1129S, 1994.

13. Snowdon, D.A. Animal product consumption and mortality because of all causes combined, coronary heart disease, stroke, diabetes, and cancer in Seventh-Day Adventists. Am. J. Clin. Nutr. 48(suppl):739S–748S, 1988.
14. Sanders, T.A.B. and Reddy, S. Vegetarian diets and children. Am. J. Clin. Nutr. 59(suppl):1176S–1181S, 1994.
15. Herbert, V. and Das, K.S. Vitamin B_{12} and folic acid. In *Modern Nutrition in Health and Disease*, 8th ed. Shils, M.E., Olson, J.A., and Shike, M., eds. Philadelphia: Lea and Febiger, 1994, pp. 402–425.
16. Weaver, C.M. and Plawecki, K.L. Dietary calcium: adequacy of a vegetarian diet. Am. J. Clin. Nutr. 59(suppl):1238S–1241S, 1994.
17. Dwyer, J.T. Nutritional consequences of vegetarianism. Annu. Rev. Nutr. 11:61–91, 1991.
18. Haddad, E.H. Development of a vegetarian food guide. Am. J. Clin. Nutr. 59(suppl):1248S–1254S, 1994.
19. Segal, M. Fat substitutes: a taste for the future? FDA Consumer 24:25–29, 1990.
20. Nelson, J.K., Moxness, K.E., Jensen, M.D., and Gastineau, C.F. *Mayo Clinic Diet Manual, A Handbook of Nutritional Practices*, 7th ed. St. Louis: Mosby, 1994.
21. Koch, R. and de la Cruz, F. The danger of birth defects in the children of women with phenylketonuria. J. NIH Res. 3:61–63, 1991.
22. Trefz, F., de Sonneville, L., Matthis, P. et al. Neuropsychological and biochemical investigations in heterozygotes for phenylketonuria during investigation of high dose aspartame (a sweetener containing phenylalanine). Hum. Genet. 93:369–374, 1994.
23. Fernstrom, J.D. Dietary amino acids and brain function. J. Am. Diet. Assoc. 94:71–77, 1994.

Energy Balance and Weight Management

CHAPTER CONCEPTS

1. Energy is the ability to do work. Energy in food and the body is measured in kcalories or kjoules.
2. Body weight is maintained by balancing energy intake with output—the principle of energy balance.
3. Energy to fuel the body comes from carbohydrate, fat, protein, and alcohol.
4. Energy is needed for three major functions: maintaining basal metabolic needs, fueling activity, and processing the nutrients in food.
5. Energy consumed in excess of needs is stored primarily as fat.
6. Excess body fat increases the risk of developing many chronic diseases.
7. There is a desirable level of body fat at which the risk of chronic disease is reduced.
8. The propensity for storing excess body fat may be determined by genetics, but environmental influences such as food intake and activity level affect what we actually weigh.
9. Approaches to weight loss include reducing intake, increasing activity, and changing eating habits.
10. The overall goal of weight management is to reduce weight to a healthy level and maintain that weight throughout life.
11. Eating disorders are psychological disorders with nutritional manifestations.

JUST A TASTE

Do overweight people eat more than thin people?

Is there an obesity gene?

Do you need to exercise to lose weight?

Bioelectric Impedance Analysis   **Bioelectric impedance analysis** estimates body fat by measuring the rate of current flow through the body. A painless, low-energy electrical current is directed through the body by electrodes placed on the hands and feet. The rate of the current flow through the body is measured. Since fat is a poor conductor of electricity, it offers resistance to the current. The percentage of the body that is water and allows current flow is estimated and the remainder is assumed to be body fat. Because bioelectric impedance depends on body water, it is most accurate in individuals who have an empty bladder and have not exercised, which causes water loss in sweat, or eaten, which adds fluid to the gastrointestinal tract, for several hours.

High-Technology Methods   Many other methods are available for measuring body composition; but for most, a laboratory or hospital setting and expensive equipment are required. One method relies on the principle of dilution. Since water is present primarily in lean tissue and not in fat, a water soluble compound can be injected into the bloodstream and allowed to mix in the water throughout the body. The amount of the compound in a sample of body fluid, such as blood, can then be measured. The extent to which the compound has been diluted can be used to calculate the amount of lean tissue. Another dilution technique measures a naturally occurring isotope of potassium. Since potassium is found primarily in lean tissue, measuring the amount of this isotope in the body can be used to determine the total amount of body potassium, which can then be used to estimate the amount of lean tissue.

Recently, a variety of newer technologies have been used to assess body composition. For example, DEXA, dual energy x-ray absorptiometry, and MRI, magnetic resonance imaging, use low-dose x-rays to visualize fat and lean tissue in the body.

Changes in Body Composition Throughout Life   Body composition changes throughout life. The percentage of body fat increases in the first year of life. During childhood muscle mass increases and body fat decreases. During adolescence females gain proportionately more fat, and males gain more muscle mass. With aging, lean body mass decreases, so there is an increase in the percentage of body fat even if body weight remains the same.[16] Some of this change may be prevented by physical activity.

Pregnancy also causes dramatic changes in body composition. An increase in blood volume and the production of amniotic fluid cause an increase in total body water. The amount of body fat increases to provide energy stores for the mother and fetus. There is also an increase in body protein due to the growth of the uterus and breasts, an increase in the number of blood cells in the mother, and an increase in fetal tissue.

WHY ARE SOME OF US FAT AND SOME OF US NOT?

The accumulation of excess body fat is a disorder of energy balance. It occurs when energy intake chronically exceeds energy output. Traditionally, external factors such as excessive food intake or lack of exercise have been used to explain why some people are fat and others are not. At the same time, however, it was noted that children had body shapes, sizes, and compositions similar to their parents. Some of us inherit tall, slender bodies with long, thin bones (Figure 7-11). Others inherit stocky bodies with short bones, wide hips, and stubby fingers. Recently, the contribution of genetics to obesity has received more attention. A number of genes in mice have now been identified that, when defective, result in

Bioelectric impedance analysis–A technique for estimating body composition that measures body water by directing current through the body and calculating resistance to flow.

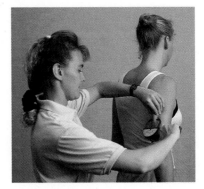

FIGURE 7-10
The triceps skinfold is measured at the midpoint of the back of the arm. This measure of the thickness of the fat layer under the skin can be used to estimate body fat. (David Young-Wolff/PhotoEdit)

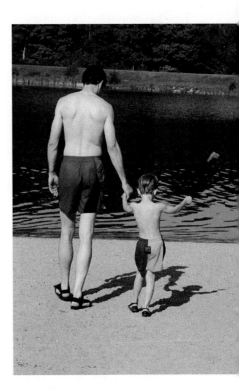

FIGURE 7-11
The genes we inherit from our parents are important determinants of our body size and shape. (Lori Smolin)

obesity.[17,18] Most likely, similar mechanisms regulate body fat in humans. This is not to say that body fat and weight are determined purely by genetics. The amount we eat and how much exercise we get are still matters of choice.

THE ROLE OF GENETICS

The importance of genetics in energy balance was demonstrated by a study that overfed pairs of identical twins.[12] Some individuals in the study gained only 9 pounds, whereas others gained as much as 29 pounds, indicating that different people have different abilities to expend the extra energy taken in. When the sets of identical twins were compared, it was found that each set of twins tended to gain the same amount of weight and that the fat was deposited in the same parts of their bodies. Because identical twins have the same genetic makeup, these results suggest that heredity determines the way we use energy and gain weight. In another study researchers compared twins who were raised in separate households with those raised together to contrast the effect of environment with that of genetics on body weight.[19] They concluded that about 70% of the weight differences between people were the result of genetic influences on metabolic rate, thermic effect of food, and the energy cost of activity.

The Obesity Genes   A child with two obese parents has an 80% chance of being obese himself.[20] The reason that obesity is passed from parent to child is because the information that regulates energy balance, body size, and body shape is contained in genes. A **gene** is a segment of DNA that provides the blueprint for the synthesis of or codes for a protein. A number of genes involved in regulating body weight have been identified in mice.[17,18] The proteins coded by the obesity genes are required to keep weight in the normal range, possibly by sending signals to the brain, particularly a region called the **hypothalamus**.[21] These signals are monitored, integrated, and organized, and then messages are sent to other parts of the body to control food intake and energy balance.[22] When a gene is defective or one of these proteins is not made, or is made incorrectly, the signal to decrease energy intake and/or increase energy expenditure is not received correctly, and weight gain results. The protein that is missing in one strain of mice that are genetically obese is leptin. Leptin is a protein hormone produced by the fat cells and released into the circulation where it travels to the hypothalamus. The hypothalamus responds by decreasing energy intake and increasing energy expenditure. There are many steps that occur between the production of leptin and alterations in food intake and energy expenditure. A defect at any step along the way will interfere with the regulation of food intake, energy expenditure, and ultimately body weight.

Humans have been found to have a gene that codes for leptin; but defects in this gene have thus far not been found to contribute to human obesity.[18] Our understanding of the signals that regulate body fat content is increasing, and it is clear that differences in the genes that code for these factors affect body fat stores. Most human obesity is not likely to be due to a single abnormal gene but rather to many genes that interact with one another and the environment to regulate body shape and size and energy intake and expenditure.[23]

Regulation of Body Fatness   It has been recognized for some time that in most people body fat and weight remain remarkably constant over long periods despite fluctuations in food intake and activity level. The existence of a **set or settling point** around which body weight is regulated is supported by studies in which individuals were fed huge amounts of energy to force weight gain, or underfed to force weight loss. After the feeding regimens were stopped, their weight returned to its original level.[24] It is hypothesized that body mechanisms strive to

Gene–A length of DNA that contains the instructions for making a protein.

Hypothalamus–The region of the brain that regulates food intake and energy expenditure.

Set or settling point–A level at which body fat or body weight seems to resist change despite changes in energy intake or output.

regulate body weight around this settling point. When energy intake or activity level changes, the body compensates metabolically to prevent a significant change in weight.[25] For instance, an increase in food intake and resulting weight gain may signal to increase energy expenditure. An increase in activity that draws on fat stores may send messages to increase food intake or decrease energy expenditure.

Many of the signals that regulate energy balance and body weight over long periods of time are likely to originate from the adipose tissue itself. These long-term signals about body fat content may act by changing the sensitivity to short-term signals that influence energy intake from meal to meal and alter energy expenditure.[26]

Signals from Fat Cells   **Adipocytes** regulate energy balance by sensing levels of energy stores and producing substances that cause changes in energy intake and expenditure.[27] This supports the idea that the size and number of adipocytes may be an important determinant of body fatness (Figure 7-12). Normally when excess energy is consumed and stored as fat, it increases the size of existing fat cells. Therefore, the more fat cells an individual has, the greater the ability to store fat. Most of the adipocytes an individual has are formed early in life. The number of fat cells increases from infancy until adolescence. In adulthood, only excessive weight gain can cause the production of new fat cells. With weight loss, fat cells shrink but rarely disappear. There also seems to be some mechanism that resists reduction in fat cell size below a certain point. If adipocytes become too small, signals may be sent to the brain that cause body mechanisms to act to increase their fat content. For example, shrunken fat cells may release less leptin, causing food intake to increase and energy expenditure to decrease. Another mechanism that may be involved in maintaining fat cells at a preset level involves the enzyme lipoprotein lipase. This enzyme promotes fat storage. If lipoprotein lipase activity is high, fat storage is efficient. In some obese individuals who have lost weight, there is an increase in the production and activity of the enzyme lipoprotein lipase, which enhances the storage of fat, making further fat loss more difficult and weight gain more probable.[28] The activity of lipoprotein lipase may also affect hunger because it can alter the levels of fat metabolites in the blood.

Regulation of Food Intake   The consumption of food sends signals to the brain to stop food intake. Some of these are sensory signals that come directly from the gastrointestinal tract, and some relay information about the availability of nutrients by using hormones or changes in blood nutrient levels.[29]

The simplest type of signal about food intake occurs when the ingestion and digestion of food cause the stomach to stretch. Nerves in the stomach and small intestine sense pressure and send a "stop eating" message to the brain. The presence of glucose, fat, and/or amino acids in the gastrointestinal tract also sends information directly to the brain. In addition, the presence of these nutrients triggers the release of gastrointestinal hormones that cause satiety. One of these, cholecystokinin, helps limit the size of meals both by affecting organs outside the brain, such as the stomach where it slows emptying, and by directly signaling control centers in the brain.[30]

After nutrients are absorbed, the brain continues to receive information that it uses to signal hunger or satiety. Circulating nutrients, including glucose, amino acids, ketones, and fatty acids, may be monitored by the brain and signal us to eat or not to eat.[29] Nutrients that are taken up by the brain may affect neurotransmitter concentrations, which then affect the amount and type of nutrients consumed. For example, when brain serotonin is low carbohydrate is craved, but when it is high protein is preferred.[29]

Other organs are also thought to be involved in signaling hunger and satiety. The pancreas releases insulin when blood glucose levels rise. Insulin limits meal size by directly signaling the brain. In addition to its role in meal-to-meal food intake, insulin is believed to be important in long-term regulation of body fat. The

Adipocytes–Fat-storing cells.

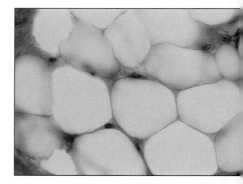

FIGURE 7-12
Fat cells contain a droplet of fat surrounded by other cell components. As body fat is gained, the size of the fat droplet increases. (Ed Reschke/Peter Arnold, Inc.)

liver is also important in food intake regulation. It is in a unique position to monitor changes in fuel metabolism because absorbed water soluble nutrients go directly there. Changes in liver metabolism, in particular the amount of ATP, are believed to trigger eating behavior.[5]

Regulation of Energy Expenditure   Genetics appears to play a role in energy expenditure. Since metabolic rate is the largest component of energy expenditure, even a small difference in metabolic rate could mean the difference between weight gain and weight maintenance over a lifetime. For example, the inheritance of a "thrifty metabolic rate" is believed to play a role in the development of obesity among the Pima Indians of the southwestern United States, among whom the incidence of obesity is greater than 75%.[31]

The role of changes in energy expenditure in maintaining body weight have been demonstrated by examining energy expenditure during underfeeding and overfeeding. During food restriction basal metabolic rate declines, and during overconsumption energy expenditure increases in both lean and obese subjects.[32] Changes in the amount of energy expended in response to changes in circumstance, such as over- or underfeeding, changes in ambient temperature, or trauma, are referred to as **adaptive thermogenesis**. Energy loss through adaptive thermogenesis may prevent some of the weight gain that accompanies an increase in energy intake.[33,34] Several biochemical mechanisms have been proposed to explain this change in energy expenditure. The first, referred to as substrate cycling or futile cycling, wastes energy by allowing opposing biochemical reactions, such as the formation and breakdown of the same molecule, to occur simultaneously. The result is that energy is consumed but there is no net change in the number of molecules in the body and therefore no storage of energy as fat.

A second way that excess energy might be dissipated is by separating or uncoupling the electron transport chain from the production of ATP. When this occurs energy is lost as heat. The increase in metabolism in mice that is caused by leptin is hypothesized to be due to the stimulation of receptors on adipose tissue that cause the cells to waste energy. It is known that a specialized type of adipose tissue, called **brown adipose tissue**, can waste energy as heat. Brown adipose tissue contains many more mitochondria than other adipose tissue, and these mitochondria can be uncoupled from the electron transport chain to release the energy in food as heat. In rats, brown adipose tissue generates heat to prevent weight gain during overfeeding and to provide warmth when the ambient temperature is low. Although brown adipose tissue is believed to be present in humans of all ages,[35] its contribution to energy expenditure has not been determined.[36]

THE ROLE OF ENVIRONMENT: IS THERE HOPE FOR THE FAT TO BE THIN?

If so much of our energy balance and body weight is determined by our genes, is there any hope for the fat to be thin? Yes. Although part of the reason for being overweight can be traced to one's genes, influences from our environment and our personal choices are also important determinants of body weight. Having obese parents increases the risk of obesity not only genetically but also because obese families typically consume more energy and use less through exercise than leaner families.[37] Living in a household where high-kcalorie foods, such as potato chips and ice cream, are always available increases the probability that they will be consumed. Socioeconomic status can also affect body weight. Education, income, and occupation influence behaviors that affect energy consumption and expenditure.[38] Personal choices are important because the genes you inherit from

Adaptive thermogenesis–The change in energy expenditure induced by factors such as changes in ambient temperature and food intake.

Brown adipose tissue–A type of fat tissue that has a greater number of mitochondria than the more common white adipose tissue. It can waste energy by producing heat and is believed to be responsible for some of the change in energy expenditure in adaptive thermogenesis.

your parents don't determine whether you eat the potato chips that are in the cupboard, whether you walk or take the bus, or how much ice cream you have for dessert. A genetic predisposition to obesity makes maintaining desirable body weight more difficult but not impossible. Given the seriousness of the health risks associated with obesity, battling our genetic predisposition is worth the fight in terms of long-term health (Figure 7-13).

Do Heavier People Eat More?   Overweight individuals consume more energy than they burn. But it is unclear whether they eat more than their lean counterparts. A number of studies have suggested that food consumption in overweight populations is not higher than in lean ones;[13] however, these studies relied on records of food intake, which can underrepresent actual intake. Obese individuals tend to underreport their food intake to a greater extent than nonobese individuals.[39]

Food intake in obese individuals may also be affected to a greater extent by sensory and environmental stimuli. While we all eat in response to external cues such as the sight and smell of food, research suggests that overweight people respond more to these cues than their leaner counterparts.[40] Obese individuals may be more influenced by cravings for specific foods, such as sweet or salty items,[41] and research has found that overweight individuals tend to choose high-fat foods.[42] Dietary fat is stored as body fat more efficiently than protein or carbohydrate, so fat kcalories can produce more body fat.

Do Heavier People Expend Less Energy?   The amount of energy an individual expends depends primarily on metabolic rate and activity. Genetics determines our metabolic rate, but activity can be changed by individual choices.

The amount of physical activity an individual gets is largely a matter of choice. When the energy expended for physical activity is compared with the amount of body fat, it is found that individuals with the most body fat have the lowest levels of physical activity, supporting the hypothesis that obesity is associated with a lower level of physical activity.[43] This does not mean that reduced physical activity necessarily causes obesity. The reduction in activity may occur as a result of the obesity. Excess weight makes it more difficult to exercise or even to perform simple daily activities. The obese carry extra weight with every action. A 230-pound man walking a mile is carrying the same weight as a 200-pound man walking a mile carrying a 30-pound suitcase. This extra burden reduces the inclination to increase activity. In addition to the physical stress, obese individuals often shy away from exercise because they don't want to be compared with their leaner counterparts. This is a particular problem for obese children who may avoid group activities to escape being teased about their weight. Inactivity reduces energy expenditure regardless of whether it is a cause of obesity or the result of it.

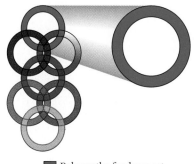

■ Balance the food you eat with physical activity; maintain or improve your weight

FIGURE 7-13
The *Dietary Guidelines for Americans* recommend that you balance the food you eat with physical activity to maintain or improve your weight. (USDA, DHHS, 1995)

CRITICAL THINKING
Is She Destined to Be Obese?

April is unhappy about the 10 pounds she gained during her freshman year at college. Her parents are both obese, and she is worried that she too will become obese. She is 5 feet 4 inches tall, 23 years old, and weighs 140 pounds. She would like to weigh 130 pounds.

In analyzing why she gained weight, she realizes that with her busy college schedule she gets less exercise than she used to and often eats candy bars from the vending machine while studying late at night. By recording and analyzing her food intake for three days, she determines that she eats about 2650 kcalories per day. By keeping an activity log, she estimates that a typical day includes 8 hours of sleep, 14 hours of very light activity such as studying, and 2 hours of light activity such as walking. To determine her expenditure, she estimates the energy she needs for RMR, activity, and the thermic effect of the food.

What is her energy expenditure?

RMR + Activity =

Thermic Effect of Food =

Total Energy Needs =

April decides to increase her activity level. She loves to play tennis and so plans to try to add 2 hours of tennis a day to her schedule.

How much additional energy will this burn?

Answer:

Is this a reasonable plan?

Although April loves tennis, she probably won't play for 2 hours each day. A more reasonable approach might be to plan on playing tennis three days a week while also increasing daily activity by riding her bike to the store, using the stairs instead of the elevator, and going dancing some evenings with friends. She may not lose the weight as quickly as she would have with 2 hours of tennis every day, but she is more likely to keep up this schedule.

April's diet contains a number of high-kcalorie, high-fat foods such as cheese danish, chicken nuggets, and macaroni and cheese. To decrease her energy intake by about 190 kcal she could have a bagel instead of a cheese danish.

APPLICATIONS

These exercises are designed to help you apply your critical thinking skills to your own nutrition choices. Many are best performed using a diet analysis software program. If you do not have access to a computer program, the exercises can be hand calculated using the information in this text and its appendices.

1. Find your desirable body weight in the Metropolitan Life Insurance table and the table of Healthy Weight Ranges for Men and Women in Appendix B.
   a. There are differences between these tables. Does your actual body weight fall within the desirable range in both tables?
   b. Calculate your body mass index. How does it compare with standards?
2. Using the three-day food record you kept in Chapter 1, calculate your average energy intake.

3. Keep an activity log for one day.
   a. Determine your average energy expenditure using your RMR (Table 7-2), activity factors (Table 7-3), and the thermic effect of food based on the energy intake calculated in question 2. (See Table 7-4.)
   b. How does your energy expenditure compare with your calculated energy intake?
   c. If you consumed and expended the amounts of energy calculated every day, would your weight increase, decrease, or stay the same?
   d. If intake does not equal output, how much would you gain or lose in a month?
   e. If your energy intake does not equal your energy expenditure, list some specific changes you could make in your diet or the amount of activity you get to make the two balance.

REFERENCES

1. Cassell, J.A. Social anthropology and nutrition: a different look at obesity. J. Am. Diet. Assoc. 95:424–427, 1995.
2. Kuczmarski, R.J., Flegel, K.M., Campbell, S.M., et al. Increasing prevalence of overweight among U.S. adults. J.A.M.A. 272:205–211, 1994.
3. National Institutes of Health. Technology Assessment Conference Statement. Methods for voluntary weight loss and control. March 30–April 1, 1992. Nutr. Rev. 50:340–345, 1992.
4. Committee to Develop Criteria for Evaluating Outcomes of Approaches to Prevent and Treat Obesity. Food and Nutrition Board, Institute of Medicine, National Academy of Sciences. Criteria for Evaluating Outcomes and Approaches to Obesity. J. Am. Diet. Assoc. 95:1–10, 1995.
5. Friedman, M.I. Control of energy intake by energy metabolism. Am. J. Clin. Nutr. 62(suppl):1096S–1100S, 1995.
6. Wadden, T.A., Foster, G.D., Letizia, K.A., and Muller, J.L. Long term effects of dieting on resting metabolic rate in obese patients. J.A.M.A. 264:707–711, 1990.
7. Devlin, J.T. and Horton, E.S. Energy requirements. In *Present Knowledge in Nutrition*, 6th ed. Brown, M.L., ed. Washington, DC: International Life Sciences Institute–Nutrition Foundation, 1990, pp. 1–6.
8. Horten, T.S., Drougas, H., Brachey, A., et al. Fat and carbohydrate overfeeding in humans: different effects on energy storage. Am. J. Clin. Nutr. 62:19–29, 1995.
9. Seale, J.L. Energy expenditure measurements in relation to energy requirements. Am. J. Clin. Nutr. 62(suppl):1042S–1046S, 1995.
10. Conway, J.M. Ethnicity and energy stores. Am. J. Clin. Nutr. 62(suppl):1067S–1071S, 1995.
11. *Healthy People 2000: National Health Promotion and Disease Prevention Objectives*. Washington, DC: U.S. Department of Health and Human Services, 1990.
12. Bouchard, C., Tremblay, A., Després, J.-P., et al. The response to long term feeding in identical twins. N. Engl. J. Med. 322:1477–1482, 1990.
13. Bray, G.A. Obesity. In *Present Knowledge in Nutrition*, 6th ed. Brown, M.L., ed. Washington, DC: International Life Sciences Institute–Nutrition Foundation, 1990, pp. 23–38.
14. Casper, R.C. Nutrition and its relation to aging. Exp. Gerontol. 30:294–314, 1995.
15. Arena, B., Maffulli, N., Maffulli, N., et al. Reproductive hormones and menstrual changes with exercise in female athletes. Sports Med. 19:278–287, 1995.
16. Roberts, S.B., Young, V.R., Fuss, P., et al. What are the dietary energy needs of elderly adults? Int. J. Obes. 16:969–976, 1992.
17. Zhang, Y., Proenca, R., Maffee, M., et al. Positional cloning of the mouse obese gene and its human homologue. Nature 372:425–432, 1994.
18. Ezzell, C. Fat times for obesity research: tons of new information, but how does it all fit together? J. NIH Res. 7:39–43, 1995.
19. Stunkard, A.J., Jennifer, M.D., Harris, R., et al. The body-mass index of twins who have been reared apart. N. Engl. J. Med. 322:1483–1487, 1990.
20. Anonymous. Obesity: nature or nurture? Nutr. Rev. 49:21–22, 1990.
21. Marx, J. Obesity gene discovery may help solve weighty problem. Science 226:1477–1478, 1994.
22. Harris, R.B.S. Role of setpoint theory in regulation of body weight. FASEB J. 4:3310–3318, 1990.
23. Friedman, J. Weight reducing effects of leptin, the plasma protein encoded by the *obese* gene. 3rd Annual H.G. Hewitt Symposium. The discovery of disease genes and their therapeutic implications. Presented at the University of Connecticut, Storrs, CT, Nov. 9, 1995.
24. Pasquet, P. and Apfelbaum, M. Recovery of initial body weight and composition after long term massive overfeeding in men. Am. J. Clin. Nutr. 60:861–863, 1994.
25. Leibel, R.L., Rosenbaum, M., and Hirsch, J. Changes in energy expenditure resulting from altered body weight. N. Engl. J. Med. 332:622–628, 1995.
26. Kaiyala, K.J., Woods, S.C., and Schwartz, M.W. New model for the regulation of energy balance and adiposity

by the central nervous system. Am. J. Clin. Nutr. 62(suppl):1123S–1134S, 1995.

27. Flier, J.S. The adipocyte: storage depot or node on the energy information superhighway? Cell 80:15–18, 1995.

28. Kern, P.A., Ong, J.M., Saffari, B., and Carty, J. The effect of weight loss on the activity and expression of adipose-tissue lipoprotein lipase in very obese humans. N. Engl. J. Med. 322:1053–1059, 1990.

29. Anderson, G.H. Regulation of food intake. In *Modern Nutrition in Health and Disease*, 8th ed. Shils, M.E., Olson, J.A., and Shike, M., eds. Philadelphia: Lea & Febiger, 1994, pp. 524–536.

30. Reidelberger, R.D. Cholecystokinin and control of food intake. J. Nutr. 124:1327S–1333S, 1994.

31. Ravussin, E. and Bogardus, C. Energy expenditure in the obese: is there a thrifty gene? Infusions Therapy 17:108–112, 1990.

32. Leibel, R.L., Rosenbaum, M., and Hirsch, J. Changes in energy expenditure resulting from altered body weight. N. Engl. J. Med. 332:622–628, 1995.

33. Tremblay, A., Després, J-P., Thriault, G., et al. Overfeeding and energy expenditure in humans. Am. J. Clin. Nutr. 56:857–862, 1992.

34. Diaz, E.O., Prentice, A.M., Goldberg, G.R., et al. Metabolic response to experimental overfeeding in lean and overweight healthy volunteers. Am. J. Clin. Nutr. 56:641–655, 1992.

35. Lean, M. Brown adipose tissue in humans. Proc. Nutr. Soc. 48:243–256, 1989.

36. Himms-Hagen, J. Brown adipose tissue thermogenesis: interdisciplinary studies. FASEB J. 4:2890–2898, 1990.

37. Moore, L.L., Lombardi, D.A., White, M.J., et al. Influence of parents, physical activity levels on young children. J. Pediatr. 118:215–219, 1991.

38. Sobal, J. Obesity and socioeconomic status: a framework for examining relationships between physical and social variables. Med. Anthropol. 13:231–247, 1991.

39. Heymsfield, S.B., Darby, P.C., Muhlheim, L.S., et al. The calorie: myth, measurement, and reality. Am. J. Clin. Nutr. 62(suppl):1034S–1041S, 1995.

40. Rodin, J., Schank, D., and Striegel-Moore, R. Psychological features of obesity. Med. Clin. North Am. 73:47–66, 1989.

41. Drewnowski, A., Krahn, D.D., and Demitrack, M.A. Naloxone, an opiate blocker, reduces the consumption of high-fat foods in obese and lean binge eaters. Am. J. Clin. Nutr. 61:1201–1206, 1995.

42. Rolls, B.J. and Hammer, V.A. Fat, carbohydrate and the regulation of food intake. Am. J. Clin. Nutr. 62(suppl):1086S–1095S, 1995.

43. Lisette, C.P., de Groot, G.M., and van Staveren, W.A. Reduced physical activity and its association with obesity. Nutr. Rev. 53:11–18, 1995.

44. Lissner, L., Odell, P.M., D'Agostino, R.B., et al. Variability of body weight and health outcomes in the Framingham population. N. Engl. J. Med. 324:1839–1844, 1991.

45. National Task Force on the Prevention and Treatment of Obesity. Weight cycling. J.A.M.A. 272:1196–1202, 1994.

46. Robison, J.I., Hoeer, S.L., Petersmarck, K.A., and Anderson, J.V. Redefining success in obesity intervention: the new paradigm. J. Am. Diet. Assoc. 4:422–423, 1995.

47. Rolls, B.J., Kim-Harris, S., Fischman, M.W., et al. Satiety after preloads with different amounts of fat and carbohydrate: implications for obesity. Am. J. Clin. Nutr. 60:476–487, 1994.

48. Stubbs, R.J., Harbron, C.G., Murgatroyd, P.R., and Prentice, A.M. Covert manipulation of dietary fat and energy density: effect on substrate flux and food intake in men eating ad libitum. Am. J. Clin. Nutr. 62:316–329, 1995.

49. Position of the American Dietetic Association: Very-low-calorie weight loss diets. J. Am. Diet. Assoc. 90:722–726, 1990.

50. Wood, P.D., Stefanick, M.L., Williams, P.T., and Haskell, W.L. The effect on plasma lipoproteins of a prudent weight-reducing diet with or without exercise in overweight men and women. N. Engl. J. Med. 325:461–466, 1991.

51. Atkinson, R.L. and Hubbard, V.S. Report on the NIH workshop on pharmacologic treatment of obesity. Am. J. Clin. Nutr. 60:153–156, 1994.

52. Goldstein, D.J. and Potvin, J.H. Long term weight loss: the effect of pharmacologic agents. Am. J. Clin. Nutr. 60:647–657, 1994.

53. Weintraub, M. and Bray, G.A. Drug treatment for obesity. Med. Clin. North Am. 73:237–250, 1989.

54. Consensus Statement. NIH Consensus Development Conference. Gastrointestinal surgery for severe obesity. vol 9, no 1, March 25–27, 1991.

55. American Psychiatric Association. *Diagnostic and Statistical Manual*, 4th ed. Washington, DC: American Psychiatric Association, 1994.

56. Kerr, J.K. Characteristics common to females who exhibit anorexic or bulimic behavior: a review of current literature. J. Clin. Psychol. 47:846–853, 1991.

57. Anonymous. Revised diagnostic subgroupings for anorexia nervosa. Nutr. Rev. 52:213–215, 1994.

58. Practice guidelines for eating disorders. Am. J. Psychiatry 150:212–218, 1993.

59. Strober, M. Family-genetic studies of eating disorders. J. Clin. Psychiatry 52(suppl):9S–12S, 1991.

60. Weltzin, T.E., Fenstrom, M.H., and Kaye, W.H. Serotonin and bulimia nervosa. Nutr. Rev. 52:399–408, 1994.

61. Lucas, A.R., Beard, C.M., O'Fallon, W.M., and Kurlan, L.T. 50-Year trends in the incidence of anorexia nervosa in Rochester, Minn.: a population-based study. Am. J. Psychiatry 148:917–922, 1991.

62. Farley, D. Eating disorders require medical attention. FDA Consumer, 26:27–29, March, 1992.

63. Crandall, C.S. Societal contagion of binge eating. J. Pers. Soc. Psychol. 55:589–599, 1988.

64. Position of the American Dietetic Association: Nutrition intervention in the treatment of anorexia nervosa, bulimia nervosa, and binge eating. J. Am. Diet. Assoc. 94:902–907, 1994.

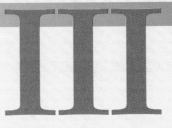

WATER AND THE MICRONUTRIENTS

III

LIFE CYCLE

A Vitamin Primer and the Water Soluble Vitamins

CHAPTER CONCEPTS

1. Vitamins are essential organic nutrients that provide no energy but are needed in small amounts in the diet to promote and regulate body functions.

2. The amount of a vitamin that is available to the body depends on intake, absorption, transport, activation, storage, and excretion. Too little will result in a deficiency, and an excess can be toxic.

3. The eight B vitamins function as coenzymes in a variety of metabolic reactions.

4. Thiamin, riboflavin, niacin, biotin, and pantothenic acid are needed in reactions that produce energy from carbohydrate, fat, and protein.

5. Vitamin B_6 is essential for amino acid metabolism, so its requirement is affected by protein intake.

6. Folate is needed for cell division, so it is particularly important for rapidly dividing cells.

7. Vitamin B_{12} is needed to maintain nerve cells and for the metabolism of folate and methionine. It is found almost exclusively in animal products.

8. Vitamin C is needed for the synthesis of collagen, neurotransmitters, and hormones. It also functions as an antioxidant.

JUST A TASTE

Do vitamins give you energy?

Are high doses of water soluble vitamins toxic?

Does taking high doses of vitamin C prevent common colds?

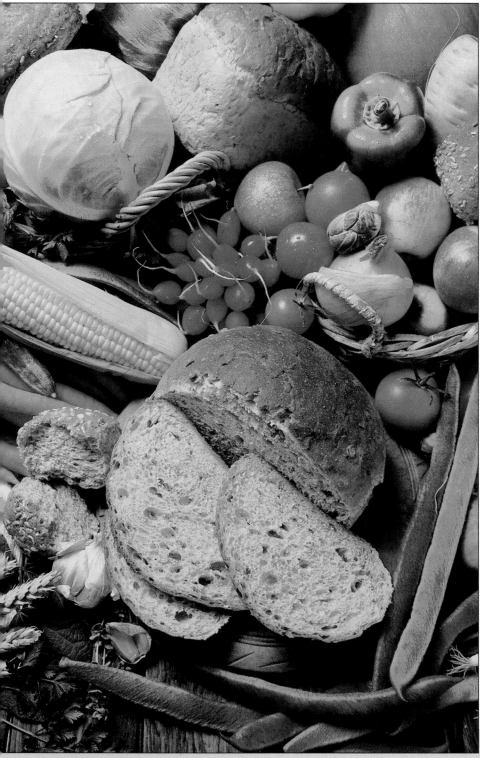

(Tony Craddock/Tony Stone Images)

CHAPTER OUTLINE

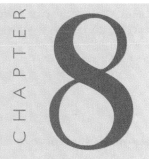

CHAPTER 8

Vitamins were discovered not because of their presence in the diet but because of their absence. The first clues to the existence of these essential nutrients were recognized when deficiency diseases were cured by changes in diet. For instance, in 1753, James Lind reported that consuming oranges and lemons cured scurvy, a disease that had plagued sailors for centuries and that we now know is due to a deficiency of vitamin C. Discoveries such as this helped scientists make connections between specific diseases and the lack of certain nutrients in the diet. With this understanding came the ability to cure debilitating, life-threatening diseases with simple dietary modifications.

As the study of vitamins progressed and nutrients were chemically isolated, the curative powers of food could be concentrated into pills and potions. The miracle cures first associated with foods began to be associated with vitamin supplements. As scientists recognized the essentiality of vitamins, salespeople recognized their marketability. As long ago as the 1920s, products ranging from health potions to chocolate bars were promoted as vitamin-rich cure-alls. Supplements containing multiple vitamins appeared as "cures" for high blood pressure and kidney disease. By the 1940s, more than 40 essential nutrients had been identified. This meant more supplements were available for sale. Today many people consume vitamin supplements in attempts to not only prevent deficiencies but to optimize health, prevent chronic disease, improve athletic performance, prevent depression, enhance sexual potency, encourage hair growth, and provide a host of other benefits. Some of these reasons for taking vitamin supplements are valid, but others are claims made to promote sales. A knowledge of what vitamins do and how much we need is necessary to evaluate the information promoting vitamins as the magic bullets of the 1990s.

The first section of this chapter is a primer on vitamins:

- What are vitamins?
- How do they function?
- What amounts are necessary?

The second section addresses the water soluble vitamins by discussing:

- Where are water soluble vitamins found in the diet?
- What do they do in the body?
- How much of each do we need?

WHAT ARE VITAMINS?

Vitamins–Organic compounds needed in the diet in small amounts to promote and regulate the chemical reactions and processes of the body.

Vitamins are a group of organic compounds that do not provide energy but are needed in small amounts in the diet to promote and regulate chemical reactions in the body. If the lack of such a compound in the diet results in deficiency symptoms that are relieved by its addition to the diet, the compound is classified as a vitamin. Although vitamins do not provide energy, many aid in the reactions that produce energy from carbohydrate, fat, and protein.

Vitamins have traditionally been grouped based on their solubility in water or fat. This solubility determines how they are absorbed, transported, excreted, and stored in the body. The **water soluble vitamins**, vitamin C and the B vitamins (thiamin, riboflavin, niacin, biotin, pantothenic acid, vitamin B_6, folate, and vitamin

Water soluble vitamins–Vitamins that dissolve in water.

B_{12}) are discussed in this chapter. The **fat soluble vitamins**, A, D, E, and K, will be discussed in Chapter 9.

The name "vitamin" was coined in 1911 by Polish biochemist Casimir Funk, who cured the thiamin deficiency disease, beriberi, with an extract of rice husks. He named the extract "vitamine" because he thought it was an amine (a compound containing an amino group) vital to life (vital + amine). Today the term "vitamin" refers to all these vital substances. Initially, the vitamins were named alphabetically in approximately the order in which they were identified: A, B, C, D, and E. The B vitamins were first thought to be one chemical substance but were later found to be many different substances, so the alphabetical name was broken down by numbers. Vitamins B_6 and B_{12} are the only ones that are still commonly referred to by their numbers; however, thiamin, riboflavin, and niacin were originally referred to as vitamin B_1, B_2, and B_3, respectively.

VITAMINS IN THE DIET

Almost all foods contain some vitamins (Figure 8-1). Grains are good sources of thiamin, niacin, riboflavin, pantothenic acid, and biotin. Meat and fish are good sources of all of the B vitamins. Milk provides riboflavin and vitamin D; leafy greens provide folate, vitamin A, and vitamin K; citrus fruit provides vitamin C; and vegetable oils are high in vitamin E.

Food processing can either increase or decrease vitamin content. The vitamins naturally found in foods can be washed away or destroyed by processing. To replace losses or enhance nutrient content, foods can be **enriched** or **fortified**. The addition of nutrients to a food for the purpose of restoring those lost in processing to the same or higher level than originally present is technically referred to as enrichment. Enrichment of grain products adds back the vitamins thiamin, niacin, and riboflavin and the mineral iron, but not all the nutrients lost in processing are restored by enrichment. Figure 8-2 illustrates the effect of milling and enrichment on the nutrient content of wheat flour. Fortification is the addition of any nutrients to foods. These nutrients may or may not have been present in the original product. Foods that are staples of the diet are often fortified to prevent deficiencies in the population—for example, the fortification of milk with vitamin D. Some foods are fortified because they are used in place of other foods that are good sources of an essential nutrient. For example, margarine is fortified with vitamin A because it is often used instead of butter.

Fat soluble vitamins–Vitamins that dissolve in fat.

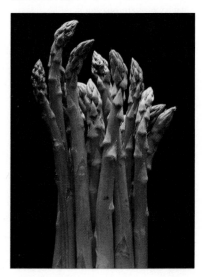

FIGURE 8-1
Vegetables are good sources of vitamins. (Lewis Harrington/FPG International Corporation)

Enriched–A term used to describe foods to which nutrients have been added to restore those lost in processing to a level equal to or higher than originally present.

Fortified–A term used to describe foods to which nutrients have been added, such as milk with added vitamin D.

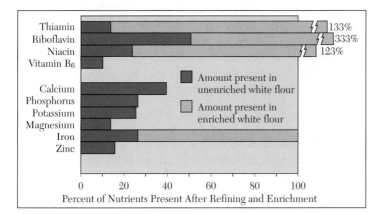

FIGURE 8-2
Many of the nutrients in whole grains are lost in refining, but only a few are added back in enrichment. This figure compares the amounts of some nutrients found in enriched and unenriched white flour with the amount in the whole wheat grain. The nutrients present in whole durum wheat are represented as 100%.

FIGURE 8-3
B vitamins serve as coenzymes necessary to activate enzymes.

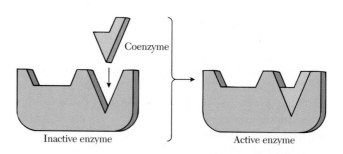

Coenzyme

Inactive enzyme

Active enzyme

Supplements are another source of vitamins and other nutrients. While these provide specific nutrients, they do not contain all of the health-promoting components such as phytochemicals found in foods. Phytochemicals and the wise use of supplements are discussed in Chapter 9.

VITAMINS IN THE BODY

Coenzymes–Small nonprotein organic molecules that act as carriers of electrons or atoms in metabolic reactions and are necessary for the proper functioning of many enzymes.
Collagen–The major protein in connective tissue.

Vitamins promote and regulate chemical reactions in the body. The B vitamins act as **coenzymes**, which are nonprotein substances that bind to enzymes to promote their activity (Figure 8-3). As coenzymes, B vitamins are essential to the proper functioning of numerous enzymes involved in the metabolism of the energy-containing nutrients. Vitamin C is essential for the synthesis of neurotransmitters, hormones, and the protein **collagen**, which provides structure to connective tissue. Each of the fat soluble vitamins serves a very different function: vitamin A for vision, vitamin D for bone health, vitamin E to protect membranes, and vitamin K for blood clotting.

Vitamins in the Digestive Tract Unlike carbohydrate, fat, and protein, vitamins do not need to be broken down into smaller units to be absorbed. About 40 to 90% of ingested vitamins are absorbed, primarily in the small intestine (Figure 8-4). The composition of the diet and conditions in the body, however, may influence **bioavailability**—the amount of a nutrient that can be absorbed and utilized by the body. For example, the amount of fat in the diet affects the bioavailability of fat soluble vitamins because they are absorbed along with dietary fat. They are poorly absorbed when the diet is very low in fat. Bioavailability may also be reduced when nutrients are bound to other substances. For instance, the niacin in corn is poorly absorbed because it is chemically bound to a protein. How a vitamin is absorbed also determines the amount that enters the body. Some vitamins are easily absorbed by simple diffusion. Others depend on energy-requiring transport systems, binding molecules, or specific conditions in the gastrointestinal tract. For example, vitamin C is easily absorbed at any dose, whereas vitamin B_{12} must be bound to a protein produced in the stomach before it can be absorbed.

Bioavailability–A general term that refers to how well a nutrient can be absorbed and used by the body.

Delivering Vitamins to Cells Once absorbed, vitamins must be transported to the cells. Many of the vitamins are bound to proteins for transport in the blood. For example, vitamin A must be bound to a specific carrier protein for transport; therefore, the amount delivered to the tissues depends on the availability of the carrier protein. In protein deficiency, vitamin A cannot be delivered to the cells where it is needed, even if it is adequate in the diet. Some vitamins are absorbed in **provitamin** or **precursor** forms that must be converted into active forms once inside the cells. How much of each provitamin can be converted into the active vitamin and the rate at which this occurs determine the amount of a vitamin available to the body.

Provitamin or **vitamin precursor**–Compounds that can be converted into the active form of a vitamin in the body.

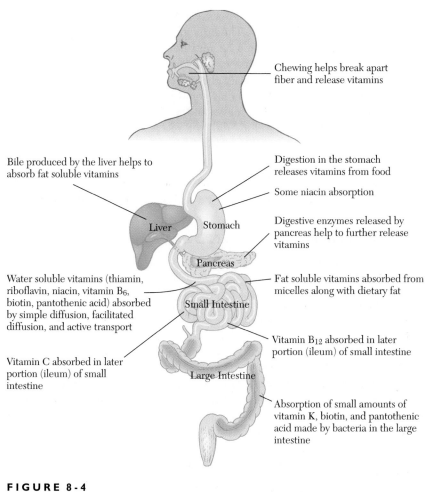

Chewing helps break apart fiber and release vitamins

Bile produced by the liver helps to absorb fat soluble vitamins

Digestion in the stomach releases vitamins from food

Some niacin absorption

Liver

Stomach

Digestive enzymes released by pancreas help to further release vitamins

Pancreas

Water soluble vitamins (thiamin, riboflavin, niacin, vitamin B$_6$, biotin, pantothenic acid) absorbed by simple diffusion, facilitated diffusion, and active transport

Fat soluble vitamins absorbed from micelles along with dietary fat

Small Intestine

Vitamin B$_{12}$ absorbed in later portion (ileum) of small intestine

Vitamin C absorbed in later portion (ileum) of small intestine

Large Intestine

Absorption of small amounts of vitamin K, biotin, and pantothenic acid made by bacteria in the large intestine

FIGURE 8-4
An overview of vitamins in the digestive tract.

Excretion of the Vitamins   The ability to store and excrete vitamins also regulates the amount present in the body. With the exception of vitamin B$_{12}$, the water soluble vitamins are easily excreted from the body in the urine. Because they are not stored to any great extent, supplies are rapidly depleted and they must regularly be included in the diet. Nevertheless, it takes more than a few days to develop deficiency symptoms even when these vitamins are completely eliminated from the diet. Fat soluble vitamins, on the other hand, are stored in the liver and fatty tissues and cannot be excreted in the urine. In general, because they are stored, it takes longer to develop a deficiency of fat soluble vitamins.

VITAMINS AND HEALTH: DEFICIENCIES AND TOXICITIES

Even though the last of the 13 compounds recognized as vitamins today was characterized in 1948, vitamin deficiencies remain a major health problem in developing countries. Children commonly go blind from vitamin A deficiency and have malformed bones from a deficiency of vitamin D. In industrialized countries where vitamins commonly lacking in the diet are supplied by fortification and enrichment, deficiency diseases have almost been eliminated. However, even in industrialized countries, deficiencies still occur in specific groups: those whose requirements are increased such as pregnant women and children, those whose intake is limited by financial or dietary restrictions, or those whose absorption or utilization is limited by a disease state.

Megavitamins–Vitamin doses in amounts greater than ten times the RDA.

In industrialized countries today, excess intakes of vitamins and minerals are as much of a concern as deficiencies. The principle of "some is good so more must be better" does not universally apply in nutrition. Just as there is a minimum amount of a vitamin necessary to prevent deficiency, so there is a maximum level above which symptoms of toxicity are likely to occur. For years it was commonly thought that only the fat soluble vitamins could build up to a toxic level in the body. It was generally believed that excesses of water soluble vitamins were merely excreted in the urine and therefore did not reach toxic levels. However, as **megavitamins**, doses in excess of ten times the recommended intake, became more popular, reports of water soluble vitamin toxicities began to appear. If the public's interest in vitamins as a "cure-all" continues, toxicity symptoms may become more common.

HOW MUCH OF EACH VITAMIN DO WE NEED?

How vitamins are used and stored in the body determines the amounts needed in the diet. Thiamin, for example, is needed to generate usable energy; therefore, the amounts needed are directly related to energy requirement. Vitamin B_6 is needed for the metabolism of amino acids, so its requirement varies with protein intake. Vitamin E protects polyunsaturated fatty acids, so its requirement varies with the intake of polyunsaturated fats.

Estimated safe and adequate daily dietary intakes (ESADDIs)–Recommended intakes of essential nutrients established when data are sufficient to estimate a range of requirements but insufficient to develop an RDA.

Determining Recommended Intakes for Vitamins
To determine vitamin requirements, their absorption, transport, metabolism, storage, and excretion must be considered. The types of experiments used to determine vitamin requirements include depletion-repletion studies, which feed experimental subjects a diet devoid of the nutrient and then refeed the nutrient until deficiency symptoms reverse; nutrient balance studies, which compare intake with excretion; biochemical and molecular biological studies that relate intake to a parameter of cellular function, such as the activity of an enzyme that requires the vitamin in question; and the extrapolation of information gathered from animal experiments. When these kinds of data are not available, epidemiological observations on nutrient intake in healthy populations are used to estimate requirements. Based on these kinds of studies, recommendations for dietary intake, such as the RDAs, are made. For some of the vitamins and minerals, the information available is not sufficient to develop an RDA. For some nutrients in this category, **estimated safe and adequate daily dietary intakes (ESADDIs)** are offered with the caution that the amounts at the upper level of the range should not be habitually exceeded. These recommendations are not minimal requirements or optimal intakes but rather recommended intakes that will prevent deficiencies in the majority of healthy individuals.

Planning a Diet to Meet Recommendations
It would be a difficult task to calculate one's intake of all 13 vitamins every day. A more realistic way to ensure an adequate intake of vitamins is to follow the serving recommendations of the Food Guide Pyramid and choose a variety of foods from each group. Food labels can be helpful in determining the vitamin content of packaged foods. Information about the content of vitamins A and C is required on food labels as a percent of the Daily Value (see Chapter 2). Although fresh vegetables and fruits, which are excellent sources of vitamins A and C, do not come with labels, nutritional information about these foods is often provided at the produce counter. Listing of other vitamins is voluntary on food labels; many foods such as breakfast cereals provide this information.

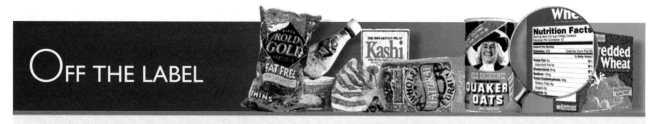

OFF THE LABEL

Micronutrients On Food Labels

Sodium, vitamin A, vitamin C, calcium, and iron are the only micronutrients that must be listed in the Nutrition Facts section of food labels. Sodium is included on food labels because the typical American diet is too high in sodium. Vitamin A, vitamin C, calcium, and iron are included because we typically don't get enough.

The information presented for sodium is similar to that given for total fat, cholesterol, and total carbohydrate. The total amount per serving is listed in milligrams (mg) and as a percent of the Daily Value. The Daily Value for sodium is the Daily Reference Value: less than 2400 mg per day, an amount that will easily meet needs but does not increase the risk of hypertension in populations. With this information, you can calculate exactly how much sodium you consume or can use the percentage to determine what proportion of the recommended intake a specific food provides.

The information given for vitamin A, vitamin C, calcium, and iron is not as explicit. Only the % Daily Value per serving of the product is given for these vitamins and minerals. The Daily Values for these vitamins and minerals are derived from the Reference Daily Intakes (RDIs). For most nutrients, the RDIs (previously called U.S. RDAs) are the highest RDA value for any age or gender group (except pregnant and lactating

women) based on the 1968 RDAs. Simplifying the RDAs into a single value for each nutrient gives one number that can be used on food labels. Although you can't calculate the amount of vitamin C, A, iron, or calcium in a food from just the information on the food label, the % Daily Value is still helpful in determining whether a food makes a significant contribution toward your needs. The amounts of these nutrients in foods can be calculated from the % Daily Value using the RDIs given in Table 2-4. For example, the vegetable juice shown here provides 140% of the RDI for vitamin C, or 140% × 60 mg = 84 mg of vitamin C.

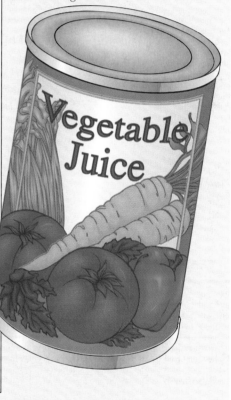

Nutrition Facts	
Serving Size 1 can (340mL)	

Amount Per Serving	
Calories 70	Calories from Fat 0

	% Daily Value**
Total Fat 0g	**0%**
Saturated Fat 0g	**0%**
Cholesterol 0mg	**0%**
Sodium 880mg	**37%**
Potassium 780mg	**22%**
Total Carbohydrate 15g	**5%**
Dietary Fiber 2g	**8%**
Sugars 11g	
Protein 2g	

Vitamin A 60% (80% as Beta Carotene)	
Vitamin C 140%•Calcium 4%•Iron 10%	

*Percent Daily Values are based on a 2,000 calorie diet. Your daily values may be higher or lower depending on your calorie needs.

	Calories:	2,000	2,500
Total Fat	Less than	65g	80g
Sat Fat	Less than	20g	25g
Cholesterol	Less than	300mg	300mg
Sodium	Less than	2,400mg	2,400mg
Potassium	Less than	3,500mg	3,500mg
Total Carbohydrate		300g	375g
Dietary Fiber		25g	30g

THE B VITAMINS

The B vitamins are often found together in food and were first thought to be a single substance needed to produce energy from food. They are now known to be eight individual nutrients with separate coenzyme functions required for various steps in metabolism. Although they each are involved in unique biochemical reactions, many of these reactions are interrelated.

Thiamin, riboflavin, niacin, pantothenic acid, and biotin do not provide energy in the diet, but all serve as coenzymes for reactions that release energy from carbohydrate, fat, and protein. Therefore, a deficiency of any one can interfere with energy metabolism and cause some common deficiency symptoms such as skin rashes, depression, and weakness. Vitamin B_6 is unique because of its importance for enzymes that metabolize amino acids from protein. Folate and vitamin B_{12} are important for the synthesis of DNA and are therefore essential for cell division.

THIAMIN

More than 4000 years ago, affluent members of Far Eastern societies began the practice of removing the outer layers of rice to produce white or "polished" rice (Figure 8-5). As polished rice became the staple of the diet, the prevalence of the disease **beriberi** increased. A connection between diet and beriberi was not made until the late 19th century, when a surgeon in the Japanese navy demonstrated that shipboard beriberi could be prevented by the addition of meat and whole grains to the diet. These foods are now known to be good sources of thiamin.

Beriberi—The disease resulting from a deficiency of thiamin.

Thiamin in the Diet   Thiamin is widely distributed in foods. A large proportion of the thiamin consumed in the United States comes from enriched grains, breakfast cereals, and bakery products. Pork, whole grains, legumes, nuts, seeds, and organ meats (liver, kidney, heart) are also good sources. The dietary sources of thiamin and the other B vitamins are summarized in Table 8-1.

Thiamin in foods may be destroyed during cooking or storage because it is sensitive to heat, oxygen, and low-acid conditions. Thiamin availability is also affected by the presence of factors in foods that destroy thiamin. For instance, there are antithiamin enzymes in raw shellfish and fresh water fish that degrade thiamin during food storage and preparation, or during passage through the gastrointestinal tract. These enzymes are only present in raw foods because they are destroyed by

TABLE 8-1   Summary of Dietary Sources of B Vitamins*

	Meat/Fish Poultry/Eggs	Dairy Products	Fruits	Vegetables	Legumes	Nuts and Seeds	Whole or Enriched Grains
Thiamin	Pork, organ meats						
Riboflavin				Asparagus, broccoli, spinach			
Niacin					Peanuts		Except corn
Biotin	Egg yolk						
Pantothenic Acid	Eggs, organ meats						
Vitamin B_6					Soybeans		
Folate	Organ meats		Oranges	Leafy greens, broccoli			Wheat bran
Vitamin B_12							

*The colored boxes indicate food categories that provide a good source of each B vitamin. Exceptional sources and exceptions within each category are noted.

cooking. Tea, coffee, betel nuts, blueberries, and red cabbage contain antithiamin factors that are not inactivated by cooking. These also destroy thiamin, making it unavailable to the body. Habitual consumption of foods containing antithiamin factors increases the risk of thiamin deficiency.[1]

Thiamin in the Body   Thiamin does not provide energy, but it is important in the energy-producing reactions in the body. The active form, thiamin pyrophosphate, is a coenzyme in reactions in which carbon dioxide is lost from larger molecules. For instance, the reaction that forms acetyl-CoA from pyruvate requires thiamine pyrophosphate. Thiamin is therefore essential to the production of energy from glucose (Figure 8-6). Thiamin is also needed for the metabolism of other sugars; the synthesis of the neurotransmitter acetylcholine; the production of the sugar ribose, which is needed to synthesize RNA; and the metabolism of alcohol.

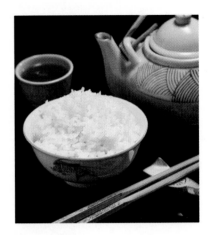

FIGURE 8-5
Unenriched white rice is a poor source of thiamin. (Charles D. Winters)

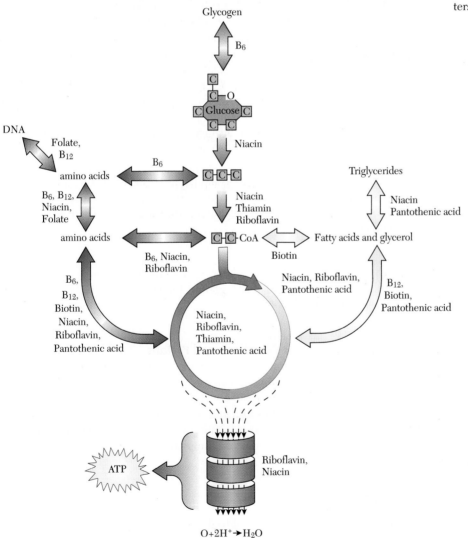

FIGURE 8-6
These examples of metabolic reactions that require B-vitamin coenzymes illustrate the widespread functions of these vitamins in the metabolism of carbohydrates, proteins, fats, and DNA.

Thiamin Deficiency   The symptoms of the thiamin deficiency disease, beriberi, are related to the role of thiamin in glucose metabolism and acetylcholine synthesis. The earliest symptoms, depression and weakness, which occur after only about ten days on a thiamin-free diet, are probably related to the inability to completely use glucose. Since brain and nerve tissue rely on glucose for energy, the inability to form acetyl-CoA will rapidly affect nervous system activity. Poor coordination and nervous tingling in the arms and legs may also be caused by the lack of acetylcholine. Advanced beriberi can result in paralysis and heart failure.

Although overt beriberi is usually thought of as a disease of 19th-century Asia, there are population groups in North America today that are at a high risk for developing thiamin deficiency. Alcoholics are particularly vulnerable because thiamin is needed for alcohol metabolism and alcohol decreases the absorption of thiamin. The risk of deficiency is also increased when thiamin requirement is increased, as it is when energy requirements are increased by strenuous physical exertion, fever, pregnancy, lactation, or adolescence.[1]

How Much Thiamin Do We Need?   The recommended intake for thiamin, as for other micronutrients, is set at a level that will satisfy the needs of 97% or more of individuals in a population. Therefore, an individual's actual requirement for thiamin may be less than or more than the recommended intake for the population. Because thiamin is important in energy production, energy intake affects thiamin requirement. The RDA for thiamin is based on 0.5 mg for every 1000 kcalories in the diet (see Table 8-2 for RDAs and Canadian RNIs). A minimum intake of 1.0 mg per day is recommended even when energy intake is less than 2000 kcalories per day. For an average individual, half of the RDA can be obtained from 3 to 4 ounces (85 to 115 g) of pork or one-quarter cup of sunflower seeds.

The requirement for thiamin is increased during pregnancy and lactation because energy requirements are increased and thiamin is secreted in milk. The recommended intake per 1000 kcalories is the same for children, adolescents, and the elderly as it is for adults.

Thiamin Toxicity   There have been no reports of thiamin toxicity even at doses as high as 500 mg per day for a month.[2] Intakes of thiamin above the RDA have not been proved to be of benefit.

Thiamin Supplements: Promises and Pitfalls   Thiamin supplements are marketed by promising to provide "more energy." Although thiamin is needed to produce energy, it does not stimulate energy production. Unless thiamin is deficient, increasing thiamin intake does not increase the ability to produce energy. Because thiamin deficiency causes mental confusion and damages the heart, supplements often promise to improve mental function and prevent heart disease. However, in the absence of a deficiency, supplements do not have these effects.

RIBOFLAVIN

The search for a cure for beriberi led to the discovery of more than just thiamin. Scientists searching for the antiberiberi factor made extracts from vegetables and grains. These extracts were found to contain two components. The one that cured beriberi contained thiamin. The other was later determined to contain riboflavin, vitamin B_6, niacin, and pantothenic acid.

the bone marrow become white blood cells, whereas others differentiate to form red blood cells. The mechanism whereby vitamin A is able to affect cell differentiation is through its ability to interact with DNA at specific target sites within the body to turn on and off various cellular functions. This is analogous to the way some hormones affect cells. The role of vitamin A in cell differentiation is important in the maintenance of epithelial tissue, growth, reproduction, and immunity.

Maintenance of Epithelial Tissue   Vitamin A is necessary for the maintenance of epithelial tissue. This type of tissue covers internal and external body surfaces and includes the skin and the linings of the eyes, intestines, lungs, bladder, and all other passages within the body. Epithelial tissue comes in direct contact with the outside environment and so is an important barrier to infection. When vitamin A is deficient, epithelial cells do not differentiate normally. For example, the epithelial tissue on many body surfaces is lubricated by mucus. When mucus-secreting cells die, new cells differentiate into mucus-secreting cells to replace them. When vitamin A is deficient, these cells are replaced by cells that secrete a protein called **keratin**. Keratin is the hard protein that makes up hair and nails. The decrease in mucus secretion and increase in keratin cause the cell surface to become hard and dry. The epithelial layer loses its protective capabilities and leaves the tissue open to infection. The risk of infection is compounded by the fact that vitamin A deficiency also decreases the activity of the immune system.

Keratin—A hard protein that makes up hair and nails.

All epithelial tissues are affected by vitamin A deficiency, but the epithelium of the eye is particularly susceptible to damage. The mucus in the eye normally provides lubrication, washes away dirt and other particles, and also contains a protein that helps destroy bacteria. When vitamin A is deficient, the lack of mucus and the buildup of keratin cause the cornea to dry and thicken and crack easily, a condition known as **xerophthalmia**, which means dry eye. Xerophthalmia leaves the eye open to infection. It can be treated by increasing vitamin A intake. If left untreated, it can result in permanent blindness (Figure 9-3).

Xerophthalmia—An eye condition resulting from vitamin A deficiency. It is characterized by a lack of mucus, which leaves the eye dry and vulnerable to cracking and infection. Xerophthalmia may lead to blindness.

Growth, Reproduction, and Immunity   The ability of vitamin A to regulate the growth and differentiation of cells makes it essential throughout life for normal growth, reproduction, and immune function. For example, vitamin A is important for bone growth, because it turns on the cells that remove old bone prior to the deposition of new bone. A vitamin A deficiency early in life can cause abnormal jawbone growth, resulting in crooked teeth and poor dental health. Poor overall growth is an early sign of vitamin A deficiency in children. In reproduction, vitamin A is hypothesized to play a role not only in cell differentiation, but in directing cells to form the shapes and patterns needed to develop into a completely formed organism.[7] It is so important that deficient animals cannot reproduce at all. In the immune system, vitamin A is needed for the differentiation that produces the different types of immune cells. When vitamin A is deficient, the activity of specific immune cells cannot be stimulated. This impaired immune function adds to the problem of infection due to abnormal epithelial tissue barriers.

Antioxidant Role of Carotenoids   Carotenoids, particularly beta-carotene, function as antioxidants. Beta-carotene, along with vitamin E, is important in protecting cell membranes from damage by free radicals. Numerous epidemiological studies have shown that people who consume diets high in fruits and vegetables containing beta-carotene or who have higher beta-carotene levels in their blood have a reduced risk of developing or dying of certain types of cancer.[8,9] Diets high in beta-carotene have been shown to protect against lung cancer in nonsmokers.[10] The effect of a beta-carotene–rich diet on cancer may be related to its antioxidant function or to the effects of other substances plentiful in such a diet.

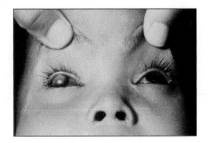

FIGURE 9-3
Vitamin A deficiency is a major cause of blindness worldwide. (Lester V. Bergman, NY)

VITAMIN A DEFICIENCY—A WORLD HEALTH PROBLEM

Vitamin A deficiency is a threat to the health, sight, and lives of millions of children in the developing world.[11] Children deficient in vitamin A grow poorly, have poor appetites, have more infections, are more anemic, are more likely to go blind, and are more likely to die in childhood than their peers.[12] As many as 5 million children yearly develop vitamin A deficiency, primarily in India, Africa, Latin America, and the Caribbean. Of these, approximately 250,000 are blinded, and within one year about half of these children will die.[13] In addition to an insufficient intake of vitamin A, a deficiency can be caused by a diet low in fat, protein, or the mineral zinc. Vitamin A cannot be absorbed without fat, so a diet very low in fat can cause a deficiency by preventing Vitamin A absorption. Protein deficiency can cause vitamin A deficiency by reducing vitamin A delivery to tissues. This is because retinol-binding protein and other proteins needed for the transport and metabolism of vitamin A cannot be made in sufficient quantities to adequately utilize vitamin A. The importance of zinc for vitamin A status is believed to be due to its role in protein synthesis. When zinc is deficient, proteins needed for vitamin A transport and metabolism are lacking.

Vitamin A deficiency is also a problem in developed countries. Here inadequate intakes of vitamin A are caused by poor food choices rather than the unavailability of good sources of vitamin A. Fresh fruits and vegetables, which are excellent sources of beta-carotene, are available to most people in developed countries, but vitamin A intake is below what is recommended. A common meal choice that is notoriously low in vitamin A is a fast-food meal of a hamburger and french fries. To increase the population's vitamin A intake, milk is fortified with vitamin A, and in the United States the vitamin A content of packaged foods must be listed on food labels.

HOW MUCH VITAMIN A DO WE NEED?

Retinol equivalents (RE)–A unit of measure for vitamin A, equal to the amount of any form of vitamin A that provides the function of 1 μg of retinol.

The recommended intake of vitamin A is expressed in **retinol equivalents (RE)**—the amount of any form of vitamin A that provides the function of 1 μg of retinol. For example, 6 μg of beta-carotene and 12 μg of other provitamin A carotenoids provide 1 RE. The recommended intake of vitamin A can be supplied by one carrot or a third of an ounce of beef liver (Table 9-1).

Although the RDA has been expressed in REs since 1980, many food tables and vitamin supplement labels still use the older measure of international units (IU). Ten IU of beta-carotene or 3.3 IU of preformed vitamin A is equal to 1 RE.

VITAMIN A TOXICITY

Acute or chronic overconsumption of preformed vitamin A can result in toxicity symptoms. Acute toxicity, whether from supplements or food sources, occurs with doses of 100 times the RDA and can result in coma and death. This has been reported in arctic explorers after consumption of polar bear liver, which contains about 100,000 RE of vitamin A in just 5 ounces. Though polar bear liver is not a common dish at most dinner tables, vitamin A supplements can be toxic. Signs of acute toxicity include nausea, vomiting, headache, dizziness, blurred vision, and lack of muscle coordination. Chronic toxicity occurs when preformed vitamin A doses as low as ten times the RDA are consumed for a period of months to years. The symptoms of chronic toxicity include weight loss, muscle and joint pain, liver damage, bone abnormalities, visual defects, dry scaling lips, and skin rashes.

 High dietary intakes of preformed vitamin A are known to cause birth defects in humans and animals. In a recent study it was found that women

TABLE 9-1	A Summary of the Fat Soluble Vitamins

Vitamin*	Sources	Recommended Intake for Adults		Major Functions	Deficiency	Groups at Risk	Toxicity
		RDA	RNI				
Vitamin A (vitamin A acetate, vitamin A palmitate, retinol, retinal, retinoic acid, retinyl palmitate, provitamin A, carotene, β-carotene, carotenoids)	Liver, carrots, peaches, leafy greens, fortified milk, sweet potatoes, broccoli	800–1000 RE	800–1000 RE	Vision, growth, cell differentiation, reproduction, immune function	Night blindness, xerophthalmia, poor growth, dry skin	Those who live in poverty (particularly children and pregnant women), those consuming very lowfat or low-protein diets	Headache, vomiting, hair loss, liver damage, skin changes, birth defects, bone pain
Vitamin D (cholecalciferol, ergocalciferol)	Egg yolk, liver, fish oils, tuna, salmon, fortified margarine and milk, sunlight	5 μg	2.5 μg	Absorption of calcium and phosphorus, maintenance of bone	Rickets in children, osteomalacia in adults	Breast-fed infants, children and elderly (especially with dark skin and little sun exposure), people with kidney disease	Calcium deposits in the soft tissues, growth retardation, kidney damage
Vitamin E (alpha-tocopherol acetate, alpha-tocopherol, mixed tocopherols)	Vegetable oils, leafy greens, nuts, peanuts	8–10 α-TE	6–9 α-TE	Antioxidant, protects cell membranes	Hemolyzed red blood cells, nerve damage	Those with poor fat absorption, premature infants	Inhibition of vitamin K activity
Vitamin K (phylloquinone, menaquinone)	Beef liver, leafy greens, intestinal bacteria	65–80 μg		Blood clotting	Hemorrhage	People on long-term antibiotics, newborns (especially premature)	Anemia, brain damage

*Additional names for a vitamin are given in parentheses.

who consumed more than 3000 RE, about four times the RDA, of preformed vitamin A as supplements were about five times more likely to have a baby with birth defects than women who consumed 1500 RE or less.[14] Since 3000 RE of vitamin A is easily obtained from supplements, it is recommended that if supplements are taken during pregnancy they contain only carotenoids, which have not been found to cause birth defects.

Unlike preformed vitamin A, carotenoids are nontoxic. This is because their absorption from the diet decreases at high doses, and once in the body, their conversion to active vitamin A is limited. High intakes do, however, lead to a condition known as **hypercarotenemia**. In this condition, the carotenoid levels become high enough to color body fat, including that just beneath the skin. This causes the skin to appear yellow. It can occur as a result of large daily intakes of carotenoids—usually in the form of carrot juice or beta-carotene supplements. It is not known to be dangerous, and when intake decreases, skin returns to its normal color.

Hypercarotenemia–A condition caused by an accumulation of carotenoids in the adipose tissue, causing the skin to appear yellow.

VITAMIN A SUPPLEMENTS: PROMISES AND PITFALLS

Vitamin A's role in vision and the maintenance of epithelial tissue has led to claims that supplements will improve vision and promote healthy skin. Although this is true in a vitamin A deficiency, the consumption of vitamin A above the recommended intake has not been shown to improve vision or make skin healthier. Vitamin A is being studied for the treatment of certain skin diseases and cancer. Beta-carotene supplements have been theorized to have a protective effect against cancer.

Retin-A and Accutane: The Anti-acne Drugs   The function of vitamin A in maintenance of epithelial tissue, particularly skin, has been employed medically as a treatment for acne. The drug called Retin-A is a derivative of vitamin A that is used topically to treat acne. It also tightens the skin and reduces wrinkles, effects that have led to its popularity with individuals who seek to reduce the wrinkles of aging. Retin-A, however, is not a fountain of youth. Continuous use does give the skin a tighter appearance, but it also makes the skin very sensitive to the sun, and users must contend with dry, peeling skin.[15]

Another derivative of vitamin A—isotretinoin, marketed as Accutane—is used orally to treat severe acne. The chemical modifications made to produce Accutane reduce its toxicity, so higher doses can be taken than would be possible with unmodified vitamin A. The user still walks a fine line between toxicity and therapy. Accutane causes some of the same symptoms seen with vitamin A toxicity, such as dryness of the mouth, eyes, and other mucous membranes; changes in liver function; and high blood lipid levels. Accutane is a drug that must be prescribed by a physician. Large doses of vitamin A from supplements are dangerous and should not be used as a self-cure for acne. Unmodified vitamin A will cause toxicity long before it cures acne. Even though Accutane is less toxic than unmodified vitamin A, it should not be used during pregnancy because it causes fetal malformations. Even Retin-A, which is applied topically, should not be used right before or during pregnancy.[15]

The Cancer Connection   Both preformed vitamin A and beta-carotene have been studied for their role in preventing or treating cancer. A number of the functions of preformed vitamin A suggest a cancer connection. First, vitamin A regulates cell differentiation, and the failure to differentiate is a basic feature of cancerous cells. Vitamin A's role in maintaining epithelial tissue may also be important, since most human cancers arise from rapidly dividing epithelial cells.[16] And vitamin A's importance in the immune system suggests that it could be beneficial in cancer prevention and possibly treatment. The role of beta-carotene is believed to be primarily preventive because of its antioxidant properties.

Preformed Vitamin A and Cancer   The use of different forms of preformed vitamin A called synthetic retinoids to treat cancer in animals has been encouraging, but the doses needed to stop cancer cells are usually toxic to normal cells as well.[17] More recent research has focused on the use of synthetic retinoids to prevent precancerous cells from becoming cancerous. These vitamin A drugs work by stimulating immature cells to mature normally rather than becoming out-of-control cancer cells. For example, they are able to reverse or prevent certain types of skin cancer and may prevent the recurrence of head and neck cancer.[15,18] These vitamin A derivatives are drugs and are not found in either food or over-the-counter supplements.

Beta-carotene and Cancer   Beta-carotene has been studied widely as a promising chemopreventive agent in reducing the risk of cancer in humans. Studies in which beta-carotene has been supplemented have been inconsistent. Beta-carotene has been shown to reduce the incidence of cancers of the oral cavity, head and neck, and colon;[9] however, a study of the effect of beta-carotene supplements on the incidence of lung cancer in smokers found that those taking the supplements had a higher incidence of lung cancer.[19] One reason supplements may not have the same effect as foods high in beta-carotene is that the protection offered by foods may be due to components other than beta-carotene. For example, broccoli, which is high in beta-carotene, also contains sulforaphane, which stimulates the production of enzymes that protect against cancer-causing molecules.[20]

VITAMIN D: THE SUNSHINE VITAMIN

There is a long-standing debate about whether vitamin D is a vitamin or a hormone. By definition, vitamins are substances that are essential in the diet. Vitamin D can be formed in the skin by exposure to sunlight, so when sunlight is available it is not a dietary essential and doesn't fit the definition of a vitamin. Further, vitamin D functions like a hormone because it is produced in one organ, the skin, and affects other organs, primarily the intestine and bone. However, when exposure to sunlight is limited, vitamin D becomes essential in the diet and, therefore, is considered a vitamin. As the human race became more civilized—began to wear clothes, live in cities, and generate smog, all of which block sunlight—dietary vitamin D became much more important.

VITAMIN D IN THE DIET

Only a few foods are naturally good sources of vitamin D. These include animal products such as liver, fatty fish, and egg yolks (Figure 9-4). These foods contain **cholecalciferol**, or vitamin D_3. Dietary vitamin D can also be obtained from foods such as milk and margarine that have been fortified with vitamin D. Fortified foods may contain vitamin D_3 or vitamin D_2, another active form of the vitamin. Cholecalciferol is the form of vitamin D that is made in the skin of animals by the action of sunlight on a form of cholesterol called 7-dehydrocholesterol.

Cholecalciferol—The chemical name for vitamin D_3. It can be formed in the skin of animals by the action of sunlight on a form of cholesterol called 7-dehydrocholesterol.

Food	Percent of RDA
Salmon, canned (3 oz)	105%
Tuna, canned in oil (3 oz)	
Butter (1 Tbsp)	
Milk, fortified (1 cup)	
Corn flakes, fortified (1 cup)	
Egg yolk (1 medium)	
Margarine, fortified (1 Tbsp)	
Hot dog (1)	
Mayonnaise (1 Tbsp)	
Whole wheat bread (1 slice)	
Orange (1 medium)	
Carrot (1 medium)	

Percent of RDA for Adult Men
(5 μg)

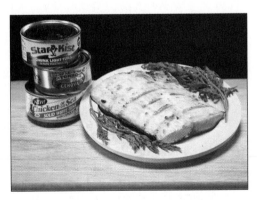

FIGURE 9-4
The vitamin D content of foods as a percent of the RDA for adult men. (Right, Charles D. Winters)

VITAMIN D IN THE BODY

Vitamin D from the diet and from synthesis in the skin is inactive until it has been chemically altered in the liver and then the kidney. In the liver, a hydroxyl group (—OH) is added to vitamin D to form 25-hydroxy vitamin D, which then travels to the kidney where another hydroxyl group is added to make the active form of vitamin D: 1,25-dihydroxy vitamin D (Figure 9-5). The activation of vitamin D by the kidney is regulated by **parathyroid hormone**.

The principal function of vitamin D is to maintain calcium levels within the normal range. Calcium is essential to the formation and maintenance of bone, as well as to other functions including the generation of nerve impulses, and the contraction of muscle. Activated vitamin D regulates calcium and phosphorus balance by acting at the bone and intestine. At the intestine, vitamin D increases calcium and phosphorus absorption. At the bone, it enhances the release of calcium and phosphorus when blood calcium levels are low. Vitamin D aids bone

Parathyroid hormone—A hormone produced by the parathyroid gland that stimulates the release of calcium from bone to help maintain blood calcium levels.

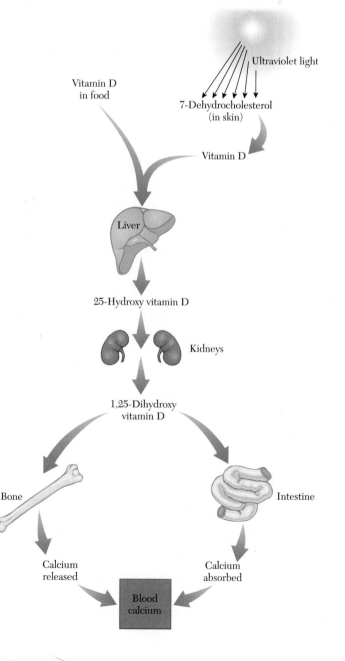

FIGURE 9-5
Vitamin D comes from food and from a chemical reaction in the skin. In order to function, it must have hydroxyl groups (—OH) added at the liver and kidney. Active vitamin D then functions in maintaining calcium balance by stimulating the release of calcium from bone and the absorption of calcium from the intestine.

mineralization by keeping blood levels of calcium and phosphorus in a range that allows bone formation.[21] If calcium levels in the blood drop too low, parathyroid hormone stimulates the kidney to activate vitamin D. The increase in active vitamin D increases the amount of calcium absorbed by the intestine, and acts with parathyroid hormone to release calcium from bones (see Chapter 10). In addition to bone and intestine, a number of other tissues in the body, such as kidney, pancreas, pituitary, breast, placenta, and skin, have been found to contain receptors for active vitamin D. The effect of vitamin D in these tissues is under investigation.

VITAMIN D DEFICIENCY

When vitamin D is deficient, dietary calcium cannot be absorbed in sufficient amounts to maintain bone structure. In children who are deficient in vitamin D, there is not enough calcium and phosphorus deposited in the bones, and as a result, the bones are weak. This syndrome, called **rickets**, is characterized by bowed legs, narrow rib cages known as pigeon breasts, and other deformities (Figure 9-6). Rickets was common in 17th- to 19th-century Europe. The incidence increased during the Industrial Revolution when large numbers of poorly nourished children lived under a layer of smog in the newly industrialized cities. Even though the fortification of milk with vitamin D has helped to greatly reduce rickets in most developed countries, it is still a problem in inner-city children who have a poor diet and whose exposure to sunlight is limited by tall buildings and smog. Dark-skinned children are more likely to be vitamin D deficient because the pigment in their skin blocks the sun, thereby reducing the formation of vitamin D in the skin. Rickets is also seen in children with disorders that affect fat absorption and in vegetarian children who do not drink milk.

In adults, the vitamin D deficiency disease comparable to rickets is called **osteomalacia**. It results in the weakening of bones because excessive calcium is released from the bone to maintain normal blood levels. This leads to fractures of the weight-bearing bones such as those in the hips and spine. It is common in adults with diseases, such as kidney disease, that affect vitamin D metabolism. Although sunscreens prevent the formation of vitamin D in the skin, children and active adults usually spend enough time outdoors without sunscreens to provide for their vitamin D requirement. The elderly are at risk for vitamin D deficiency because they typically spend less time in the sun than their younger counterparts and their ability to produce vitamin D in the skin is decreased.[22] Bones may also become weakened and fracture easily because of a condition called osteoporosis, which is discussed in Chapter 10.

Rickets–A vitamin D deficiency disease in children that is characterized by poor bone development because of inadequate calcium deposition.

Osteomalacia–A vitamin D deficiency disease in adults that causes weak bones and an increase in bone fractures.

HOW MUCH VITAMIN D DO WE NEED?

An exact adult requirement for vitamin D has never been established because vitamin D is a dietary essential only when exposure to sunlight is limited. Dietary requirements are affected by skin color, climate and season, clothing, the application of sunblocking skin creams, and the presence of pollution and tall buildings that block sunlight.

The RDA for vitamin D is expressed as micrograms (μg) or International Units (IU). One IU is equal to 0.024 μg of vitamin D_3. The recommended intake of vitamin D for adults can be obtained by drinking about 2 cups of vitamin D–fortified milk (see Table 9-1).

Since vitamin D is especially important in bone development, the requirement is highest during periods of rapid growth. Thus, infants and children require a greater amount of vitamin D per unit of body weight than do adults. The RDA for pregnancy and lactation is increased to ensure adequate calcium absorption.

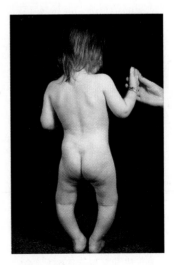

FIGURE 9-6
Bowed legs are characteristic of rickets. (Biophoto Associates/Photo Researchers, Inc.)

VITAMIN D TOXICITY AND SUPPLEMENTS

Vitamin D is the most toxic of all the vitamins. Toxicity has been reported with doses of only four to five times the RDA. Toxicity does not occur from dietary sources or exposure to sunlight because the amounts found naturally in the diet are too small to be toxic and the formation of vitamin D by the action of sunlight is carefully regulated. Toxic amounts of vitamin D can be ingested from supplements. Toxicity is more likely to occur in young children. It was reported in individuals who consumed milk that was erroneously fortified with 580 times the amount normally added per quart of milk (400 IU per quart).[23] Symptoms include high blood and urine calcium, deposition of calcium in soft tissues such as the blood vessels, and kidney and cardiovascular damage.

No specific claims have been made about vitamin D supplements. Because of the potential for toxicity, supplements containing more than 100% of the RDI or 10 μg of vitamin D_3 per dose are not recommended.

VITAMIN E: FROM FERTILITY AID TO ANTI-AGING

Vitamin E was first identified as a fat soluble component of grains that was necessary for fertility in laboratory rats. It then took almost 30 years to identify and isolate this vitamin and to determine that it is also necessary for reproduction in humans. The chemical name for vitamin E, **tocopherol**, is from the Greek *tos*, meaning childbirth, and *phero*, to bring forth. Today, vitamin E is promoted as a cure for infertility, an anti-scar medication, a defense against air pollution, and a fountain of youth.

Tocopherol–The chemical name for vitamin E.

VITAMIN E IN THE DIET

Alpha-tocopherol (α-tocopherol)– The form of tocopherol that is most common and has the greatest biological activity.

There are several forms of vitamin E. The most common one is **alpha-tocopherol (α-tocopherol)**, which provides more than twice the amount of vitamin E activity of other tocopherols. Dietary sources of vitamin E include nuts and peanuts; plant oils, such as soybean, corn, and sunflower oils; leafy green vegetables; and wheat germ and fortified breakfast cereals (Figure 9-7). Since vitamin E is sensitive to

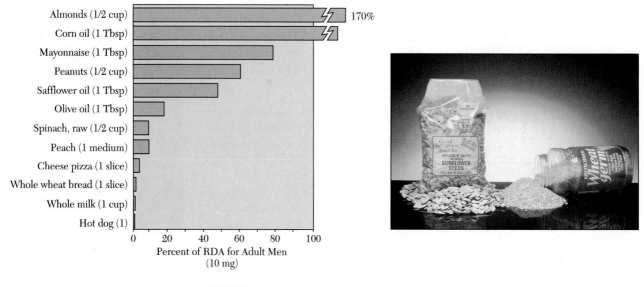

FIGURE 9-7
The vitamin E content of foods as a percent of the RDA for adult men. (Right, Charles D. Winters)

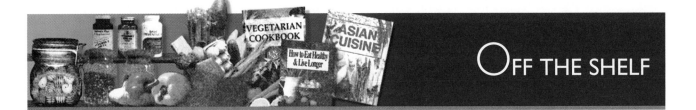

They Aren't Vitamins But . . .

The labels of vitamin supplements often list substances that do not fit the definition of a vitamin. Some of them, such as lipoic acid, carnitine, and ubiquinone, are important in energy metabolism. Others, such as choline, inositol, and PABA, are a part of larger molecules that are important in cellular activities. What are these substances and why are they included in vitamin supplements?

Lipoic acid is a coenzyme in the same reactions that require the active coenzyme form of thiamine, the conversion of pyruvate, the 3-carbon product of glycolysis, into acetyl-CoA and a reaction of the citric acid cycle. Although essential to energy production, lipoic acid can be synthesized in adequate amounts by human cells.

Carnitine is important for the utilization of fat for energy because it is needed to move fatty acids and the breakdown products of some amino acids into the mitochondria of cells, where they can be used for energy. Carnitine is made in the body from the amino acids lysine and methionine in a reaction that requires vitamin B_6. Dietary sources of carnitine include meat and dairy products. Although vegetarian diets are low in carnitine, vegetarians have normal blood levels of carnitine, suggesting that synthesis is adequate to meet needs. Dietary carnitine may be necessary under certain conditions such as rapid growth, pregnancy, lactation, or medical conditions that increase its requirement or decrease synthesis.[1]

Ubiquinone, or coenzyme Q, is important for the production of energy from carbohydrate, fat, and protein because it is one of the electron carriers in the electron transport chain. As its name implies, it is present ubiquitously, in animals, plants, and microorganisms, and is made in

the human body. Supplements have been reported to improve reproductive performance in rats fed a diet deficient in vitamin E, but there is no evidence that it is needed in the diet of healthy humans.

Choline is required to make several phospholipids that are essential components of cell membranes. It is also required to make the neurotransmitter acetylcholine, and it is an important source of carbons for biochemical reactions. Although it can be synthesized by humans and is not currently classified as essential, there is a great deal of evidence that suggests that it is an essential nutrient.[2,3] It is required by human cells grown in culture, and humans given TPN without choline or fed a choline-deficient diet show signs of liver dysfunction.[4] Prolonged deficiency in animals leads to fat accumulation in the liver and may contribute to liver cancer. Choline is also a dietary essential in a number of animal species including the dog, cat, and rat. Choline deficiency in humans is unlikely because it is widely distributed in foods. Particularly good sources include egg yolks, organ meats, spinach, nuts, and wheat germ. Average daily choline intake is estimated to be about 600 to 1000 mg per day.

Inositol, like choline, is a component of phospholipids in cell membranes where it plays a role in relaying messages to the inside of the cell. It is found in the diet in both plant and animal foods. In plants, it is part of phytic acid, which, when consumed in the diet, binds calcium and iron, interfering with their absorption. Inositol can be synthesized from glucose and has not been shown to be essential in the human diet, but it may have some clinical value in treating diseases such as diabetes and kidney failure.[5]

Para-aminobenzoic acid (PABA) is a part of the folic acid molecule but has no vitamin activity on its own and cannot be used by humans to make folate. It is, however, used in topical sunblock products to protect the skin from damage due to ultraviolet radiation. There is no evidence that oral PABA offers protection from the sun or anything else, and in large doses it may cause liver damage.

Lipoic acid, carnitine, ubiquinone, choline, inositol, and PABA are not currently considered dietary essentials. Manufacturers may include them in supplements because they serve vitamin-like roles in the body. Although unnecessary, in moderate doses they are unlikely to be harmful. There are also other substances sold as nutritional supplements. Some are natural sources of vitamins. For instance, evening primrose oil, a plant source of vitamin C, is marketed as a cure for hot flashes and PMS. For others, like pangamic acid, also called vitamin B_{15}, which is sold to enhance exercise performance, the actual compound has not even been defined.

[1] Broquist, H.P. Carnitine. In *Modern Nutrition in Health and Disease*, 8th ed. Shils, M.E., Olson, J.A., and Shike, M., eds. Philadelphia: Lea & Febiger, 1994, pp. 459–465.

[2] Zeisel, S.H., Da Costa, K.A., Franklin, P.D., et al. Choline, an essential nutrient for humans. FASEB J. 5:2093–2098, 1991.

[3] Canty, D.J. and Zeisel, S.H. Lecithin and choline in human health and disease. Nutr. Rev. 52:327–339, 1994.

[4] Zeisel, S.H. Choline. In *Modern Nutrition in Health and Disease*, 8th ed. Shils, M.E., Olson, J.A. and Shike, M., eds. Philadelphia: Lea & Febiger, 1994, pp. 449–458.

[5] Aukema, H.M. and Holub, B.J. Inositol and pyrroloquinoline quinone. In *Modern Nutrition in Health and Disease*, 8th ed. Shils, M.E., Olson, J.A. and Shike, M., eds. Philadelphia: Lea & Febiger, 1994, pp. 449–458.

inhibits their blood from clotting, and they bleed to death from minor cuts and scratches. Within a few years of its discovery, dicumarol was widely used to treat heart attack victims and others at risk for blood clots. Further work with this anticoagulant led Link to propose the use of a more potent derivative, called warfarin, as rat poison. When rats consume the odorless, colorless warfarin, their blood fails to clot, and they bleed to death. Warfarin is now also used as a blood thinner in humans.

HOW MUCH VITAMIN K DO WE NEED?

The RDA for vitamin K is set at about 1 μg per kilogram of body weight per day (see Table 9-1). Typical intakes in North America are well above this.[32] Additional vitamin K is provided by bacteria in the gastrointestinal tract. Although the form of vitamin K produced by intestinal bacteria is less well absorbed than that from plant sources, it does contribute to needs.

VITAMIN K TOXICITY AND SUPPLEMENTS

Vitamin K toxicity occurs only as a result of supplement overuse. Excessive doses result in the clotting and breaking of blood cells. This causes anemia and releases the yellow pigment bilirubin into the circulation, which can cause brain damage at high levels. The treatment for vitamin K toxicity is to give dicumarol, which interferes with vitamin K activity and prevents blood from clotting. Supplements are typically administered before surgery to aid in blood clotting.

MEETING YOUR VITAMIN NEEDS

The prospect of designing your diet to meet your need for all of the vitamins can be overwhelming. It may seem easier to just take a supplement and not be concerned with diet. However, consuming a balanced diet from a variety of foods can meet all vitamin needs in most individuals. In addition, such a diet is likely to provide health-promoting substances for which recommendations have not been made, reduce the risk of consuming a toxic amount of any one vitamin, and provide the sensory pleasures that accompany a well-prepared meal.

PHYTOCHEMICALS

Phytochemicals—Chemicals found in plants that are not essential nutrients for humans but may be important for preventing chronic diseases, particularly cancer.

In addition to the nutrients discussed here and in other chapters of this text, foods contain many physiologically relevant molecules that are not currently considered essential in the diet of healthy adults, but that may play a role in human health. One group of substances is called **phytochemicals**. "Phyto" is derived from the Greek word for plant, so this term refers to the hundreds, perhaps thousands, of chemicals found in plants. In plants they serve as protection from sunlight and as a defense against predators. They are not essential nutrients for humans, so deficiencies will not occur if they are eliminated from the diet. But scientists are finding that phytochemicals may be important for preventing chronic diseases, particularly cancer.

Although no long-term study to date can say that any particular phytochemical retards or prevents cancer in humans, there are hundreds of studies linking diets rich in fruits and vegetables with a lower incidence of human cancers. This reduced disease incidence cannot be reproduced by providing supplements of the essential nutrients in these foods. This may be because the nonessential phytochemicals are also important in disease prevention. Many of the health-promoting properties that have long been recognized for particular foods are now being attributed to

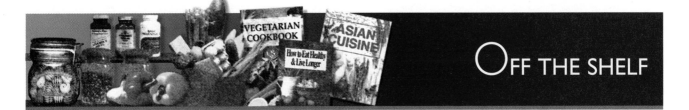

OFF THE SHELF

Should You Choose Fresh, Frozen or Canned?

To optimize the nutrient content of your diet, grow vegetables yourself and pick them as you need them or choose produce that is in season locally and use it the same day you buy it. Although ideal, these options are not always realistic or even possible. Not everyone has the time, location, or desire for a vegetable garden. Transportation and time considerations may limit trips to the store, storage at home may be limited, and cost is always a factor.

When selecting among fresh, frozen, or canned foods, it is important to weigh the nutrient content of the food and its contribution to the total diet against convenience and availability. For example, fresh-picked vegetables provide more nutrients than frozen or canned vegetables. However, if the "fresh vegetable" has actually been a week in transport and another week in your refrigerator, frozen vegetables may actually supply more vitamins to your diet. Manufacturers of frozen vegetables often freeze their produce right in the fields where it is grown, thereby maintaining most of the nutrients. Vitamin losses are generally higher when produce is canned than when other methods of preserving fruits and vegetables are used, because the high temperatures involved in canning destroy many of the water soluble vitamins. However, since canned foods keep for a long time, don't require refrigeration, and are often less expensive than fresh or frozen, they provide an available, affordable source of nutrients that may be the best choice in some situations.

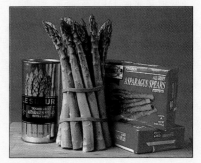

(Dennis Drenner)

---

phytochemicals. Garlic, for example, has been used medicinally for centuries, but more recent work has pointed to the role of its phytochemicals in protecting against cancer and heart disease. The phytochemicals in soy products are also hypothesized to protect against heart disease and cancer.[33,34] Green tea has recently been in the news for its anticancer properties, and similar compounds in red wine are believed to contribute to its protective effect against heart disease.[35] A number of phytochemicals have been promoted in supplements. For example, bioflavonoids, rutin, hesperidin, and vitamin P are marketed as cures for arthritis, heart disease, high blood pressure, and colds. Although these marketing promises are exaggerated, our emerging understanding of the phytochemicals indicates that they may have a significant impact on human health. Researchers are beginning to identify and isolate them and determine how they function.

Some phytochemicals may protect against disease because they are antioxidants,[36] but many are anticarcinogens due to their ability to inhibit the metabolic activation of carcinogens, stimulate enzymes that help eliminate carcinogens, or act at some other stage of cancer development. The phytochemicals in green tea increase the activity of antioxidant enzymes and enzymes that help eliminate carcinogens. Sulforaphane, found in broccoli, cauliflower, brussel sprouts, turnips, and kale, boosts the synthesis of anticancer enzymes and has now been shown to protect animals from breast cancer.[37] P-coumaric acid and chlorogenic acid, found in tomatoes, green peppers, pineapples, strawberries, and carrots, prevent the formation of cancer-causing nitrosamines in the digestive tract.[38] Phenethyl isothiocyanate stops the formation of carcinogens by blocking enzymes that transform harmless chemicals into carcinogens that bind DNA. Ellagic acid found in strawberries, grapes, and raspberries neutralizes carcinogens before they can bind to

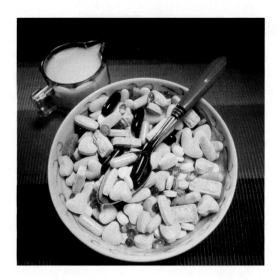

FIGURE 9-12
Vitamin supplements cannot take the place of a balanced diet. (Charles D. Winters)

DNA. Onions and garlic contain substances that stimulates enzymes that detoxify carcinogens. Capsaicin in hot peppers prevents carcinogens from binding to DNA. Flavonoids, found in almost all fruits and vegetables, prevent cancer-causing substances from binding to cells. Genistein in soybeans inhibits the growth of cancer cells.[39] In addition to the phytochemicals that have been identified, many remain to be discovered. Although the biological importance of these substances for humans has not been fully defined, current evidence suggests that consuming a diet high in plant foods is beneficial.

MEETING YOUR NEEDS WITH FOOD

Nutritionists have been saying it for years and mothers for even longer—eat your vegetables. Having a multivitamin pill with your donut and coffee doesn't make it a healthy breakfast. You can't cover up a poor diet with a pill (Figure 9-12). Food provides nutrients in infinite combinations and with unlimited variety. It can provide all the things in a pill and in addition contains factors that affect absorption, protect against spoilage, influence nutrient utilization, and protect you from disease. The benefits of these substances can be obtained by consuming a diet that provides at least 5 servings of fruits and vegetables daily as recommended by the Food Guide Pyramid.[2] Despite the strong incentive to consume a diet high in fruits and vegetables, studies estimate that 11% of the population still does not consume fruits or vegetables on a daily basis[2] (Figure 9-13).

Choosing a Nutrient-Dense Diet   The first step toward consuming a diet that meets all of your needs is to select foods with high nutrient density. Nutrient-dense foods are high in essential nutrients relative to the energy they contain. For instance, you can get 50% of your RDA for thiamin and niacin from a Big Mac or from a turkey sandwich. The Big Mac contains over 500 kcalories, whereas the turkey sandwich contains about 300 kcalories. Choosing the turkey sandwich, which is more nutrient dense, allows you to eat more of other foods, which contain other nutrients, without exceeding your energy requirements. Using the serving recommendations and the selection tips in the Food Guide Pyramid can help obtain adequate nutrients from food without exceeding energy needs (Figure 9-14). Such a diet will also include plenty of grains, vegetables, and fruits rich in phytochemicals. Since vitamin losses can occur through processing, storage, and

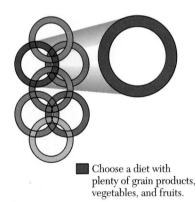

■ Choose a diet with plenty of grain products, vegetables, and fruits.

FIGURE 9-13
The *Dietary Guidelines for Americans* recommend choosing a diet with plenty of grain products, vegetables, and fruits. A diet that follows this recommendation will be rich in vitamins and phytochemicals. (USDA, DHHS, 1995)

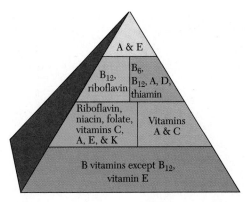

FIGURE 9-14
A diet that follows the recommendations of the Food Guide Pyramid provides many sources of vitamins.

cooking, the vitamin-conscious consumer must also consider these factors when purchasing and preparing food.

Minimizing Vitamin Losses   Proponents of vitamin supplements argue that modern agricultural methods produce vitamin-deficient crops; transportation, storage, refining, and processing further deplete vitamin content; and cooking practices destroy what is left. Some of this is true. Vitamin losses occur because of the passage of time; exposure to oxygen, light, or heat; changes in acidity (pH); and the physical separation of the vitamins from the food (Table 9-2). Such losses,

TABLE 9-2	Vitamin Losses in Handling
Vitamin	**Causes of Loss**
Vitamin A and beta-carotene	Losses occur with exposure to air, light, and acid. Fairly stable in cooking.
Vitamin D	Some losses occur with exposure to air, light, heat, and low-acid conditions. Stable in cooking.
Vitamin E	Losses occur in high-temperature frying and with exposure to light, air, and freezing.
Vitamin K	Losses occur with exposure to light and low- or high-acid conditions.
Vitamin C	Losses occur with exposure to light and heat and contact with iron or copper cooking utensils. More stable in the presence of acid than in neutral or low-acid conditions, so citrus fruits maintain their vitamin C content longer than other sources. One of the most easily destroyed vitamins.
Thiamin	Losses occur with exposure to heat and air and neutral- or low-acid conditions.
Riboflavin	Most losses occur as a result of exposure to light, especially in moist and low-acid environments. Also destroyed by heat. When it is dry or in a high-acid food, it is more stable.
Niacin	Stable.
Vitamin B_6	Losses occur with exposure to heat and light.
Vitamin B_{12}	Losses occur with exposure to air, light, and vitamin C.
Folate	Losses occur with exposure to heat, air, light, and acid conditions.
Biotin	Losses occur with exposure to heat.
Pantothenic acid	Losses occur with exposure to heat and low- or high-acid conditions.

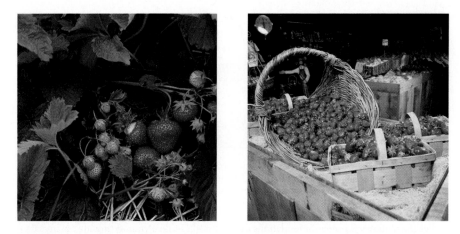

FIGURE 9-15
By the time fresh produce arrives in our kitchen, it may have lost a significant proportion of the vitamins that it contained in the field. (Left, Thomas Hovland/Grant Heilman Photography, Inc. Right, Charles D. Winters)

however, do not necessarily result in a vitamin-deficient food supply. Careful choices and proper preparation and storage techniques can significantly enhance the nutrient content of the foods in your diet.

Food on the Move   The soil in which plants are grown can affect their mineral content, but the vitamin content of foods depends on the type of food, not the growing location. Packaging and transportation conditions can seriously affect the vitamin content of food. Since riboflavin is destroyed by light, milk should be packaged in opaque containers. Folate and vitamin C are destroyed by heat and exposure to oxygen, so losses are minimized at low temperatures and by packaging that excludes oxygen. Foods that spend a long time in transit also lose nutrients. The longer it takes food to move from the field to your plate, the more nutrients may be lost. So, for example, strawberries grown in California, loaded on a truck and driven to New Jersey, displayed in a grocery store for a few days, and then held for a few more days at home provide less vitamin C than strawberries picked fresh and eaten that evening for dessert (Figure 9-15).

Despite some losses in transit, the year-round variety of food that is available because of shipping is a dietary plus that was not enjoyed by our ancestors and is not available to many people in developing nations. To minimize further losses, try to use fresh produce as soon as possible. Another day in your refrigerator means more losses.

The Effect of Food Processing   Refining and processing can affect nutrient content. The story of the discovery of thiamin is an excellent example of the impact of refining on nutrient content. Whole grain brown rice is a good source of thiamin. However, when the outer layers are removed and the rice is polished to a pearly white color, the part of the kernel containing thiamin is discarded, and therefore, thiamin is lost. Other processing procedures such as cutting, chopping, blending, and heating also cause nutrient losses. When foods are cut and chopped into smaller pieces, more surfaces are exposed to oxygen and light, increasing losses. When food is heated, as in canning, heat-sensitive vitamins are destroyed. Therefore, the more a food is handled, the more nutrients are lost. Keep this in mind when choosing between a whole cantaloupe and one that has been cut and packaged for sale. The whole fruit has less exposure to light and oxygen and, therefore, contains more of its original nutrients.

Processing can also add to foods. These additions may affect the nutrient content of a food in a positive or a negative way. Processing can add back nutrients that were lost in refining, as with the enrichment of flour to replace iron and some of the B vitamins. Or it can add nutrients that were never present in the food to begin with, as with the vitamin A fortification of margarine. Food additives may preserve quality and prevent the loss of some nutrients. However, some additives, like salt and sugar that are used as preservatives and flavor enhancers, add nutrients that are already in excess in the typical American diet. For instance, unflavored oatmeal is a high-carbohydrate food low in simple sugars. But when you buy instant oatmeal flavored with maple and brown sugar, you are getting a product that is high in added simple sugars.

To minimize processing and refining losses, choose brown rice and whole grain cereals and breads. If these are not available, enriched and fortified foods provide more nutrients than unenriched refined ones.

Storage: Save It Right   Nutrient losses over time cannot be avoided, but proper storage and preservation techniques at home can minimize them. Treatment of food at home is as important as proper selection at the store. Keep freezer temperatures at 0°F or below to minimize losses. Even at low temperatures, the longer frozen foods are stored, the greater their losses. It is recommended that frozen foods be used within a month or two. Even canned foods continue to lose vitamins on the shelf, especially at high temperatures. Try to store cans at about 65°F to minimize losses. Fresh vegetables like kale, spinach, broccoli, chard, and salad greens keep their nutrients best when stored at low temperatures and high humidity. They should, therefore, be refrigerated in a crisper or a moisture-proof bag. Leave peas in the pod until you are ready to use them. Store roots and tubers such as sweet potatoes, potatoes, and carrots in a place that is cool and moist enough to prevent withering. When tomatoes are picked green, they should be ripened away from the sun at about 60 to 75°F. More nutrients are lost when they are placed in the refrigerator or on a hot, sunny windowsill. Keep milk and bread away from strong light to protect riboflavin, and wrap and refrigerate all cut-up foods.

Avoiding Cooking Losses   Cooking can account for major vitamin losses from our food. However, unlike losses in production and transportation, cooking losses can be controlled by the consumer. Do not soak vegetables or wash rice before cooking, because water soluble B vitamins and vitamin C will go down the drain. Do not cut up or cook vegetables until the last minute. Moreover, the smaller the pieces into which vegetables are cut before cooking, the greater the losses. The best cooking method depends on the food. Since longer cooking times increase vitamin losses, cabbage and beans that require longer cooking times may retain more vitamins when cooked in a pressure cooker than when steamed. Foods that need short cooking times like spinach lose less when steamed.[40] Stir-frying and steaming broccoli are equivalent in terms of vitamin C losses. In general, to minimize the nutrients lost in cooking, steam vegetables and cook them minimally so they remain slightly crisp. Potatoes lose fewer nutrients when cooked whole in their skins. Frozen vegetables should not be thawed or washed first, and baking soda should not be added to the cooking water. Meats retain more vitamins if broiled or roasted than if braised or stewed. The nutrients lost from braised or stewed meat can be reclaimed by consuming the broth. Cooking water from vegetables can also be reused to make soups and sauces. Microwave cooking is another option. Microwave cooking times are shorter and minimal water is used, both of which help preserve nutrients. For this reason, vitamin retention in microwaved vegetables is often higher than in conventionally cooked vegetables. For example, vitamin C, which is very unstable, is 50 to 100% retained in microwave cooking compared with 40 to 60% in conventional cooking. Only 77% of the folate in spinach is retained during conventional cooking, but 100% is retained when spinach is cooked in a microwave.[41] In meats, microwaving causes a greater loss of thiamin, but riboflavin and niacin losses are comparable to those that occur with

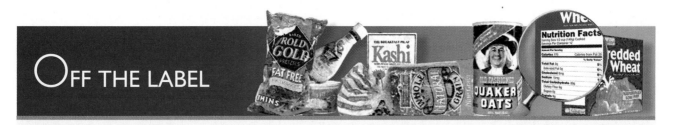

OFF THE LABEL

Supplement Labels

Are supplements foods or are they drugs? Health food and supplement industries believe their products are unique and should be regulated under different rules than either foods or drugs. The public wants supplements to be readily available and relatively affordable, and the FDA wants to make sure they don't represent a health hazard. The Dietary Supplement Health and Education Act of 1994 provides a compromise between the desires of the manufacturers, the demands of the public, and the safety concerns of the FDA. This act defines supplements and establishes regulations for labeling and advertising.[1]

According to this act, a dietary supplement is defined as a product added to the diet that contains one or more of the following ingredients: a vitamin; a mineral; an herb or other botanical; an amino acid; another dietary substance used to supplement the diet; or a metabolite, constituent, extract, or combination of any ingredient described above. Dietary supplements are considered foods, and as such do not need to be approved by the FDA unless they contain a dietary ingredient that was not marketed in the United States before October 15, 1994. Before a drug can be marketed, the FDA requires that the manufacturer prove its safety and effectiveness for the prescribed use. The marketing of food, however, requires no such testing. The fact that supplements are categorized as foods, not drugs, makes it difficult for the FDA to challenge products of concern. Challenging a product is made more difficult by the fact that the burden of proving a product unsafe is on the FDA, not the manufacturer.

The Dietary Supplement Health and Education Act also regulates health claims on supplement labels. Food labels are permitted to mention only eight specific FDA-approved claims about the relationship between a nutrient or a food and the risk of a specific disease or health-related condition (see Chapter 2). In addition to the claims approved for food labels, supplement manufacturers are allowed to make claims that address classic nutrient-deficiency diseases however, such a claim must be followed by: "This statement has not been evaluated by the Food and Drug Administration. This product is not intended to diagnose, treat, cure, or prevent any disease." Although this new regulation limits the claims manufacturers can use on labels, products may still be promoted by using information in the form of articles, book chapters, and scientific abstracts that are displayed separately from the products. This information must not be false or misleading or promote a particular brand of supplement, and must be presented in a balanced fashion.

The Dietary Supplement Health and Education Act also specifies new regulations for dietary supplement labels that will be enforced beginning in 1997. Labels must list the name and quantity of each ingredient per serving and the source of the ingredient. Ingredients present in a significant amount, and for which there is a Daily Value, must be listed first. Those not present in significant amounts need not be listed. Although supplements are required to list all ingredients on the label, consumers may not get 100% of what is listed on the

label. There are two reasons for this. First, because the manufacturing of supplements is not standardized, the exact contents of each tablet may vary. Secondly, the dissolvability of the tablet is not regulated. If the pills don't dissolve, the nutrients may not be absorbed. For example, if it takes a multivitamin and mineral supplement 3 hours to dissolve, only a small percentage of the nutrients may be in solution and therefore available for absorption when they reach the small intestine. In response to concerns about supplement safety and nutritional value, the Pharmacopoeial (USP) Convention, which sets the standards for drugs, is setting standards for supplements. These standards will not be mandatory, but many companies will adopt them. Such standards would protect the consumer from the inconsistencies in supplement composition but would also increase the cost of nutritional supplements.

The debate over whether nutritional supplements should be bound by pharmaceutical standards is ongoing. Opponents argue that in many cases such inconsistencies in nutritional supplements are of little consequence. However, proponents argue that the lack of standards could have serious nutritional consequences. Consumers may want a product that meets USP standards, but if it means a more expensive pill, the power of the purse may win out over concern for a more uniform product.

[1] Anonymous. Dietary supplements: recent chronology and legislation. Nutr. Rev. 53:31–36, 1995.

TABLE 9-3	Storage and Preparation to Reduce Vitamin Losses from Foods

Eat foods as soon as possible after harvesting or purchasing.

Refrigerate fresh produce and wrap tightly to retain moisture and decrease exposure to air.

For longer storage, freezing is best. Blanch first to retain flavor and stop enzymes that destroy vitamins.

Wait as long as possible before cutting up food for a meal. The smaller the pieces that food is cut into, the greater the nutrient losses due to exposure to light and oxygen.

The higher the temperature and the longer heat is applied, the greater the losses. Use as low a temperature for as short a time as possible, but you must cook hot enough and long enough to ensure the safety of what you are preparing. Microwaving uses shorter cooking times, so may in some cases result in greater nutrient retention.

Water soluble nutrients are lost in water, so avoid soaking, and cook vegetables in their skins.

Cook frozen vegetables without thawing.

Do not add baking soda to vegetable cooking water.

Use cooking techniques that don't bring food into direct contact with water, such as steaming and pressure cooking, or dry heat, such as roasting, grilling, stir-frying, or baking.

cooking in a conventional oven. In general, the differences in vitamin losses between microwaved and conventionally cooked meats are small.

Some storage and preparation suggestions for reducing vitamin losses are listed in Table 9-3.

USING SUPPLEMENTS WISELY

It is estimated that 70% of adults in the United States take vitamin and mineral supplements.[1] In general, these supplements are not taken by people at risk for deficiency. Studies indicate that people who take supplements tend to eat more fruits and vegetables and have higher intakes of nutrients from foods than people who don't use supplements.[1] Supplement use is usually related more closely to personal perceptions of health and well-being and food beliefs than it is to nutritional needs. People take supplements to energize themselves, to protect themselves from disease, to cure their illnesses, to replace what they don't get in food, or simply to ensure against deficiencies. Some people feel that today's eating patterns widen the gap between intake and needs or that the RDAs underestimate what is needed to maintain health. Supplements provide insurance against deficiency. Whether we actually need this insurance is still open to debate (Figure 9-16).

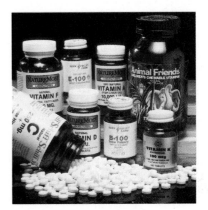

FIGURE 9-16
The variety of nutritional supplements seems limitless. (Charles D. Winters)

Do Modern Lifestyles Increase Need or Decrease Intake?   Modern lifestyles that include fast-food meals, eat-and-run and eat-on-the-run eating habits, and the stress of modern society are often cited as reasons to take vitamin supplements. Although the eating habits of Americans are not always good, they don't necessarily breed vitamin deficiencies. For example, eating on the run may not be relaxing, but it doesn't decrease the vitamin content of the foods consumed. Fast food is not necessarily lacking in vitamins but it is usually high in energy, fat, and salt. As for stress, we all live with it, but unless it is stress associated with physical trauma, it is unlikely to significantly alter your nutrient needs. Even if our needs are slightly increased and meals are occasionally skipped, a carefully planned diet including healthy snacks and a greater variety of foods at other meals can meet nutrient needs.

Do the Recommended Intakes Underestimate Our Vitamin Needs?   The current RDAs are designed to prevent deficiency diseases rather than to optimize health and protect against chronic disease. As our understanding of the roles of certain nutrients in preventing chronic disease and maximizing immune function has grown so has the attitude that the recommendations of the RDAs should be expanded to consider not only the amounts of nutrients needed to prevent deficiencies but also the amounts needed to optimize biological performance and reduce chronic disease risk.[42] However, even if the RDAs considered disease prevention they are still designed as general guidelines for a healthy population, not as requirements for individuals. Individual needs may vary depending on genetics, lifestyle, and health considerations; some individuals require more of some nutrients, whereas others require less.

Who Needs Vitamin Supplements?   Even though it is recommended that people obtain their vitamins from food rather than supplements, there are groups of individuals who cannot or do not meet their nutrient needs with the foods they consume and therefore need vitamin supplements. Groups who typically need vitamin supplements include dieters, vegans, chronic drug and alcohol users, people with chronic disorders, people at certain stages of life, and individuals in the general population who do not eat an adequate diet for various reasons.

Dieters   Individuals following weight-loss diets are restricting their intake of energy and consequently reducing their intake of micronutrients. It is difficult to meet the recommended intakes for vitamins and minerals if energy intake is less than 1200 kcalories per day, no matter how well planned the diet is. Therefore, it is important to supplement your diet if you are restricting kcalories below that level.

Vegans   Although vegetarian diets are generally high in micronutrients, a vegan diet, which excludes all animal products, will be deficient in vitamin B_{12}. Vitamin B_{12} is found almost exclusively in animal products. Vegans need to obtain vitamin B_{12} from fortified foods or from supplements. Another vitamin that may need to be supplemented in the vegan diet is vitamin D, which is obtained primarily from milk or synthesized in the skin when exposed to sunlight. In areas with little sunlight, vegans may not synthesize enough vitamin D to meet their needs.

Drug and Alcohol Users   The use of certain drugs and alcohol affects vitamin requirements. Heavy cigarette smokers, for instance, require more vitamin C to maintain the blood levels of vitamin C found in nonsmokers. The extra vitamin C may be needed to protect lung cells from cigarette smoke.[43] Heavy drinkers have a higher requirement for thiamin, niacin, vitamin B_6, and folate because alcohol inhibits their absorption and may affect their metabolism. Consumers of certain prescription drugs may also need additional vitamins. Antibiotics interfere with the production of vitamin K in the intestine, and anticonvulsant medication can cause vitamin D deficiency. Individuals who routinely take medications should discuss nutrient-drug interactions with their doctor or pharmacist (see Chapter 15).

Nutritionally Vulnerable Populations   Individuals with diseases that increase nutrient needs or decrease the body's ability to absorb or utilize vitamins require supplements. For example, people with kidney disease cannot convert vitamin D to its active form. Without supplements, these individuals develop vitamin D deficiencies. Individuals who are lactose intolerant may not be able to consume enough dairy products to meet their need for calcium and vitamin D and may benefit from fortified foods and supplements.

Vitamin and mineral supplements are commonly prescribed for infants and pregnant women. Breast-fed infants are sometimes supplemented with vitamin D and the mineral fluoride, both of which are low in breast milk. After four to six months, infants who are still breast fed often need supplemental iron, since by that time the iron stored at birth is depleted. During pregnancy, the mother's intake of vitamins and minerals must meet both her needs and those of the growing child. Although a well-planned diet can meet the needs of pregnancy and lactation, supplements of iron and folate are generally recommended and multivitamin and mineral supplements are usually prescribed.

A vitamin and mineral supplement may also be beneficial for elderly individuals. There may be some reduction in the capacity to absorb or utilize vitamins with aging. However, the most common reason for vitamin deficiencies in the elderly is limited food intake caused by lack of resources and transportation to purchase food, lack of interest in preparing meals, dental problems, and other diseases. A vitamin supplement is a good insurance policy for the elderly when food choices are limited.

General Population   The importance of supplements in these special groups is clear, but deciding on the benefits of supplements for the population at large is more difficult. Eating a variety of foods is the best way to meet nutrient needs. This can ensure a balance of nutrients as well as provide food components for which essentiality has not been established. Individuals who are concerned about their nutrient intake should have their nutritional status assessed.[1] For individuals with limited dietary intakes, a multivitamin and mineral supplement that supplies no more than 100% of the RDI may provide some benefit. Megavitamin supplements of individual nutrients are unwarranted and potentially dangerous.

Selecting a Supplement   If you decide to take a vitamin supplement, choose with care. Because vitamins are classified as foods rather than drugs, the strict laws controlling manufacturing, dosage, and usage that regulate the drug industry do not apply to vitamin supplements. This allows ready access to supplements at a modest price; however, it also allows potentially harmful doses of vitamins to be sold. The pros and cons of specific vitamin supplements and the risks of toxicity have been reviewed with each vitamin in this and the preceding chapter. Before selecting a supplement, read the label carefully. Compare the amounts of vitamins in the supplement with the RDIs, and consider the possibilities of toxicity. Supplements of individual nutrients should be taken with care to avoid toxicity and imbalances in nutrient intake. One of the most important arguments against the use of supplements is that it gives people a false sense of security, causing them to pay less attention to the nutrient content of the foods they choose. If you choose to take a supplement, don't ignore the food you eat.

CRITICAL THINKING
Evaluating Vitamin Supplements

Miquel had been feeling run down after a busy semester at school, so he went to the local health food store and asked for some advice. He bought several different types of supplements he was told would help him withstand the stresses of school and prevent him from getting sick. These included a vitamin C supplement, a Stress Pack, Prevention Plus, and Brain Booster. The contents of these are shown here. After taking these for several months, he enrolled in a nutrition class. He is now beginning to wonder if he really needs all these and if some could actually be harmful.

Vitamin C:	Vitamin C	600 mg
Stress Pack:	Thiamin	45 mg
	Niacin	57 mg
	Vitamin B$_6$	500 mg
	Riboflavin	30 mg
Prevention Plus:	Vitamin E	1000 IU
	Beta-carotene	5000 RE
	Vitamin C	1 g
Brain Booster:	Choline	100 mg
	Niacin	50 mg

To evaluate the benefits and risks of these supplements, Miquel asks himself the following questions:

How do the amounts of these vitamins compare with the RDAs?

The total dose of vitamin C is more than 25 times the RDA. The B vitamins in Stress Pack are 3 to 250 times the RDA. Prevention Plus contains 100 times the RDA of vitamin E, 5 times the RDA of vitamin A as beta-carotene. Brain Booster has more than twice the RDA for niacin, and there is no RDA for choline because it is not currently considered a dietary essential.

Have any of these vitamins been shown to be toxic?

Although thiamin and riboflavin are well in excess of the RDAs, there is no known toxicity.

The dose of vitamin B$_6$ (250 times the RDA) may cause nerve changes.

The total dose of niacin (over 5 times the RDA) has been shown to cause flushing and other side effects if it is in the nicotinic acid form.

The dose of vitamin C is high and may cause diarrhea, but no toxicity has been found at this level.

Vitamin E and beta-carotene have not been shown to be toxic.

Since there is no RDA for choline, he decides to investigate by reading about it.

Is choline essential?

Choline is important in human health as a part of a number of phospholipids found in cell membranes and as a component of the neurotransmitter acetylcholine. Humans fed TPN solutions lacking choline and humans fed a choline-deficient diet both developed liver abnormalities. This indicated to Miquel that even though choline can be made by the body, not enough is made to satisfy needs when there is no choline in the diet. This seemed to fit the definition of an essential nutrient that Miquel learned in his nutrition class. Despite Miquel's belief that choline is essential, his reading indicated Dthat it is widely distributed in foods and is unlikely to be deficient in the diet of a healthy college student.

What are the risks and benefits of taking these supplements?

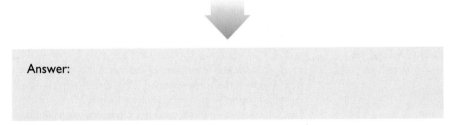

Answer:

SUMMARY

1. Vitamin A is needed for vision and for the growth and differentiation of cells. It is particularly important for the health of epithelial tissue, reproduction, and proper immune function. It is found in the diet both preformed as retinoids and in precursor forms, carotenoids, the most potent of which is beta-carotene. Although carotenoids are not toxic, preformed vitamin A can be toxic at doses as low as ten times the RDA and causes birth defects at doses only four times the RDA. The major food sources of preformed vitamin A include liver, eggs, fish, and fortified dairy products. Carotenoids are found in fruits and vegetables such as mangos and carrots. Beta-carotene functions as an antioxidant, a role that is independent of its conversion to vitamin A.

2. Vitamin D can be made in the skin by exposure to sunlight, so the dietary requirement varies depending on the amount synthesized. Vitamin D is essential for maintaining proper levels of calcium in the body. It promotes calcium and phosphorus absorption from the intestines and release from bone. Vitamin D is found in fish oils and fortified milk. A deficiency in children results in a condition called rickets; in adults, vitamin D deficiency causes osteomalacia.

3. Vitamin E functions primarily as a fat soluble antioxidant. It is necessary for reproduction and protects cell membranes from oxidative damage. Since polyunsaturated fats are particularly susceptible to oxidative damage, the requirement

for vitamin E increases as the polyunsaturated fat content of the diet increases. It is found in nuts, plant oils, green vegetables, and fortified cereals.

4. Vitamin K is essential for blood clotting. It is found in plants and is synthesized by bacteria in the gastrointestinal tract. A deficiency of vitamin K results in a failure of blood to clot. Since this is a problem in newborns, they are routinely given vitamin K injections at birth. Dicumarol, a substance that inhibits vitamin K activity, is used medically as an anticoagulant.

5. Foods contain essential nutrients and other substances, such as the phytochemicals in plant foods, that may play a role in human health. When nutrients come from foods, they come with these substances that help protect against disease. When nutrients come from supplements, they come without phytochemicals and other food components.

6. Nutrients are lost when foods are transported, stored, processed, and cooked. By choosing a diet rich in a variety of nutrient-dense foods and minimizing vitamin losses by appropriate selection, storage, and cooking techniques, most healthy individuals can meet their vitamin needs with food alone.

7. Vitamin supplements are recommended for some groups of individuals such as dieters, vegetarians, drug and alcohol users, and nutritionally vulnerable groups.

SELF-TEST

1. What is beta-carotene?
2. List three functions of performed vitamin A.
3. Is vitamin A toxic?
4. Is vitamin A deficiency a common problem?
5. List three food sources of preformed vitamin A and three food sources of beta-carotene.
6. Why is vitamin D called the sunshine vitamin?
7. Name two sources of vitamin D in the diet.
8. What is the function of vitamin D?
9. How does vitamin E protect cell membranes?
10. What is the main function of vitamin K?
11. What are the benefits of meeting micronutrient needs with foods rather than supplements?
12. List five groups of people for whom vitamin supplements might be needed to meet nutritional needs.
13. Are fresh fruits and vegetables always higher in vitamins than frozen ones?

APPLICATIONS

These exercises are designed to help you apply your critical thinking skills to your own nutrition choices. Many are best performed using a diet analysis software program. If you do not have access to a computer program, the exercises can be hand calculated using the information in this text and its appendices.

1. Using the three-day food intake record you kept in Chapter 1:
   a. Calculate your average daily intake of vitamin A.
   b. How does your vitamin A intake compare to the RDA for someone of your age and sex?
   c. What are three major food sources of vitamin A in your diet?
   d. Do the major food sources of vitamin A in your diet contain preformed vitamin A or beta-carotene?
2. Look at the label of a vitamin supplement containing vitamin A.
   a. How much and what form of vitamin A does it contain?
   b. If you took the recommended dose of this supplement, would you be at risk for vitamin A toxicity?
3. List the cooking methods used to prepare the foods in one day of your food record. How could these be modified to minimize vitamin losses?

REFERENCES

1. American Dietetic Association. Position paper of the American Dietetic Association: vitamin and mineral supplementation. J. Am. Diet. Assoc. 96:73–77, 1996.
2. American Dietetic Association. Position paper on phytochemicals and functional foods. Am. J. Diet. Assoc. 95:493–496, 1995.
3. Mangels, A.R., Holden, J.M., Beecher, G.R., et al. Carotenoid content of fruits and vegetables: an evaluation of analytic data. J. Am. Diet. Assoc. 93:284–296, 1993.
4. Olson, J.A. Needs and sources of carotenoids and vitamin A. Nutr. Rev. 52:S67–S73, 1994.
5. Blomhoff, R. Transport and metabolism of vitamin A. Nutr. Rev. 52:S13–S23, 1994.
6. Mangelsdorf, D.J. Vitamin A receptors. Nutr. Rev. 52:S32–S44, 1994.
7. Maden, M. Vitamin A in embryonic development. Nutr. Rev. 52:S3–S12, 1994.
8. van Poppel, G. Carotenoids and cancer: an update with emphasis on human intervention studies. Eur. J. Cancer 29A:1335–1344, 1993.
9. Toma, S., Losardo, P.L., Vincent, M., and Palumbo, R. Effectiveness of beta-carotene in cancer chemoprevention. Eur. J. Cancer Prev. 4:213–224, 1995.
10. Mayne, S.T., Janerich, D.T., Greenwald, P., et al. Dietary beta carotene and lung cancer risk in U.S. nonsmokers. J. Natl. Cancer Inst. 86:33–38, 1994.
11. Sommer, A. Vitamin A: its effect on childhood sight and life. Nutr. Rev. 52:S60–S66, 1994.
12. Sommer, A. Bellagio brief on vitamin A deficiency. J. Indian Pediatr. 29:1025–1027, 1992.
13. Olson, J.A. Vitamin A, retinoids, and carotenoids. In *Modern Nutrition in Health and Disease*, 8th ed. Shils, M.E., Olson, J.A., and Shike, M., eds. Philadelphia: Lea & Febiger, 1994, pp. 287–307.
14. Rothman, K.J., Moore, L.L., Singer, M.R., et al. Teratogenicity of high vitamin A intake. N. Engl. J. Med. 333:1369–1373, 1995.
15. Futoryan, T. and Gilchrest, B.A. Retinoids and the skin. Nutr. Rev. 52:299–310, 1994.
16. De Luca, L.M., Darwiche, N., Celli, G., et al. Vitamin A in epithelial differentiation and skin carcinoma. Nutr. Rev. 52:S45–S52, 1994.
17. Willett, W.C. Vitamin A and lung cancer. Nutr. Rev. 48:201–211, 1990.
18. Hong, W.K., Lippman, S.M., Itri, L.M., et al. Prevention of second primary tumors with isotretinoin in squamous-cell carcinoma of the head and neck. N. Engl. J. Med. 323:795–801, 1990.
19. The Alpha-Tocopherol, Beta-Carotene Cancer Prevention Study Group. The effect of vitamin E and beta-carotene on the incidence of lung cancer and other cancers in male smokers. N. Engl. J. Med. 330:1029–1035, 1994.

MINERALS IN NUTRITION

Minerals perform a wide range of vital structural and regulatory roles in the body. The amounts of both the **major minerals** and the trace elements in the body are regulated by absorption and excretion. Both excesses and deficiencies cause changes in body function that can be detrimental to overall health. For example, excess sodium in the diet may contribute to high blood pressure, and a deficiency of calcium may result in decreased bone density.

The bioavailability of minerals is affected by a number of factors, including the composition of the diet and the body's need for that mineral. Dietary fiber and other organic compounds found in foods decrease mineral absorption. **Phytic acid**, or **phytate**, is an organic compound containing phosphorus that is found in whole grains, bran, and soy products. It binds calcium, magnesium, zinc, and iron, limiting their absorption. Phytic acid does not affect mineral absorption in yeast-leavened breads because it is broken down.[1] **Tannins**, found in tea and some grains, can interfere with iron absorption; and **oxalates**, which are organic acids found in spinach, rhubarb, beet greens, and chocolate, have been found to interfere with calcium and iron absorption (Figure 10-6).

The electrical charge carried by minerals can also affect their bioavailability. Mineral ions that carry the same charge compete for absorption in the gastrointestinal tract. For example, calcium, magnesium, zinc, and iron all carry a 2^+ charge, and compete with one another for absorption. A high intake of one mineral in the diet may increase the need for another. For example, a diet high in calcium is known to decrease the absorption of magnesium, zinc, and iron. For this reason, taking a supplement containing an individual mineral such as calcium may affect the absorption of other minerals. Other interactions enhance absorption. For example, when vitamin C is present, absorption of the trace element iron is improved.

Once inside the body, minerals continue to interact, usually by complementing each other's function. Sodium and potassium ions, which both carry a 1^+ charge, are exchanged across membranes to regulate fluid balance and the electrical charge of the membrane. Calcium and phosphorus are both needed to mineralize bone, and blood levels of one can influence the use and excretion of the other.

The interactions of the major minerals with one another and with body water make it difficult to discuss one without including the roles of others. Therefore, the major electrolytes—sodium, potassium, and chloride—will be discussed together, as will calcium and phosphorus. Magnesium and sulfur, also major minerals of nutritional importance, are discussed separately.

Minerals–Elements needed by the body as structural components and regulators of chemical reactions and body processes.

Major minerals–Minerals needed in the diet in amounts greater than 100 mg per day or present in the body in amounts greater than 0.01% of body weight.

Phytic acid or **phytate**–A substance found in the husks of grains, legumes, and seeds that can bind minerals and decrease their absorption.

Tannins–Substances found in tea and some grains that can bind certain minerals and decrease their absorption.

Oxalates–Organic acids found in spinach, rhubarb, and other leafy green vegetables that can bind certain minerals and decrease their absorption.

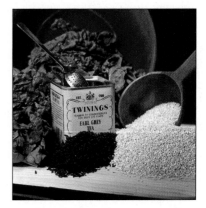

FIGURE 10-6
Compounds such as phytic acid, oxalates, and tannins found in these foods decrease mineral absorption. (Charles D. Winters)

THE ELECTROLYTES: SALTS OF THE INTERNAL SEA

Electrolytes are elements that conduct electricity. In nutrition, the term generally refers to sodium, potassium, and chloride. In North America today, most individuals consume a diet that is high in sodium and chloride, mostly from table salt added to processed foods, and low in potassium, from fresh fruits and vegetables. Throughout history, however, salt was scarce in most parts of the world. Archaeological and anthropological studies have shown that the diets of prehistoric hunter-gatherers consisted of foods high in potassium and low in sodium. Salt was highly prized by ancient cultures in Asia, Africa, and Europe, where it was used in rituals and in the preservation of food. Roman soldiers were paid in *sal*, the Latin word for salt from which we get our word salary. Today, our high intake of dietary sodium is associated with the high incidence of **hypertension**, making sodium a nutrient that we attempt to restrict in the modern diet.

Hypertension–Elevated blood pressure.

ELECTROLYTES IN THE DIET

In the diet, sodium and chloride are generally consumed together as sodium chloride, or table salt. The typical American diet contains about 9 grams of salt (almost 2 tsp). By weight, salt is 40% sodium and 60% chloride, so a person who consumes 9 grams of salt is consuming 3.6 grams of sodium. Chloride intakes parallel those of sodium. About 5.4 grams of chloride per day are consumed as sodium chloride. Most of the salt in the Western diet comes from processed foods. Only 10% comes from salt found naturally in food, 15% is from that added in cooking and at the table, and 75% is from that added during processing and manufacturing. The sodium in processed foods is added as a preservative and flavor enhancer. Most often sodium is added to processed foods as sodium chloride, but other sodium salts, such as sodium bicarbonate, sodium citrate, and sodium glutamate, also contribute to the sodium content of the diet. Drinking water from community water supplies contributes less than 10% of our intake.[2] Softened water or mineral water is often higher in sodium than tap water and if consumed in large quantities can contribute significantly to daily sodium intake.

In contrast to sodium and chloride, the richest sources of potassium are unprocessed foods such as fruits, vegetables, whole grains, and fresh meats. Bananas, oranges, potatoes, and tomatoes are some of the best sources. Processed foods are generally low in potassium (see Table 10-2).

ELECTROLYTES IN THE BODY

Almost all of the sodium, chloride, and potassium consumed in the diet is absorbed. Despite large variations in dietary intake, homeostatic mechanisms act to regulate the concentrations of these electrolytes in the body. For example, in northern China, sodium chloride intake is greater than 13.9 grams per day; in the Kalahari Desert, it is less than 1.7 grams per day; and in an Indian population in Brazil, consumption may be less than 0.06 gram of salt per day, yet blood levels of sodium are not different among these groups.[2]

Functions of Electrolytes   In the body, electrolytes help regulate fluid balance and are important for nerve conduction and muscle contraction. Electrolytes and other solutes cannot move freely back and forth across cell membranes but water can pass freely. Therefore, water moves between compartments depending

TABLE 10-2	Sodium and Potassium in Foods		
Food	**Amount**	**Sodium (mg)**	**Potassium (mg)**
Roast pork	3 oz (85 g)	55	333
Ham	3 oz	1010	243
2% Milk	1 cup (240 ml)	122	376
American cheese	1 oz	405	46
Whole wheat bread	1 slice	185	88
Biscuit from mix	1	271	53
Potato, baked	1 medium	6	477
Potato chips	1 oz	168	362
Fresh tomato	1 medium	11	273
Spaghetti sauce	½ cup	657	565
Orange	1 medium	0	237
Orange drink	1 cup	8	0

on the concentrations of sodium and potassium and other solutes in the various compartments. For example, if the concentration of electrolytes is high in the extracellular fluid, water is drawn into this compartment by osmosis to dilute the electrolytes, reducing their concentration.

Sodium and potassium are important for the conduction of nerve impulses (see Table 10-1). Nerve impulses are created by a change in the electrical charge across cell membranes. Sodium is the most abundant positively charged electrolyte in the extracellular fluid. Chloride is the principal negatively charged ion in the extracellular fluid. Potassium is the principal positively charged ion inside cells, where it is 30 times more concentrated than outside. The electrical charge, or membrane potential, exists because the number of negative ions inside the cell membrane is greater than the number outside. Stimuli, like neurotransmitters, change the permeability of the cell membrane to sodium, allowing it to rush into the cells. This reverses, or depolarizes, the charge of the cell membrane at that location, and an electrical current is generated. The nerve impulse travels as an electrical current. Once the nerve impulse passes, the original membrane potential is rapidly restored by another change in permeability, and then the original distribution of sodium and potassium ions across the cell membrane is restored by a sodium/potassium pump in the cell membrane (the sodium-potassium ATPase). A similar mechanism causes the depolarization of the muscle cell membranes, leading to muscle contraction.

Regulation of Electrolyte Balance   Sodium and chloride homeostasis is regulated to some extent by the intake of both water and salt. When salt intake is high, thirst is stimulated to increase water intake. When salt intake is very low, a salt appetite causes the individual to seek out salt. These mechanisms help ensure that appropriate proportions of salt and water are taken in. The kidneys, however, are the primary regulator of sodium and chloride concentration in the body.

Urinary excretion of sodium is decreased when sodium intake is low and increased when intake is high. Because water follows sodium by osmosis, the ability of the kidneys to conserve sodium provides a mechanism to conserve body water. When sodium concentration increases, water follows, causing an increase in the volume of extracellular fluid, primarily in the blood. Changes in blood volume can change **blood pressure**, the pressure of the blood against the arterial walls. Changes in blood pressure trigger the production and release of proteins and hormones that affect the amount of sodium, and hence water, retained by the kidney. For example, when blood pressure decreases, the kidneys release the enzyme renin, which begins a series of events leading to the production of **angiotensin II**. Angiotensin II increases blood pressure both by causing the blood vessel walls to constrict and by stimulating the release of the hormone **aldosterone**, which acts on the kidneys to increase sodium reabsorption. Water follows the reabsorbed sodium, resulting in an increase in blood volume and consequently blood pressure. The increase in blood pressure then inhibits the release of renin and aldosterone so that blood pressure does not continue to rise (Figure 10-7).

As with sodium and chloride, the kidneys regulate potassium excretion to maintain a relatively constant amount of potassium in the body. If blood levels begin to rise, aldosterone is released, which causes the kidney to excrete potassium and retain sodium. Most excess potassium is excreted by the kidney. Some is lost in the secretions of the gastrointestinal tract, and a very small amount is lost in sweat.

Blood pressure—The amount of force exerted by the blood against the artery walls.

Angiotensin II—A compound that causes blood vessel walls to constrict and stimulates the release of the hormone aldosterone.

Aldosterone—A hormone that increases sodium reabsorption and therefore enhances water reabsorption by the kidney.

ELECTROLYTES AND HEALTH: HYPERTENSION

Electrolytes in the body are carefully regulated and, in turn, regulate fluid volume. As the extracellular fluid volume increases, blood pressure increases. A certain level of blood pressure is necessary to ensure that blood is delivered to all tissues.

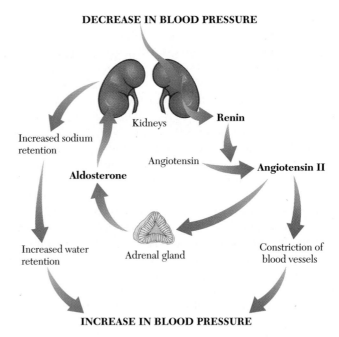

DECREASE IN BLOOD PRESSURE

Kidneys

Renin

Increased sodium retention

Angiotensin

Aldosterone

Angiotensin II

Increased water retention

Adrenal gland

Constriction of blood vessels

INCREASE IN BLOOD PRESSURE

F I G U R E   1 0 - 7
When blood pressure decreases, a series of events returns blood pressure to normal by constricting blood vessels and increasing sodium and water retention by the kidney.

A healthy blood pressure is 120/80 mm mercury or less. However, an increase in blood volume or a narrowing of the blood vessels can cause high blood pressure, or hypertension, generally defined as a blood pressure over 140/90 mm mercury. Hypertension has been called the silent killer because hypertension itself has no symptoms but can cause cardiovascular disease, strokes, kidney disease, and early death. Approximately 50 million Americans are at increased risk of illness and early death because of hypertension.[3]

What Causes Hypertension?   Most people with high blood pressure have essential hypertension, hypertension with no obvious external cause. It is a complex disorder, most likely resulting from disturbances in one or more of the mechanisms that control body fluid and electrolyte balance. High blood pressure that occurs as a result of some other disorder is referred to as secondary hypertension. It is frequently caused by a condition such as atherosclerosis, which narrows blood vessels, or kidney disease, which increases blood pressure to deliver more blood to the kidney.

There is a genetic predisposition to hypertension, so a family history of high blood pressure increases one's risk of developing this disorder. It is more common in African Americans than in whites.[4] It occurs frequently in individuals with diabetes and obesity, particularly those with excess abdominal fat, and decreases with weight loss.[5] A lack of physical activity, heavy alcohol consumption, and stress can also increase blood pressure.[6] In addition, blood pressure may be affected by the amounts of sodium, chloride, potassium, calcium, and magnesium in the diet.

Diet and Hypertension   Epidemiological studies have found that populations with high salt intakes have a higher incidence of hypertension. For example, the Intersalt study, which examined the incidence of hypertension in different populations, found that in populations consuming less than 4.5 grams of salt per day, average blood pressure was low, and hypertension was rare or absent. In populations consuming 5.8 grams of salt or more per day, blood pressure increased with sodium intake.[7]

here, labeled "light in sodium," contains 50% less sodium than regular spaghetti sauce. In addition to these nutrient claims, the health claim that diets low in sodium may reduce the risk of high blood pressure is an authorized claim that may appear on food labels. Foods may have this claim if they meet the definition of a low-sodium food and provide 20% or less of the Daily Value for fat, saturated fat, and cholesterol per serving.[1] This is to ensure that a food claiming to reduce blood pressure will not contribute to heart disease in other ways.

Medications can also be a source of sodium in the diet. Pain relievers, antacids, cough medicines, and laxatives frequently contain large amounts of sodium. For example, Alka-Seltzer with Aspirin contains over 1000 mg per dose. Again, check the label. Many of these over-the-counter medications list the sodium content on the label, and some are available in low-sodium forms.

[1] Kurtzweil, P. Scouting for sodium and other nutrients important to blood pressure. FDA Consumer, 28:18–22, Sept., 1994.

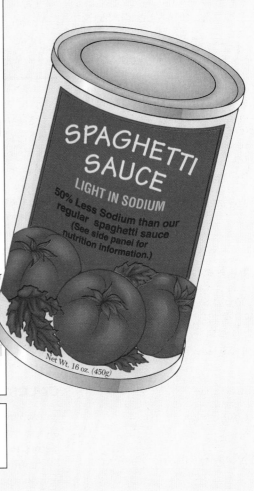

Nutrition Facts

Serving Size 1/2 cup (125g)
Servings Per Container about 3½

Amount Per Serving

Calories 50	Calories from Fat 10

	%Daily Value**
Total Fat 1g	**2%**
Saturated Fat 0g	**0%**
Cholesterol 0mg	**0%**
Sodium 250mg	**10%**
Potassium 530mg	**15%**
Total Carbohydrate 9g	**3%**
Dietary Fiber 1g	**4%**
Sugars 7g	
Protein 2g	

Vitamin A 10%	•	Vitamin C 25%
Calcium 2%	•	Iron 10%

*Percent Daily Values are based on a 2,000 calorie diet. Your daily values may be higher or lower depending on your calorie needs.

	Calories:	2,000	2,500
Total Fat	Less than	65g	80g
Sat Fat	Less than	20g	25g
Cholesterol	Less than	300mg	300mg
Sodium	Less than	2,400mg	2,400mg
Potassium		3,500mg	3,500mg
Total Carbohydrate		300g	375g
Dietary Fiber		25g	30g

Light Spaghetti Sauce, 250 milligrams (mg) per serving
Regular Spaghetti Sauce, 500mg per serving

CALCIUM AND PHOSPHORUS IN THE DIET

The main source of calcium in the North American diet is dairy products such as milk, cheese, and yogurt. Fish, such as sardines, that are consumed with the bones are also a good source, as are some green vegetables, like broccoli and kale (see Table 10-5). Some other vegetables are high in calcium, but the calcium is not well absorbed because it is bound by oxalates. For example, only about 5% of the calcium in spinach is absorbed.[21] The rest is bound by oxalates and excreted in the feces. Chocolate also contains oxalates, but chocolate milk is still a good source of calcium because the amount of chocolate added is small.

TABLE 10-5	Calcium and Phosphorus in Food		
Food	**Amount**	**Calcium (mg)**	**Phosphorus (mg)**
Plain yogurt	1 cup (240 ml)	448	353
Sardines	3 oz (85 g)	325	417
2% milk	1 cup	298	232
Cheddar cheese	1 oz	204	145
Salmon, canned	3 oz	181	280
Ice cream	1 cup	169	139
Tofu	3 oz	89	82
Mustard greens	½ cup	52	29
Kale	½ cup	47	18
Broccoli	½ cup	36	46

Some of the calcium in the diet is added during food processing. Baked goods, like breads, rolls, and crackers, to which nonfat dry milk powder has been added, provide calcium. Tofu is a good source when calcium is used in its processing. Since not all tofu is processed using calcium, check the label to select a brand that provides calcium. There are also several products on the market, such as orange juice, that are fortified with calcium.

Phosphorus is more widely distributed in the diet than calcium. Like calcium, it is found in dairy products such as milk, yogurt, and cheese; but in addition, meat, cereals, bran, eggs, nuts, and fish are good sources of dietary phosphorus. Food additives used in baked goods, cheeses, processed meats, and soft drinks also provide phosphorus. Because phosphorus is so widely distributed, dietary deficiencies do not usually occur. Marginal phosphorus deficiencies most commonly occur in premature infants, vegans, alcoholics, and the elderly. Chronic diarrhea and chronic use of aluminum-containing antacids, which prevent phosphorus absorption, can cause marginal phosphorus status.

CALCIUM AND PHOSPHORUS IN THE BODY

One quarter to one half of the calcium contained in foods is absorbed, depending on the composition of the diet and the physiology of the body. The presence of lactose in the diet enhances calcium absorption. Calcium absorption is decreased by tannins, fiber, phytates, and oxalates. Absorption is also decreased by the polyphosphate form of phosphorus found in many processed foods. Polyphosphates bind calcium in the gastrointestinal tract, preventing its absorption. Some calcium is absorbed by diffusion, so the more calcium in the diet, the more calcium is absorbed.[22] Most calcium is absorbed by active transport, which is regulated by the active form of vitamin D. When vitamin D is deficient, absorption decreases. Absorption decreases with age due to a decline in blood levels of the active form of vitamin D.[23] An additional decrease in calcium absorption occurs in women after menopause due to the drop in levels of the hormone estrogen, which enhances absorption. During pregnancy, when calcium need is high, absorption increases.

Phosphorus is more readily absorbed than calcium. Phosphorus can be absorbed when vitamin D is deficient but its absorption is reduced.

Functions of Calcium and Phosphorus   Calcium and phosphorus are important in the maintenance of bones and teeth (see Table 10-1). Bone is com-

What changes could Laura make at breakfast to increase her calcium content intake?

1. She could switch from toast to cereal with milk.
2. She could _____.

What choices could Laura make to increase her calcium intake at lunch?

1. She could choose a cheeseburger instead of a hamburger—the cheese contains calcium.
2. She might switch to lemon-lime soda because the cola contains a type of phosphorous that increases calcium losses.
3. She could _____.

How do the changes in Laura's dinner and snacks increase her calcium intake?

1. Having milk instead of tea increases her calcium intake. In addition, the tannins in tea may be reducing the absorption of the calcium in her meal.
2. Having broccoli would _____.

These changes increase Laura's calcium intake to meet the RDA. How could she meet her needs if she were lactose intolerant?

Answer:

MAGNESIUM

Magnesium is a mineral that affects the metabolism of calcium, sodium, and potassium. Magnesium is found in greens because it is a component of chlorophyll. The germ and bran of whole grains, nuts, seeds, and bananas are also good sources, but fruits, fish, meat, and milk are poor sources. In areas with hard water, the water supply may provide a significant amount of magnesium.

MAGNESIUM IN THE BODY

About 30 to 40% of the magnesium in the diet is absorbed. The active form of vitamin D can enhance magnesium absorption, and the presence of phytate and fiber may decrease absorption. As calcium in the diet increases, the absorption of magnesium decreases, so the use of calcium supplements can reduce the absorption of magnesium.

Most of the magnesium in the body is in bone where it is essential for the maintenance of structure. It prevents bone fragility by affecting the formation of hydroxyapatite crystals.[44] Low blood magnesium can result in low blood calcium and resistance to the effects of vitamin D and parathyroid hormone.[45] Magnesium is a positively charged ion involved in the maintenance of electrical potentials across nerve and muscle membranes and the transmission of impulses from nerves to muscles. It is therefore essential for proper functioning of the nerves and muscles including the heart. It is necessary for the utilization of ATP and is therefore an important activator of enzymatic reactions involving ATP. Such reactions are important in the metabolism of carbohydrate, lipid, and protein and the synthesis of DNA (see Table 10-1).

Blood levels of magnesium are closely regulated by the kidney. When magnesium intake is low, excretion in the urine is decreased. As intake increases, urinary excretion increases to maintain normal blood levels. This efficient regulation permits homeostasis over a wide range of dietary intakes.

MAGNESIUM DEFICIENCY

Magnesium deficiency is rare in the normal population. However, it does occur in those with alcoholism, general malnutrition, kidney disease, and gastrointestinal disease, as well as in those who use diuretics that increase magnesium loss in the urine. Deficiency symptoms include nausea, muscle weakness, irritability, mental derangement, and changes in heartbeat. Since low blood magnesium levels are accompanied by low blood calcium and potassium, some of the symptoms of magnesium deficiency may be due to alterations in the levels of these other minerals.

Diets low in magnesium have been associated with atherosclerosis in animal studies.[46] Epidemiological evidence suggests that humans with good magnesium status are at a lower risk of atherosclerosis, and supplements improve blood lipid levels.[47] Experiments in rats suggest that magnesium may protect against atherosclerosis by preventing the oxidation of lipids in lipoproteins and body tissues.[48]

HOW MUCH MAGNESIUM DO WE NEED?

The RDA for magnesium is 350 mg per day for men and 280 mg per day for women. A serving of whole grain breakfast cereal, spinach, or legumes contains about 100 mg.

There is no evidence that large intakes of magnesium are harmful to people with normal kidney function. Magnesium toxicity has been reported in elderly patients with impaired kidney function who frequently use laxatives and antacids. Magnesium-containing laxatives or antacids (magnesium hydroxide or milk of magnesia) are the most common form of added magnesium in the diet. Magnesium toxicity is characterized by nausea, vomiting, low blood pressure, and other cardiovascular changes.

SULFUR

Sulfur in the diet comes from organic molecules such as sulfur-containing amino acids in proteins and the sulfur-containing vitamins, as well as from some inorganic food preservatives such as sulfur dioxide, sodium sulfite, and sodium and potassium bisulfite, which are used as antioxidants. In the body, the sulfur-containing amino acids methionine and cysteine are needed for protein synthesis. Cysteine is also part of the compound glutathione, which is important in detoxifying drugs and protecting cells from oxidative damage. The vitamins thiamin and biotin, essential for energy production, also contain sulfur. Sulfur-containing ions are a part of an important buffer system that regulates acid–base balance.

There is no recommended intake for sulfur, and no deficiencies are known when protein needs are met (see Table 10-1).

SUMMARY

1. Water is an essential nutrient that constitutes about 60% of the adult human body. It is consumed in beverages and food, and a small amount is produced by metabolism. Fluid intake is stimulated by the sensation of thirst, which occurs in response to a decrease in body water.

2. Body water is distributed between intracellular and extracellular compartments. The amount in each compartment depends largely on the concentration of solutes. Since water will diffuse from a compartment with a lower concentration of solutes to one with a higher concentration by osmosis, the body regulates the distribution of water by adjusting the concentration of electrolytes and other solutes in each compartment.

3. In the body, water helps transport other nutrients and waste products within the body and out of the body. It also helps to protect the body, to regulate body temperature, and to lubricate areas such as the eyes and the joints. Its polar structure allows it to function as a solvent for the molecules involved in metabolism.

4. Water is lost from the body in urine and feces and through evaporation from the skin and lungs. The kidney is the primary regulator of water output. If water intake is low, antidiuretic hormone will cause the kidney to conserve water. If water intake is high, more water will be excreted in the urine. Dehydration can occur if water intake is too low or output is excessive.

5. The amount of water required by the body, about 1 ml per kcalorie of intake, may vary depending on environmental conditions and activity level.

6. Minerals are elements needed by the body to regulate chemical reactions and provide structure. Their bioavailability is affected by interactions with other minerals, vitamins, and other dietary components such as fiber, phytates, oxalates, and tannins.

7. The minerals sodium, chloride, and potassium are electrolytes important in the maintenance of fluid balance and the formation of membrane potentials. The North American diet is abundant in sodium and chloride from processed foods and table salt but generally low in potassium, which is high in unprocessed foods such as fruits and vegetables.

8. Electrolyte and fluid homeostasis is regulated primarily by the kidney. A decrease in blood pressure or blood volume signals the release of the enzyme renin, which helps form angiotensin II. Angiotensin II causes blood vessels to constrict and the hormone aldosterone to be released. Aldosterone causes the kidneys to reabsorb sodium and hence water, thereby increasing blood volume. Failure of these regulatory mechanisms may be a cause of hypertension.

9. Hypertension is common in the adult population of the United States. Although the causes of most hypertension are not known, some individuals have a form that is sensitive to sodium intake. For these individuals, a reduction in sodium intake helps reduce blood pressure.

10. There are no RDAs for sodium, chloride, or potassium. Public health recommendations suggest an increase in potassium intake and a decrease in sodium intake.

11. Most of the calcium and phosphorus in the body is in bone. Calcium not found in bone is essential for nerve transmission, muscle contraction, blood clotting, and blood pressure regulation. Phosphorus is part of a buffer that helps prevent changes in pH and is an essential component of phospholipids, ATP, and DNA.

12. Blood levels of calcium are regulated by controlling the amounts that are absorbed from the intestine, excreted by the kidney, and released from or deposited in bone. When blood calcium drops, parathyroid hormone is released. It stimulates the release of calcium from bone, decreases calcium excretion by the kidney, and activates vitamin D to increase the amount of calcium absorbed from the gastrointestinal tract and released from bone. When calcium levels increase, calcitonin is secreted, blocking calcium release from bone.

13. The RDA for calcium and phosphorus ranges from 800 to 1200 mg per day for adults. Sources of calcium in the American diet include dairy products, fish consumed with bones, and leafy green vegetables. The typical Ameri-

can does not consume a diet that meets the RDA for calcium. It is suggested that an increase in calcium intake will reduce the incidence of osteoporosis. Good sources of phosphorus include dairy products, meats, and grains.

14. Osteoporosis is a condition in which loss of bone mass results in easily fractured bones. The risk of osteoporosis is related to the peak bone mass achieved and the rate of bone loss. These are affected by race and sex as well as diet and exercise. Women are at particular risk for developing osteoporosis because of low peak bone mass and rapid bone loss after menopause.

15. Magnesium is important for bone health and is needed in reactions involving ATP and for nerve and muscle conductivity. Homeostasis is regulated by the kidney. Deficiency is rare, and the best dietary sources are whole grains and green vegetables.

16. Sulfur is needed in the diet as preformed organic molecules including the amino acids methionine and cysteine, needed to synthesize proteins and glutathione, and the vitamins thiamin and biotin, needed for energy metabolism. Sulfur is also part of a buffer that regulates acid–base balance. A dietary deficiency is unknown in the absence of protein malnutrition.

SELF-TEST

1. How is the amount of water in the body regulated?
2. List the functions of water in the body.
3. What is the recommended water intake for adults?
4. List three factors that increase water needs.
5. What are the functions of sodium, potassium, and chloride in the body?
6. What types of foods contribute the most sodium to the North American diet?
7. What types of foods are good sources of potassium?
8. Does a high-salt diet cause high blood pressure?
9. What is the major source of calcium in the North American diet?
10. How are blood calcium levels regulated?
11. How is calcium intake related to the risk of osteoporosis?
12. What factors other than calcium are related to the risk of osteoporosis?
13. What is the function of phosphorus in the body?
14. Name some food sources of phosphorus.
15. What is the function of magnesium in the body?
16. Where is sulfur found in the body?

APPLICATIONS

These exercises are designed to help you apply your critical thinking skills to your own nutrition choices. Many are best performed using a diet analysis software program. If you do not have access to a computer program, the exercises can be hand calculated using the information in this text and its appendices.

1. Keep a log of all the fluids you consume in one day.
   a. Calculate your fluid intake by totaling the volume of water, beverages, and foods that are liquid at room temperature, such as soup and ice cream, that you consumed.
   b. How does your intake on this day compare with your estimated requirement?
2. Calculate your sodium intake. Don't forget to include salt added at the table.
   a. How does it compare with the Daily Value?
   b. Make a list of the processed foods that contain more than 10% of the Daily Value for sodium (2400 mg) per serving.
   c. If your diet contains more sodium than recommended, modify it to reduce your sodium intake to the Daily Value or less.
3. Using the food record you kept in Chapter 1, calculate your average calcium intake.
   a. How does your intake compare with the RDA for calcium for someone of your age and sex?
   b. Modify your diet to increase your calcium consumption without significantly increasing your energy intake?

REFERENCES

1. King, J.C. and Keen, C.L. Zinc. In *Modern Nutrition in Health and Disease*, 8th ed. Shils, M.E., Olson, J.A., and Moshe, S., eds. Philadelphia: Lea & Febiger, 1994, pp. 214–230.
2. National Research Council, Food and Nutrition Board. *Recommended Dietary Allowances*, 10th ed. Washington, DC: National Academy Press, 1989.
3. *The Fifth Report of the Joint National Committee on Detection, Evaluation, and Treatment of High Blood Pressure*, Washington, DC: U.S. Dept. of Health and Human Services, National Heart, Lung, and Blood Institute; 1993. NIH publication 93-1088.
4. Weinberger, M.H. Racial differences in renal sodium excretion: relationship to hypertension. Am. J. Kidney Dis. 21:41–45, 1993.
5. Kochar, M.S. Hypertension in obese patients. Postgrad. Med. 93:199–200, 1993.
6. Perry, I.J., Whincup, P.H., and Shaper, A.G. Environmental factors in the development of essential hypertension. Br. Med. Bull. 50:246–259, 1994.
7. Carvalho, J.J., Baruzzi, R.G., Howard, P.F., et al. Blood pressure in four remote populations in the Intersalt study. Hypertension 14:238–246, 1989.
8. Weinberger, M.H. Salt sensitivity as a predictor of hypertension. Am. J. Hypertens. 4:615S–616S, 1991.
9. Boegehold, M.A. and Kotchen, T.A. Relative contributions of dietary Na$^+$ and Cl$^-$ to salt-sensitive hypertension. Hypertension 14:579–583, 1989.

10. Young, D.B., Lin, H., and McCabe, R.D. Potassium's cardiovascular protective mechanisms. Am. J. Physiol. 268:R825–837, 1995.

11. Gillman, M.W., Cupples, A., Gagnon, D., et al. Protective effect of fruits and vegetables on development of stroke in men. J.A.M.A. 273:1113–1117, 1995.

12. Haddy, F.J. Roles of sodium, potassium, calcium and natriuretic factors in hypertension. Hypertension 18:PIII 179–183, 1991.

13. Barger-Lux, M.J. and Heaney, R.P. The role of calcium intake in preventing bone fragility, hypertension, and certain cancers. J. Nutr. 124:1406S–1411S, 1994.

14. Hamet, P. The evaluation of the scientific evidence for a relationship between calcium and hypertension. J. Nutr. 125:311S–343S, 1995.

15. Mikamo, H., Ogihara, T., and Tabuchi, Y. Blood pressure response to dietary calcium interventions in humans. Am. J. Hypertens. 3:147S–151S, 1990.

16. The Trials of Hypertension Prevention Collaborative Research Group. The effects of nonpharmacologic interventions on blood pressure of persons with high normal levels. Results of the trials of hypertension prevention, phase I. J.A.M.A. 267:1213–1220, 1992.

17. *The Fifth Report of the Joint National Committee on Detection, Evaluation, and Treatment of High Blood Pressure.* Arch. Intern. Med. 153:154–183, 1993.

18. Sacks, F.M., Obarzanek, E., Windhauser, M.M., et al. Rational and design of the Dietary Approaches to Stop Hypertension trial (DASH). A multicenter controlled-feeding study of dietary patterns to lower blood pressure. Ann. Epidemiol. 5:108–118, 1995.

19. National Research Council. *Diet and Health: Implications for Reducing Chronic Disease Risk.* Washington, DC: National Academy Press, 1989.

20. Committee on Nutritional Status During Pregnancy and Lactation, National Academy of Sciences. *Nutrition During Pregnancy.* Washington, DC: National Academy Press, 1990.

21. Heaney, R.P., Weaver, C.M., and Recker, R.R. Calcium absorption from spinach. Am. J. Clin. Nutr. 47:707–709, 1988.

22. Allen, L.H. and Wood, R.J. Calcium and phosphorus. In *Modern Nutrition in Health and Disease*, 8th ed. Shils, M.E., Olson, J.A., and Shike, M., eds. Philadelphia: Lea & Febiger, 1994, pp. 144–163.

23. Weaver, C.M. Age-related calcium requirements due to changes in absorption and utilization. J. Nutr. 124:1418S–1425S, 1994.

24. Sowers, J.R., Zemel, M.B., Zemel, P.C., and Standley, P.R. Calcium metabolism and dietary calcium in salt-sensitive hypertension. Am. J. Hypertens. 4:557–563, 1991.

25. Beatty, D. and Finn, S.C. Position of the American Dietetic Association and the Canadian Dietetic Association: Women's health and nutrition. J. Am. Diet. Assoc. 95:362–366, 1995.

26. Reeker, R.R., Davies, K.M., Hiners, S.M., et al. Bone gain in young adult women. J.A.M.A. 268:2403–2408, 1992.

27. Toss, G. Effect of calcium intake and other lifestyle factors in bone loss. J. Int. Med. Res. 231:181–186, 1992.

28. Hu, J.F., Zhao, X.H., Parpia, B., and Campbell, T.C. Dietary intakes and urinary excretion of calcium and acids: a cross-sectional study of women in China. Am. J. Clin. Nutr. 58:398–406, 1993.

29. Nordin, B.E.C., Need, A.G., Morris, H.A., and Horowitz, M. The nature and significance of the relationship between urinary sodium and urinary calcium in women. J. Nutr. 123:1615–1622, 1993.

30. Calvo, M.S. The effects of high phosphorus intake on calcium homeostasis. Adv. Nutr. Res. 9:183–207, 1994.

31. Harris, S.S. and Dawson-Hughes, B. Caffeine and bone loss in healthy postmenopausal women. Am. J. Clin. Nutr. 60:573–578, 1994.

32. Bunker, V.W. The role of nutrition in osteoporosis. Br. J. Biomed. Sci. 51:228–240, 1994.

33. Dawson-Hughes, B. Calcium supplementation and bone loss: a review of controlled clinical trials. Am. J. Clin. Nutr. 54(suppl.):272S–280S, 1991.

34. Heaney, R.P. Nutritional factors in osteoporosis. Ann. Rev. Nutr. 13:287–316, 1993.

35. Prince, R.L., Smith, M., Dick, I.M., et al. Prevention of postmenopausal osteoporosis. A comparative study of exercise, calcium supplementation and hormone replacement therapy. N. Engl. J. Med. 325:1189–1195, 1991.

36. Stendig-Lindberg, G., Tepper, R., and Leicher, I. Trabecular bone density in a two-year controlled trial of peroral magnesium in osteoporosis. Magnesium Res. 6:155–163, 1993.

37. Pak, C.Y. Sakhaec, K., Adams-Huet, B., et al. Treatment of postmenopausal osteoporosis with slow-release sodium fluoride. Final report of a randomized trial. Ann. Intern. Med. 123:401–408, 1995.

38. Volpe, S.L., Taper, L.J., and Meacham, S. The relationship between boron and magnesium status and bone mineral density in the human: a review. Magnesium Res. 6:291–296, 1993.

39. NIH Consensus Conference. Optimal calcium intake. J.A.M.A. 272:1942–1948, 1994.

40. Levenson, D.I. and Bockman, R.S. A review of calcium preparations. Nutr. Rev. 52:221–232, 1994.

41. Heaney, R.P., Weaver, C.M., and Fitzsimmons, M.L. Influence of calcium load on absorption fraction. J. Bone Min. Res. 5:1135–1138, 1990.

42. Blumsohn, A., Herrington, K., Hannon, R.A., et al. The effect of calcium supplementation on the circadian rhythm of bone resorption. J. Clin. Endocrinol. Metab. 79:730–735, 1994.

43. Bourgoin, B.P., Evans, D.R., Cornett, J.R., et al. Lead content in 70 brands of dietary calcium supplements. Am. J. Public Health 83:1155–1160, 1993.

44. Bigi, A., Foresti, E., Gregorini, R., et al. The role of magnesium on the structure of biological apatites. Calcif. Tissue Int. 50:439–444, 1992.

45. Sojka, J.E. Magnesium supplementation and osteoporosis. Nutr. Rev. 53:71–80, 1995.

46. Altura, B.T., Brust, M., Bloom, S., et al. Magnesium dietary intake modulates blood lipid levels and atherogenesis. Proc. Natl. Acad. Sci. USA 87:1840–1844, 1990.

47. Dreosti, I.E. Magnesium status and health. Nutr. Rev. 53:S23–S27, 1995.

48. Rayssiguier, Y., Gueux, E., Durlach, J., et al. Dietary magnesium affects susceptibility of lipoproteins and tissues to peroxidation in rats. J. Am. Coll. Nutr. 12:133–137, 1993.

The Trace Minerals: Our Elemental Needs

CHAPTER CONCEPTS

1. Trace elements are required by the body in small amounts and are vital to human health.

2. Interactions among the elements and other dietary components affect the bioavailability of trace elements.

3. Iron is important for the delivery of oxygen to cells. Iron deficiency anemia is the most common nutritional deficiency worldwide.

4. Zinc is needed for tissue growth and repair, sexual development, and immune function.

5. Copper is needed to prevent anemia. High intakes of zinc can interfere with copper absorption.

6. Selenium, copper, zinc, and manganese are all involved in antioxidant enzyme systems.

7. Iodine is essential for the synthesis of the thyroid hormones. Deficiency is a problem worldwide, but the use of iodized salt has virtually eliminated iodine deficiency in North America.

8. Fluoride is essential for dental health.

9. Chromium is needed for the transport of glucose into cells.

10. Molybdenum is needed for the activity of several enzymes involved in uric acid production.

11. Our understanding of the functions of other trace elements is still limited.

JUST A TASTE

Can a supplement of one trace element cause a deficiency of another?

How does fluoride protect against tooth decay?

Can taking chromium supplements change body composition?

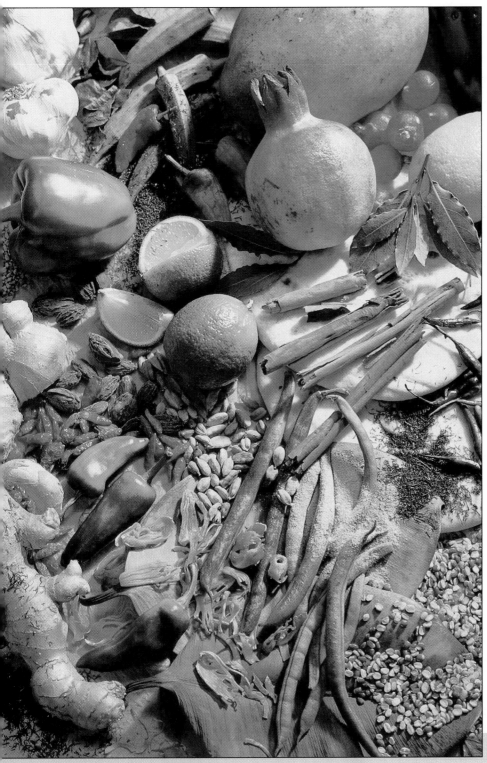

(Trevor Wood/Tony Stone Images)

CHAPTER OUTLINE

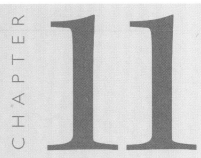

CHAPTER

11

319

Trace minerals are the most recently recognized of the essential nutrients. Like the major minerals, they are a group of elements needed by the body to maintain health. The terms trace minerals and trace elements are used interchangeably to refer to iron, zinc, copper, manganese, selenium, iodine, fluoride, chromium, molybdenum, boron, arsenic, nickel, silicon, cadmium, lead, lithium, aluminum, bromine, rubidium, and vanadium. They are grouped together not because of similar functions but because they are all required in very small amounts.

As our knowledge of the trace elements has evolved, so has our thinking about their role in human health. The methods traditionally used to establish the essentiality of substances and determine requirements for nutrients have not been effective for studying many of the trace elements. The requirements for these elements are so small and interactions among the elements are so great that isolated deficiencies of trace elements have not always been possible to create, even in the laboratory. This has caused researchers to focus not only on the needs for individual nutrients, but on the balanced interactions of nutrients within the whole diet.[1]

In this chapter we will address properties shared by the trace elements and the unique roles of individual elements by discussing:
- Where are the trace elements found in the diet?
- What are their functions in the body?
- How are their needs determined?
- How much of each do we need?

TRACE ELEMENTS IN NUTRITION

Trace elements–Minerals required in the diet in amounts less than 100 mg per day or present in the body in amounts less than 0.01% of body weight.

By definition, the **trace elements** are the minerals required by the body in an amount of 100 mg or less per day (Figure 11-1). Iron, zinc, copper, manganese, and fluoride are required in milligram amounts, while selenium, iodine, chromium, and molybdenum are needed in microgram quantities. The total amount of all of the trace elements in the body is only about 25 to 30 grams. When compared with calcium—which alone constitutes 1 to 2 kg of body weight—the amounts seem insignificant, but the functions of the trace elements as factors needed for enzyme activity or as components of protein molecules make their significance for human life far from trivial.

TRACE ELEMENTS IN THE DIET

Trace elements are found in foods from both plant and animal sources. Many of the trace elements in animal products are present as regulated components of the animal body. For instance, iron is a component of muscle tissue; therefore, it is found in consistent amounts in meat. In plants, trace elements may be present as regulated components or as contaminants from soil and water. Because soil concentrations of trace elements vary greatly, the amounts plants absorb from the soil and, ultimately, the trace element content of plants also vary (Figure 11-2). For example, the soil content of iodine is high near the ocean but usually quite low in

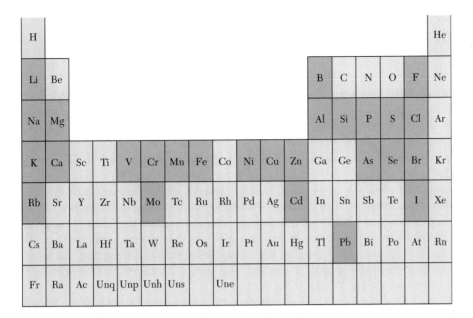

FIGURE 11-1
The minerals are chemical elements found in the periodic table. The major minerals are shown in purple and the trace elements are shown in blue.

inland areas. Therefore, foods grown near the ocean are better sources of iodine than those grown inland. In developed countries, modern transportation provides a diet that includes foods produced in many locations, so the diet is unlikely to be deficient in trace elements. In countries where the diet consists predominantly of locally grown foods, individual trace element deficiencies and excesses are more likely to occur.

TRACE ELEMENTS IN THE BODY

The bioavailability of trace elements can be affected by an individual's health and nutritional status as well as the composition of the total diet. The amount available for utilization at the tissues can be varied by increasing or decreasing the amount delivered by transport proteins. For example, when iron stores are low, the ability to transport iron to cells increases. When an individual's need for a trace element is increased, the utilization of the element from the diet may increase and excretion may decrease.

In addition to individual needs, interactions among trace elements and between trace elements and other components of the diet can affect their absorption and transport. For example, zinc intake affects copper absorption, so copper requirements are affected by the amount of zinc in the diet. The presence of vitamin C increases iron absorption; therefore, iron requirements are more easily met when the diet is high in vitamin C. Phytates, oxalates, and tannins all inhibit trace element absorption. Although North Americans generally do not consume enough of any of these to interfere with trace element nutrition, this is a problem in developing countries. For example, since zinc absorption is decreased by phytates, the amount of zinc that meets needs in a population consuming a diet low in phytates might result in a deficiency in a population that consumes a diet high in phytates. The complexity of the interactions among the trace elements and other components of the diet as well as the effect of an individual's needs has made it difficult to determine specific requirements.

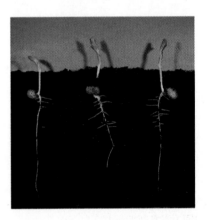

FIGURE 11-2
The mineral content of some plants varies with the mineral content of the soil in which they are grown. (Stephen J. Krasemann/Peter Arnold, Inc.)

HOW MUCH OF EACH TRACE ELEMENT DO WE NEED? DETERMINING REQUIREMENTS

Determining trace element needs is difficult. The first step is usually to remove the element from the diet of laboratory animals and monitor the animals for signs of deficiency. An element is considered essential if a deficiency consistently results in less than optimal biological function and is preventable or reversible by supplementation of the element at levels similar to those found normally in the diet. Because trace elements already in the body can meet requirements for months or even years, these studies are very costly and take years to complete. Because of the many potential interactions among trace elements and other dietary components, the need for an element must be studied within the context of the total diet. Each element must be studied along with known amounts of other dietary components that interact with it. Because the amounts needed are so small, contamination from the environment may supply enough of a trace element to meet needs. Therefore, when studying trace elements in animals, everything that comes in contact with the animals, including food, water, air, cages, and keepers, must be kept cleansed of the elements.

Once an element has been determined to be essential in animals, needs in humans can be studied. Balance studies can be used to determine the level of intake that replaces losses. Again, these studies must consider the amounts of other dietary components to evaluate the need of a specific element. One approach that avoids some of these problems has been to study diseases that affect trace element utilization. For example, much of our knowledge about copper comes from studying Menkes' kinky hair syndrome, an inherited condition in which copper absorption and metabolism are abnormal. The symptoms of this syndrome are those of a copper deficiency. Another way in which trace element needs have been studied is by observing people being fed TPN solutions for long periods of time. The nutrient intake of an individual receiving TPN is entirely dependent on the composition of the TPN solution (Figure 11-3). Only elements known to be essential are provided. Occasionally, elements not known previously to be essential become deficient. For example, selenium was determined to be essential when a patient was given TPN without selenium. The patient developed symptoms that resolved when selenium was added to the solution. Trace element needs can also be studied by determining the functions of elements using biochemical and molecular biological techniques. If no other evidence is available, trace element needs can be estimated by evaluating the typical intake of an element in a healthy population. It is assumed that if there are no deficiency symptoms, the diet must meet the requirement for that nutrient. One problem with this approach is that deficiency symptoms may be recognized only when the deficiency is severe. Subtle signs of a deficiency in a population may be difficult to detect.

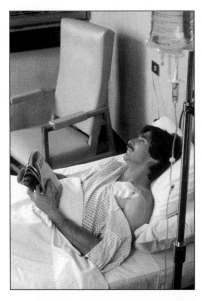

FIGURE 11-3
Trace element deficiencies occur when incomplete TPN solutions are administered. (© L. Steinmark/Custom Medical Stock)

TRACE ELEMENTS AND HEALTH: DEFICIENCY AND TOXICITY

With the exception of iron and iodine, which are commonly deficient worldwide, deficiencies of trace elements are rare, occurring only when the food supply is particularly limited. For example, in certain rural areas of China, selenium deficiency is common because the selenium content of the soil is extremely low and the diet is based on locally grown food. In industrialized nations, trace element intake is affected by the refining and processing of food. As the skins of produce and the bran and germ of grains are removed, trace elements are lost. For example, iron, selenium, zinc, and copper are lost when flour is refined. Only iron is replaced by enrichment. Trace elements are also inadvertently added to food through processing and handling. For example, the iodine content of dairy products is increased by contamination with the cleaning solutions used in milking machines.

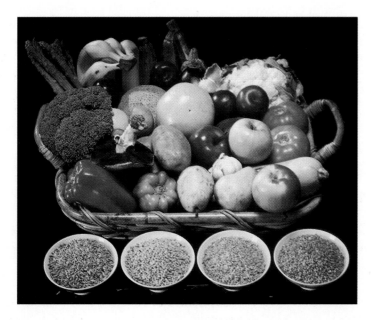

FIGURE II-4
The trace element content of the diet can be maximized by eating a variety of nutrient-dense foods. (Charles D. Winters)

The trace element content of the diet can be maximized by eating a variety of foods, including many unprocessed or less processed foods such as fresh fruits, vegetables, and whole grains and cereals (Figure 11-4).

Trace element toxicity is also a concern, mostly as a result of environmental pollution or excessive supplementation. For example, environmental lead from old chipped lead paint, lead pipes, and soil and air contamination is a risk to small children. Chronic exposure can cause growth retardation and learning disabilities (see Chapter 14: *Off the Shelf:* "Getting the Lead Out"). Trace element supplements may pose a risk of toxicity because elements that are essential in small doses may be toxic at high intakes. For instance, iron is essential yet can be deadly at very high doses. Supplementing trace elements may also cause problems because of the complex interactions among elements. Taking high doses of one trace element can compromise the bioavailability of others, creating a mineral imbalance, which can interfere with functions essential to human health. The body's regulatory mechanisms control the absorption and excretion of trace elements but have evolved to deal with small amounts of these elements as they occur in the diet. Large doses of supplements may override this regulation and toxicity can occur.

CLASSIFYING TRACE ELEMENTS

The trace elements can be classified in a number of ways. One way is based on the amounts needed in the diet—milligram (mg) versus microgram (μg) amounts. Another way is based on what is known about them. Those that have been well studied and for which an RDA has been established include iron, zinc, iodine, and selenium. Those that are known to be essential for humans, and for which an estimated safe and adequate daily dietary intake (ESADDI) has been set include copper, manganese, fluoride, chromium, and molybdenum. Those that are known to be essential in other mammals or have been identified as part of normal human enzyme systems but for which a deficiency has not been identified in humans include boron, arsenic, nickel, silicon, cadmium, lead, lithium, aluminum, bromine, rubidium, and vanadium.

A third way of classifying trace elements for study is to group them according to their functions and interactions. In the discussion that follows, iron, zinc, and copper are addressed sequentially because of their interactions in absorption and transport. Copper, zinc, manganese, and selenium are also discussed sequentially because they function in antioxidant enzymes.

CRITICAL THINKING
Is This Trace Element Essential?

The Amecht research group is conducting studies to determine whether a trace element called "R" is essential for humans. Can the results from these be used to establish the essentiality of this element for humans?

Experiment 1

A group of 50 rats were housed under strict laboratory conditions. Half of them were fed a diet deficient in R; the other half received the identical diet with the addition of 25 μg per day of R. After two months, the R-deficient group was growing and reproducing poorly compared with the R-supplemented group. When 25 μg per day of R was added back to the deficient diet, the animals began to grow and reproduce normally.

Can these results be used to establish essentiality for humans?

No. This study demonstrates that deficiency symptoms occur in rats depleted of R and that repletion alleviates these symptoms. It gives no information about the need for R in humans. The amount that alleviates deficiency symptoms in rats may be unrelated to the human requirement. Time, cost, ethics, and the need for strict laboratory conditions make this type of depletion-repletion difficult to do using humans.

Experiment 2

An analysis of human blood indicates that R is consistently present but at low levels.

Can these results be used to establish essentiality for humans?

No. The presence of an element in the blood or other body tissues does not mean it is essential. Some substances are present in the body because they have a physiological role; others are present because they are contaminants from the environment.

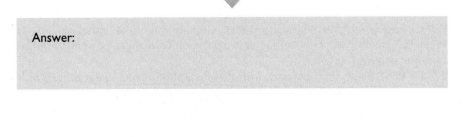

Experiment 3

A balance study done in humans shows that when the intake of R is 500 μg per day, R excretion equals R intake, suggesting that there is adequate R to meet body needs.

Can these results be used to establish essentiality for humans?

Not necessarily. A balance study indicates the amount that will replace body losses. It does not prove that R is required in the body. Balance information can be obtained for minerals that are present in the body but serve no function. Even if R is essential, the information obtained from balance studies may not help determine the amount of R needed to prevent deficiency symptoms or maintain optimal health.

Experiment 4

Epidemiological surveys of four different apparently healthy population groups show that dietary consumption of R ranges from 50 to 700 μg per day.

Can these results be used to establish essentiality for humans?

Answer:

IRON (Fe)

Iron was the first of the trace elements to be recognized. It was identified as a major constituent of blood in the 18th century. By 1832, iron tablets were used to treat young women for whom "coloring matter" was lacking in the blood. Today we know that the red color in blood is due to the iron-containing protein **hemoglobin**, and that a deficiency of iron decreases hemoglobin production. Despite the fact that iron is one of the best understood of the trace elements, iron deficiency remains the most common nutritional deficiency in North America and the world.

IRON IN THE DIET

Iron in the diet comes from both plant and animal sources. Much of the iron in animal products is **heme iron**, a form of iron found in proteins, such as the **myoglobin** in muscle and hemoglobin in blood. Heme iron is absorbed more than

Hemoglobin–An iron-containing protein in red blood cells that binds oxygen and transports it to cells.

Heme iron–A readily absorbed form of iron found in animal products that is chemically associated with proteins such as hemoglobin and myoglobin.
Myoglobin–An iron-containing protein in muscle cells that binds oxygen.

TABLE 11-1	Iron Content of Foods	
Food	**Amount**	**Iron (mg)**
All Bran cereal	1 cup (200 mg)	6.8
Beef liver	3 oz (85 g)	5.4
Garbanzo beans	½ cup	4.8
Tofu	3 oz	4.6
Spinach, cooked	½ cup	3.2
Roast beef	3 oz	2
Enriched white rice	1 cup	1.8
Chicken thigh	3 oz	1.1
Brown rice	1 cup	0.8
Salmon	3 oz	0.5
Raisins	2 Tbsp	0.4
Dried apricots	2 halves	0.3

Nonheme iron–A poorly absorbed form of iron found in both plant and animal products that is not part of the iron complex found in hemoglobin and myoglobin.

twice as efficiently as **nonheme iron**. Meat, poultry, and fish are good sources of heme iron. Leafy green vegetables, legumes, whole or enriched grains, and dried fruit are good sources of nonheme iron (see Table 11-1). Another source of nonheme iron in the diet is iron cooking utensils. Iron leaches from these utensils into food. This process is enhanced by acidic foods. For example, spaghetti sauce cooked in a glass pan contains about 3 mg of iron, and the same sauce cooked in an iron skillet may contain more than 80 mg, depending on how long it is cooked.

The absorption of nonheme iron is enhanced by a number of dietary factors. Acidity enhances iron absorption because it helps keep iron in the ferrous (Fe^{2+}) form, which is better absorbed than the ferric (Fe^{3+}) form. Vitamin C enhances the absorption of iron for two reasons. First, it is an acid; and second, vitamin C prevents iron from forming complexes in the gastrointestinal tract that cannot be absorbed.[2] Consuming meats, such as beef, fish, or poultry, that are sources of heme iron also has a beneficial effect on the absorption of nonheme iron. So, for example, a small amount of hamburger in a pot of chili will enhance iron absorption from the beans.

Dietary factors that interfere with the absorption of nonheme iron include fiber, phytates found in cereals, tannins found in tea, and oxalates found in some leafy greens such as spinach. These prevent absorption by binding iron in the gastrointestinal tract. The presence of other minerals may also decrease iron absorption. For instance, calcium supplements decrease iron absorption, particularly when both are consumed at the same meal.[3]

IRON IN THE BODY

Iron is essential for the delivery of oxygen to cells. It is a component of two oxygen-carrying proteins, hemoglobin and myoglobin. Most of the iron in the body is part of hemoglobin. Hemoglobin, in red blood cells, transports oxygen to body cells and carries carbon dioxide away from cells for elimination by the lungs. Myoglobin is found in the muscle, where it stores oxygen for use in muscle contraction. Iron is also a part of several proteins involved in the electron transport chain, drug metabolism, and the immune system. The iron-containing enzyme catalase functions as an antioxidant.

Iron from the diet is absorbed into the intestinal mucosal cells. The amount of iron transported from the mucosal cells depends on body needs. If body stores of iron are high, less of the iron in the mucosal cells is transported. If iron stores are low, a greater percentage of the iron that has been absorbed into the mucosal cells is transported to body tissues. The transport and delivery of iron is regulated

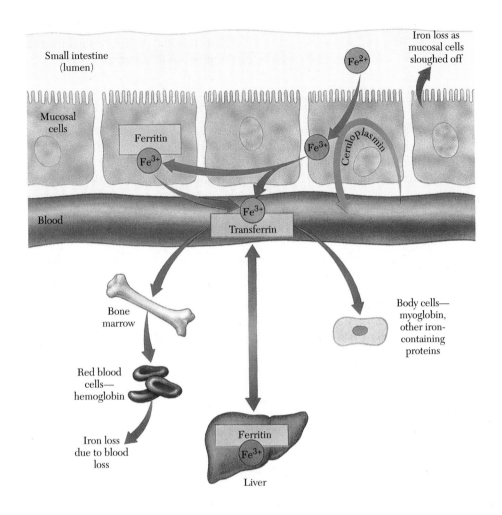

FIGURE 11-5

Ferrous iron (Fe^{2+}) is absorbed and converted to ferric iron (Fe^{3+}) by ceruloplasmin. Excess remains in mucosal cells and is excreted when the cells die. Iron is transported in the blood bound to transferrin. It is delivered to bone, where it is needed to synthesize hemoglobin for red blood cells, and to other body cells, where it is used to synthesize myoglobin and other iron-containing proteins. Excess is stored primarily in the liver, bound to ferritin.

by several proteins. The copper-containing protein **ceruloplasmin** is needed to convert absorbed iron to the form that binds the iron transport protein **transferrin** and the iron storage protein **ferritin** (Figure 11-5). Transferrin picks up iron from the mucosal cells and transports it in the blood to the liver, bones, and other body tissues. Transferrin receptors on cell membranes allow the transferrin-iron complex into the cell, where the iron is released for use. When iron is in short supply, the amount of transferrin and number of transferrin receptors increase, allowing more iron to be transported into the cells.[4] When iron is plentiful, transferrin and transferrin receptors decrease, so the capacity to pick up iron from the mucosal cells and transport it into body cells is reduced. Iron that is not picked up from mucosal cells is excreted in the feces when the mucosal cells die.

Iron that is absorbed in excess of immediate needs can be stored in the protein ferritin primarily in the liver, spleen, and bone marrow. Levels of ferritin in the blood can be used to estimate iron stores. If ferritin concentrations in the liver become high, some is converted to an insoluble storage protein called hemosiderin. Iron can be mobilized from body stores as needed, and deficiency signs will appear only after stores are depleted.

Ceruloplasmin–A copper-containing protein that converts iron to the ferric form, which can bind to iron storage and iron transport proteins.

Transferrin–An iron transport protein in the blood.

Ferritin–The major iron storage protein.

In healthy individuals, iron loss occurs through blood loss, including that lost during menstruation and small amounts lost from the gastrointestinal tract, and through the shedding of cells from the intestine, skin, and urinary tract.[2]

IRON DEFICIENCY

Iron deficiency anemia—A condition that occurs when the oxygen-carrying capacity of the blood is decreased because there is insufficient iron to make hemoglobin.

Pica—The compulsive ingestion of non-food substances such as clay, laundry starch, and paint chips.

When the diet is low in iron and body stores have been depleted by blood loss or rapid growth, hemoglobin cannot be produced. When not enough hemoglobin is available, the red blood cells that are formed are small and pale and are unable to deliver adequate oxygen to the tissues. This is known as **iron deficiency anemia** (Figure 11-6). The symptoms include fatigue, weakness, headache, decreased work capacity, an inability to maintain body temperature in a cold environment, changes in behavior, impaired development in infants, decreased resistance to infection, and an increased risk of lead poisoning in young children. One strange symptom that has been hypothesized to be related to iron deficiency is **pica**. This is a compulsion to eat nonfood items such as clay, ice, paste, laundry starch, paint chips, and ashes. Pica can cause the consumption of substances containing toxic minerals such as lead-based paints, and it can introduce substances into the diet that inhibit mineral absorption (see Chapter 13).

In the United States and Canada, about 8% of women and 10 to 20% of low-income children have iron deficiency anemia.[5] Among minority women and children, the incidence is even greater. In addition, about 30% of women, while not anemic, have low or no iron stores. When iron stores are low, blood loss or a change in diet that reduces iron intake is more likely to lead to anemia.

LABORATORY REPORT

Diagnosis: Iron Deficiency Anemia

Measurement	Value	Normal Range
Hematocrit	33ml/100ml	men 40-45 women 36-47
Hemoglobin	10.6g/100 ml	men 14-18 women 12-16
Serum iron	55 ug/100ml	men 75-175 women 65-165
Ferritin	16 ng/ml	men 20-300 women 20-120

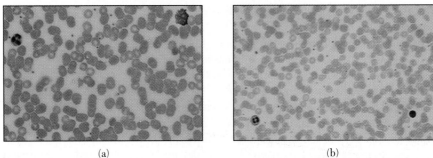

(a)   (b)

FIGURE 11-6

Iron deficiency anemia is diagnosed by low levels of cells or proteins containing iron. It causes the red blood cells to become small and pale. (a) Normal red blood cells. (b) Iron deficiency anemia. (*a*, B & B Photos/Custom Medical Stock; *b*, Custom Medical Stock)

COPPER IN THE DIET

The richest sources of copper in the diet are organ meats such as liver and kidney. Seafood, nuts and seeds, whole grain breads and cereals, and chocolate are also good sources. As with other trace elements, soil content affects the amount of copper in plant foods (Table 11-3).

COPPER IN THE BODY

The absorption of copper is affected by the presence of other minerals and vitamins in the diet. The zinc content of the diet can have a major impact on copper absorption. When zinc intake is high, it stimulates the synthesis of metallothionein in the mucosal cells; however, metallothionein preferentially binds copper rather than zinc. This prevents the copper from being moved out of mucosal cells into the blood.[20] The antagonism of copper absorption by zinc is so great that phytates, which inhibit zinc absorption, actually increase the absorption and utilization of copper. Other factors that affect copper absorption include vitamin C, which decreases absorption,[21] and large doses of antacids, which inhibit copper absorption and over the long term can cause copper deficiency.

Once absorbed, copper binds to albumin, a protein in the blood, and travels to the liver, where it binds to ceruloplasmin for delivery to other tissues. Copper can be removed from the body by secretion in the bile and subsequent elimination in the feces.

Copper functions in a number of important proteins and enzymes that are involved in iron and lipid metabolism, connective tissue synthesis, maintenance of heart muscle, and function of the immune and central nervous systems. It is an

TABLE 11-3   A Summary of Good Dietary Sources of Trace Elements*

	Meat/Fish/ Poultry	Dairy Products	Fruit	Vegetables	Legumes	Nuts/ Seeds	Whole or Enriched Grains	Other
Iron			Dried fruits					Iron cookware
Zinc								
Copper	Organ meats							Chocolate
Manganese								
Selenium	Seafood, organ meats							Eggs
Iodine	Fish, seafood							Iodized salt
Fluoride	Fish with bones							Water, tea, toothpaste
Chromium	Organ meats							Brewer's yeast
Molybdenum	Organ meats							
Boron								Cider, wine, beer
Arsenic	Fish							
Nickel								Chocolate
Silicon				Root vegetables				

*The colored boxes indicate food categories that provide a good source of the mineral.
Exceptional sources within each category are noted. For some minerals, such as iodine and selenium, the amount in plant food depends on the amount in the soil where they were grown.

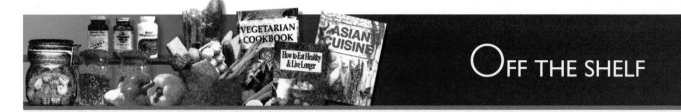

Will Antioxidant Supplements Keep Us Healthy?

Many vitamins, minerals, and enzymes are marketed as antioxidant supplements. These are suggested to boost our antioxidant defenses and keep us healthy. Although antioxidant nutrients are an important part of our defense systems, more is not always better.

The rationale for needing extra antioxidants is based on the fact that we are constantly bombarded with damaging reactive oxygen molecules, such as free radicals, peroxides, and superoxides that come from reactions inside our body or from environmental sources such as air pollution or cigarette smoke. The cumulative effect of these over time plays a role in the aging process and the development of chronic disease.[1] To protect us from oxidative damage, the body is equipped with antioxidant defenses. Some of these are vitamins—vitamin C, beta-carotene, and vitamin E. Others are enzymes—catalase, glutathione peroxidase, and superoxide dismutase. These enzyme systems rely on minerals including zinc, copper, manganese, and selenium for activity. Can supplements of nutrients or enzymes boost our antioxidant defenses?

Each antioxidant in the body acts under specific conditions to destroy particular types of reactive oxygen compounds. Vitamin E, vitamin C, and beta-carotene directly pick up free radicals. Selenium is a part of the antioxidant enzyme glutathione peroxidase, which neutralizes peroxides before they can form dangerous free radicals. The molecule glutathione, which is made of three amino acids, plays an antioxidant role by participating in this reaction. Catalase is an iron-containing enzyme that can also destroy peroxides. Zinc, copper, and manganese are necessary for forms of the enzyme superoxide dismutase, which destroys superoxide free radicals.

Each antioxidant also acts at a specific location inside the body or cell. Antioxidant enzymes are located primarily inside cells, where each patrols a specific cellular compartment. For example, zinc/copper–superoxide dismutase and glutathione peroxidase police the cytoplasm, along with vitamin C. Glutathione peroxidase also acts inside the mitochondria, along with manganese–superoxide dismutase. Catalase acts inside another or-

ganelle, the peroxisome. Vitamin E and beta-carotene are fat soluble nutrients that protect cell membranes. The antioxidant vitamins and the copper-containing protein ceruloplasmin function outside the cells by inactivating free radicals circulating in the blood and body fluids (see figure).

Although scientific evidence confirms the role of certain nutrients as antioxidants, we do not know the optimum dose of each for maximum antioxidant protection. The amounts needed will vary depending on environmental conditions and the health and genetic makeup of the individual. In addition, many of the antioxidant nutrients interact. Therefore a deficiency of one of these nutrients could increase the need for another, and an excess of one may create a deficiency of another. For instance, vitamin C is necessary to regenerate the active form of vitamin E, and vitamin E in turn can spare beta-carotene by protecting it from oxidation. Vitamin E can also help prevent selenium deficiency and vice versa. And excesses of zinc can cause copper deficiency.

If antioxidant vitamins and minerals are deficient in the diet, increas-

essential component of the antioxidant enzyme superoxide dismutase. It plays a role in cholesterol metabolism, and high blood cholesterol levels occur in copper deficiency. It is also needed for the synthesis of the neurotransmitters norepinephrine and dopamine, and may be involved in the synthesis of myelin, which is necessary for transmission of nerve signals.

COPPER DEFICIENCY

A copper deficiency results in anemia. This is due in part to the fact that the copper-containing protein ceruloplasmin is needed for iron transport. In copper deficiency, even if iron is sufficient in the diet, iron cannot be transported out of the intestinal mucosa. Another reason that copper deficiency causes anemia is that the copper-containing enzyme superoxide dismutase protects red blood cells from free radical damage. The third connection between copper and anemia is copper's role in the synthesis of the connective tissue protein collagen. Connective tissue

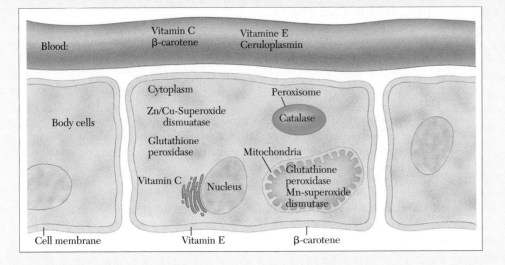

Each of the antioxidant nutrients functions under specific conditions in specific locations.

ing their intake will enhance antioxidant defenses. But whether consumption of these nutrients above the recommended intake will further improve the body's antioxidant defenses is still under investigation. Taking a supplement that contains an antioxidant enzyme like catalase, superoxide dismutase, or glutathione peroxidase will not boost antioxidant defenses because it will not increase the amount of enzyme in the body. Enzymes supplied in the diet,

whether in food or in supplements, are broken down to amino acids and peptides in the gastrointestinal tract.

The total diet is probably more important in health promotion than these nutrients alone. Other components of the diet, such as total fat and fiber intake and other substances in food such as phytochemicals, may be just as important as vitamins and minerals at protecting us from oxidative damage and chronic disease. Based on our current understanding, it is

probably best to boost antioxidant nutrients by eating more fruits and vegetables that are high in beta-carotene and vitamin C and by including foods containing vitamin E, iron, copper, selenium, manganese, and zinc in your diet.

[1]Block, G. The data support a role for antioxidants in reducing cancer risk. Nutr. Rev. 50:207–213, 1992.

cannot form properly when copper is deficient. Because connective tissue strengthens blood vessels, when copper is deficient they are weakened and may rupture, causing blood loss and consequently anemia. Copper's role in the synthesis of connective tissue may also explain the skeletal changes, degeneration of the heart muscle, degeneration of the nervous system, and changes in hair color and structure seen in copper deficiency. A diet low in copper may also decrease the immune response.[22]

HOW MUCH COPPER DO WE NEED?

There is no RDA for copper. The ESADDI is 1.5 to 3.0 mg per day for adults.

The American Academy of Pediatrics recommends that formula-fed newborns consume about 0.4 mg of copper per day. Needs increase throughout childhood until they reach adult levels. Specific recommendations have not been made for pregnancy, lactation, or the elderly.

COPPER TOXICITY

Copper toxicity from dietary sources is extremely rare. No toxicity has been reported from intakes up to 0.5 mg per kilogram of body weight, or about 3.5 mg per day. An occasional intake of up to 10 mg per day is probably safe, but acute doses of greater than 10 to 15 mg may cause vomiting.[23]

MANGANESE (Mn)

Manganese, like copper and zinc, functions in a form of the antioxidant enzyme superoxide dismutase, which protects against damage by free radicals.

The best dietary sources of manganese are whole grains and nuts. Fruits and vegetables are fair sources. Meat, fish, and poultry are poor sources (see Table 11-3).

The absorption of manganese is not well regulated. Instead, body levels are regulated by the excretion of manganese into the intestinal tract in bile. Manganese is involved in carbohydrate and lipid metabolism and brain function. It functions as a constituent of some enzymes and an activator of others.

MANGANESE DEFICIENCY

Manganese deficiency in animals results in growth retardation; reproductive problems; congenital malformations in the offspring; and abnormalities in brain function, bone formation, glucose regulation, and lipid metabolism. Although a naturally occurring manganese deficiency has never been reported in humans, a man participating in a study of vitamin K was inadvertently fed a diet deficient in manganese for 17 weeks.[23] He lost weight, his black hair turned a red color, and he developed dermatitis. Manganese deficiency was further studied in young male volunteers fed a manganese-deficient diet for 39 days. These men developed dermatitis and had altered blood levels of cholesterol, calcium, and phosphorus.[23]

HOW MUCH MANGANESE DO WE NEED?

The ESADDI for manganese is 2 to 5 mg per day for adults. It was established based on the typical intake of manganese, since deficiency does not appear to be a nutritional problem in the United States.

Breast-fed infants consume about 2 μg per day of manganese during the first month of life. This level of intake results in decreases in tissue levels of manganese, but no deficiency symptoms have been reported. Once solid foods are introduced into the infant diet, manganese intake increases.

It is not known if the manganese requirement is increased by pregnancy, but absorption of manganese triples during pregnancy. Since very little manganese is lost in breast milk, it is unlikely that lactation increases needs.

MANGANESE TOXICITY

Toxic levels of manganese result in damage to the nervous system. In humans, toxicity has been reported in manganese mine workers exposed to high concentrations of inhaled manganese dust. Dietary intakes of up to 10 mg per day are considered safe.[23]

SELENIUM (Se)

Like zinc, copper, and manganese, selenium functions in an antioxidant enzyme system. Selenium interacts with vitamin E in protecting the body from oxidative damage. Because of the similar roles of selenium and vitamin E, it has been difficult to separate symptoms of selenium deficiency from those of vitamin E deficiency.

SELENIUM IN THE DIET

Seafood, kidney, liver, and eggs are excellent sources of selenium (see Table 11-3). Fruits, vegetables, and drinking water are generally poor sources of selenium. Grains and seeds can be good sources depending on the selenium content of the soil where they were grown. For example, wheat grown in Kansas has a different selenium content from wheat grown in Michigan. An analysis of bread from different metropolitan areas found a threefold difference in the selenium content.[24] Soil selenium content can have a significant impact on the selenium intake of populations consuming primarily locally grown food.

SELENIUM IN THE BODY

Once selenium is absorbed, homeostasis is maintained by regulating its excretion in the urine. Selenium is an essential part of the enzyme **glutathione peroxidase**. Glutathione peroxidase neutralizes peroxides so they no longer form free radicals, which cause oxidative damage. Selenium can spare some of the requirement for vitamin E, since vitamin E acts by stopping the action of free radicals once they are produced (Figure 11-9). Selenium is also needed for the synthesis of thyroid hormones.[25]

SELENIUM DEFICIENCY

A role for selenium was first recognized by studying animals deficient in vitamin E. Selenium deficiency was not identified in humans until the late 1970s when it was observed in patients fed TPN solutions inadvertently deficient in selenium and in individuals living in a region of China where the soil is selenium deficient. Symptoms of deficiency include muscular discomfort and weakness. A form of heart disease called Keshan's disease may also occur with selenium deficiency. Although selenium is not the only factor involved, symptoms of the disease are relieved by selenium supplementation.[23] Selenium deficiency is not likely to be a problem when the diet includes foods grown in many different locations.

HOW MUCH SELENIUM DO WE NEED?

The RDA for selenium is 55 μg per day for women and 70 μg per day for men. The average adult intake of selenium in the United States exceeds this recommendation but is well within the range considered safe and adequate.[24]

An increase in selenium intake is recommended during pregnancy and lactation. The RDA for infants is 10 μg per day for the first six months of age and 15 μg per day after six months.

SELENIUM SUPPLEMENTS

Selenium supplements are marketed with claims that they will protect against environmental pollutants, prevent cancer and heart disease, slow the aging process, and improve immune function. Although selenium does play a role in these processes, supplements of selenium have not been demonstrated to be of additional benefit. The hypothesis that selenium protects against cancer is based primarily on the increased incidence of certain human cancers in regions where selenium intake is low. Currently there are no data on the effect of selenium supplementation above the recommended intake in preventing cancer.[26] The suggestion that

Glutathione peroxidase—A selenium-containing enzyme that protects cells from oxidative damage by neutralizing peroxides.

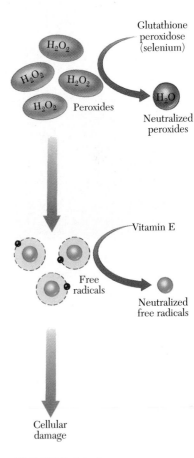

FIGURE II-9
Selenium is a part of the enzyme glutathione peroxidase, which neutralizes peroxides before they form free radicals. This can spare some of the need for vitamin E.

poor selenium status is associated with an increased risk of developing heart disease is also based on epidemiological studies.[27] The mechamism whereby selenium deficiency affects heart disease risk is not known. It is known, however, that selenium status does not increase the risk of cardiovascular disease by affecting serum lipid levels, blood pressure, and body mass index.[28]

SELENIUM TOXICITY

In a region of China with very high selenium soil an intake of 5 mg per day resulted in fingernail changes and hair loss. Selenium toxicity has also been reported in the United States because of a manufacturing error that created mineral supplements containing a dose of 27 mg of selenium per day. Symptoms include nausea, diarrhea, abdominal pain, fingernail and hair changes, nervous system abnormalities, fatigue, and irritability.[23]

IODINE (I)

Iodine is needed for the synthesis of thyroid hormones. One hundred years ago, iodine deficiency was common in the central United States and Canada but it has virtually disappeared due to the addition of iodine to table salt.

IODINE IN THE DIET

Most of the iodine in our diets comes from the sea. There are high concentrations of iodine in seawater, and seafood (Figure 11-10). Plants grown close to the sea are high in iodine. The amount of iodine in plants grown inland depends on the iodine content of the soil.

Iodine in our diet also comes from contaminants and additives in foods. Dairy products accumulate iodine because of the iodine-containing additives used in cattle feed and the use of iodine-containing disinfectants on cows, milking machines, and storage tanks. Iodine-containing sterilizing agents are also used in fast-food restaurants, and iodine is used in dough conditioners and some food colorings. Most of the iodine in the North American diet comes from salt fortified with iodine, referred to as iodized salt. It is commonplace in the United States, and only iodized salt is sold in Canada. Iodized salt should not be confused with sea salt, which is a poor source of iodine because the iodine is lost in the drying process.

IODINE IN THE BODY

Iodine is an essential component of the thyroid hormones, which regulate basal metabolic rate, growth and development, and promote protein synthesis. Iodine along with selenium is essential for the synthesis of the thyroid hormones. If blood levels of the thyroid hormones drop, thyroid-stimulating hormone is released. This hormone signals the thyroid gland to take up iodine and synthesize thyroid hormones. When the supply of iodine is adequate, thyroid hormones can be made and their presence turns off the synthesis of thyroid-stimulating hormone.

IODINE DEFICIENCY

When iodine is deficient, not enough of the thyroid hormones are made to shut off the synthesis of thyroid-stimulating hormone, so it continues to be released and causes the thyroid gland to enlarge, forming a **goiter** (Figure 11-11). Since metabolic rate slows with insufficient thyroid hormone, an iodine deficiency causes fatigue and weight gain.

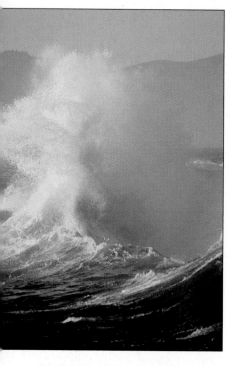

FIGURE 11-10
Most of the iodine in our diet comes from the sea. (Darrell Gulin/Tony Stone Images, Inc.)

Goiter—An enlargement of the thyroid gland that is caused by a deficiency of iodine.

A number of other iodine deficiency disorders occur because of the effect of iodine on growth and development. If iodine is deficient during pregnancy, it increases the risk of stillbirth and spontaneous abortion and can result in a condition in the offspring called **cretinism**. There are a number of forms of cretinism characterized by symptoms such as mental retardation, deaf mutism, and growth failure.[29] Iodine deficiency during childhood and adolescence can result in goiter and impaired mental function.

The risk of iodine deficiency is increased by consuming **goitrogens**, substances in food that interfere with the utilization of iodine or with thyroid function. Goitrogens are found in turnips, rutabaga, cabbage, and cassava. Most are destroyed in cooking or are present in foods that do not play an important role in human diets. However, in countries where cassava is a dietary staple, high goitrogen intake plays a role in the developmental iodine deficiency disorders.[30]

Since it was first used in Switzerland in the 1920s, iodized salt has been the major means of combating iodine deficiency. Because of the fortification of table salt with iodine, cretinism and goiter are now rare in North America, though more than 1 billion people worldwide are still believed to be at risk of iodine deficiency.[29] Problems in producing iodized salt and convincing people to use it have limited its effectiveness in the prevention of iodine deficiency in some areas.[31] For example, the people in certain provinces in China won't use iodized salt, since they prefer to use desert salt. Other forms of iodine supplementation, such as injections of iodized oil, may be more effective in these populations.

HOW MUCH IODINE DO WE NEED?

The current intake of iodine in North America exceeds the RDA of 150 μg per day. This amount is considered safe, but it is recommended that no new sources of iodine be introduced into the American diet.[23]

Iodine needs are increased during pregnancy and lactation. The recommended intake for infants is 40 μg, an amount that is easily obtained from breast milk or formula. The recommended intake is not different for the elderly.

IODINE TOXICITY

Acute toxicity can occur with very large doses of iodine. Intakes between 200 and 500 mg per kilogram of body weight have caused death in laboratory animals.[23] Chronically high intakes of iodine can cause an enlargement of the thyroid gland that resembles goiter. This can also occur if iodine intake changes drastically. For example, in a population with a marginal intake, a large increase in intake due to supplementation can cause thyroid enlargement even at levels that would not be toxic in a healthy population. Generally, doses of 2 mg or less per day have no toxic effects.

FLUORIDE (F)

The importance of fluoride for dental health has been recognized since the 1930s, when an association between the fluoride content of drinking water and the prevalence of dental caries was noted.

FLUORIDE IN THE DIET

Fluoride is present in small amounts in almost all soil, water, plants, and animals. The richest dietary sources of fluoride are water, tea, and marine fish consumed with their bones (Figure 11-12). In countries that consume large amounts of tea, it contributes significantly to total fluoride intake. In the United States, most of the fluoride in the diet comes from toothpaste and from fluoride added to the

Cretinism–A condition resulting from poor maternal iodine intake during pregnancy that causes stunted growth and poor mental development in offspring.

Goitrogens–Substances that interfere with the utilization of iodine or the function of the thyroid gland.

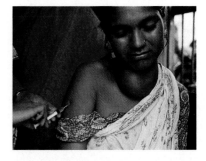

FIGURE 11-11
Iodine deficiency causes enlargement of the thyroid gland, a condition called goiter. (John Paul Kay/Peter Arnold, Inc.)

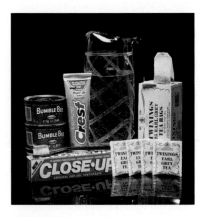

FIGURE 11-12
Dietary sources of fluoride include water, tea, fish eaten with bones, and toothpaste. (Charles D. Winters)

Iodine: Can Environmental Iodine Meet Our Needs?

Should you buy iodized salt? Do you get enough iodine in the foods you eat? Currently most people in the United States consume more than enough iodine. Yet 100 years ago, goiter was endemic in the central United States and Canada. Do we still need iodized salt?

The iodine in our food and in our bodies comes from the earth's soil and the sea. After the earth was formed, soil was high in iodine. Over time large amounts of iodine have been washed out of the soil in some regions by glaciers, snow, rain, and flood waters. The iodine washed from the soil has accumulated in the oceans of the world. Therefore, mountainous areas, such as the Himalayas, Andes, and Alps, and river valleys that repeatedly flood, such as the Ganges in India, have little iodine left in the soil. Soils in coastal regions are richer in iodine.

The iodine in soil and water is present as iodide ions. When these come in contact with sunlight, they are oxidized to form iodine, which can escape into the air. Every year ap-

proximately 400,000 tons of iodine escapes into the atmosphere from the ocean surface. The iodine in the atmosphere is returned to the soil in rain, but the return is slow and the amounts returned to the soil are small. In areas where the forces of nature have resulted in iodine-deficient soil, the iodine deposited from rain will be washed away again by these same forces. Therefore iodine-deficient soil will remain deficient. The iodine content of plants grown in iodine-deficient soil may be 100 times less than those grown in iodine-rich soil.[1] Areas where the soil is depleted of iodine and that rely primarily on locally grown food, such as parts of Asia, have a high incidence of iodine deficiency. In such areas iodine deficiency will continue to be a problem unless iodine is supplemented or the diet is diversified to include foods grown outside the iodine-deficient area.

In the United States, iodine deficiency is now rare. We consume a variety of foods from across the country and around the world. In addition to

iodine from plants grown in iodine-rich soils, we get iodine from the contamination of foods with iodine-containing food additives, food processing, and cleaning solutions. Does this mean that we are getting enough iodine from our environment without iodized salt? Should you choose iodized or non-iodized salt in the grocery store? In Canada there is no choice; all salt is iodized. In the United States, if you live inland where the soil is deficient in iodine, eat little seafood, and consume primarily foods grown locally, iodized salt is the best choice. If you live on the coast and buy your food in a supermarket, you are unlikely to be iodine deficient even if you choose non-iodized salt. But because the risks of consuming the amounts of iodine added to salt are small, if you are not sure, choose iodized.

[1] Clugston, G.A. and Hertzel, B.S. Iodine. In *Modern Nutrition in Health and Disease*, 8th ed. Shils, M.E., Olson, J.A. and Shike, M., eds. Philadelphia: Lea & Febiger, 1994, pp. 252–263.

water supply—usually 0.7 to 1.2 mg per liter. Since food readily absorbs the fluoride in cooking water, the fluoride content of food can be significantly increased when it is handled and prepared using fluoridated water. Cooking utensils also affect food fluoride content. Foods cooked with Teflon utensils can pick up fluoride from the Teflon, whereas aluminum cookware can decrease fluoride content. Fluoride is absorbed into the body in proportion to its content in the diet.

FLUORIDE IN THE BODY

The mechanism whereby fluoride reduces cavities is not fully understood, but it is thought to be related to the incorporation of fluoride into the tooth enamel. Fluoride forms the compound **fluoroapatite**, which is more resistant to acid than the hydroxyapatite crystals it replaces. Fluoride has its greatest effect on caries prevention early in life during maximal tooth development (up to the age of eight), but it has been shown to have some effect in adults.[23] It has also been suggested that fluoride strengthens bones in adults. A slow-release fluoride supplement ad-

Fluoroapatite—Fluoride-containing mineral deposits in the tooth enamel that are resistant to acid.

ministered with calcium has been found to increase bone mass and prevent new fractures.[32]

HOW MUCH FLUORIDE DO WE NEED?

For adults, an ESADDI of 1.5 to 4 mg per day has been established. For children the maximum intake should be 2.5 mg per day.

Breast milk is low in fluoride, and ready-made infant formulas are prepared with unfluoridated water. Unless infant formula is prepared at home with fluoridated water, it contains little fluoride. The American Academy of Pediatrics suggests a supplement of 0.25 mg per day for infants and children up to the age of two years who are receiving less than 0.3 mg per liter of fluoride in the water supply. Swallowed toothpaste can account for much of the fluoride consumed by children under the age of four.[33]

The fluoridation of public drinking water to prevent dental caries began in Grand Rapids, Michigan, in 1945. Today, about half of all the drinking water in the United States is fluoridated. Despite epidemiological evidence showing that the risks of consuming these small amounts of fluoride are slight, some people believe that it represents a public health hazard. A federal study has shown a very weak association between fluoride and bone cancer in male rats.[34] However, a Public Health Service review of epidemiological studies over the past 40 years found no evidence linking the levels of fluoride in water to bone cancer in humans.[34]

FLUORIDE TOXICITY

Fluoride can be toxic in high doses. Fluoride intakes of 2 to 8 mg per day can cause mottled teeth in children. A recent increase in the prevalence of this condition in the United States has occurred due to the chronic ingestion of toothpaste containing fluoride.[33] Doses of 20 to 80 mg per day in adults can result in changes in bone health, kidney function, and possibly nerve and muscle function. Death was reported with an intake of 5 to 10 grams per day.

CHROMIUM (Cr)

Chromium is essential for the transport of glucose into cells.

CHROMIUM IN THE DIET

Dietary sources of chromium include liver, brewer's yeast, nuts, and whole grains. Milk, vegetables, and fruit are poor sources. Refined carbohydrates such as white breads, pasta, and white rice are also poor sources because chromium is lost in milling and not added back in the enrichment process. Chromium intake can be increased by cooking in stainless steel cookware, because chromium leaches from the steel into the food.

CHROMIUM IN THE BODY

In general, chromium is poorly absorbed; however, absorption increases when chromium intake is low.

Chromium is part of a glucose tolerance factor necessary for the transport of glucose into cells, but the exact mechanism is not known. A role for chromium in the development of noninsulin-dependent diabetes and glucose intolerance has been suggested but has not been firmly established.[35]

CHROMIUM DEFICIENCY

Deficiencies have been reported in patients on long-term TPN not containing chromium and in malnourished children. Symptoms include impaired glucose tolerance with diabetes-like symptoms, such as elevated blood glucose levels and increased insulin levels. Chromium deficiency may also be associated with elevated blood cholesterol and triglyceride levels, but the role of chromium in lipid metabolism is not fully understood.[35]

HOW MUCH CHROMIUM DO WE NEED?

The ESADDI for chromium is 50 to 200 μg per day for adults.[23] This level is recommended based on the fact that no deficiency signs have been reported in American populations consuming around 50 μg, and likewise no adverse affects have been reported in studies with daily intakes of 200 μg.

CHROMIUM SUPPLEMENTS

Chromium supplements, marketed as chromium picolinate, have been promoted recently to reduce body fat and increase lean body tissue. This appeals to individuals wanting to lose weight as well as to athletes trying to build muscle. Since chromium is needed for insulin action and insulin promotes protein synthesis, it is likely that chromium is necessary for an increase in lean body mass. However, research in humans has not shown chromium picolinate supplements to affect muscle strength or body composition.[36] No dietary toxicity has been reported in humans, but with the increased popularity of chromium supplements, toxicity symptoms may become evident.[37]

MOLYBDENUM (Mo)

Like many other trace elements, molybdenum is needed to activate enzymes. The molybdenum content of food varies with the molybdenum content of the soil where the food is produced. The most reliable sources include milk, milk products, organ meats, breads, cereals, and legumes.

Molybdenum is readily absorbed from foods. The amount in the body is regulated by excretion in the urine and bile. Molybdenum is necessary for the production of uric acid and the oxidation and detoxification of various other compounds.

Although molybdenum deficiency in humans has been reported as a result of long-term TPN, a naturally occurring deficiency has never been reported. Deficiency has been induced in laboratory animals by feeding high doses of tungsten, which inhibits molybdenum absorption. The resulting deficiency caused growth retardation, decreased food intake, impaired reproduction, and decreased life expectancy.

Based on estimates of molybdenum intake in the American diet, the ESADDI has been set at 75 to 250 μg per day for adults.[22]

In a region with high environmental molybdenum, intake is 10 to 15 mg per day. This high intake has been associated with goutlike symptoms such as arthritis and inflammation of the joints. Molybdenum also interacts with copper, and levels of 500 μg per day have been associated with increased excretion of copper in the urine.[22]

A summary of the sources, recommended intakes, functions, deficiencies, and toxicities of the trace elements is given in Table 11-4.

9. Give two reasons why a deficiency of copper can contribute to anemia.
10. What is the role of selenium in the body?
11. Why does selenium decrease the need for vitamin E?
12. What is a goiter and what causes it?

13. How does fluoride help prevent dental caries?
14. What is the role of chromium in the body?
15. How are needs estimated for trace elements for which no function has yet been identified?

APPLICATIONS

These exercises are designed to help you apply your critical thinking skills to your own nutrition choices. Many are best performed using a diet analysis software program. If you do not have access to a computer program, the exercises can be hand calculated using the information in this text and its appendices.

1. Using the three-day food intake record you kept in Chapter 1.
   a. Calculate your average daily intake of iron?
   b. How does your iron intake compare with the recommendation for someone of your age and sex?
   c. If your intake is low, modify your diet to meet your RDA for iron.
   d. If your diet already meets the recommendations for iron, make a list of foods you like that are high in iron.
   e. Identify the major food sources of iron in your diet and indicate whether they contribute heme iron.
2. Using your food record, calculate your zinc intake.
   a. If you eliminated meat from your diet, would you meet the RDA for zinc?
   b. What foods could you substitute for meat that would allow you to meet the RDA?
3. Does your water supply contain fluoride?

REFERENCES

1. Mertz, W. Essential trace metals: new definitions based on new paradigms. Nutr. Rev. 51:287–295, 1993.
2. Bothwell, T.H. Overview and mechanisms of iron regulation. Nutr. Rev. 53:237–245, 1995.
3. Whiting, S.J. The inhibitory effect of dietary calcium on iron bioavailability: a cause for concern? Nutr. Rev. 53:77–80, 1995.
4. Chesters, J.K. Trace element–gene interactions. Nutr. Rev. 50:217–223, 1992.
5. *Healthy People 2000: National Health Promotion and Disease Prevention Objectives.* Washington, DC: U.S. Department of Health and Human Services, 1991.
6. Weaver, C. and Rajaram, S. Exercise and iron status: nutrition and exercise symposium. J. Nutr. 122:782–787, 1992.
7. Lynch, S.R. Iron overload: prevalence and impact on health. Nutr. Rev. 53:255–260, 1995.
8. Gordeuk, V., Mukiibi, J., Hasstedt, S.J., et al. Iron overload in Africa. Interaction between a gene and dietary iron content. N. Engl. J. Med. 326:95–100, 1992.
9. Salonen, J.T., Nyyssonen, K., Korpela, H., et al. High stored iron levels are associated with excess risk of myocardial infarction in Eastern Finnish men. Circulation 86:803–811, 1992.
10. Baer, D.M., Tekawa, I.S., and Hurley, L.B. Iron stores are not associated with acute myocardial infarction. Circulation 89:2915–2918, 1994.
11. Sempos, C.T., Looker, A.C., Gillum, R.F., and Makuc, D.M. Body iron stores and the risk of coronary heart disease. N. Engl. J. Med. 330:1119–1124, 1994.
12. Stampfer, M.J., Colditz, G.A., Willett, W.C., et al. Postmenopausal estrogen therapy and cardiovascular disease—ten-year follow up from the Nurses' Health Study. N. Engl. J. Med. 325:756–762, 1991.
13. Ascherio, A., Walter, C.W., Rimm, E.B., et al. Dietary iron intake and risk of coronary disease among men. Circulation 89:969–974, 1994.
14. King, J.C. and Keen, C.L. Zinc. In *Modern Nutrition in Health and Disease*, 8th ed. Shils, M.E., Olson, J.A., and Shike, M., eds. Philadelphia: Lea & Febiger, 1994, pp. 214–230.
15. Prasad, A.S. Discovery of human zinc deficiency and studies in an experimental human model. Am. J. Clin. Nutr. 53:403–412, 1991.
16. Aggett, P.J. and Comerford, J.G. Zinc and human health. Nutr. Rev. 53:S16–S22, 1995.
17. Boukaiba, N., Flament, C., Acher, S., et al. A physiologic amount of zinc supplementation: effects on nutritional, lipid, and thymic status in an elderly population. Am. J. Clin. Nutr. 57:566–572, 1993.
18. Bogden, J.D. Studies on micronutrient supplements and immunity in older people. Nutr. Rev. 53:S59–S65, 1995.
19. Fosmire, G.J. Zinc toxicity. Am. J. Clin. Nutr. 51:225–227, 1990.
20. Turnlund, J.R. Copper. In *Modern Nutrition in Health and Disease*, 8th ed. Shils, M.E., Olson, J.A., and Shike, M., eds. Philadelphia: Lea & Febiger, 1994, pp. 231–241.
21. O'Dell, B.L. Dietary carbohydrate source and copper bioavailability. Nutr. Rev. 48:425–434, 1990.
22. Kelley, D.S., Daudu, P.A., Taylor, P.C., et al. Effects of low-copper diets on human immune response. Am. J. Clin. Nutr. 62:412–416, 1995.
23. National Research Council, Food and Nutrition Board. *Recommended Dietary Allowances*, 10th ed. Washington, DC: National Academy Press, 1989.
24. Levander, O.A. Scientific rationale for the 1989 Recommended Dietary Allowance for selenium. J. Am. Diet. Assoc. 91:1572–1576, 1991.
25. Arthur, J.R., Nicol, F., and Beckett, G.J. Selenium deficiency, thyroid hormone metabolism and thyroid hormone deiodinases. Am. J. Clin. Nutr. 57:236–239, 1993.

26. Barber, D.A. and Harris, S.R. Oxygen free radicals and antioxidants: a review. Am. Pharm. 34:26–35, 1994.

27. Oster, O. and Prellwitz, W. Selenium and cardiovascular disease. Biol. Trace Elem. Res. 24:91–103, 1990.

28. Bukkens, S.G., deVos, N., Koh, F.J., et al. Selenium status and cardiovascular disease risk factors in healthy Dutch subjects. J. Am. Coll. Nutr. 9:128–135, 1990.

29. Clugston, G.A. and Hetzel, B.S. Iodine. In *Modern Nutrition in Health and Disease*, 8th ed. Shils, M.E., Olson, J.A., and Shike, M., eds. Philadelphia: Lea & Febiger, 1994, pp. 252–263.

30. Delange, F. The disorders induced by iodine deficiency. Thyroid 4:107–128, 1994.

31. Hetzel, B.S. Iodine deficiency: an international public health problem. In *Present Knowledge in Nutrition*, 6th ed. Brown, M.L., ed. Washington, DC: International Life Sciences Institute—Nutrition Foundation, 1990, pp. 308–313.

32. Pak, C.Y., Sakhaee, K., Adams-Huet, B., et al. Treatment of postmenopausal osteoporosis with slow-release sodium fluoride. Final report of a randomized trial. Ann. Intern. Med. 123:401–408, 1995.

33. Newbrun, E. Current regulations and recommendations concerning water fluoridation, fluoride supplements, and topical fluoride agents. J. Dent. Res. 71:1255–1265, 1993.

34. Anonymous. Government assesses fluoride. FDA Consumer 25:4, May, 1991.

35. Mertz, W. Chromium in human nutrition: a review. J. Nutr. 123:626–633, 1993.

36. Clancy, S.P., Clarkson, P.M., DeCheke, M.E., et al. Effects of chromium picolinate supplementation on body composition, strength, and urinary chromium loss in football players. Int. J. Sport Nutr. 4:142–153, 1994.

37. Huszonek, J. Over-the-counter chromium picolinate. Am. J. Psychiatry 150:1560–1561, 1993.

38. Mertz, W. Risk assessment of essential trace elements: new approaches to setting recommended dietary allowances and safe limits. Nutr. Rev. 53:179–185, 1995.

39. Volpe, S.L., Taper, L.J., and Meacham, S. The relationship between boron and magnesium status and bone mineral density in the human: a review. Magnes. Res. 6:291–296, 1993.

40. Nielsen, F.H. Nutritional requirements for boron, silicon, vanadium, nickel and arsenic: current knowledge and speculation. FASEB J. 5:2661–2667, 1991.

41. Mertz, W., Abernathy, C.O., and Olin, S.S., eds. *Risk Assessment of Essential Elements*. Washington, DC: ILSI Press, 1994.

Regular aerobic exercise strengthens heart muscle and increases stroke volume, which is the amount of blood pumped with each beat of the heart. This decreases **resting heart rate**, the rate at which the heart must beat to supply blood to the tissues at rest. Resting heart rate can be estimated by measuring one's pulse (Figure 12-1). The more fit one is, the lower the resting heart rate and pulse and the more activity that can be performed before reaching **maximum heart rate**. Maximum heart rate is the maximum number of beats per minute that the heart can attain. It is dependent on age and can be estimated by subtracting one's age from 220.

Aerobic exercise also increases **maximal oxygen consumption**, or **VO_2 max**, the maximum amount of oxygen that can be consumed by the tissues during exercise. VO_2 max is dependent on the ability of the cardiorespiratory system to deliver oxygen to the cells and the ability of the cells to use oxygen to produce energy. The greater one's VO_2 max, the more intense activity one can perform before a lack of oxygen affects performance. VO_2 max can be determined in an exercise laboratory by measuring oxygen uptake during exercise, using the following equation:

$$\text{Oxygen inhaled} - \text{Oxygen exhaled} = \text{Oxygen uptake}$$

For example, to measure VO_2 max, an individual may be asked to run on a treadmill. The workload would then be increased by increasing the speed and/or grade of the treadmill until the individual can no longer continue (Figure 12-2). The amount of oxygen consumed at the highest workload achieved is the VO_2 max. A trained athlete will have a greater VO_2 max than an untrained individual.

Muscle Strength and Endurance   Muscle strength and endurance enhance the ability to perform tasks such as pushing or lifting. In daily life, this could mean lifting a bag of groceries, unscrewing the lid of a jar, or shoveling snow from your driveway. Muscle strength and endurance are increased by repeatedly using muscles in activities that require moving against a resistance. This type of exercise is called strength-training or resistance-training exercise and includes activities such as weight lifting.

Resting heart rate–The number of times that the heart beats per minute while a person is at rest.

Maximum heart rate–The maximum number of beats per minute that the heart can attain. It declines with age and can be estimated by subtracting age in years from 220.

Maximal oxygen consumption, or **VO_2 max**–The maximal amount of oxygen that can be consumed by the tissues during exercise.

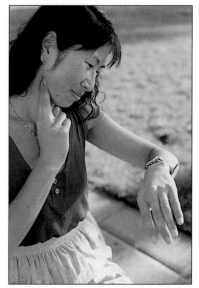

FIGURE 12-1
Heart rate can be estimated by feeling the pulse at the side of the neck just below the jaw bone. A pulse is caused by the heart beating and forcing blood through the arteries. The number of pulses per minute equals heart rate. (© Michael Newman/Photo Edit)

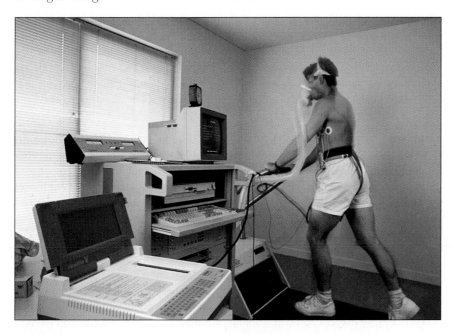

FIGURE 12-2
Maximal oxygen consumption can be estimated by measuring oxygen uptake while running to exhaustion on a treadmill. (Jon Love/The Image Bank)

Flexibility Flexibility determines range of motion—how far one can bend and stretch muscles and ligaments. If flexibility is poor, you cannot easily bend to tie your shoes or stretch to remove packages from the car. Regularly moving the limbs, neck, and torso through their full ranges of motion helps increase and maintain flexibility.

Desirable Body Composition A regular program of balanced physical activity helps to limit or reduce body fat and maintain or increase lean tissue. Individuals who are physically fit have a greater proportion of lean body tissue than unfit individuals of the same body weight.

THE HEALTH BENEFITS OF EXERCISE

In addition to making the tasks of everyday life easier, fitness through regular activity offers many health benefits. A regular exercise program can make it easier to maintain a healthy body weight. It can help to prevent or delay the onset of cardiovascular disease, hypertension, diabetes, and osteoporosis,[1,2] and may reduce the risk of certain cancers.[3] Regular exercise may improve sleep and overall mood, and it can even increase longevity.[4]

Preventing and Treating Obesity Exercise makes weight maintenance easier and is an essential component of any weight-reduction program. Exercise promotes the loss of body fat and slows the rate of lean tissue loss that occurs with energy restriction.[5] Exercise also increases energy expenditure both by increasing the amount of energy used for activity and by affecting basal metabolic rate.[6] Exercise increases metabolic rate for a number of hours after exercise stops; however, with light to moderate exercise the increase is too small to have a significant effect on energy balance or weight loss.[7] Since an increase in the proportion of lean body mass increases BMR, the long-term, and more significant, effect that regular exercise has on metabolic rate is due to increased lean body mass.[8]

Cardiovascular Disease Exercise reduces the risk of cardiovascular disease.[4] Individuals who do not exercise have an increased risk of cardiovascular disease similar to the risks incurred by elevated blood pressure, high blood cholesterol, or cigarette smoking.[9] Aerobic exercise strengthens the heart muscle, thereby reducing resting heart rate and decreasing the workload on the heart. Exercise may also lower blood pressure and increase HDL cholesterol levels in the blood.

Diabetes People with excess body fat are more likely to develop diabetes. By keeping body fat within the normal range, aerobic exercise can decrease the risk of developing diabetes. Aerobic exercise also benefits individuals with diabetes. Exercise and the reduction in body fat it promotes increase the sensitivity of tissues to insulin.[10] This may reduce or eliminate the need for medication to maintain normal blood glucose levels. People with diabetes should develop exercise programs with the help of physicians and dietitians because exercise can affect diet and any medication needs.

Osteoporosis and Joint Disorders Exercise reduces the risk of osteoporosis. One of the causes of bone loss, like muscle loss, is lack of use; therefore, weight-bearing exercise such as walking, running, and aerobic dance can prevent bone loss and even increase bone mass. Exercise can also benefit individuals with arthritis because the strength and flexibility promoted by exercise helps arthritic joints move more easily.

Cancer   Individuals who exercise regularly may be reducing their cancer risk. The evidence is strongest for colon and breast cancer. Studies have found that physically active individuals are less likely to develop colon cancer than their sedentary counterparts,[11,12] and that more physically active women have a decreased risk of breast cancer.[13] When evaluating the impact of exercise on cancer risk, diet and other lifestyle factors must be carefully considered. It is possible that some of the effect is due to the fact that people who exercise regularly are more likely to have healthier overall diets and lifestyles.

Exercise Can Slow the Changes That Occur with Age   As we age, many physiological changes occur, including a decrease in lean body mass, muscle strength and endurance, and cardiorespiratory endurance (see Chapter 15). Regular physical activity can prevent or slow some of these changes. For example, a program of regular exercise that includes strength training can prevent the reduction in lean body mass and maintain muscle strength and endurance,[14] and regular aerobic exercise can increase cardiorespiratory endurance.

Exercise Benefits Children   The health of our children tomorrow may depend on their fitness today. Healthy children should be encouraged to engage in regular physical activity, with the goal of adopting appropriate lifelong exercise behaviors. Healthy People 2000 recommends that by the year 2000, 75% of children should engage in at least 20 minutes of exercise three times per week and 50% of school-age children should participate in a physical education class every school day. To promote this amount of exercise, enjoyable activities should be stressed and competition de-emphasized. Learning by example is always best. Children who have physically active parents are the leanest and the fittest. Television is an important cause of inactivity among children. Children today spend more time watching TV than at any activity, other than sleeping.[15] Watching television takes time away from more strenuous activities and may promote the consumption of foods high in fat, salt, and refined sugars (see Chapter 14).

Psychological Benefits of Exercise   In addition to its other benefits, exercise can improve sleep patterns and overall outlook on life. During exercise, the release of chemicals called endorphins is stimulated. Endorphins are thought to be natural tranquilizers that play a role in triggering what athletes describe as an "exercise high." In addition to causing this state of exercise euphoria, endorphins are thought to aid in relaxation; improve mood, pain tolerance, and appetite control; and reduce anxiety.

AN EXERCISE PROGRAM FOR YOU

Despite the increasing popularity of exercise in recent years, too few Americans get enough exercise. It is estimated that 25% of the population gets little or no exercise, and less than 10% of people exercise enough to improve cardiorespiratory fitness. One of the goals of Healthy People 2000 is to get more people to be more active more of the time.[1]

Almost everyone can participate in some form of exercise, no matter where they live, how old they are, or what physical limitations they might have. Exercise classes are taught in retirement homes. Heart patients, amputees, the blind, and those confined to wheelchairs compete in athletic events. You are never too old to exercise, and it is never too late to start.

Components of a Good Exercise Regimen   The American College of Sports Medicine recommends structuring an exercise program to include aerobic

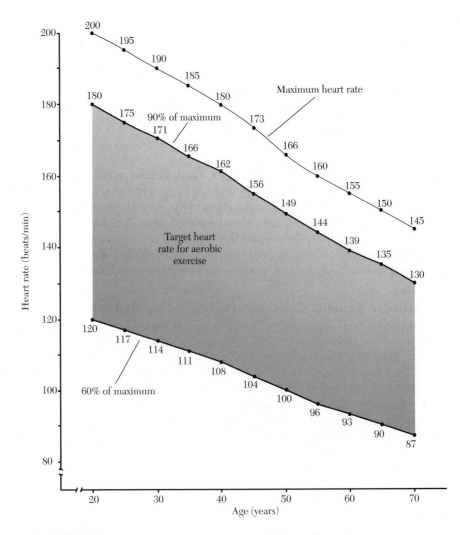

F I G U R E   1 2 - 3
The orange area represents the target heart rate for aerobic exercise—between 60 and
90% of maximum heart rate. Exercise performed at this level will benefit health.
(Adapted from McArdle, W.D., Katch, F.I., and Katch, V.L. *Exercise Physiology: Energy,
Nutrition, and Human Performance*, 3rd ed. Philadelphia: Lea & Febiger, 1991.)

exercise, which raises heart rate and therefore improves cardiorespiratory fitness;
stretching, which promotes and maintains flexibility; and strength training, which
enhances the strength and endurance of specific muscles.[5] Aerobic exercise, such
as walking, jogging, skating, swimming, or bicycling, should be performed for
about 20 to 60 minutes three to five days per week. For optimal benefit, aerobic
activity should be performed at a level that raises the heart rate to 60 to 90%
of maximum. For example, a 35-year-old would have a maximum heart rate of
220 − 35, or 185 beats per minute. For this individual, 60 to 90% of maximum is
111 to 166 beats per minute (Figure 12-3). For a sedentary individual beginning
an exercise program, mild exercise such as walking can raise heart rate into this
range. As fitness improves, exercisers must perform more intense activity to raise
their heart rates to this level.

Stretching exercises should be done at least three days a week. Muscles should
be stretched to a position of mild discomfort and held for 10 to 30 seconds. Each
stretch should be repeated three to five times. Areas that are particularly important
to stretch are the lower back and thigh areas.

Strength training, such as weight lifting, should be done two to three days a
week at the start of an exercise program, and two days a week after desired strength

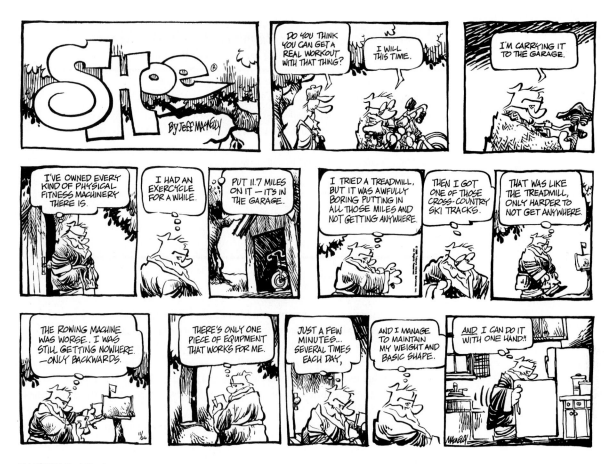

FIGURE 12-4
Many people find it difficult to maintain an exercise regimen. (Reprinted by permission: Tribune Media Services)

has been obtained. This can be done with weights or with resistance-exercise machines, which allow you to exercise specific muscles. Each session should include a minimum of 8 to 10 exercises that train the major muscle groups. Each exercise should be repeated 8 to 12 times. The weights should be heavy enough to cause the muscle to be near exhaustion after the 8 to 12 repetitions. If the weight is too light, the lifting will not build strength.

Getting Started   Incorporating exercise into day-to-day life requires a behavior change, and changing behavior is not easy. Changing exercise behavior involves recognizing the reasons for not exercising and identifying ways to overcome them. Many people don't exercise because they don't enjoy it, feel they have to join an expensive health club, don't have the motivation to do it alone, or find it inconvenient and uncomfortable (Figure 12-4). Finding a type of exercise that is enjoyable, a time for exercise that is realistic and convenient, and a place to exercise that is safe are important first steps in adopting a pattern of increased exercise. Special clothes and large amounts of time and money are not needed. Parking the car farther from the shopping mall, walking the dog more often, and taking the stairs at work are all effective ways to increase your activity level. Behavioral strategies such as those listed in Table 12-1 may help promote regular exercise.

Exercising Safely   Safety should be a concern in planning any exercise regimen. Before beginning, individuals should check with their physicians to be sure that their plans are safe, considering their medical histories. To decrease the risk of injury, each exercise session should begin with a warm-up to increase blood

TABLE 12-1	Behavior Modification for Beginning and Maintaining an Exercise Program

1. **Start slowly**—Instead of planning to run three miles a day five days a week, plan to start with a 20-minute walk three days a week.

2. **Make it fun**—Choose activities you enjoy and find a partner with whom to exercise.

3. **Set specific attainable goals**—"I will walk for 20 minutes on Mondays, Wednesdays, and Fridays."

4. **Make it convenient**—Plan to walk early in the morning, during your lunch hour at work, or after dinner.

5. **Record your progress**—Keep a record of your activity so you can track your progress and keep yourself motivated.

6. **Reward yourself**—Plan to reward yourself when you succeed at your goal: a new book, a movie.

flow to the muscles. A warm-up might include a few minutes of mild stretching and some easy walking or jogging. Other components of safety should also be considered. Busy work schedules often force people to exercise in the dark early morning or evening hours. A safe, well-lit location should be found for exercise. Exercisers who use the street for walking or jogging should wear light-colored, reflective clothing so they can be seen by motorists. Exercising with a partner is safer and more enjoyable.

Temperature is also a concern. Extreme heat or cold can cause problems for exercisers. Physical activity produces heat, which normally is dissipated to the environment by the evaporation of sweat. When the environmental temperature or humidity is high, sweat evaporates slowly, making it difficult to cool the body. Exercise should be reduced or curtailed in hot and humid conditions. Cold environments may also pose problems for the outdoor exerciser. In general, cold does not impair exercise capacity, but the numbing of exposed flesh and the bulk of extra clothing can be problems for joggers and bicyclists. Because exercise produces heat, clothing must allow for evaporation of sweat while providing protection from the cold. For swimmers, cold water can cause a deterioration in performance.

Environmental conditions can pose particular risks for young exercisers. Hot environments are of concern because children produce more heat, are less able to transfer heat from muscles to the skin, and sweat less than adults. To reduce risks to children, they should rest periodically in the shade, consume fluids frequently, and limit the intensity and duration of activities until they are acclimatized.[16] Children lose more heat in cold environments than adults because they have a greater surface area per unit of body weight. Therefore, they are more prone to **hypothermia**. Swimming in cold water can be a particular problem for young children.

Hypothermia–A condition in which body temperature drops below normal. Hypothermia depresses the central nervous system, resulting in the inability to shiver, sleepiness, and eventually coma.

CRITICAL THINKING

Incorporating Exercise into Your Life

Nicole recently turned 45 years old. Her promise to herself was to get back in shape. She is 5 feet 4 inches tall and weighs 140 pounds. Although her weight is still within the healthy weight ranges suggested by the *Dietary Guidelines*, she is above her usual weight. Currently Nicole exercises about once a month, and then suffers from a few days of sore muscles. When the family goes on outings, she finds that she tires long before her husband and children. She would like to lose a few pounds, but more importantly she would like to increase her strength and endurance.

Before beginning her exercise program she checks with her physician, who agrees that she should increase her exercise and recommends that she do stretching and strength-training exercise as well as aerobic activities that increase her heart rate to 60 to 90% of her maximum.

What is 60 to 90% of Nicole's maximum heart rate?

Maximum heart rate = 220 − age = 220 − 45 = 175 beats per minute

60% of maximum 175 × 0.6 = 105 beats per minute

90% of maximum 175 × 0.9 = 158 beats per minute

She should exercise at a heart rate of at least 105 but no more than 158 beats per minute.

Nicole's fitness plan

Nicole decides she will exercise for 90 minutes a day, 5 days a week. Her plan is to join a gym and stretch and lift weights for 30 minutes, followed by an hour of aerobic exercise outdoors, either jogging or riding a bicycle in the park.

After three days on her new schedule, a rainy day keeps Nicole indoors. She realizes that her family is angry and feels abandoned. She hasn't been able to do an hour of aerobics without exceeding her maximum heart rate. She is tired, sore, and ready to give up and accept the fact that she is just not an athletic person.

Where did she go wrong?

It is unrealistic to go from exercising one day a month to five days a week. She needs an exercise program that will fit easily into her daily routine, without drastically changing her schedule. It is unnecessary to lift weights five days a week to gain muscle strength, and she can reach 60 to 90% of her maximum heart rate by walking quickly. A more achievable goal might be a stretching routine at home, three days of walking for 20 to 60 minutes at a moderate rate and two weight-lifting sessions per week. She can increase the frequency and duration of her program as her strength and endurance improve. She also needs to make alternative plans for bad weather and allow time for warming up and cooling down in order to exercise safely.

Nicole's new fitness plan

She continues her gym membership but only goes to lift weights two evenings a week, when her husband can watch the children. As a treat afterwards she relaxes in the whirlpool before showering and returning home. She shares her story with a friend at work, and they decide to walk during their lunch hour three days a week. As their fitness improves, they walk faster to keep their heart rate between 60 and 90% of maximum to improve cardiovascular fitness.

How has this change in activity affected Nicole's energy needs for the day?

On the three days a week when she walks she replaces 1 hour of sitting with an hour of walking, increasing her energy expenditure by 223 kcalories (see Table 12-2).

$$1 \text{ hour of walking} = 307 \text{ kcal}$$

$$1 \text{ hour of sitting} = 84 \text{ kcal}$$

$$\text{Increase in energy expenditure} = 307 \text{ kcal} - 84 \text{ kcal} = 223 \text{ kcal}$$

On days that Nicole goes to the gym she spends 15 minutes weight lifting (330 kcal per hour × 0.25 hour = 82 kcal). This replaces 15 minutes of very light activity at only about 28 kcalories, so she expends an extra 54 kcalories. During the week she therefore expends an extra 777 kcalories (223 kcal × 3 days of walking + 54 kcal × 2 days of weight lifting).

If Nicole's food intake does not increase, how long will it take for her to lose 5 pounds?

Answer:

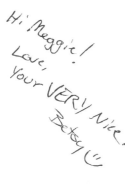

FUELING ACTIVITY

Just as an automobile engine runs on energy from gasoline, the body machine runs on energy from the carbohydrate, fat, and protein in food and body stores. These fuels are needed whether you are writing a letter, walking around the block, or running a marathon. But the amount of each of these nutrients that is used depends on the type of activity that is performed, how long it is performed, and the physical conditioning of the exerciser.

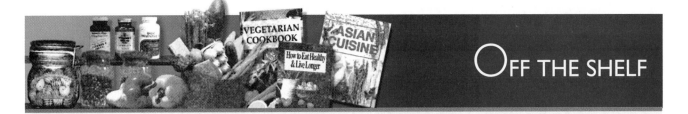

OFF THE SHELF

Power Bars and Power Beverages: Are They Worth the Cost?

Exceed, Gatorade, Power Burst, Power Bar . . . Beverages and bars claim to provide you with that extra boost that makes your workout more satisfying or your performance more competitive. They are marketed to people at all levels of activity from strollers to professional athletes. What do they actually provide?

Fluids before, during, and after exercise are important to prevent dehydration. Sports drinks such as Gatorade claim to be the fluid you need for exercise. A glance at the label finds that they are really water, sugar, and salts. Most of what athletes lose in sweat is water—so the best beverage to replace it is water. The sugar is included with the promise that it will help maintain blood glucose. For moderate exercise such as a 20-minute jog, glucose-containing beverages offer no advantage over water. And because they contain 50 to 100 kcalories per cup, they may be counterproductive if the goal of exercise is losing or maintaining body weight. During exercise that lasts longer than 60 to 90 minutes, consuming glucose does help to maintain blood glucose and has been shown to increase endurance. To be effective, the drink should contain between 6 and 10% glucose. Less than 6% may not enhance performance, and more than 10% may delay stomach emptying and cause abdominal cramps. Some beverages contain glucose polymers rather than glucose. These are short chains of glucose molecules. They leave the stomach more quickly than the same amount of glucose but have not been shown to offer

any additional benefit in terms of performance.[1]

The sodium and other electrolytes may help increase the rate of fluid and glucose absorption from the gastrointestinal tract. There is usually no need to replace electrolytes. Only small amounts are lost in sweat, and these are easily replaced from foods eaten during the next meal. An exception is during strenuous ultraendurance events lasting longer than 5 hours. During such events a fluid containing electrolytes may be of benefit because simple water replacement can dilute the blood and contribute to dehydration.[2]

A newer addition to the world of "sports foods" are power bars. They are advertised as a snack or precompetition meal that will optimize performance. A precompetition meal should contain about 300 kcalories and be high in carbohydrate and low in fat. Although toast and cereal with lowfat milk, or a stack of pancakes, will provide this, power bar products are now marketed to take the place of this meal. A typical product provides about 230 kcalories and is low in fat, about 2 grams, and high in carbohydrate, about 45 grams. Power bars differ from candy bars because they are lower in fat; provide more fiber; and contain vitamin C, vitamin E, calcium, iron, magnesium, copper, zinc, and a host of B vitamins. Although the micronutrients contained in power bars may benefit athletes with inadequate diets, these products should not take the place of the whole grains, fresh vegetables and fruits, dairy

products, and meats or meat substitutes that make up a healthy diet. Power bars do not improve performance beyond what a well-planned precompetition meal will, but their convenience may be an important advantage. They come in compact, individually wrapped packages that will fit in a pocket or bicycle pack. If convenience means the difference between consuming a power bar or no meal at all, they can be beneficial.

Power beverages and power bars may also provide a psychological edge if people believe they will enhance performance. They cost more than water or a regular meal, but if taste and convenience make them preferable, there is little reason not to use them.

[1] Puhl, S.M. and Buskirk, E.R. Nutrient beverages for exercise and sport. In *Nutrition in Exercise and Sport*, 2nd ed. Wolinski, I. and Hickson, J.F., Jr., eds. Boca Raton, FL: CRC Press, 1994, pp. 264–294.

[2] Lyle, B.J. and Forgac, T. Hydration and fluid replacement. In *Sports Nutrition for the 90s*. Berning, J.R. and Steen, S.N., eds. Gaithersburg, MD: Aspen Publishers, Inc., 1991, pp. 175–196.

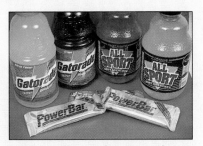

(© Trent Steffler/David R. Frazier Photolibrary)

slowly, they can sustain aerobic exercise for longer periods at higher intensities than can untrained individuals.

Living and working at high altitudes, where the air contains less oxygen, also causes adaptations that improve the capacity of the lungs and blood to transport oxygen. Therefore endurance athletes often train at high altitudes to further enhance their aerobic capacity.

EXERCISING GOOD NUTRITION: FOOD AND DRINK FOR SPORT

Adequate nutrition is essential to performance whether you are a marathon runner or a mall walker. For every exerciser, diet must provide sufficient energy from the appropriate sources to fuel activity, protein to maintain muscle mass, micronutrients to allow utilization of the energy-containing nutrients, and water to transport nutrients and cool the body.

ENERGY NEEDS

Energy needs include those required for basal metabolic rate, activity, and the thermic effect of food. For a mall walker, the energy needed for activity may be only a few hundred kcalories. An endurance athlete, such as a marathon runner, may expend an additional 2000 to 3000 kcalories per day while training, so some may require 6000 kcalories a day to maintain body weight.

Factors Affecting the Energy Needed for Activity   The amount of energy needed for activity depends on the activity, the exerciser, and even the location. The intensity, duration, and frequency of activity performed are determinants of energy need (see Table 12-2 and Appendix L). The more intense the activity, the more energy it requires. For example, riding a bicycle involves less work than running the same distance and therefore requires less energy. The more time spent exercising, the more energy it requires. Riding a bicycle for 10 minutes requires ten times the energy needed to ride for 1 minute. The body weight of the exerciser is another factor in determining energy needs. Moving a heavier body requires more energy than moving a lighter one. Therefore, it requires less energy for a 120-pound woman to walk for 5 minutes than it does for a 250-pound woman.

TABLE 12-2	**Energy Expended for Activity**						
Activity	**Energy (kcal/hr)**						
Body Weight (kg)	**50**	**57**	**64**	**70**	**77**	**84**	**91**
(lb)	**110**	**125**	**140**	**155**	**170**	**185**	**200**
Sitting	66	75	84	92	102	111	120
Cycling							
5.5 mph	192	219	246	269	296	323	349
9.4 mph	300	342	384	420	462	504	546
Aerobics	309	352	396	433	476	519	562
Rope jumping							
80 jumps/min	492	561	630	689	758	827	895
Running							
9 min/mile	579	660	741	811	892	973	1054
6 min/mile	756	862	968	1058	1164	1270	1376
Swimming							
Fast crawl	468	534	599	655	721	786	852
Slow crawl	384	438	491	538	591	645	699
Walking	240	274	307	336	370	403	437
Weight lifting	258	294	330	361	397	433	470

Adapted from McArdle, W.D., Katch, F.I., and Katch, V.L. *Exercise Physiology: Energy, Nutrition, and Human Performance*, 3rd ed. Philadelphia: Lea & Febiger, 1991.

There are also some special considerations in determining energy needs for activity. For example, although an obese woman would expend more energy jogging a mile than a lighter counterpart, when swimming the obese woman would expend less energy because the buoyancy of her adipose tissue reduces the amount of work required to swim. If a lean individual and an obese individual were in the weightlessness of space, it would require no more energy for one to leap across the room than for the other. Other special circumstances may also affect the amount of energy needed daily for activity. A paraplegic in a wheelchair may have lower energy needs because many of the major muscles of the body are always inactive. At the other extreme, people with uncontrolled muscle movements may have higher energy needs because their muscles never stop moving.

What Is the Desirable Body Weight for Athletes?   Desirable body weight and composition for nonathletes can be estimated from height-weight tables, by calculating body mass index, or by measuring the percent body fat (see Chapter 7 or Appendix B). However, what is considered desirable body weight and composition for some athletes may differ from what is viewed as optimal for the general population. For example, the desirable body weight of a runner may be less than that of an average person, whereas that of a weight lifter may be greater. But both the runner and the weight lifter are likely to have a lower percent body fat than sedentary individuals.

Athletes involved in activities where small, light bodies offer an advantage—for instance, ballet, gymnastics, and certain running events—may restrict energy intake to maintain a low body weight. While a slightly leaner physique may be beneficial, dieting to maintain an unrealistically low weight may threaten health and performance. An athlete who needs to lose weight should do so in advance of the competitive season to prevent weight loss from affecting performance. The general guidelines for healthy weight loss should be followed—reduce energy intake, increase activity, and change the behaviors that led to weight gain (see Chapter 7). This can be accomplished by reducing total energy intake by 200 to 500 kcalories per day. To preserve lean body mass and enhance fat loss, weight loss should be at a rate of about ½ to 1 pound per week and should be accompanied by an exercise program.[23] If weight gain is desired, 200 to 500 extra kcalories should be consumed per day and weight gain should be accompanied by training to promote an increase in lean as well as fat weight.

Extreme weight loss in young athletes should be discouraged. In adolescents, athletic activities combined with weight loss may affect the maturation process and increase the risks of developing anorexia or bulimia.[24] Female ballerinas and gymnasts who maintain extremely low levels of body fat often have delayed menses and delayed sexual maturation.[25] Sporadic dieting to fit into a specific weight class, which occurs in sports such as wrestling, may be detrimental to health and performance (see Chapter 14).[26]

CARBOHYDRATE, FAT, AND PROTEIN NEEDS

The source of energy used to fuel activity is often as important as the amount of energy. In general, the diet of physically active individuals should contain the same proportion of carbohydrate, fat, and protein as is recommended to the general public, about 55 to 60% of total energy as carbohydrate, less than 30% of energy as fat, and about 12 to 17% of energy as protein. For athletes in training, adequate carbohydrate is necessary to rapidly replace muscle and liver glycogen stores depleted by daily exercise. Most of the carbohydrate should come from complex carbohydrates, such as grains and starchy vegetables, as well as naturally occurring simple sugars, such as those found in fruit and milk. This type of diet provides vitamins, minerals, and fiber as well as energy.

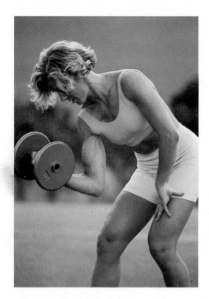

FIGURE 12-9
Muscle size is increased by exercising, not by increasing protein intake. (Marc Romanelli/The Image Bank)

Although fat is an important source of energy for exercise, excess dietary fat is unnecessary. Body stores of fat provide enough energy to support the needs of even the longest endurance events. Excess energy consumed as fat, carbohydrate, or protein can cause an increase in body fat.

The amount of protein needed by athletes has been the subject of controversy. The ancient Greek belief, still held by many, that eating muscle will give you bigger muscles is incorrect. Muscle growth is stimulated by exercise, not by increasing protein intake (Figure 12-9). The quick bursts of activity needed for weight lifting and other strength events rely on carbohydrate, not protein, as an energy source. The protein needs of most athletes can be met by consuming a diet that provides the RDA of 0.8 gram per kilogram of body weight per day. Athletes participating in endurance sports, in which protein is used for energy and to maintain blood glucose, and weight training, which requires amino acids to synthesize new muscle proteins, may benefit from slightly more protein—1 to 1.5 grams per kilogram per day.[27] This amount, however, is no more than what is contained in the typical American diet.

Protein and amino acid supplements are often marketed to athletes with the promise of enhancing muscle growth or improving performance. The most popular amino acid supplements for athletes are ornithine and arginine, which are marketed with the promise that they will stimulate the release of growth hormone and in turn enhance the growth of muscles. Although studies have shown that large doses of arginine and ornithine can stimulate growth hormone release, and may enhance fat loss associated with strength training, there is little evidence that supplements of these amino acids cause an increase in muscle strength or muscle mass.[28,29] The amino acids leucine, isoleucine, and valine are also promoted to athletes as muscle fuel. They are the predominant amino acids used for fuel during exercise, but there is no evidence that athletes need more of them.[30]

Synthetic hormones known as anabolic steroids are also commonly used by athletes to increase muscle mass. Although their use does help build muscle, they are illegal and have dangerous side effects that may impair health in both the short and long term.[31] (See *Off the Shelf*: Anabolic Steroids: Running on Roids.)

VITAMIN AND MINERAL NEEDS

Since exercise increases energy needs, it also increases the need for the vitamins and minerals involved in energy production. For instance, the RDA for thiamin is 0.5 mg per 1000 kcalories. As exercise increases energy requirement, it also increases the need for thiamin. If the extra energy required for exercise comes from nutrient-dense sources, the additional vitamin and mineral needs are usually met. This may not be true for exercisers consuming low-energy diets, such as ballerinas, gymnasts, or individuals exercising to lose weight. Their diets must be carefully planned to meet nutrient needs.

For most individuals, exercise does not increase the risk of nutrient deficiencies. Iron status, however, is commonly reduced in athletes.[32] This may be caused by inadequate dietary iron intake, increased demand for iron, increased iron losses, or a redistribution of iron due to exercise training. Iron needs are increased by exercise because it stimulates the production of red blood cells, so more iron is needed for hemoglobin synthesis. Iron is also needed for the synthesis of muscle myoglobin and iron-containing proteins needed for ATP production in the mitochondria. Iron losses may be increased by exercise due to losses in sweat. Iron deficiency anemia due to inadequate intake, increased needs, or increased losses, will affect performance.[33,34] Adolescent and female athletes are at greatest risk of iron deficiency because they have high iron needs and may consume poor diets.[35] Vegetarian athletes must also be careful to avoid iron deficiency, since they do not consume meat, an excellent source of readily absorbable heme iron. Some athletes

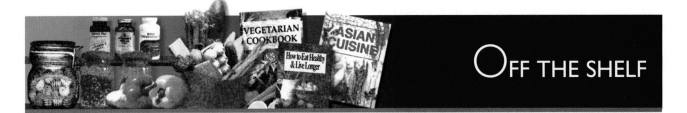

OFF THE SHELF

Anabolic Steroids: Running on Roids

When athletes from Eastern European nations began to dominate certain athletic events in the 1950s, the athletic community became aware that many of these successful athletes had taken large doses of anabolic steroids. Today the sale of steroids, known as "roids" in the jargon of the gym, is a $100-million-a-year black market.[1] While anabolic steroids build muscle quickly, they have negative side effects that may be permanent.

Steroids are fat soluble hormones. Those used by athletes are a synthetic version of the human hormone testosterone. An average man produces 2.5 to 11 mg of testosterone daily; females also produce testosterone but in much smaller amounts. Natural testosterone stimulates and maintains the male sexual organs and stimulates the development of bones and muscles, and the growth of skin and hair. Synthetic steroids have been structurally modified to maximize their effect on muscle development and minimize their other effects, such as those on sexual organs and bone.

Social pressures on young men to look strong and muscular and the "win at any cost" philosophy have encouraged the use of anabolic steroids. Medical and psychiatric journals are reporting an increasing number of body builders and athletes who abuse anabolic steroids. In a survey of weight lifters, respondents indicated that they used an average of three steroids at once, a practice known as stacking, and took 10 to 100 times the amount of testosterone produced naturally.[2]

Large doses of synthetic steroids, when taken in conjunction with exercise and an adequate diet, build muscle mass. However, they also make the body think testosterone is being produced. The perceived excess of testosterone causes a reduction in the production of natural testosterone and therefore a decrease in its other functions, such as bone growth and maintenance of sexual organs. The result is stunted growth, shrinkage of the testicles, decreased sperm production, and a host of other undesirable physiological, psychological, and behavioral side effects. Steroid use may also cause oily skin and acne, genital changes, sterility, water retention in the tissues, yellowing of the eyes and skin, coronary artery disease, liver disease, and sometimes death. Users may have violent outbursts and depression leading to suicide. The dangers of steroid use are increased by the fact that they are illegal, so their manufacturing and distribution procedures aren't regulated. Users can never be sure of the potency and purity of what they are taking.

Most professional and amateur sports organizations have sanctions against steroid use, and possession of anabolic steroids without a prescription became a federal offense in 1991. The stiff penalties associated with steroid abuse have caused some athletes to turn to alternative chemicals that are not technically classified as steroids. These include prescription, veterinary, investigational, and unapproved drugs as well as dietary supplements.[3] These steroid alternatives are often just as dangerous as steroids and in some cases more so. The prowess that steroids and other performance-enhancing drugs offer often overshadows both the legal repercussions and possible negative health effects. For example, the Canadian sprinter Ben Johnson had his 1988 Olympic gold medal revoked when he tested positive for steroids. However, the fact that he clearly outran his closest competitor, U.S. sprinter Carl Lewis, may have increased the temptation to try these drugs.

[1] Mishra, R. Steroids and sports are a losing proposition. FDA Consumer 25:25–27, Sept., 1991.

[2] Bower, B. Pumped up and strung out. Science News 140:30–31, 1991.

[3] Ropp, K.L. No-win situation for athletes. FDA Consumer 26:8–12, Dec., 1992.

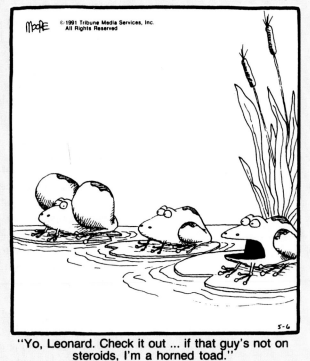

"Yo, Leonard. Check it out ... if that guy's not on steroids, I'm a horned toad."

(Reprinted by permission: Tribune Media Services)

experience a condition known as sports anemia, which is a temporary decrease in hemoglobin concentration that occurs during exercise training. It is an adaptation to training that does not seem to impair delivery of oxygen to tissues. It occurs because blood volume expands to increase oxygen delivery but the synthesis of red blood cells lags behind the increase in plasma volume. The number of red cells may be further reduced because some are broken by impact in events like running (foot-strike hemolysis) or by the contraction of large muscles.[32] The breaking of red cells stimulates the production of new ones.

Calcium status may be compromised in female athletes. A combination of nutritional factors and strenuous training regimens can cause menstruation to stop, a condition known as amenorrhea. The level of the hormone estrogen decreases in these women, reducing calcium absorption and predisposing them to bone loss. Female athletes with menstrual irregularities have spinal bones that are less dense than those of either nonathletes or athletes who menstruate regularly.[36] This can make them more vulnerable to the development of stress fractures and set the stage for osteoporosis later in life. In addition, many female athletes and females in general do not consume adequate calcium. Even if they do, neither adequate dietary calcium nor the increase in bone mass caused by weight-bearing exercise is enough to compensate for bone loss due to amenorrhea.

THE IMPORTANCE OF WATER

Water is needed to regulate body temperature and to transport oxygen and nutrients to the muscles. Water loss in sweat can be critical to even the most casual exerciser.

Water and the Regulation of Body Temperature
During exercise, heat production increases as exercise intensity increases. If heat cannot be lost from the body, body temperature rises and exercise performance as well as health may be in jeopardy. The ability to dissipate the heat generated during exercise is affected by the hydration status of the exerciser as well as by environmental conditions. At rest in a temperate environment, an individual loses about 1.1 liters (about 4.5 cups) of water per day, or 50 ml per hour, from the skin and lungs. Exercise in a hot environment can increase this tenfold. Adequate fluids should be consumed before, during, and after exercise. Since thirst is not a reliable indicator of fluid needs, it is important for anyone exercising to schedule regular fluid breaks. Strenuous exercise should be avoided if the weather is too hot or humid.

Consequences of Inadequate Hydration
The water lost in sweat and evaporation from the lungs must be replaced. Inadequate body water does not allow heat to dissipate and leads to thermal distress. Dehydration, heat cramps, heat exhaustion, and heat stroke are all types of thermal distress. Dehydration occurs when water loss is great enough for blood volume to decrease, thereby reducing the ability to deliver oxygen and nutrients to exercising muscles. Maximal oxygen consumption, exercise capacity, muscle strength, and liver glycogen content are all reduced with dehydration.[37] Even mild dehydration can impair exercise performance (Figure 12-10). Heat cramps occur when water and salt have been lost during extended exercise. They are involuntary cramps and spasms in the muscles involved in exercise and are caused by an imbalance of the electrolytes sodium and potassium at the muscle cell membranes. Heat exhaustion occurs when fluid loss causes blood volume to decrease so much that it is not possible to both cool the skin and deliver oxygen to active muscles. It is characterized by a rapid weak pulse, low blood pressure, fainting, profuse sweating, and disorientation. Heat stroke, the most serious form of thermal distress, occurs when the

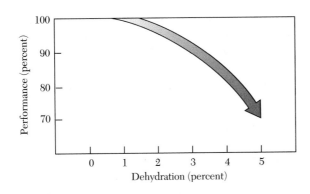

FIGURE 12-10
As dehydration increases, exercise performance declines. (Adapted from Saltin, B. and Castill, D.I. Fluid and electrolyte balance during prolonged exercise. In *Exercise, Nutrition, and Energy Metabolism*. Horton, E.S. and Tergung, R.I., eds. New York: Macmillan, 1988.)

temperature regulatory center of the brain fails. Heat stroke is characterized by elevated body temperature, hot dry skin, extreme confusion, and unconsciousness.[38] It requires immediate medical attention.

Weight Loss Through Dehydration in Young Athletes   Athletes involved in sports with weight classes, such as wrestlers and boxers, sometimes go to unhealthy extremes to keep body weight down so they can compete in lower weight classes. Being at the high end of a weight class is thought to give an advantage over smaller opponents. Frequently, rapid weight loss is accomplished by dehydration. No advantage is gained, however, if the athlete's performance and health are impaired. A loss of even 2% of body weight as water—for instance, a loss of 2 pounds in a 100-pound person—can adversely affect endurance.[39]

Fluid Intake For Exercise   To ensure adequate hydration, drink freely (about 16 oz) during the 2 hours before exercise and consume 14 to 20 ounces of fluid about 30 minutes before exercising. During exercise, competitive or otherwise, 3 to 6 ounces of fluid should be consumed every 10 to 15 minutes, and immediately after exercise each pound of weight lost should be replaced with 16 ounces of fluid (see Table 12-3).[40] A good way to prevent dehydration is to consume enough fluid during exercise to minimize weight loss (Figure 12-11).

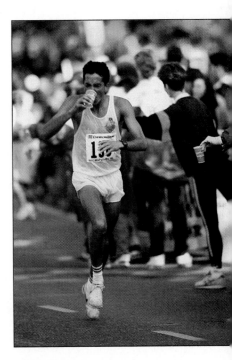

FIGURE 12-11
Fluids should be consumed before, during, and after exercise. (John Kelly/The Image Bank)

TABLE 12-3	Recommended Fluid Intake for Exercise

Before Exercise
Begin exercise well hydrated by consuming fluids during the 2 hours before exercise.
Consume 14 to 20 oz of fluid during the 30 minutes before exercise.

During Exercise
Consume 3 to 6 oz of fluid every 15 minutes.
For exercise lasting less than 60 to 90 minutes, water is the best fluid.
For exercise lasting longer than 60 to 90 minutes, consuming a fluid containing about 6% carbohydrate may improve endurance.
For exercise lasting longer than 5 hours, a fluid containing carbohydrate and electrolytes may be beneficial.

After Exercise
Begin fluid replacement immediately after exercise.
Consume 16 oz of fluid for each pound of weight lost.

For exercise lasting less than 60 to 90 minutes, the best fluid to drink is water.[41] The risk of dehydration can be increased if other types of fluids are consumed. Alcohol and beverages containing caffeine, such as colas, iced tea, and coffee, act as diuretics, substances that cause fluid to be lost through the kidneys, and therefore do little to maintain hydration. Fluids high in sugars slow gastric emptying, causing fluid to be trapped in the stomach so it cannot enter the blood. For exercise lasting longer than 60 to 90 minutes, depletion of body carbohydrate stores is a concern. The addition of carbohydrate to fluid replacements has been found to enhance endurance.[41] The added carbohydrate delays fatigue by preventing a drop in blood glucose and providing a source of glucose for the muscle.

Because small amounts of minerals, including sodium, are also lost in sweat, many sports drinks are marketed with the promise of providing glucose and replacing these lost electrolytes (see *Off the Shelf*: Power Bars and Power Beverages). The combination of sodium and glucose enhances fluid absorption in the intestine, but for most exercise, replacing electrolytes is not a primary concern. Sweat is mostly water. The amounts of sodium and other minerals lost in sweat during exercise lasting even as long as 5 hours do not affect health or performance and can easily be replaced by food eaten after the exercise has stopped. For ultraendurance events such as iron-man triathlons and events lasting longer than 8 hours, there are significant losses of sodium as well as small amounts of other minerals in the sweat, and replacement becomes important. If, during an endurance event, an athlete were to drink water without electrolytes, the water would dilute the sodium remaining in the blood. When the blood is diluted, it signals the brain to stop the thirst sensation and it stimulates the production of urine by the kidneys, increasing water losses and resulting in dehydration. The consumption of fluids containing electrolytes will prevent blood from becoming too dilute in ultraendurance events.[37] The belief that salt pills are necessary to replace the sodium lost in sweat and prevent dehydration is a common misconception. Their use is unnecessary and dangerous because the salt will draw water away from the tissues and may cause dehydration, nausea, and vomiting.

MEALS FOR COMPETITION

For most of us, a trip to the gym requires no special nutritional planning beyond that needed to consume a balanced diet and plenty of water. For competitive athletes, however, meals eaten in preparation for competition may give or take away the extra seconds that can mean victory or defeat. Thus far there is no magic pill to maximize performance, but there are a number of sound sports nutrition recommendations.

Carbohydrate loading–A regimen of diet and exercise training designed to maximize muscle glycogen stores before an athletic event.

Carbohydrate Loading: Maximizing Glycogen Stores   For the serious endurance athlete, larger glycogen stores allow exercise to continue for a longer period. One way to maximize glycogen stores before an event is to follow a **carbohydrate-loading** regimen. This regimen involves depleting glycogen stores by exercising strenuously and then replenishing glycogen by consuming a high-carbohydrate diet for a few days before competition, during which time only light exercise is performed. Current practice is to decrease training during the six days before competition while increasing the carbohydrate content of the diet to 70% of energy intake during the three days before competition.[42] Since consuming this much carbohydrate can be difficult, there are a number of high-carbohydrate supplements available. These drinks contain 20 to 25% carbohydrate (200 to 250 grams per liter) and should not be confused with sports drinks designed to be consumed during competition, which contain only about 6 to 10% carbohydrate. A carbohydrate-loading regimen will increase glycogen stores to more than one and a half times the level they would be on a typical diet.[43]

Although carbohydrate loading is beneficial to endurance athletes, for those exercising for periods less than 90 minutes it will provide no benefit and has some disadvantages. For every gram of glycogen in the muscle, 3 grams of water are also deposited. This water will cause a 2- to 7-pound weight gain and may cause some muscle stiffness. As the glycogen is used, the water is released. This can be an advantage when exercising in hot weather, but the extra weight is a disadvantage for those competing in events of short duration.

The Precompetition Meal   Muscle glycogen is used as an energy source for exercising muscle, so once muscle glycogen stores have been filled, only exercise will deplete them. Liver glycogen, however, is used to supply blood glucose, and so is depleted even during rest if no food is ingested. To ensure that liver glycogen stores are full, a high-carbohydrate meal should be eaten 2 to 4 hours before the event. The meal should be high in carbohydrate, low in fat, and moderate in protein content, and provide about 300 kcalories—for example, a cup of pasta with tomato sauce and a slice of bread or a turkey sandwich and a cup of juice. High-fiber foods should be avoided to prevent feeling bloated during competition. In addition to nutritional clout, a precompetition meal including "lucky" foods may impart an added psychological advantage.

Attitudes about what and when to eat before an event have changed. Past recommendations opposed carbohydrate intake immediately before competition. It was hypothesized that carbohydrate would raise insulin levels. This would decrease blood glucose and inhibit the release of fatty acids, thereby reducing the fuel available to muscles. It is now known, however, that for most individuals, a small carbohydrate meal or beverage, consumed from 4 hours to a few minutes before an event, will not have a detrimental effect on performance and may enhance endurance.[44] The effect of such a meal may be different for different individuals, so athletes should test the effect of precompetition meals during training, not during competition.

Postcompetition Meals   When exercise ends, the body must shift from the catabolic state of exercise to the anabolic state of restoring muscle and liver glycogen, depositing lipids, and synthesizing muscle proteins. These needs make postcompetition meals just as important as precompetition meals. First, fluid losses should be replaced. Sodium intake should be minimal until this is complete. To maximize glycogen replacement, a high-carbohydrate meal or drink should be consumed as soon as possible after the event and again every 2 hours for 6 hours after the event.[45] Ideally the meals should provide about 1 gram of carbohydrate per kilogram of body weight, the equivalent of two pancakes with syrup and a glass of fruit punch for a 70-kg person.[42]

DO SUPPLEMENTS ENHANCE ATHLETIC PERFORMANCE?

For competitive athletes, the diet must provide the optimal mix of nutrients to fuel their special needs. The idea that specific nutrients might enhance athletic performance and confer athletic prowess is not new. In ancient Greece, the wrestler Milo of Croton was said to have subsisted on a daily diet of 20 pounds of bread, 20 pounds of meat, and 18 pints of wine.[46] Today, many nutritional supplements are marketed as **ergogenic aids**, or performance-enhancing aids. The use of carnitine, protein and amino acid supplements, and anabolic steroids as ergogenic aids has already been discussed. Although these supplements are generally unnecessary, expensive, or illegal, and most have not been shown to improve performance, athletes are susceptible to their enticements. Some of the supplements marketed to athletes as ergogenic aids are essential nutrients such as vitamins and minerals; others are nonessential substances (see Table 12-4).

Ergogenic aids—Substances that enhance work or exercise performance.

TABLE 12-4   Claims, Effectiveness, and Risks of Popular Ergogenic Aids

Ergogenic Aid	Claim	Effectiveness	Risk
Arginine and ornithine	Cause the release of growth hormone, which stimulates muscle development and decreases body fat.	Most studies show no increase in growth hormone or lean body mass with supplementation.	High levels of one amino acid may interfere with the absorption of others.
Bee pollen	Causes faster recovery from training workouts, which enables a higher level of training.	No evidence that it improves training level or other parameters of performance.	Some individuals have allergic reactions.
Bicarbonate (sodium bicarbonate, baking soda)	Helps buffer lactic acid produced during exercise, which delays fatigue.	Supplements increase blood pH and may enhance performance and strength in intense anaerobic activities but not in aerobic exercise.	Bloating, diarrhea, high blood pH.
Caffeine	Increases the release of fatty acids from adipose tissue, spares glycogen, and enhances endurance.	Research supports claims of increased endurance but the effect depends on the individual.	Dehydration, jitters, digestive discomfort; delirium and death with excessive amounts.
Carnitine	Enhances the utilization of fatty acids and spares glycogen.	Most studies show no increase in fatty acid utilization or improvement in exercise performance.	L-carnitine has little risk but D, L-carnitine and D-carnitine can be toxic.
Chromium (chromium picolinate)	Increases lean body mass, decreases body fat, delays fatigue.	Chromium affects glucose utilization, protein synthesis, and lipid metabolism via its effect on insulin action, but supplements will not affect these processes unless a deficiency exists.	Little information on toxicity.
Creatine (creatine phosphate)	Increases energy production and speeds recovery after high-intensity exercise like power lifting.	Creatine phosphate is rapidly converted into ATP for muscle contraction. Supplements increase muscle creatine and creatine phosphate synthesis after exercise, and enhance strength, performance, and recovery from high-intensity exercise.	Stomach pain.
Ginseng	Spares glycogen, increases fatty acid oxidation, reduces fatigue.	No human research to support these claims.	Nervousness, confusion, depression.
Medium-chain triglycerides	Provide energy to body builders without promoting fat deposition; reduce muscle protein breakdown during prolonged exercise.	Provide energy and must be metabolized before they can be stored as body fat. They increase endurance and fatty acid oxidation in mice, but there is no evidence of a benefit in humans.	None known.
Vanadium (vanadyl sulfate)	More rapid and intense muscle pumping for body builders.	No evidence to support a benefit for body builders.	Little information on toxicity. Reduces insulin production.

Vitamin Supplements   Many of the promises made about vitamin supplements are extrapolated from their biochemical functions. For example, thiamin, riboflavin, niacin, and pantothenic acid are all involved in muscle energy metabolism. Thiamin and pantothenic acid are needed for carbohydrate to enter the citric acid cycle for aerobic metabolism. Riboflavin and niacin are needed to shuttle electrons to the electron transport chain so ATP can be formed. A deficiency of one or more of these would interfere with energy metabolism and impair athletic performance, but there is no evidence that consuming more than the recommended intake will enhance physical performance.

Other B vitamins are marketed for improving aerobic metabolism because of their roles in oxygen transport and delivery. For example, vitamin B_6 assists in the synthesis of hemoglobin and other proteins involved in oxygen transfer and utilization. Folic acid and vitamin B_{12} are both involved in the synthesis of red blood cells needed for oxygen transport and delivery.

The claims for vitamin E, vitamin C, and beta-carotene focus on their antioxidant functions. Since exercise increases oxidative processes, it increases the production of free radicals. Free radicals can damage tissues and have been associated with fatigue during exercise.[47] Antioxidant supplements have been hypothesized to prevent free radical damage and delay fatigue. Vitamin E is particularly important in maintaining muscle function by protecting muscle cell membranes from free radical damage. Although the data on the effect of vitamin E supplements on exercise performance are contradictory, high doses of vitamin E (200 to 400 mg per day) have been shown to prevent exercise-induced oxidation of muscle cell membranes.[48] Studies with vitamin C supplementation are also equivocal, with about half showing an increase in performance and half showing no effect.[49] Supplementation with mixtures of antioxidants prevents free radical damage but has not been shown conclusively to enhance performance.[29] Active individuals should consume plenty of fruits and vegetables to ensure adequate intakes of vitamin E, vitamin C, and beta-carotene.

Mineral Supplements   Some of the minerals advertised as endurance enhancers include electrolytes, chromium, selenium, zinc, and iron. Electrolyte replacements are marketed to restore losses in sweat. They can be useful in prolonged exercise. Chromium supplements, as chromium picolinate, claim to stimulate protein synthesis and delay fatigue because of chromium's role in insulin metabolism and glucose utilization. Since exercise increases chromium losses, the risk of chromium deficiency is increased in active individuals.[29] It is possible that the effects observed from supplements are due to repletion of a marginally deficient state. In controlled human studies, chromium supplements have not been found to affect muscle strength or body composition.[50] Selenium is marketed for its antioxidant properties and zinc for its role in protein synthesis and tissue repair. Selenium and zinc supplements have not been found to improve athletic performance in healthy individuals with no mineral deficiencies. Iron is also marketed as an ergogenic mineral because it is needed for hemoglobin synthesis. If a deficiency exists, as it frequently does in athletes, supplements can be of benefit.

Nonessential Substances as Ergogenic Aids   Some of the nonessential substances marketed as ergogenic aids include bicarbonate and caffeine, which can have an ergogenic effect for some types of activity and bee pollen, wheat germ oil, brewer's yeast, ginseng, royal jelly, and DNA and RNA, which have not been found to be ergogenic. (Figure 12-12).

Bicarbonate supplements have been hypothesized to neutralize the lactic acid produced by anaerobic exercise and therefore delay fatigue and increase performance. Bicarbonate ions are an important buffering system in the body. Bicarbonate administration before exercise has been found to be of benefit for exhaustive exercise lasting 1 to 7 minutes, such as sprint cycling, but it is of no benefit for lower intensity aerobic exercise.[29]

Some athletes may try to enhance endurance by consuming caffeine before an event. Caffeine ingestion prior to exercise has been found to enhance perfor-

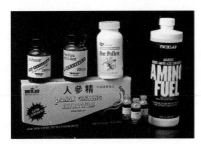

FIGURE 12-12
Many types of supplements are marketed to athletes as ergogenic aids. (Dennis Drenner)

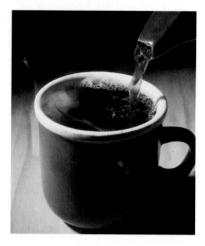

FIGURE 12-13
For some athletes, caffeine consumption prior to exercise increases performance, but the use of large amounts of caffeine is illegal in athletic competition. (Jorge's Estudio/The Image Bank)

mance during prolonged moderate-intensity endurance exercise and short-term intense exercise.[51,52] This is hypothesized to occur because caffeine enhances the release of fatty acids, and when fatty acids are used as a fuel source, glycogen is spared, delaying the onset of fatigue. The effect may vary, depending on the type of activity and the athlete. Athletes who are unaccustomed to caffeine respond better than those who routinely consume it. In some athletes caffeine may impair performance by increasing water loss in the urine or by causing gastrointestinal upset. Regardless of its effectiveness, athletes should know that excess caffeine is illegal. The International Olympic Committee prohibits athletes with urine caffeine levels of 12 μg per ml or greater from competing. This doesn't mean that coffee will not be served in the Olympic village (Figure 12-13). The consumption of 1 cup of coffee brewed in the United States only raises the urine caffeine level to 1.5 μg per ml within 2 hours.[53] For the urine caffeine level to reach 12 μg per ml, an individual would need to drink 6 to 8 cups of coffee within about a 2-hour period. Caffeine is also found in pill form in products such as No Doz, which contains about 100 mg of caffeine per tablet—about the same amount as in a cup of coffee (Table 12-5).

Bee pollen is a mixture of the pollen of flowering plants, plant nectar, and bee saliva. It contains no extraordinary factors and has not been shown to have any performance-enhancing effects.[54] In addition, ingesting or inhaling bee pollen can be hazardous to individuals allergic to various pollens.[55] Brewer's yeast, while a source of B vitamins and some minerals, has not been demonstrated to have any ergogenic properties. Likewise, there is no evidence to support claims that wheat germ oil will aid endurance. As an oil it is high in fat, but it is no better as an energy source than any other fat. Royal jelly is a substance produced by the worker bee to feed to the queen bee. It helps the queen bee grow to twice the size of worker bees and live 40 times longer, but royal jelly does not appear to enhance athletic capacity in humans. Ginseng is promoted to be ergogenic. It can cause nervousness, confusion, and depression. The results of human studies on its effectiveness have been mixed.[29] Finally, DNA and RNA are genetic material marketed to aid in tissue regeneration. In the body they carry genetic information and are needed to synthesize proteins. DNA and RNA are not required in the diet, and supplements do not help replace damaged cells.

TABLE 12-5	The Caffeine Content of Commonly Consumed Foods and Medications	
Food	**Amount**	**Caffeine (mg)**
Coffee, regular	1 cup (240 ml)	139
Coffee, decaffeinated	1 cup	3
Tea, brewed	1 cup	45
Cola	12 oz (1 can)	46
Mountain Dew	12 oz	54
Hot chocolate	1 cup	7
Brownie	1	14
Chocolate bar	1 oz	15
No Doz	1 tablet	100
Excedrin	1 tablet	65
Empirin, Anacin	1 tablet	32

CRITICAL THINKING
Analyzing an Athlete's Diet

Hector is on the college track team. He recently decided to change his diet to increase his carbohydrate intake. Since beginning the new diet, his performance has gotten worse. Now he wants to start taking amino acids and some other nutritional supplements. He reviews his plans with a nutritionist. Hector is 20 years old, 5 feet 10 inches tall, and has weighed between 150 and 160 pounds for the last year or so. His one-day food record includes:

Hector's Current Diet		Modified Diet	
Food	**Serving**	**Food**	**Serving**
Breakfast			
Orange juice	1 cup	Orange juice	1 cup
~~Whole milk~~	1 cup	Lowfat milk	1 cup
~~Croissants~~	2	Whole wheat toast	2 slices
Butter	2 tsp	Butter	2 tsp
		Oatmeal	1 cup
Snack			
Candy bar	1	Candy bar	1
~~Whole milk~~	1 cup	Lowfat milk	1 cup
Lunch			
~~Breaded chicken~~	1	Plain hamburger	1
on roll	1	on roll	1
~~with mayonnaise~~	2 tsp	with cheese	1 oz
~~French fries~~	small order	Green salad	1 cup
		Carrot	1
		Italian dressing	1 Tbsp
Sparkling water	12 oz	Sparkling water	12 oz
Apple	1 medium	Apple	1 medium
Orange	1 medium	Orange	1 medium
Snack			
~~Potato chips~~	2 oz	Bagel	1
~~Onion dip~~	4 Tbsp	Banana	1 medium
~~Diet soda~~	12 oz	Apple juice	12 oz
Dinner			
Spaghetti	2 cups	Spaghetti	2 cups
~~Alfredo cream sauce~~	3 oz	Marinara sauce	1 cup
		Zucchini	1 cup
Italian bread	2 slices	Italian bread	2 slices
Butter	1 tsp	Butter	1 tsp
~~Whole milk~~	1 cup	Lowfat milk	1 cup
~~Ice cream~~	1 cup	Sherbet	1½ cups
		Chocolate chip cookies	3
Supplements			
~~Bee pollen~~		None	
~~Amino acids arginine and ornithine~~		None	

Analysis of Hector's diet shows an intake of 3350 kcalories, 90 grams of protein, 22 grams of dietary fiber, with 43% of energy from fat and 47% from carbohydrate. It meets the RDAs for all micronutrients.

What changes would you recommend in Hector's macronutrient intake?

Energy	No change is needed. His intake exceeds the RDA but meets his needs, since he is neither gaining nor losing weight.
Carbohydrate	**Answer:**
Fat	**Answer:**
Protein	**Answer:**
Fiber intake	**Answer:**

What foods could Hector change to meet these recommendations?

Instead of potato chips he could have pretzels.
Instead of croissants he could have _____.
Instead of pasta he could have _____.
Instead of a breaded chicken patty he could have _____.
Instead of ice cream he could have _____.

What are the potential risks and benefits of Hector taking the amino acid supplements and bee pollen?

Answer:

SUMMARY

1. Fitness, which is the ability to perform routine physical activity without undue fatigue, involves cardiorespiratory endurance, muscle strength and endurance, flexibility, and desirable body composition.

2. Regular exercise improves fitness in individuals of all ages and can reduce the risk of chronic diseases such as obesity, heart disease, diabetes, and osteoporosis. Exercise can also delay some of the changes in body composition and metabolism that occur with age.

3. A well-designed fitness program involves aerobic exercise, stretching, and strength training and is carried out in a safe environment. Aerobic exercise improves endurance and cardiovascular fitness by decreasing resting heart rate and increasing maximal oxygen consumption. Stretching improves flexibility, and strength training improves muscle strength and endurance.

4. Activity is fueled by energy in the form of ATP. ATP is generated from carbohydrate, fat, and protein. The proportion of each utilized depends on whether oxygen is available. When oxygen is limited, anaerobic glycolysis, which produces ATP from carbohydrate, predominates. When oxygen is plentiful, aerobic metabolism can proceed. It generates ATP more efficiently than anaerobic glycolysis and can utilize carbohydrate, fatty acids, and amino acids as energy sources.

5. The availability of oxygen and the proportion of carbohydrate and fat used as fuel for a given activity depend on the intensity and duration of the activity and the training of the exerciser. For short-term, high-intensity activity, ATP is generated primarily from the anaerobic metabolism of glucose from muscle glycogen stores. For lower intensity exercise of longer duration, aerobic metabolism predominates, and glucose and free fatty acids delivered to the tissues by the blood become important fuel sources.

The proportion of energy generated from fatty acids increases with the duration of low-intensity exercise.

6. The daily diet of an active individual should provide sufficient energy to fuel activity. It should be high in carbohydrate to ensure that glycogen stores are replenished after daily exercise. Fat intake should be low. Protein intake should be adequate, and excess protein provides no benefits.

7. Water intake must be sufficient to ensure that the body can be cooled and that nutrients and oxygen can be delivered to body tissues. Intake during exercise must replace water lost in sweat and evaporation through the lungs. If water intake is inadequate, exercise performance will decrease and thermal distress may occur. Plain water is the best fluid except during exercise lasting longer than 60 to 90 minutes, when athletes might benefit from fluids containing glucose. Electrolyte replacement is only necessary during ultraendurance events.

8. Sufficient micronutrients are needed to generate ATP from macronutrients and to transport oxygen and wastes to and from the cells. Some athletes are at risk for deficiencies of iron and calcium.

9. Competitive endurance athletes may utilize carbohydrate-loading regimens to maximize glycogen stores before an event. Meals eaten before competition should provide about 300 kcalories; should be high in carbohydrate, low in fat, moderate in protein, and low in fiber; and should satisfy the psychological needs of the athlete.

10. Postcompetition meals should replace lost fluids and electrolytes and begin restoring muscle and liver glycogen.

11. Many types of ergogenic aids are marketed to improve athletic performance. Some are beneficial for certain types of activity, but most of these offer little or no benefit.

SELF-TEST

1. List the health benefits of fitness.
2. What is aerobic exercise?
3. What is strength training?
4. How does aerobic exercise affect resting heart rate?
5. What is maximal oxygen consumption and how is it affected by aerobic exercise?
6. How does aerobic exercise help to prevent cardiovascular disease?
7. What fuels are used to produce ATP in anaerobic metabolism?
8. Which is more efficient, aerobic or anaerobic metabolism?
9. What fuels are used in exercise of long duration such as marathon running?
10. What factors affect the availability of oxygen and the type of fuel used during exercise?
11. What are the recommendations for fluid intake during exercise?
12. How does exercise affect protein needs?
13. Does activity change the proportions of carbohydrate, fat, and protein recommended in the diet?
14. What is carbohydrate loading?
15. Can ergogenic acids enhance exercise performance?

APPLICATIONS

These exercises are designed to help you apply your critical thinking skills to your own lifestyle choices. They can be calculated using information in this text and its appendices.

1. Keep a log of your activity for one day.
   a. Note the number of hours you spend in (1) sleep, (2) very light, (3) light, (4) moderate, and (5) heavy activity.
   b. What is your RMR per hour? (Use Table 7-2 or Appendix B.)
   c. What are your energy needs for activity? (Use Table 7-3, Table 12-3, or Appendix L.)
   d. If you added a 1-hour jog to your day, what would your new energy expenditure be?

e. Make a list of foods that you could add to your diet to balance the added expenditure of the jog.

2. Taking into consideration your typical weekly schedule of activities and events, design a reasonable exercise program for yourself. Include the types of activities, the times during the week you will be involved in each activity, and the length of time you will engage in each activity.

a. Have you chosen activities you enjoy, scheduled them for reasonable lengths of time and at reasonable frequencies?

b. Which activities are aerobic, which improve flexibility, and which are strength-training?

c. Can each of these activities be performed all year round? Suggest alternative activities and locations for inclement weather.

REFERENCES

1. *Healthy People 2000: National Health Promotion and Disease Prevention Objectives*. Washington, DC: U.S. Department of Health and Human Services, 1990.

2. Kujala, U.M., Kaprio, J., Taimla, S., and Sarna, S. Prevalence of diabetes, hypertension, and ischemic heart disease in former elite athletes. Metabolism 43:1255–1260, 1994.

3. Shephard, R.J. and Shek, P.N. Cancer, immune function, and physical activity. Can. J. Appl. Physiol. 20:1–25, 1995.

4. Paffenbarger, R.S., Hyde, P.H., Wing, A.L., et al. The association of changes in physical-activity level and other lifestyle characteristics with mortality among men. N. Engl. J. Med. 328:538–545, 1993.

5. American College of Sports Medicine. *ACSM's Guidelines for Exercise Testing and Prescription*, 5th ed. Baltimore: Williams & Wilkins, 1995.

6. Svendsen, O.L., Hassager, C., and Christiansen, C. Effect of an energy-restrictive diet, with or without exercise, on lean tissue mass, resting metabolic rate, cardiovascular risk factors, and bone in overweight postmenopausal women. Am. J. Med. 95:131–140, 1993.

7. Zelasko, C.J. Exercise for weight loss: what are the facts? J. Am. Diet. Assoc. 95:1414–1417, 1995.

8. Horton, T.J. and Geissler, C.A. Effect of habitual exercise on daily energy expenditure and metabolic rate during standardized activity. Am. J. Clin. Nutr. 59:13–19, 1994.

9. Powell, K.E., Caspersen, C.J., Koplan, J.P., and Ford, E.S. Physical activity and chronic diseases. Am. J. Clin. Nutr. 49:999–1006, 1989.

10. Martin, I.K., Katz, A., and Wahren, J. Splanchnic and muscle metabolism during exercise in NIDDM patients. Am. J. Physiol. 269:583–590, 1995.

11. Giovannucci, E., Ascherio, A., Rimm, E.B., et al. Physical activity, obesity and the risk of colon cancer. Ann. Intern. Med. 122:327–334, 1995.

12. Macfarlane, G.J. and Lowenfels, A.B. Physical activity and colon cancer. Eur. J. Cancer Prev. 3:393–398, 1994.

13. Friedenreich, C.M. and Rohan, T.E. A review of physical activity and breast cancer. Epidemiology 6:311–317, 1994.

14. Fiatarone, M.A., O'Neill, E.F., Ryan, N.D., et al. Exercise training and nutritional supplementation for physical frailty in very elderly people. N. Engl. J. Med. 330:1769–1775, 1994.

15. Gortmaker, S.L., Dietz, W.H., and Cheung, L.W. Inactivity, diet, and the fattening of America. J. Am. Diet. Assoc. 90:1247–1252, 1990.

16. Steen, S.N. Nutritional assessment and management of the school-aged child athlete. In *Sports Nutrition for the 90s*. Berning, J.R. and Steen, S.N., eds. Gaithersburg, MD: Aspen Publishers, Inc., 1991, pp. 229–250.

17. Vukovich, M., Costill, D., and Fink, W. Carnitine supplementation: effect on muscle carnitine and glycogen content during exercise. Med. Sci. Sports Exerc. 26:1122–1129, 1994.

18. Trappe, S.W., Costill, D.L., Goodpaster, B., et al. The effect of L-carnitine supplementation on performance during interval swimming. Int. J. Sports Med. 15:181–185, 1994.

19. Brass, E.P., Hoppel, C.L., and Hiatt, W.R. Effect of intravenous L-carnitine on carnitine homeostasis and fuel metabolism during exercise in humans. Clin. Pharmacol. Ther. 55:681–692, 1994.

20. Horton, E.S. Metabolic fuels, utilization and exercise: panel summary statements. Am. J. Clin. Nutr. 49:931–937, 1989.

21. Layzer, R.B. How muscles use fuel. N. Engl. J. Med. 324:411–412, 1991.

22. Coleman, E. Carbohydrates: the master fuel. In *Sports Nutrition for the 90s*. Berning, J.R. and Steen, S.N., eds. Gaithersburg, MD: Aspen Publishers, Inc., 1991, pp. 31–52.

23. U.S. Department of Agriculture, U.S. Department of Health and Human Services. *Nutrition and Your Health: Dietary Guidelines for Americans*, 4th ed. Home and Garden Bulletin No. 232. Hyattsville, MD: U.S. Government Printing Office, 1995.

24. Sundjot-Borgen, J. Risks and trigger factors for the development of eating disorders in female elite athletes. Med. Sci. Sports Med. 26:414–419, 1994.

25. Arena, B., Maffulli, N., Maffulli, F., and Morleo, M.A. Reproductive hormones and menstrual changes with exercise in female athletes. Sports Med. 19:278–287, 1995.

26. Horswill, C.A. Applied physiology of amateur wrestling. Sports Med. 14:114–143, 1992.

27. Position of the American Dietetic Association and The Canadian Dietetic Association: Nutrition for physical fitness and athletic performance for adults. Am. J. Diet. Assoc. 93:691–695, 1993.

28. Jacobson, B.H. Effect of amino acids on growth hormone release. Physician Sports Med. 18:63–70, 1990.

29. Bucci, L.R. Nutritional ergogenic aids. In *Nutrition in Exercise and Sport*, 2nd ed. Wolinski, I. and Hickson, J.F., Jr., eds. Boca Raton, FL: CRC Press, 1994. pp. 296–346.

30. Slavin, J.L., Lanners, G., and Engstrom, M.A. Amino acid supplements: beneficial or risky? Physician Sports Med. 16:221–225, 1988.

31. Ropp, K.L. No-win situation for athletes. FDA Consumer, 26:8–12, Dec, 1992.

32. Weaver, C.M. and Rajaram, S. Exercise and iron status. J. Nutr. 122:782–787, 1992.

33. Eichner, E.R. Sports anemia, iron supplements, and blood doping. Med. Sci. Sports Exerc. 24(suppl):315S–318S, 1993.

34. Weight, L.M., Jacobs, P., and Noakes, T.D. Dietary iron deficiency and sports anemia. Br. J. Nutr. 68:253–260, 1992.

35. Rowland, T.W. Iron deficiency in the young athlete. Pediatr. Clin. North Am. 37:1153–1163, 1990.

36. Snead, D.B., Weltman, A., Weltman, J.Y., et al. Reproductive hormones and bone density in women runners. J. Appl. Physiol. 72:2149–2156, 1992.

37. Lyle, B.J. and Forgac, T. Hydration and fluid replacement. In *Sports Nutrition for the 90s*. Berning, J.R. and Steen, S.N., eds. Gaithersburg, MD: Aspen Publishers, Inc., 1991, pp. 175–196.

38. Bross, M.H., Nash, B.T., Jr., and Carlton, F.B., Jr. Heat emergencies. Am. Fam. Physician 50:389–396, 398, 1994.

39. Pichan, G., Sridharan, K., and Gauttam, R.K. Physiological and metabolic responses to work in heat with graded hypohydration in tropical subjects. Eur. J. Appl. Physiol. 58:214–218, 1988.

40. Hoffman, C.J. and Coleman, E. An eating plan and update on recommended dietary practices for the endurance athlete. J. Am. Diet. Assoc. 91:325–330, 1991.

41. Puhl, S.M. and Buskirk, E.R. Nutrient beverages for exercise and sport. In *Nutrition in Exercise and Sport*, 2nd ed. Wolinski, I. and Hickson, J.F., Jr., eds. Boca Raton, FL: CRC Press, 1994, pp. 264–294.

42. Liebman, M. and Wilkinson, J.G. Carbohydrate metabolism and exercise. In *Nutrition in Exercise and Sport*, 2nd ed. Wolinski, I. and Hickson, J.F., Jr., eds. Boca Raton, FL: CRC Press, 1994, pp. 15–47.

43. Miller, G.D. Carbohydrates in ultra-endurance exercise and athletic performance. In *Nutrition in Exercise and Sport*, 2nd ed. Wolinski, I. and Hickson, J.F., Jr., eds. Boca Raton, FL: CRC Press, 1994, pp. 49–64.

44. Sherman, W.M. and Wright, D.A. Preevent nutrition for prolonged exercise. In *The Theory and Practice of Athletic Nutrition: Bridging the Gap. Report of the Ross Symposium*. Grandjean, A.S. and Storlie, J., eds. Columbus, OH: Ross Laboratories, 1989, pp. 30–46.

45. Clark, N., Tobin, J., and Ellis, C. Feeding the ultraendurance athlete: practical tips and a case study. Am. J. Diet. Assoc. 92:1258–1262, 1992.

46. Harris, H.A. Nutrition and physical performance: the diet of Greek athletes. Proc. Nutr. Soc. 25:87–90, 1966.

47. Singh, V.N. A current perspective on nutrition and exercise. J. Nutr. 122:760S–765S, 1992.

48. Kagan, V.E., Spirichev, V.B., Serbinova, E.A., et al. The significance of vitamin E and free radicals in physical exercise. In *Nutrition in Exercise and Sport*, 2nd ed. Wolinski, I. and Hickson, J.F., Jr., eds. Boca Raton, FL: CRC Press, 1994, pp. 186–213.

49. Keith, R.E. Vitamins and physical activity. In *Nutrition in Exercise and Sport*, 2nd ed. Wolinski, I. and Hickson, J.F., Jr., eds. Boca Raton, FL: CRC Press, 1994, pp. 160–183.

50. Clancy, S.P., Clarkson, P.M., DeCheke, M.E., et al. Effects of chromium picolinate supplementation on body composition, strength, and urinary chromium loss in football players. Int. J. Sports Nutr. 4:142–153, 1994.

51. Dodd, S.L., Herb, R.A., and Powers, S.K. Caffeine and exercise performance. An update. Sports Med. 15:14–23, 1993.

52. Spriet, L.L. Caffeine and performance. Int. J. Sports Nutr. 5(suppl):84S–99S, 1995.

53. U.S. Olympic Committee, Drug Control Program, Committee on Substance Abuse Research and Education. Copyright 1990.

54. Williams, M.H. Ergogenic aids. In *Sports Nutrition for the 90s*. Berning, J.R. and Steen, S.N., eds. Gaithersburg, MD: Aspen Publishers, Inc., 1991, pp. 101–127.

55. Mirkin, G. Bee pollen: living up to its hype? Physician Sports Med. 13:159–160, 1989.

In the Beginning: Nutrition for Mothers and Infants

CHAPTER CONCEPTS

1. Nutrient intake during pregnancy and lactation must meet the needs of both the mother and baby.

2. During normal gestation, a single cell grows and differentiates into a 3- to 4-kilogram baby.

3. In order to support pregnancy and prepare for lactation, a pregnant woman's body undergoes many changes including the development of a placenta and an amniotic sac, an increase in blood volume, the enlargement of the breasts and uterus, and the accumulation of body fat.

4. Energy, protein, water, vitamin, and mineral needs increase during pregnancy.

5. Regardless of prepregnancy weight, adequate weight gain during pregnancy is essential to the health of the mother and unborn baby.

6. The age, health, and nutritional status of the mother and her use of drugs and alcohol during pregnancy can affect the development of her child.

7. A newborn infant's energy and protein needs are higher per unit of body weight than at any other time of life.

8. Breast feeding is the ideal way to nourish infants. Infant formula can also provide adequate nutrition.

9. Monitoring growth rate is the best way to tell if infants are receiving adequate nutrients.

10. After four to six months of age, semisolid and solid foods can gradually be introduced into the infant's diet.

JUST A TASTE

Do pregnant women need vitamin and mineral supplements to meet their needs?

Should overweight women gain weight during pregnancy?

Is it safe to drink alcohol during pregnancy?

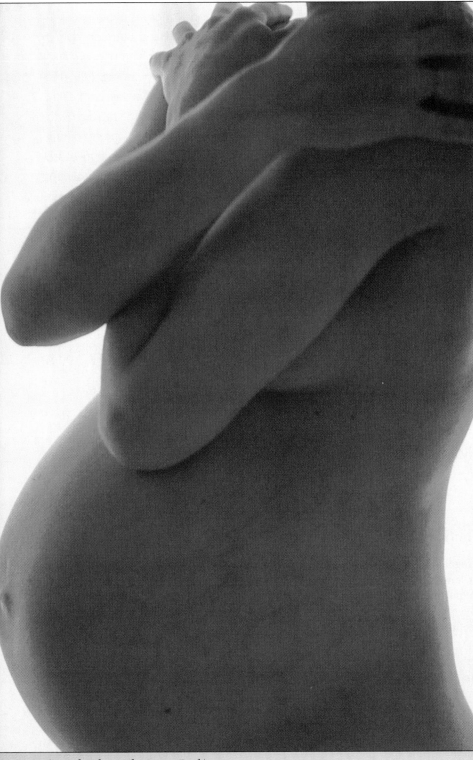

(*David Delossy/The Image Bank*)

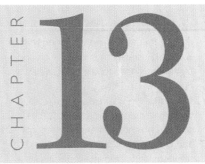

CHAPTER 13

Having a baby can be one of the most exciting and wondrous experiences in life. Most women pay special attention to their health and nutrition during pregnancy to help ensure the health of their babies. A woman's nutritional status is one of the most important factors affecting pregnancy outcome. Her diet must be carefully planned to supply the nutrients needed to maintain her health, support the physiological changes in her body, and provide for the rapid growth and development of her unborn baby. A deficiency or excess of nutrients during pregnancy, as well as the use of alcohol, illicit drugs, and cigarettes, may cause birth defects and low birth weights. Although good nutrition cannot always prevent these problems, adequate nutrition and consistent prenatal care can reduce the number of babies born too soon and too small.

Once the child is born, she must be adequately nourished to continue her rapid growth. Breast-fed infants continue to depend on nutrients from the mother to meet their needs. Lactation has high nutrient costs and the composition of breast milk can be affected by maternal intake, so a nursing woman's diet must be selected carefully. Formula-fed infants rely on the nutrients in infant formulas to meet their needs.

In this chapter, nutrition during pregnancy and early postnatal life will be addressed by discussing:

* What physiological changes occur during pregnancy?
* What are women's nutritional needs during pregnancy and lactation?
* What nutritional factors affect the risks to mother and child?
* What are the nutritional needs of breast-fed or bottle fed-infants?

THE PHYSIOLOGY OF PREGNANCY

Pregnancy, from conception to birth, usually lasts 40 weeks, or about nine months in humans. During pregnancy, the unborn child grows from a single cell to an infant that is ready for life outside the womb. Many physical changes also take place in the mother to support her developing offspring and prepare her for **lactation**.

PRENATAL GROWTH AND DEVELOPMENT

Reproduction requires the **fertilization** of an egg, or ovum, from the mother by a sperm from the father. Fertilization, which occurs in the **fallopian tube (oviduct)**, produces a single-celled **zygote**. The zygote travels down the mother's fallopian tube into the uterus. Along the way the zygote divides many times to form a ball of smaller cells. In the uterus it attaches to the uterine lining in a process known as **implantation**. Once implantation has occurred, two new organs, the **amniotic sac** and **placenta**, develop to protect and nourish the developing offspring (Figure 13-1). The amniotic sac is a fluid-filled membrane that surrounds the unborn baby and protects it from the bumps and bruises of the outside world. The placenta secretes hormones necessary to maintain pregnancy and allows nutrients and waste products to be transferred between the mother's blood and the blood of the developing baby.

Lactation–Milk production and secretion.

Fertilization–The union of sperm and egg.

Fallopian tubes (oviducts)–Narrow ducts leading from the ovaries and to the uterus.

Zygote–The cell produced by the union of sperm and ovum during fertilization.

Implantation–The process by which the zygote embeds in the uterine lining.

Amniotic sac–A membrane surrounding the fetus that contains the amniotic fluid.

Placenta–An organ produced from both maternal and embryonic tissues. It secretes hormones, transfers nutrients and oxygen from the mother's blood to the fetus, and removes wastes.

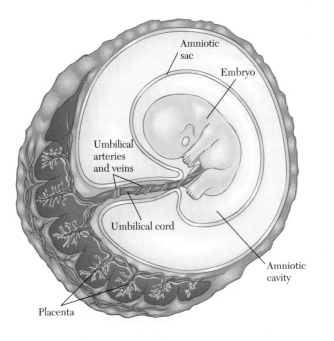

Amniotic sac

Embryo

Umbilical arteries and veins

Umbilical cord

Amniotic cavity

Placenta

FIGURE 13-1
During pregnancy, the amniotic sac protects the fetus, and the placenta allows nutrients and wastes to be transferred between mother and baby.

As these structures develop, the ball of cells continues to grow. The cells differentiate to form the multitude of specialized cell types that make up the body, and arrange themselves in the proper shapes and locations to form body organs and structures. About two weeks after fertilization, the developing offspring is known as an **embryo**. The embryonic stage of development lasts until the eighth week after fertilization, by which time rudimentary organ systems have been formed. The embryo is approximately 3 cm long (a little more than an inch) and has a beating heart. All major external and internal structures have been formed. Beginning at the ninth week of development and continuing until birth, the unborn baby is known as a **fetus** (Figure 13-2). During the fetal period of development, structures that appeared during the embryonic period continue to

Embryo–The developing human from two to eight weeks after fertilization. All organ systems are formed during this time.

Fetus–The developing human from the ninth week to birth. Growth and refinement of structures occur during this time.

FIGURE 13-2
At 16 weeks the fetus is about 16 cm (6.4 inches) long. (Custom Medical Stock)

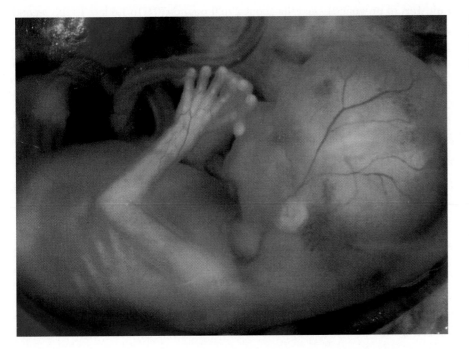

Spontaneous abortion, or **miscarriage**–Interruption of pregnancy prior to the seventh month.
Gestation–The time between conception and birth, which lasts about nine months in humans.
Low birth weight infant–An infant born weighing less than 2.5 kg (5.5 lb).
Preterm or **premature**–An infant born before 37 weeks of gestation.
Small for gestational age–An infant born at term weighing less than or equal to 2.5 kg (5.5 lb).

grow and mature. Anything that interferes with development can result in birth defects. If the damage to the embryo or fetus is severe, it may result in a **spontaneous abortion**, or **miscarriage**.

The fetal period usually ends after 40 weeks of **gestation** with the birth of an infant weighing about 3 to 4 kilograms (6.6 to 8.8 lb).[1] **Low birth weight infants**, those weighing less than 2.5 kg (5.5 lb) at birth, are at increased risk for illness and early death. Low birth weight can occur when the child is **preterm** or **premature**, born before 37 weeks of gestation. Preterm infants are born before their organ systems are fully developed for life outside the uterus, so they are at risk of early death from a variety of causes. Low birth weight may also occur when infants have suffered growth failure in the uterus. These infants are called **small for gestational age** and are also at risk. Today, with advances in medical and nutritional care, infants born as early as 25 weeks of gestation and those weighing as little as 1 kg (2.2 lb) can survive. Survival improves with increasing gestational age and birthweight.

CHANGES IN THE MOTHER

A woman's body undergoes many changes during pregnancy to develop and maintain the systems necessary to support the growing fetus. The mother's blood volume increases by 50%, and her heart, lungs, and kidneys work harder to deliver nutrients and oxygen and remove wastes. The placenta develops, and the hormones produced by it orchestrate other changes. They promote uterine growth. They relax muscles and ligaments to accommodate the growing fetus and allow for childbirth. They promote breast development, and they increase fat deposition to provide the energy stores that will be needed during late pregnancy and lactation. These changes all result in weight gain and can affect the type and level of physical activity that is safe. In some cases they can also cause uncomfortable and dangerous complications.

Trimester–Each third, or three-month period, of a pregnancy.

Weight Gain During Pregnancy   The recommended weight gain during pregnancy for healthy normal weight women, those with a body mass index of 19.8 to 26, is 25 to 35 pounds (11 to 15 kg). The rate of weight gain is as important as the total weight gain. Little gain is expected in the first three months, or **trimester**, of pregnancy—usually about 2 to 4 pounds (0.9 to 1.8 kg). In the second and third trimesters, when the fetus grows from less than a pound to 6 to 8 pounds, the recommended maternal weight gain is about 1 pound (0.45 kg) per week. Women who are underweight or overweight at conception should also gain weight at a slow, steady rate (Figure 13-3). Weight gains of up to 40 pounds (18 kg) are recommended for women who begin pregnancy with a body mass index of less than 19.8. Women with a body mass index of greater than 26 should gain less, only about 15 to 25 pounds (6.8 to 11.4 kg) over the course of pregnancy. Too little weight gain during pregnancy is associated with an increased risk of low birth weight infants.[1]

Maternal weight gain is due to the growth of both the mother and the fetus. On average the fetus represents 25% of total weight gain, the placenta 5%, and the amniotic fluid 6%. Expansion of maternal tissues accounts for most of the weight gained during pregnancy. This includes increases in the size of the uterus and breasts, expansion of blood volume, extracellular fluid, and fat stores (Figure 13-4). Some women are concerned that weight gained during pregnancy will be permanent. Typically within a year of delivery, women lose all but about 2 pounds of the weight.[2] Approximately 10 pounds are lost at birth from the weight of the baby, amniotic fluid, and placenta. In the week after delivery, another 5 pounds of fluid are typically lost. Once this initial fluid and tissue weight is lost, weight loss requires that energy intake be less than energy output. After the mother has

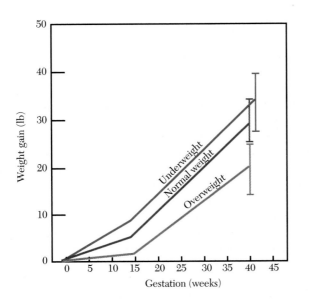

FIGURE 13-3
The same pattern of weight gain is recommended for women who are normal weight, underweight, or overweight at the start of pregnancy; but the recommendations for total weight changes are different. (Adapted from Committee on Nutritional Status During Pregnancy and Lactation. *Nutrition During Pregnancy*. Washington, DC: National Academy Press, 1990.)

recovered from delivery, a balanced, low-energy diet combined with moderate exercise will encourage weight loss and the return of muscle tone.

Physical Activity During Pregnancy   Physical activity can benefit the pregnant woman by improving her overall fitness, reducing stress, preventing excess weight gain, preventing low back pain, preventing gestational diabetes, improving mood and body image, and speeding recovery from childbirth. The phys-

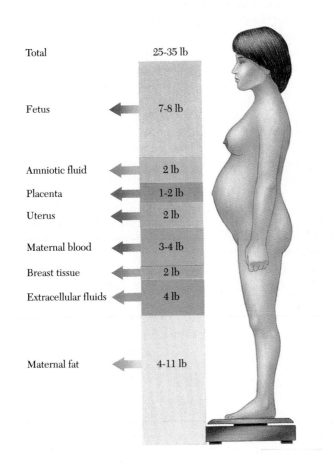

FIGURE 13-4
The weight gained by the mother during pregnancy includes increases in the weight of her tissues as well as the weight of the infant, placenta, and the amniotic fluid.

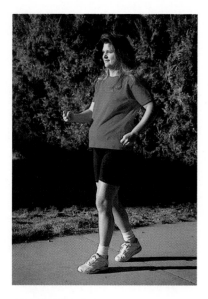

FIGURE 13-5
Exercise can usually be continued during pregnancy as along as a few safety rules are followed. (Trent Steffler/David R. Frazier Photolibrary)

Morning sickness–Nausea and vomiting that affects some women during the first few months of pregnancy.

iological changes of pregnancy affect the type and level of physical activity that is recommended. Too much exercise that is too intense could harm the fetus by reducing the amount of oxygen and nutrients it receives or by increasing body temperature. This is a concern for pregnant athletes as well as pregnant women whose jobs require prolonged physical activity. Some studies suggest that women in physically demanding jobs may be at increased risk of having a preterm or low birth weight infant.[3]

All pregnant women should check with their physicians before engaging in an exercise program. For women who were physically active before becoming pregnant, moderate exercise is usually safe during a healthy pregnancy (Figure 13-5). There is less information about the risks and benefits of an exercise program that is initiated during pregnancy.[4] Previously inactive women should therefore increase exercise frequency and intensity very gradually. Exercise guidelines have been developed to minimize the risks and maximize the benefits of exercise during pregnancy.[5] These guidelines are summarized in Table 13-1. Because women weigh more during pregnancy and carry that weight in the front of their bodies where it can interfere with balance and place stress on the bones, joints, and muscles, non–weight-bearing activities like swimming and cycling are recommended. Intense exercise should be limited during pregnancy, and exercise outdoors in hot humid weather should be avoided.

Digestive Discomforts of Pregnancy   Many of the physiological changes that occur during pregnancy affect the digestive tract and may cause discomfort for the mother. Most of these problems are minor, but in some cases they may endanger the mother and the fetus.

Morning sickness is a syndrome of nausea and vomiting that occurs during pregnancy. In most cases symptoms decrease significantly after the first trimester. The term morning sickness is somewhat of a misnomer because symptoms can occur anytime during the day or night. It is thought to be related to the hormonal changes of pregnancy and may be alleviated to some extent by eating small, frequent snacks of dry, starchy foods, such as plain crackers or bread. In some cases the symptoms last for the entire pregnancy and, in severe cases, may require medical intervention to assure that nutrient needs can be met.

Heartburn, a burning sensation caused by stomach acid leaking up into the esophagus, is another common digestive complaint during pregnancy. Heartburn is common in pregnancy because the hormones produced to relax the muscles of the uterus also relax the muscles of the gastrointestinal tract. Relaxation of the lower esophageal sphincter allows the acidic stomach contents to back up into the esophagus, causing irritation. The problem gets more severe as pregnancy pro-

TABLE 13-1 Guidelines for Physical Activity During Pregnancy
Obtain medical permission before exercising.
If inactive before pregnancy, increase activity very gradually.
Stop exercising when fatigued and do not exercise to exhaustion.
Participate in non–weight-bearing activities like cycling and swimming rather than weight-bearing activities such as jogging.
Avoid exercising in the supine position after the first trimester.
Avoid strenuous exertion during the first trimester, and at other times strenuous exercise should not be continued for more than 15 minutes.
Avoid exercising in hot or humid environments.
Drink plenty of liquids before, during, and after exercise.

Modified from Dewey, K.G. and McCrory, M.A. Effects of dieting and physical activity on pregnancy and lactation. Am. J. Clin. Nutr. 59(suppl):446S–453S, 1994.

gresses because the growing baby crowds the stomach. The fuller the stomach, the more likely that its contents will reflux into the esophagus. Therefore, heartburn can be reduced by consuming small meals throughout the day rather than several large meals. Because high-fat foods, such as fried foods, rich sauces, and desserts, leave the stomach slowly, a lowfat diet of grains, fruits, plain meats and vegetables, and lowfat dairy products is less likely to cause heartburn. Because a reclining position makes it easier for acidic juices to flow into the esophagus, remaining upright after eating also reduces heartburn. Avoiding substances that are known to cause heartburn such as caffeine and peppermint can also be helpful.

Constipation is a common complaint during pregnancy. The hormones of pregnancy that cause muscles to relax decrease intestinal motility and slow transit time. Constipation becomes more of a problem late in pregnancy when the weight of the uterus puts pressure on the gastrointestinal tract. In addition, iron supplements often prescribed during pregnancy cause constipation. Maintaining a moderate level of physical activity and consuming at least one-half gallon of water and other fluids, as well as high-fiber foods such as whole grains, vegetables, and fruits, is recommended to prevent constipation. Hemorrhoids are also more common during pregnancy, as a result of both constipation and physiological changes in blood flow.

Complications of Pregnancy
Occasionally, abnormal hormonal changes occur during pregnancy causing complications for the mother.

Gestational Diabetes
Consistently elevated blood glucose during pregnancy is known as **gestational diabetes**. It occurs in 1 to 3% of all pregnancies and is most common in obese women.[6] This form of diabetes usually disappears when the pregnancy is completed, although the mother remains at higher risk for developing adult-onset diabetes.

High levels of glucose in the mother's blood can adversely affect the fetus. Glucose in the mother's blood passes freely across the placenta, so high blood sugar in the mother provides extra energy to the fetus. This extra energy can produce a baby who is **large for gestational age** and consequently at increased risk of complications. The treatment of gestational diabetes, as with other types of diabetes, involves consuming a carefully planned diet that is eaten at consistent intervals throughout the day.

Edema
The hormonal changes of pregnancy allow blood volume to expand to nourish the fetus, but the expansion of blood volume may also cause the accumulation of extracellular fluid in the tissues, known as **edema**. Edema is characterized by puffiness and swelling, particularly in the feet and ankles. Treatment involves restricting activity and keeping the feet and legs elevated. Restriction of dietary sodium below the recommendation for the general population is not recommended. Edema increases medical risks only if it is accompanied by a rise in blood pressure.

Pregnancy-Induced Hypertension
Another complication of pregnancy is a rise in blood pressure referred to as **pregnancy-induced hypertension**. The onset of pregnancy-induced hypertension may be signaled by the gain of several pounds within a few days. Mild symptoms include an increase in blood pressure, edema, and protein in the urine. Severe pregnancy-induced hypertension can cause convulsions and be life threatening. It is most common in mothers under 20 or over 35 years of age, those in low-income groups, and those who are underweight. The cause of pregnancy-induced hypertension is not known, but research suggests that low calcium intake may be involved.[7] Treatment includes bed rest and careful medical attention. Dietary sodium intake should be moderate, but sodium restriction does not cure the syndrome. The condition usually resolves after the baby is born.

Gestational diabetes—A consistently elevated blood glucose level that develops during pregnancy and returns to normal after delivery.

Large for gestational age—An infant weighing greater than 4 kg (8.8 lb) at birth.

Edema—Swelling due to the buildup of extracellular fluid in the tissues.

Pregnancy-induced hypertension—A condition during pregnancy that is characterized by an increase in body weight, elevated blood pressure, protein in the urine, and edema. It can be life threatening to mother and fetus.

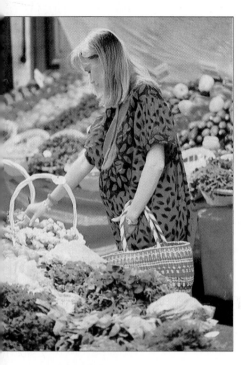

FIGURE 13-6
The diet must be carefully selected to meet all the needs of pregnancy.
(© J. DaCunha/Petit Format/Photo Researchers, Inc.)

THE NUTRITIONAL NEEDS OF PREGNANCY

Nutrition is important both before and during pregnancy. During pregnancy, a woman's nutrient intake and body stores must provide all the nutrients needed to support the growth and development of the baby while continuing to meet the mother's needs. Because the increased need for energy is proportionately smaller than the increased need for protein, vitamins, and minerals, a well-balanced, nutrient-dense diet is required (Figure 13-6).

THE IMPORTANCE OF NUTRITION BEFORE PREGNANCY

A woman's nutritional status before she becomes pregnant may affect her ability to conceive a child or successfully complete a pregnancy. For example, starvation diets, anorexia nervosa, and excessive athletic activity, such as marathon running, can interfere with ovulation and therefore make conception difficult. Obesity can also alter hormone levels and decrease fertility. Deficiencies or excesses of nutrients can affect pregnancy outcome. For instance, a deficiency of folic acid or an excess of vitamin A early in pregnancy can cause birth defects.[8,9]

Nutritional status can be affected by some birth control methods, and these can therefore have an impact on a subsequent pregnancy. For example, intrauterine devices (IUDs) increase menstrual blood loss and therefore increase the likelihood of iron deficiency anemia. Oral contraceptives can interfere with the metabolism of folic acid and decrease blood levels of vitamin B_6, vitamin B_{12}, vitamin C, and beta-carotene.[10] If conception occurs soon after oral contraceptive use stops, these levels will not have time to return to normal before pregnancy begins. The use of drugs—whether over-the-counter, prescribed, or illicit—can also affect both fertility and pregnancy outcome. A woman who is considering pregnancy should discuss her plans with her physician in order to determine the risks of any medication she is taking.

ENERGY, PROTEIN, AND WATER NEEDS DURING PREGNANCY

A typical pregnancy has been estimated to require an additional 55,000 kcalories.[1] Although this number may seem staggering, it amounts to only about an extra sandwich and glass of milk, or about 300 kcalories, per day during the second and third trimesters of the pregnancy (Table 13-2). During the first trimester the additional energy required is small, and the RDA is not increased. The composition of the diet during pregnancy should be about the same as in a nonpregnant diet, 55 to 60% of energy coming from carbohydrate and about 30% from fat. If carbohydrate intake is less than 100 grams per day, ketosis may occur. Prolonged ketosis may be harmful to the fetus, even though some ketone production occurs normally after an overnight fast, and the fetus can metabolize ketones.[11]

Protein needs are also increased during pregnancy. Protein is needed for the structure of all new cells in both the mother and the fetus. An increase of 10 grams of protein per day is recommended throughout pregnancy to provide for the increase in maternal blood volume; the development of the placenta, breasts, uterus, and uterine muscles; and the development and growth of all fetal structures. For a woman weighing 62 kg, this increases protein needs to about 60 grams per day. Many nonpregnant women already consume this amount or more.

The need for water is increased during pregnancy because of the increase in blood volume, the production of amniotic fluid, and the needs of the fetus. This requires the consumption of only an extra 30 ml per day. However, adequate fluid consumption, about 2 liters per day, throughout pregnancy is important in preventing constipation.

TABLE 13-2	Recommended Nutrient Intakes for a 25-Year-Old Woman During Pregnancy and Lactation					
	Nonpregnant		Pregnant*		Lactating (0–6 months)	
Nutrient	RDA	RNI[†]	RDA	RNI[†]	RDA	RNI
Energy (kcal)	2200	1900	2500	2200	2700	2350
Protein (g)	50	51	60	75	65	71
Vitamin A (RE)	800	800	800	800	1300	1200
Vitamin D (μg)	5	2.5	10	5	10	5
Vitamin E (α-TE)	8	6	10	8	12	9
Vitamin K (μg)	65	—	65	—	65	—
Vitamin C (mg)	60	30	70	40	95	55
Thiamin (mg)	1.1	0.8	1.5	0.9	1.6	1.0
Riboflavin (mg)	1.3	1.0	1.6	1.3	1.8	1.4
Niacin (mg)	15	14	17	16	20	17
Vitamin B_6 (mg)	1.6	0.8	2.2	1.1	2.1	1.1
Folate (μg)	180	185	400	385	280	285
Vitamin B_{12} (μg)	2.0	1.0	2.2	1.2	2.6	1.2
Calcium (mg)	800	700	1200	1200	1200	1200
Phosphorus (mg)	800	850	1200	1050	1200	1050
Magnesium (mg)	280	200	320	245	355	265
Iron (mg)	15	13	30	23	15	13
Zinc (mg)	12	9	15	15	19	15
Iodine (μg)	150	160	175	185	200	210
Selenium (μg)	55	—	65	—	75	—

*Values represent the recommendations for the third trimester.
[†]Canadian Recommended Nutrient Intakes.

MICRONUTRIENT NEEDS DURING PREGNANCY

The need for many vitamins and minerals is increased during pregnancy (see Table 13-2). Since energy intake increases, the requirements for the micronutrients needed for energy utilization, such as thiamin, niacin, riboflavin, and magnesium, increase. Since protein needs are higher, the requirements for vitamin B_6 and zinc, needed for protein metabolism, increase. The needs for micronutrients involved in the growth and development of bone and connective tissue and the synthesis of new cells are also greater.

Micronutrient Needs for the Development of Bone and Connective Tissue   Bone formation requires calcium and phosphorus, vitamin D for proper calcium absorption and metabolism, and vitamin C for connective tissue formation.

Calcium and Phosphorus   The fetus retains about 30 grams of calcium over the course of gestation. Most of the calcium is deposited in the last trimester when the fetal skeleton is growing most rapidly and the teeth are forming.[12] Pregnant women absorb more of the calcium they consume and lose less calcium in the urine than do nonpregnant women.[1] Despite this improved efficiency, the recommended intake for calcium is increased during pregnancy. The RDA is 1200 mg per day and a recent NIH Consensus Conference on Optimal Calcium Intake recommends between 1200 and 1500 mg per day.[13] These needs can be met by consuming 3 servings of milk or other dairy products daily. Women who are lactose intolerant may be able to meet their calcium needs with yogurt, cheese, reduced-lactose milk, and calcium-rich vegetables such as collard greens. Additional phosphorus is recommended to keep phosphorus in balance with calcium.

Vitamin D   In order to ensure efficient calcium absorption, the recommended intake for vitamin D is increased to 10 μg per day. If exposure to sunlight is limited and sufficient vitamin D is not consumed in the diet, supplements should be considered. Inadequate vitamin D is a particular problem in African American women because darker skin pigmentation reduces vitamin D synthesis and lactose intolerance is common, so the intake of dairy products is typically low.[14]

Vitamin C   Vitamin C is important for bone and connective tissue formation. It is needed for the synthesis of collagen, which forms connective tissue in the skin, tendons, and the protein matrix of bones. The RDA for vitamin C is increased to 70 mg per day during pregnancy.

The RDA for vitamin C can easily be met with foods such as citrus fruit, and supplements are generally not necessary. If large doses of vitamin C are taken during pregnancy, the fetus becomes adapted to a high intake of vitamin C. At birth, when the vitamin is no longer available from the mother's blood, symptoms of vitamin C deficiency may develop even if the diet provides the amount typically recommended.

Micronutrient Needs for Increased Cell Division
To form new fetal and maternal cells, additional folic acid, vitamin B_{12}, and zinc are required. The synthesis of new red blood cells for the fetus and for the increase in maternal blood volume during pregnancy also requires additional iron.

Folic Acid and Vitamin B_{12}   Folic acid and vitamin B_{12} are essential for cell division. Adequate folate intake is crucial even before conception because rapid cell division occurs in the first days and weeks of pregnancy. Folate is believed to be essential for proper formation of the **neural tube**. The neural tube is a portion of the embryo that develops into the brain and spinal cord. If it does not develop normally the infant can be born with a neural tube defect such as spina bifida, a defect of the spinal column that can cause varying degrees of physical and intellectual disability (Figure 13-7). The incidence of neural tube defects can be re-

Neural tube—A portion of the embryo that develops into the brain and spinal cord.

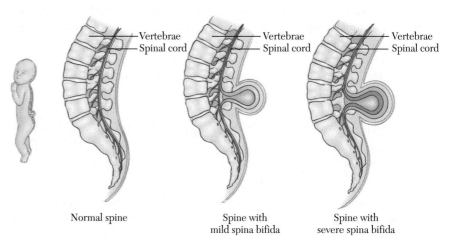

Normal spine

Spine with mild spina bifida

Spine with severe spina bifida

FIGURE 13-7
The brain and spinal cord develop from the neural tube. When the neural tube fails to close, spina bifida may result. Compared with the normal spine on the left, the spine of a baby with spina bifida has a noticeable sac (middle), and in more severe cases the spinal cord protrudes through the spine into the sac (right). (FDA Consumer, May 1994.)

but it does not address the need for good nutrition for women planning a pregnancy.

More than 50% of the women who give birth every year in the United States are in the workforce.[10] Women with the greatest job stress have an increased risk of spontaneous abortion, low birth weight infants, stillbirth, and infant mortality.

SUBSTANCES THAT AFFECT THE HEALTH OF THE UNBORN CHILD

Many substances can affect the health of the child during pregnancy. Some of these are environmental toxins, some are dietary, and others are the result of maternal behaviors such as smoking and drug use (Figure 13-10).

The Developing Child Is Particularly Vulnerable   The rapidly dividing cells of the embryo and fetus are sensitive to many substances that might normally be a part of a woman's daily routine. Any chemical, biological, or physical agent that causes birth defects is called a **teratogen**. The placenta prevents some teratogens from passing from the mother's blood to the embryonic or fetal blood, but it cannot prevent the passage of all hazardous substances.

The developing embryo and fetus are particularly vulnerable to assault because both cell division and differentiation occur rapidly early in development. Times during development when teratogens are particularly damaging are called **critical periods** of development. Anything that interferes with development during a critical period causes irreversible damage. Critical periods correspond to times when cells are dividing, differentiating, and moving to form structures and organs. Because each organ system develops at a different rate and time, when a nutritional, chemical, or other insult occurs determines which organ system is primarily affected. The majority of cell differentiation occurs during the embryonic period, so this is the time when exposure to teratogens can do the most damage, but vital body organs can still be affected during the fetal period (Figure 13-11). Severe damage to an embryo or fetus usually results in a spontaneous abortion.

Nutrients as Teratogens   Deficiencies or excesses of some nutrients can have teratogenic effects. As discussed previously, inadequate folate intake may affect neural tube development. Excess vitamin D can cause mental retardation, and vitamin E, in high doses, increases the incidence of spontaneous abortions. Vitamin A is of particular concern because kidney problems and central nervous system abnormalities can occur in the offspring even when the maternal dose is not extremely high. Consumption by the mother of supplements containing 3000 RE or more of preformed vitamin A, about four times the RDA, causes a fivefold increase in the risk of birth defects.[9] Supplements consumed during pregnancy should therefore contain beta-carotene, which is not teratogenic. The RDA for vitamin A is not increased during pregnancy.

Alcohol   Alcohol impairs fetal growth and development in a number of ways. It is a toxin that directly affects fetal development and it reduces blood flow to the placenta, which decreases the delivery of oxygen and nutrients to the fetus. The use of alcohol can also impair maternal nutritional status, further increasing the risk to the embryo or fetus. Alcohol consumption during pregnancy is the leading cause of preventable birth defects and mental retardation.[27] Alcohol-related birth defects occur in 0.1% of live births in the United States and in 4.3% of babies born to heavy drinkers. They are more common in minority women and in women of lower socioeconomic status.[28] Alcohol can cause a spectrum of abnor-

Teratogen–A chemical, biological, or physical agent that causes birth defects.

Critical periods–Times in growth and development when an organism is more susceptible to harm from poor nutrition or other environmental factors.

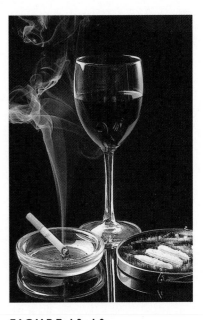

FIGURE 13-10
Women who smoke, drink alcohol, or use illicit drugs during pregnancy put their babies at risk. (Dennis Drenner)

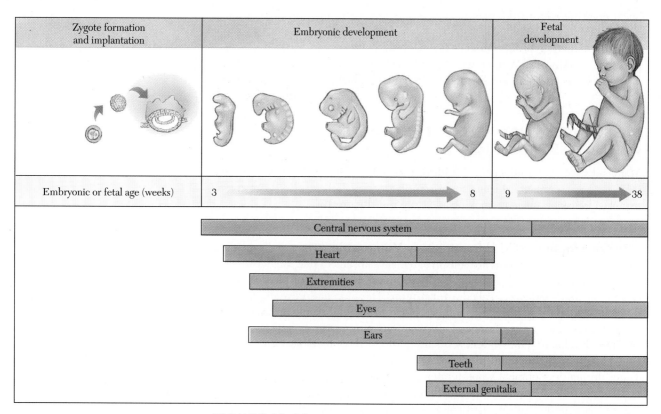

FIGURE 13-11

Critical periods of development are different for different body systems. The orange bars indicate when injury to the fetus from teratogens is likely to be the greatest. The purple bars indicate when damage may be less severe. (Adapted from Moore, K. and Persuad, T. *The Developing Human*, 5th ed. Philadelphia: W.B. Saunders Company, 1993.)

Fetal alcohol syndrome—A characteristic group of physical and mental abnormalities in an infant resulting from alcohol consumed by the mother during pregnancy.

malities. Less severe effects such as learning disabilities and behavioral abnormalities are referred to as alcohol-related birth defects or fetal alcohol effects. More severe alcohol-related damage during pregnancy is called **fetal alcohol syndrome** (Figure 13-12).

Fetal alcohol syndrome is a pattern of facial deformities, growth retardation, and permanent brain damage that causes problems throughout the child's lifetime.[27] The most notable physical features of fetal alcohol syndrome involve the face, eyes, and upper lip. Growth retardation either during gestation or after birth is common. Newborns with the syndrome may be shaky and irritable, and have poor muscle tone and withdrawal symptoms. Other symptoms include heart and urinary tract defects, impaired vision and hearing, and delayed language development. Mental retardation is the most common and most serious deficit.

Adolescents and adults diagnosed with fetal alcohol syndrome are plagued by debilitating behavioral problems, such as poor concentration, and poor socialization and communication skills. These problems interfere with their abilities to hold jobs and live independently.[29] Since alcohol consumption in each trimester has been associated with abnormalities, and there is no level of alcohol consumption that is known to be safe during pregnancy, complete abstinence from alcohol during pregnancy is recommended (see Figure 13-12).

Cigarettes   Exposure to cigarette smoke during gestation affects the baby before birth and throughout life. Compounds in tobacco smoke bind to hemoglobin and reduce oxygen delivery to fetal tissues. In addition, nicotine constricts arteries and limits blood flow, which reduces both oxygen and nutrient delivery to the

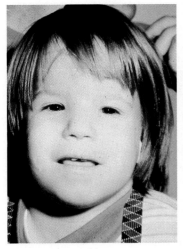

(a)

(b)

GOVERNMENT WARNING: (1) ACCORDING TO THE SURGEON GENERAL, WOMEN SHOULD NOT DRINK ALCOHOLIC BEVERAGES DURING PREGNANCY BECAUSE OF THE RISK OF BIRTH DEFECTS. (2) CONSUMPTION OF ALCOHOLIC BEVERAGES IMPAIRS YOUR ABILITY TO DRIVE A CAR OR OPERATE MACHINERY, AND MAY CAUSE HEALTH PROBLEMS.

FIGURE 13-12
(a) Children with fetal alcohol syndrome have common facial characteristics including a low nasal bridge, a short nose, distinct eyelids, and a thin upper lip. (b) Alcoholic beverage packages include a warning against alcohol consumption during pregnancy. (a, Dennis Drenner; b, courtesy of A.P. Streissguth, University of Washington, Seattle.)

fetus. A full day of smoking may cause a 20 to 25% reduction in oxygen delivery to the fetus.[30] A woman who smokes is twice as likely to give birth to a small-for-gestational-age baby. The birth weight of the baby is correlated with how much the mother smokes, so any time spent by the mother during the pregnancy without smoking will benefit the baby. The risks of miscarriage, stillbirth, premature birth, **sudden infant death syndrome (crib death)**, and respiratory problems are all increased in mothers who smoke.[31] The risks of sudden infant death syndrome and respiratory problems are also increased in children exposed to environmental cigarette smoke after birth.[32] The effects of maternal smoking follow children throughout life. Children whose mothers smoked while pregnant may have impaired intellectual development and a greater risk of developing cancer in their youth.[33]

Sudden infant death syndrome (crib death)—The unexplained death of infants, usually during sleep.

Caffeine   Although caffeine has been found to cause fetal abnormalities in animals, similar effects have not been found in humans.[34] Caffeine has been found to enhance the teratogenic effect of substances such as tobacco, alcohol, and drugs that constrict blood vessels, but when caffeine consumption is moderate and spread out over the day these interactions do not appear to affect pregnancy outcome.[35] Large amounts of caffeine during pregnancy (greater than 7 cups of coffee per day) can cause decreases in birth weight. It is therefore recommended that pregnant women limit their caffeine intake to no more than 300 mg of caffeine or the equivalent of 2 to 3 cups of coffee per day.[36] Caffeine is a natural component of coffee, tea, and chocolate and is added to soft drinks and certain medications. Table 12-5 lists the caffeine content of some commonly consumed foods, beverages, and medications.

Illicit Drug Abuse   About one in every ten newborns in the United States is exposed to one or more illicit drugs before birth. In major cities, the percentage of newborns showing the effects of drugs is 16% or higher. Fetal exposure to cocaine, phenylcyclidine hydrochloride (PCP), and other drugs that affect the central nervous system produces low birth weight infants who have difficulty interacting with others and responding to changes in their environment.[37]

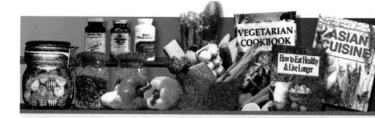

Prenatal Supplements

Most pregnant women leave their first prenatal doctor's visit with a prescription for a prenatal vitamin and mineral supplement. Yet, public health agencies only recommend routine supplementation of iron and folate.[1,2] The supplements prescribed by physicians contain iron and folate, but they also contain about 15 other vitamins and minerals. Should women take these supplements?

There is nothing wrong with taking a multivitamin and mineral supplement during pregnancy as long as the recommended dosage is not exceeded. The concern of public health agencies is that individuals taking supplements may ignore other components of their diet, thinking that the supplement will meet all their needs. Even when a prenatal supplement is taken, a woman's diet must be carefully planned to satisfy all of the requirements of pregnancy.

Prenatal vitamin and mineral supplements supply many nutrients at levels that meet or slightly exceed the recommended intake for pregnancy, but some are present in amounts that do not meet the needs of pregnancy, and others are missing altogether. For example, the tablet shown in the table contains only 200 mg of calcium, which is less than 20% of the recommended intake. The reason it does not contain more is that the tablet would have to be very large to provide the recommendation of 1200 mg. To meet her needs a pregnant woman would need to consume this tablet plus the amount of calcium in three glasses of milk. For similar reasons,

the tablet doesn't meet the recommendation for magnesium. Even if all the calcium and magnesium needed for pregnancy could be packed into a little pill, it still would not provide an adequate diet. Prenatal supplements do not contain the protein needed for tissue synthesis or the complex carbohydrates needed for energy. They lack fiber, which helps prevent constipation, and they do not contain fluid for expanding tissues and blood volume. They are also lacking in food components such as the phytochemicals that are supplied by a diet rich in whole grains, fruits, and vegetables.

Prenatal supplements are not absolutely necessary to meet the nutrient needs of pregnancy, but a very carefully planned diet is necessary to provide all the nutrients needed to produce a healthy baby. If a prenatal supplement is taken, it must be part of a healthy diet.

[1]Committee on Nutritional Status During Pregnancy and Lactation, National Academy of Science. *Nutrition During Pregnancy*. Washington, DC: National Academy Press, 1990.

[2]U.S. Public Health Service. Recommendations for the use of folic acid to reduce the number of cases of spina bifida and other neural tube defects. Morb. Mortal. Wkly. Rep. 41:1–7, 1992.

Nutrients Commonly Contained in a Prenatal Supplement

Nutrient	Amount per Tablet	Recommendations for Pregnancy RDA	Recommendations for Pregnancy RNI†
Vitamin A (RE)	800	800	800
Vitamin D (ergocalciferol) (µg)	10	10	5
Vitamin E (α-TE)	11–15	10	8
Vitamin C (mg)	80–120	70	40
Folic acid (µg)	400–1000	400	385
Thiamin (mg)	1.5	1.5	0.9
Riboflavin (mg)	1.6–3.0	1.6	1.3
Niacin (mg)	17–20	17	16
Vitamin B_6 (mg)	2.6–10	2.2	1.1
Vitamin B_{12} (µg)	2.5–12	2.2	1.2
Biotin (mg)	0.03	0.03–0.1°	—
Pantothenic acid (mg)	7	4–7°	—
Calcium (mg)	200	1200	1200
Iron (mg)	60–65	30	23
Magnesium (mg)	100	320	245
Copper (mg)	2–3	1.5–3°	—
Zinc (mg)	25	15	15

°Estimated safe and adequate daily dietary intake
†For third trimester

The most commonly used illicit drug among pregnant women is cocaine. During pregnancy, cocaine use is associated with a high rate of miscarriages, premature labor and delivery, intrauterine growth retardation, low birth weight infants, birth defects, and sudden infant death syndrome.[38] The risk of maternal complications is also increased. This drug easily crosses the placenta and causes damage by constricting blood vessels, thereby reducing the flow of oxygen and nutrients to the rapidly dividing fetal cells.[39] At birth, these babies are small and overly excitable. They have a small head circumference, which is associated with lower IQ scores. Cocaine also affects brain chemistry by altering the action of neurotransmitters. This may cause the impulsiveness and moodiness characteristic of some cocaine-exposed children. Some of these babies have physical deformities, and most suffer from behavioral problems severe enough to sabotage their education and social development.

Marijuana also crosses the placenta and enters fetal blood. Thus far, studies have not shown a relationship between marijuana use during pregnancy and birth weight, prematurity, or birth defects.[40] Some babies born to marijuana users have been shown to have a poor visual response and an increased tremor and startle reflex.[30]

LACTATION

The nutrient requirements of pregnancy include those needed to prepare for lactation. After childbirth, the breast-feeding mother's nutrient intake must support milk production and can influence the nutrient composition of milk.

THE PHYSIOLOGY OF LACTATION

During pregnancy, changes occur in the breasts to prepare for milk production, and body fat is deposited to ensure that energy is available for lactation. After birth the suckling of the infant causes the release of the pituitary hormone prolactin, which stimulates milk production. The more the infant suckles, the more milk is produced. Once produced, the milk must move from storage lobules in the breast to the nipple, a process known as **let-down** (Figure 13-13). The let-down of milk is caused by oxytocin, a hormone produced by the pituitary gland. Oxytocin release is also stimulated by the suckling of the infant, but as nursing becomes more automatic, oxytocin release and the let-down of milk may occur in response to the sight or sound of an infant. It can be inhibited by nervous tension, fatigue, or embarrassment, as may occur in the United States where public breast feeding is sometimes frowned upon. This let-down response is essential for successful breast feeding and makes suckling easier for the child. If let-down is slow, the child can become frustrated and difficult to feed.

Let-down—A reflex triggered by the infant's suckling that causes milk to be released from the milk ducts and flow to the nipple.

MATERNAL NUTRIENT NEEDS DURING LACTATION

The need for energy and many nutrients is even greater during lactation than during pregnancy. This is because the mother is still providing for all of the nutrient needs of the infant who is growing faster and is more active than the fetus. The newborn also has greater energy and nutrient needs for processes like temperature regulation and digestion that were partially or completely managed by the mother when the fetus was still in the womb.

Energy and Protein Needs During Lactation
During the first six months of lactation, approximately 600 to 900 ml, or 3 cups, of milk is produced daily. The amount is increased or decreased depending on the amount that the infant consumes. Producing a cup (240 ml) of breast milk requires about 225 kcalories. The milk itself contains approximately 175 kcalories, and the additional 50 kcalories are needed to synthesize the components of the milk. Providing an infant with 750 ml of milk would require approximately 700 kcalories from the

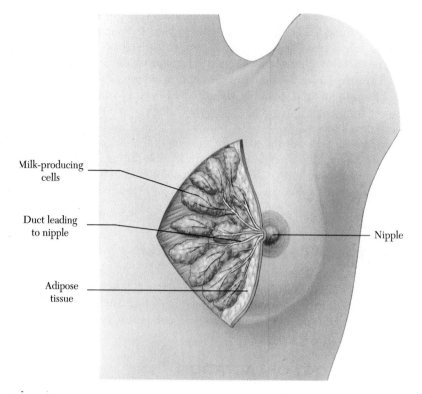

Milk-producing cells

Duct leading to nipple

Adipose tissue

Nipple

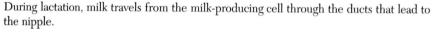

FIGURE 13-13
During lactation, milk travels from the milk-producing cell through the ducts that lead to the nipple.

mother. It is estimated that fat stored during pregnancy will provide 200 to 300 kcalories per day during the first 3 months of lactation. The remainder must be supplied in the diet. Therefore, an increase of about 500 kcalories per day over nonpregnant needs is recommended during early lactation.

The protein needed to produce milk increases maternal protein needs, and therefore recommended protein intake, by about 15 to 20 grams per day above nonpregnant needs.

Many women are concerned about losing weight after pregnancy. It is normal to lose weight during the first six months after delivery. Some studies report that breast feeding does not affect the amount of weight lost,[41] whereas others suggest it does so initially[42] or if breast feeding continues for at least six months.[43] Beginning one month after birth, most lactating women lose 0.5 to 1 kilogram (1 to 2 lb) per month for six months. Some women will lose more and others may maintain or even gain weight regardless of whether they breast feed.[44] Rapid weight loss is not recommended because it can decrease milk production. Regular exercise may speed weight loss and still allows adequate milk production.[44]

Water Needs During Lactation When fluid intake is low, the mother's urine will become more concentrated to conserve water for milk production. To avoid dehydration and ensure adequate milk production, fluid intake should be increased by about 1 liter per day. This can be done by consuming an extra glass of milk, juice, or water at every meal and whenever the infant nurses.

Micronutrient Needs During Lactation The recommended intakes for several vitamins and minerals are increased during lactation to meet the metabolic needs of synthesizing milk and to replace the nutrients secreted in the milk itself (see Table 13-2). Maternal intake of some vitamins can affect milk composition. This is particularly true of the water soluble vitamins, C, B_6, and B_{12}, and the fat soluble vitamins, A and D. When maternal intake is low, the amounts in milk are decreased. For other nutrients such as calcium and folate, levels in the milk are maintained at the expense of maternal stores. Lactation for 6 months or more is associated with maternal bone loss, but there is evidence that the calcium lost is replaced by 12 months after birth.[45] A calcium intake of 1200 to 1500 mg per day is recommended.[13] Folate needs are increased above nonpregnant levels but are not as high as during pregnancy. Iron needs are not increased during lactation because little iron is lost in milk, and in most women losses are decreased because menstruation is absent.

Meeting Maternal Nutrient Needs During Lactation   Meeting the needs of lactation requires a varied nutrient-dense diet that follows the Food Guide Pyramid recommendations for lactating women (see Figure 13-8). The need for calcium is met by consuming 3 servings of dairy products, and additional nutrients and energy are obtained from extra servings of vegetables and grains, and a larger serving of meat or meat substitutes. Most women can meet all their needs without supplements.

CRITICAL THINKING

How to Nourish a New Baby

Chevon had her baby last week. He is a healthy 7-pound, 19-inch-long boy, named Henry. Her grandmother has come to stay for a while to help with the baby. Chevon is breast feeding, but Grandma occasionally feeds Henry a bottle with pumped breast milk or formula.

After three weeks the baby still wakes up at night to eat. Grandma says to give him a bottle with formula mixed with cereal before bed to help him sleep through the night.

Will this help?

There is no evidence that babies who consume cereal in their bottles sleep better. Henry is still too young to need any food other than breast milk or formula and may have difficulty digesting the cereal.

When Henry is six weeks old, Chevon must return to work. She would like to continue breast feeding even though Henry will be home with Grandma while she is at work across town.

What options does she have?

Even if she works full time, she will still be able to nurse at home in the morning and evening. Since there is a refrigerator in the lunch room at work, she can pump milk once or twice during the day and refrigerate it to be fed to Henry the following day while she is at work. This will allow him to consume breast milk and will ensure that her milk production remains adequate. The refrigerated milk should be used within 24 to 48 hours. If no refrigerator were available, Chevon could try nursing mornings and nights and have Grandma feed him formula during the day.

Grandma is anxious to start feeding Henry solid foods. She says he's too big to just consume breast milk.

Why should Grandma wait until Henry is four to six months old before feeding him solid food?

Answer:

NUTRITION FOR THE INFANT

When a child is born and the umbilical cord is cut, he suddenly must be actively involved in obtaining nutrients rather than being passively fed through the placenta. The infant must satisfy all of his nutrient needs with either breast milk or infant formula. Solid food is not needed until four to six months of age, and even after solid food is introduced breast milk or formula remains the basis of the diet until about one year of age.

NUTRIENT REQUIREMENTS OF THE INFANT

Adequate nutrition is extremely important for newborns. They grow more rapidly than at any other time during their life and many of their organ systems and metabolic processes are still developing. Since their digestive abilities are limited and they have no teeth, a special type of diet is required.

Energy and Macronutrients   Energy requirements per unit of body weight are about three times greater in the newborn than in adults. The RDA for infants 0 to 6 months and 6 to 12 months is 108 and 98 kcalories per kilogram of body weight, respectively, whereas adults require only 30 to 40 kcalories per kilogram. (See front cover for RDAs for infants.)

About 40 to 50% of the energy in an infant's diet should come from fat, with 3% from essential fatty acids. This high energy density allows the infant's small stomach to hold enough food to meet energy needs. Fat in the diet is also important for nervous system development. Breast milk and formulas contain approximately 50% of energy as fat.

As with energy, the infant's protein requirement is very high compared with the adult requirement; the RDA is 2.2 and 1.6 grams per kilogram of body weight for a 0- to 6-month-old infant and a 6- to 12-month-old infant, respectively, compared with 0.8 gram per kilogram for an adult. The ideal protein source for newborns is human milk. Infant formulas are designed to mimic its amino acid pattern. The more closely the protein resembles that in human milk, the better it meets needs. A diet too high in protein may lead to dehydration because the infant kidney is immature and cannot concentrate urine. The load of metabolic wastes from excess protein requires extra water for excretion.

Water   The fluid requirements of infants are also very high compared with those of adults. Infant kidneys are poorly developed and unable to reabsorb much of the water that is filtered out of the blood. Therefore, infants lose proportionately more water in their urine than adults. Infants also lose proportionately more water through evaporation than do adults because they have a large surface area compared with their total body weight. These factors, in addition to the fact that infants cannot say they are thirsty, puts them at risk for dehydration. They rely on their caregivers to provide them with enough fluid. It is recommended that infants receive 150 ml of water per kilogram of body weight. Usually the amount of water in breast milk or formula is enough to meet needs; however, hot weather, fever, diarrhea, and vomiting, which increase water losses, may require that additional water be given.

Diarrhea kills one child each day in the United States, most often an infant under one year of age. The cause of the diarrhea is usually a bacterial or viral infection, and the cause of death is dehydration. The fluid intake of infants with diarrhea should be monitored carefully, and a pediatrician should be contacted. Mixtures of sugar, water, and electrolytes are available to replace lost fluids.

Micronutrients   There are several vitamins and minerals that may be limited in the unsupplemented infant diet. Iron is the nutrient most commonly deficient in infants who are consuming adequate energy and protein. Iron deficiency is usually not a problem during the first four to six months of life because infants have iron stores at birth. In addition, the iron in human milk, though not particularly abundant, is very well absorbed, and iron-fortified infant formulas are available. After four to six months, breast-fed infants not consuming other sources of iron, such as iron-fortified cereal, should be given supplements.

Newborns are also potentially at risk for vitamin D deficiency. Breast milk is relatively low in vitamin D, and breast-fed infants have lower levels of vitamin D and lower bone mineral content than bottle-fed infants.[46] Supplementation of 5 to 7.5 µg of vitamin D is recommended for breast-fed infants, especially in climates where exposure to sunlight is limited. To synthesize adequate vitamin D, about 15 minutes per day of sun exposure is needed for light-skinned babies and longer for darker-skinned babies.

Vitamin K, important in blood clotting, is another nutrient for which newborns are at risk of deficiency. Today, most newborns are injected with vitamin K at birth to prevent the possibility of hemorrhage. This provides them with enough vitamin K to last until their intestines are colonized with bacteria that synthesize it.

Fluoride is important in the development of teeth, even before they erupt. Breast milk is low in fluoride and formula manufacturers use unfluoridated water in preparing liquid formula. Therefore, breast-fed infants, infants fed premixed formula, and those fed formula mixed with low-fluoride water are often supplemented beginning at six months. In areas where the drinking water is fluoridated, infants fed formula reconstituted with tap water should not be given fluoride supplements.

Vitamin B_{12} may be deficient in the breast-milk of vegan mothers. Therefore their infants should be supplemented with vitamin B_{12}.

All of these nutrients can be toxic at high doses; they should be supplemented only in the recommended amounts.

FEEDING THE NEWBORN

Newborns have high nutrient requirements but can eat only 2 to 4 ounces at a feeding because their stomachs are small. They therefore require frequent feedings throughout the day and night whether breast or bottle fed. Newborns should be fed on demand about eight times daily. A well-fed infant will produce enough urine to soak six to eight diapers per day. An infant not producing this much urine may not be getting adequate fluids and is at risk for dehydration.

A relatively common but not life-threatening problem in infants is **colic**. Colic involves daily periods of inconsolable crying that cannot be stopped by holding, feeding, or changing the infant. Colic usually begins at a few weeks of age and continues through the first two to three months. Although its cause is unknown, it is hypothesized that colic is related to intestinal gas caused by milk intolerance, improper feeding practices, or immaturity of the central nervous system.

Colic–Inconsolable crying that is believed to be due to pain from gas buildup in the gastrointestinal tract or immaturity of the central nervous system.

Breast Versus Bottle Feeding   "Breast-feeding is the optimal way of providing food for the health, growth, and development of human infants."[47] One of the public health goals of Healthy People 2000 is to increase the proportion of breast-fed infants to 75% of infants at hospital discharge and 50% at six months of age.[48] Breast milk provides protection against infection early in life by passing immune factors from the mother to the infant. Breast milk is less likely to cause allergies, and breast-fed babies have fewer problems with constipation. The stronger suckling required by breast feeding aids in the development of facial muscles, which help in speech development. Breast-fed babies are also less likely to be overfed, since the amount of milk consumed cannot be monitored visually. In bottle feeding, it is often tempting to encourage the baby to finish the entire bottle whether or not he is hungry. Breast feeding also has advantages for the mother. Breast milk is readily available and inexpensive. It doesn't require preparation or bottles and nipples that must be washed. It is more ecological because it doesn't require energy for manufacture or packaging that must be disposed of. Physiologically, breast feeding causes contractions that help the mother's uterus return to size more quickly and may promote weight loss in some women. Psychologically, breast feeding can be a relaxing, emotionally enjoyable interaction for both mother and infant (Table 13-3).

Although breast milk from a well-nourished mother is the ideal food for newborns, there are situations when it is not the best choice. Bottle feeding is easier for the infant; less strength is needed to consume the same nutrients. If the infant is small or weak, he may not have the strength to receive adequate nutrition from breast feeding. In this case, formula, which provides almost the same nutrients as breast milk, can be used, or pumped breast milk can be offered to the infant in a bottle (Figure 13-14).

Another advantage of bottle feeding is that it limits the transmission of disease or drugs via breast milk. Hepatitis and HIV infection, which causes AIDS, can be transmitted to the infant in breast milk, but common illnesses such as colds, flu, and skin infections should not interfere with breast feeding.[49] Women who are taking medications should check with their physician as to whether it is safe to breast feed. Since alcohol and drugs such as cocaine and marijuana can be passed to the baby in breast milk, alcoholic and drug-addicted mothers are counseled not to breast feed. Nicotine from cigarette smoke is also rapidly transferred from maternal blood to milk. Heavy smoking may decrease the supply of milk, and

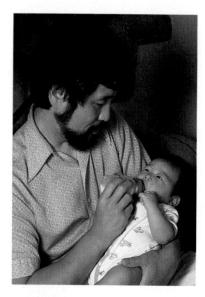

FIGURE 13-14
Bottle feeding with breast milk or formula can supplement breast feeding and in some situations is preferable. (Mary Kate Denny/Photo Edit)

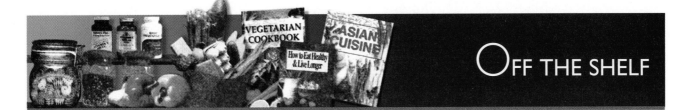

OFF THE SHELF

Infant Formula Choices

Many parents are faced with the decision of which infant formula is best. Infants are often formula fed from birth, and most are formula fed after a few months of breast feeding. Selecting an infant formula can be confusing. Is one better for the baby than another? Is a less expensive formula likely to be missing certain nutrients?

To ensure the safety of infant formulas, the American Academy of Pediatrics has published standards for the nutrient composition of infant formulas. These are based on the composition of human milk from a healthy mother. For a healthy full-term baby, the only real choices that consumers face are whether the formula is made with cow's milk protein, soy protein, or a protein hydrolysate; whether the formula is fortified with iron; how much preparation is required; and how much it costs.

For most healthy babies, formulas based on cow's milk protein are fine. If cow's milk protein is not well tolerated, a soy formula or protein hydrolysate can be tried. Since infant iron stores are depleted by four to six months of age, a formula with iron is usually recommended. Formulas are marketed in three basic forms: ready-to-feed, liquid concentrates, and powdered. Ready-to-feed formulas require no preparation and are available in sizes ranging from 4-ounce bottles to 32-ounce containers. Liquid concentrates are prepared for use by mixing equal amounts of the concentrate and water. Powdered formulas are prepared by mixing 1 tablespoon of powder for every 2 ounces of water. When properly prepared all of these provide the needed nutrients in an appropriate concentration. Problems arise when formulas are mixed incorrectly. This can result from a lack of understanding, poor measuring techniques, the addition of extra water to make the formula last longer, or the belief that a more concentrated formula will make the baby grow better.

The choice of formula may depend on cost, transportation, and food preparation facili-

ties. Ready-to-feed formulas are easiest to use but may cost more and are heavier and bulkier to carry home from the store. Liquid concentrates are a good compromise because they provide more formula for less weight, and are easy to mix. Powders are the least expensive and the easiest to transport home in a grocery bag but require more measuring and mixing. Since all of these products are nutritionally comparable, the choice depends on the needs of the caregivers.

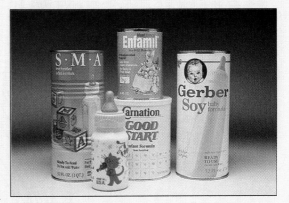

(Charles D. Winters)

HOW MUCH IS ENOUGH: ASSESSING INFANT GROWTH

Although nutrient needs for infants are fairly well defined, it is difficult to calculate an infant's actual nutrient intake. The best indicator of adequate nourishment is growth. Most healthy infants follow standard patterns of growth, so an infant's growth can be monitored by comparing length, weight, and head circumference to standard growth charts (Figure 13-18). Charts for infants 0 to 36 months and children 2 to 18 years are included in Appendix B. These charts plot typical growth patterns of infants and children in the United States. By using these charts, an infant's measurements at a particular age can be ranked with other infants of the same age. This ranking, or percentile, indicates where the infant's growth falls in relation to population standards. For example, if a newborn boy is at the 20th percentile for weight it means that 19% of newborn boys weigh less

FIGURE 13-18
Growth charts, such as this one for boys from birth to 36 months, demonstrate typical patterns of growth.
(© 1982 Ross Laboratories)

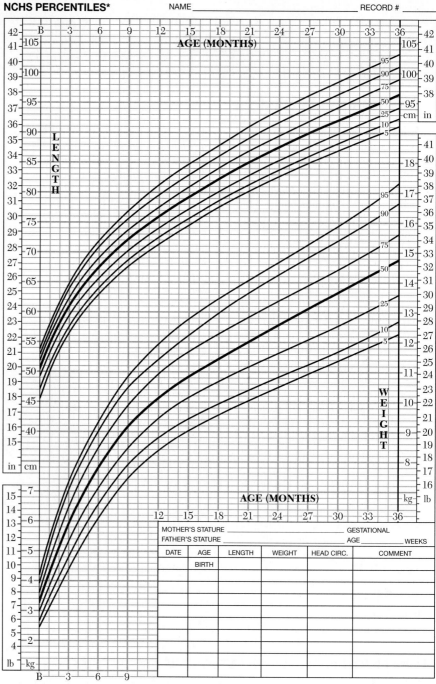

BOYS: BIRTH TO 36 MONTHS
PHYSICAL GROWTH
NCHS PERCENTILES*

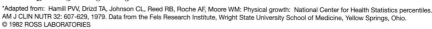

*Adapted from: Hamill PVV, Drizd TA, Johnson CL, Reed RB, Roche AF, Moore WM: Physical growth: National Center for Health Statistics percentiles. AM J CLIN NUTR 32: 607-629, 1979. Data from the Fels Research Institute, Wright State University School of Medicine, Yellow Springs, Ohio.
© 1982 ROSS LABORATORIES

and 80% weigh more. Children should continue at the same percentiles as they grow. For instance, a child who is at the 50th percentile for height and 25th percentile for weight should continue to follow these weight and height curves.

Whether an infant is 6 pounds or 8 pounds at birth, the rate of growth should be approximately the same—rapid initially and slowing slightly as the infant approaches one year of age. A rule of thumb is that an infant should double his or her birth weight by four months and triple it by one year of age. In the first year of life, most infants increase their length by 50%. Breast-fed and bottle-fed infants have similar growth for the first three to four months, but then bottle-fed infants grow at a faster rate. Small infants and premature infants often follow a pattern parallel to but below the growth curve for a period of time and then experience catch-up growth that brings them onto the growth curve in a place compatible with their genetic growth potential. Slight fluctuations in growth rate are normal, but a consistent pattern of not following the growth curve or a sudden change in growth pattern is cause for concern.

A rapid increase in weight without an increase in height may be an indicator that the infant is being overfed. Growth that is slower than the predicted pattern indicates **failure to thrive**. This is a catch-all term for growth failure for any reason in a young child. The cause may be a congenital condition, the presence of disease, poor nutrition, neglect, abuse, or psychosocial problems. Whatever the cause, the treatment is usually an individualized plan that includes adequate nutrition and careful monitoring by physicians, dietitians, and other health-care professionals. Just as there are critical periods in fetal life, there are critical periods for growth and development during infancy. For example, the brain is growing rapidly at birth, and undernutrition at this time can permanently affect brain development.

Failure to thrive—The inability of a child's growth to keep up with normal growth curves.

INTRODUCING SOLID FOOD

Solid and semisolid foods can be gradually introduced into the infant's diet starting between the fourth and sixth months of life.

When to Introduce Foods   Introducing solid food before four months is not recommended because the infant's feeding abilities and gastrointestinal tract are not mature enough to handle foods other than breast milk or formula. The young infant takes milk by a licking motion of the tongue, which strokes or milks the liquid from the nipple. Solid food placed in the mouth at an early age is usually pushed out as the tongue thrusts forward. By four to six months of age the early reflex to bring the tongue to the front of the mouth to suckle has diminished, and the tongue is held farther back in the mouth, allowing solid food to be accepted. By this age, the infant can hold her head up steadily and is able to sit, either with or without support. Internally, the digestive tract has developed. Enzymes are present for starch digestion. The kidneys are more mature and better able to concentrate urine. With all of these changes, the child is ready to begin a new approach to eating. The introduction of solid food assists in infant development, but until one year of age most nutritional needs are still met by breast milk or formula. Some suggest that the addition of infant cereal to the bottle during the first few months will help the infant sleep through the night. However, studies have shown that there is no difference in sleeping patterns based on feeding practices.

Which Foods to Offer First   The most commonly recommended first food is iron-fortified infant rice cereal mixed with formula or breast milk. Rice is the recommended first food because it is easily digested and rarely causes allergic reactions. After rice has been successfully included in the diet, other grains can then be introduced, with wheat cereal last because it is most likely to cause an allergic reaction. To monitor for food allergies, it is important to introduce new foods one at a time. Each new food should be offered for a few days without the addition of any other new foods. If an allergic reaction occurs, it can be assumed that it is caused by the newly introduced food. Foods that cause symptoms like

TABLE 13-4   Typical Meal Patterns for Infants

Food	Serving Size	Servings per Day		
		4–6 months	6–8 months	9–12 months
Formula or Breast milk°	8 oz	4	4	4
Dry infant cereal	2 Tbsp	2	4	4
Vegetables	2–3 Tbsp	—	2	3
Fruits	2 Tbsp	—	2	4
Fruit juice	4 oz	—	—	1 (by cup)
Meats (or egg yolk)	1 Tbsp	—	2–4 (strained)	4–6 (chopped)
Finger foods			1†	4‡

° Includes that added to cereal
† Dry toast, teething biscuits
‡ Table foods except hot dogs, carrots, and other "choking" foods

rashes, digestive upsets, or respiratory problems should be discontinued before any other new foods are added. After cereals are introduced, puréed fruits or vegetables can be tried. Some suggest that vegetables should be offered before fruits so that the child will learn to enjoy food that is not sweet before being introduced to sweet foods. Once teeth have erupted, foods with more texture can be added. For the 6- to 12-month-old child, small pieces of soft or ground fruits, vegetables, and meats are appropriate (see Table 13-4).

Offer Developmentally Appropriate Choices   As the child becomes familiar with more variety, food choices should be made from each of the food groups. At one year of age whole milk should be offered and continued until two years of age. Lowfat milk should not be used until after the age of two years because before this age children need enough dietary fat to fuel their rapid growth and development.

To avoid choking, foods that can easily lodge in the throat, such as carrots, grapes, and hot dogs, should be avoided. As children become more independent, they will want to feed themselves. Although this is not always a neat and clean process, it is important for their development (Figure 13-19). By eight or nine months infants can hold a bottle and self-feed finger food such as crackers. Avoid offering salty foods, since added salt is not necessary. By ten months most infants can drink from a cup so fruit juices can be offered. Juice should not be given in a bottle because it may contribute to nursing bottle syndrome. Naturally occurring sugars from milk and fruits are an important energy source for infants and come with other essential nutrients like calcium and vitamin C. Excess quantities of apple and pear juice should be avoided, since they contain sorbitol, a poorly absorbed sugar alcohol, which can cause diarrhea. Added sugars are not harmful but should be used in moderation to ensure a nutrient-dense diet. Honey and corn syrup should be avoided in children less than a year old because these foods may contain spores of the bacterium *Clostridium botulinum*. The spores can germinate in the infant gastrointestinal tract and cause botulism poisoning (see Chapter 16).

Food Allergies   Allergic reactions to food, or food allergies, occur when an **allergen** consumed in the diet is absorbed from the intestine and enters the lymph and bloodstream. Most food allergens are incompletely digested proteins that squeeze through gaps between the intestinal cells. Foods that commonly cause allergies include wheat, peanuts, eggs, milk, nuts, seafood, soy products, and some

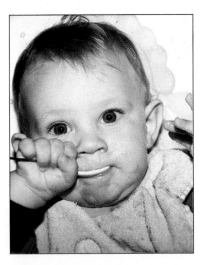

FIGURE 13-19
Self-feeding is important in infant development, but it is not a tidy process. (Gregory Smolin)

Allergen—A foreign protein that stimulates an immune response.

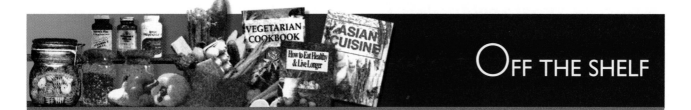

Choosing Foods for Babies

Commercially prepared baby foods are big business. There are endless varieties—junior or strained, jars or dehydrated, even organic. What is in these little jars? Are they better or worse than what you can make at home?

The ideal diet for an infant is varied, nutritious, and safe. Providing a variety of foods ensures that a variety of nutrients are consumed. Offering foods without added fats, sugars, or salt provides a nutrient-dense diet. To be safe, infant food should be free of contaminants and prepared in a manner that is appropriate for the infant's development and minimizes the risk of choking. For example, an eight-month-old could be offered puréed steamed carrots, but raw carrots would not be appropriate.

Commercial baby food fulfills these criteria and has the advantage of convenience. Being able to buy small jars of vegetables, fruits, meats, and mixed dishes enables parents to provide babies with more variety than is possible when all food is prepared at home. In the same meal, a small child can be offered three or four different fruits and vegetables, two different cereals, and meat. Many baby foods have no added ingredients. A jar of carrots simply contains puréed carrots. Added ingredients that are still common are modified food starch, which

is often added to maintain consistency in mixed dishes, and sugar, which is added to most desserts. Read the labels to determine which foods contain these additives. Commercial baby food also has safety advantages. The food is sterile and ready to eat. It comes in jars small enough to be finished in one meal or during the course of one day. Leftovers not finished the day they are opened should be discarded.

Although most commercial baby food sold in North America comes in jars, dehydrated baby foods are available in some locations. These foods are generally comparable to baby food in jars and can offer even greater convenience. Since they can be reconstituted in small serving-size portions, they may be more economical.

Organic baby foods are also available. They are generally more expensive than the standard variety. Although these foods may be free of additives and pesticides, they are not fortified, so extra care must be taken to meet infants' needs, especially for iron and vitamin C.

Homemade baby food allows the caregivers to control exactly what goes into a meal, and it is more economical than buying prepared foods. However, care must be taken to ensure the nutrient content and safety of foods made at home. Baby food can be

made from the foods prepared for the rest of the family. These foods should be cooked in ways that maintain their nutrient content. For example, vegetables should be steamed or boiled in a very small amount of water, and meats should be broiled or roasted. The baby's portion should be removed before salt or other seasonings are added.

It is safest to prepare and serve homemade baby food immediately. A portion should be removed from the family meal and ground, mashed, blended, or diced. For convenience, a large amount may be puréed ahead of time and frozen in small portions. To ensure safety, leftovers should not be reheated more than once, and if food is left at room temperature for more than 30 minutes it should be discarded. Baby food should not be made from canned fruits, meats, and vegetables that contain added salt or sugar.

Decisions on commercial versus homemade baby foods depend on time and money. Homemade baby food is cheaper than commercial baby food. However, it takes more time to prepare and it is often difficult to offer the same variety that can be purchased in individual servings. Whichever is chosen, care should be taken to minimize the risk of contamination during handling and storing.

meats. Exposure to an allergen for the first time causes the immune system to produce antibodies to that allergen. When the allergen is encountered again by eating the same food, allergy symptoms such as vomiting, diarrhea, asthma, hives, eczema, hay fever, and general cramps and aches may result as the immune system battles the allergen. The symptoms may occur almost immediately or take up to 24 hours to appear.

Food allergies are common in infants because their digestive tracts are not fully mature. After about three months of age, the risk of developing food allergies

Elimination diet–A diet that eliminates potential allergy-causing foods from an allergic individual's diet and then systematically adds them back one at a time.

is reduced because whole proteins are less likely to be absorbed. The best treatment for a food allergy is to avoid the offending food. Food allergies can be diagnosed by several laboratory methods. Such tests may identify foods that are likely to cause problems, but they cannot determine the source of the problem with 100% reliability. The cause of a food allergy can be confirmed by using an **elimination diet**. This diet involves removing all foods suspected of causing an allergic reaction from the diet. The information on food labels can be of great help. (See Chapter 6 *Off the Label*: Identifying Protein Sources.) When a diet that causes no symptoms has been established, it should be followed for two to four weeks. After that, foods that do not cause severe reactions can be reintroduced one at a time in small amounts under a doctor's supervision. If no reaction to the food occurs, then increasing amounts can be introduced until a normal portion is offered. If there is still no reaction, then the food can be ruled out as an allergen and another food can be tested.

Many children who develop food allergies before the age of three will outgrow them. Therefore, unless the allergic reaction is severe, an offending food may be reintroduced under a doctor's supervision every six months after the age of one year to see if tolerance to it has increased. Allergies that appear after three years are more likely to be a problem for life. If certain foods must be avoided in the diet, care must be taken to ensure that nutrient needs are met without these foods.

Food intolerance–An adverse reaction to a food that does not involve the immune system.

Food Intolerances   True food allergies are relatively rare; more frequently symptoms are caused by **food intolerances**. Food intolerances do not involve antibody production by the immune system. In individuals with food intolerances, foods cause problems because they are difficult or impossible to digest or because they cause other drug-like reactions. For instance, some people report adverse reactions after consuming the food coloring FD&C Yellow No. 5 (see Chapter 16).

SUMMARY

1. Pregnancy begins with the fertilization of an egg by a sperm, producing a zygote. About three weeks after fertilization, the embryonic period of development begins. The embryo grows and the cells differentiate and move to form the organs and structures of the body. At nine weeks the embryo enters the fetal period of development, which continues until birth, about 40 weeks after fertilization.

2. During pregnancy, maternal physiology changes to support the pregnancy and prepare for lactation. The amniotic sac and the placenta develop; maternal blood volume increases; the uterus and supporting muscles expand; body fat is deposited; the heart, lungs, and kidneys work harder; and the breasts enlarge.

3. Recommended weight gain during pregnancy is 25 to 35 pounds. If too little weight is gained, the infant may be small at birth and at increased risk for illness and death. Too much weight gain can also place both mother and baby at risk, but weight loss should never be attempted during pregnancy. Normal-weight, underweight, and overweight mothers should all experience a slow, steady weight gain during pregnancy.

4. For healthy pregnancies, non–weight-bearing, moderate-intensity activities are beneficial and safe.

5. The hormones that direct changes in maternal physiology and the growth and development of the fetus sometimes cause unwanted side effects. Digestive system discomforts that are common in pregnancy include morning sickness, heartburn, constipation, and hemorrhoids. Changes in glucose utilization can cause gestational diabetes, and changes in fluid balance can cause edema and high blood pressure. When a rise in blood pressure is accompanied by edema and protein in the urine, it is known as pregnancy-induced hypertension and can be life threatening.

6. Nutritional status is important before, during, and after pregnancy. Poor nutrition before pregnancy can decrease fertility and lead to a poor pregnancy outcome. During pregnancy the requirements for energy, protein, water, vitamins, and minerals increase. B vitamins are needed to support increased energy and protein metabolism; calcium, phosphorus, and vitamins C and D are needed for bone and connective tissue growth; protein, folic acid, vitamin B$_{12}$, and zinc are needed for cell replication; and iron is needed for red blood cell synthesis.

7. Because the embryo is rapidly developing and growing, it is susceptible to permanent damage from poor nutrition and physical, chemical, or other environmental agents.
8. Factors that increase the risks of pregnancy include maternal age that is under 20 or over 35; a short interval between pregnancies or a history of poor reproductive outcomes; poverty; and behaviors such as smoking, alcohol use, and illicit drug use.
9. During lactation the need for energy, protein, fluid, and many vitamins and minerals is even greater than during pregnancy.
10. Newborns are growing more rapidly and require more energy and protein per kilogram of body weight than at any other time in life. Fat and fluid needs are also higher than in adults. A diet that meets energy, protein, and fat needs may not necessarily meet the need for iron, fluoride, and vitamins D and K.
11. Breast milk is the ideal food for new babies. It is designed specifically for the human newborn, is always available, requires no mixing or sterilization, and provides immune protection. If breast feeding is not chosen, there are many infant formulas on the market that are patterned after human milk and provide adequate nutrition to the baby.
12. Formulas are the best option when the mother is ill or is taking prescription or illicit drugs, or when the infant has special nutritional needs. The major disadvantages of bottle feeding are the potential for errors in mixing formula and the risk of bacterial contamination.
13. Introducing solid foods between four and six months of age adds iron and other nutrients to the diet and aids in development. Newly introduced foods should be appropriate to the child's development and offered one at a time to monitor for food allergies.
14. Food allergies are caused by the absorption of allergens, most of which are proteins. Food allergies are more common in infancy because the infant's immature gastrointestinal tract is likely to absorb whole proteins. Specific foods that cause allergies can be identified by an elimination diet. Food intolerances do not involve the immune system.

SELF-TEST

1. How does a fetus receive nutrients while in the uterus?
2. List three physiological changes that occur in the mother's body during pregnancy.
3. How do the requirements for energy and protein change during pregnancy?
4. Why does the mother's recommended intake for iron double during pregnancy?
5. What is the recommended weight gain during pregnancy?
6. How do the recommendations for weight gain differ for overweight and underweight women?
7. Are vegetarian diets safe for pregnant women?
8. How does alcohol consumed by the mother during pregnancy affect the unborn child?
9. How does maternal age affect nutrient requirements during pregnancy?
10. How do maternal energy and protein requirements change during lactation?
11. What are the advantages and disadvantages of breast and bottle feeding?
12. When should solid and semisolid foods be introduced into an infant's diet?
13. How should new foods be introduced to monitor for the development of food allergies?

APPLICATIONS

These exercises are designed to help you apply your critical thinking skills to your own nutrition choices. Many are best performed using a diet analysis software program. If you do not have access to a computer program, the exercises can be hand calculated using the information in this text and its appendices.

1. Assume that one day of the food record you kept in Chapter 1 is the record of a 25-year-old pregnant woman.
   a. Does this diet meet her energy and protein needs? If not, what foods would you add to the diet to meet the needs of pregnancy?
   b. Does this diet meet the iron and calcium needs for a 25-year-old pregnant woman? List three foods that are good sources of each and show where these could be added to the diet to increase calcium and iron intake.
   c. Does this diet meet the folate needs for a 25-year-old pregnant woman? What foods could you add to the diet to meet the need for folate without supplements?
2. For each of the following nutrients, describe how the needs for nonpregnant, pregnant, and lactating women differ. Explain why the needs for pregnancy and lactation might differ from those of the nonpregnant state.
   a. Energy
   b. Protein
   c. Calcium
   d. Iron
   e. Folate

REFERENCES

1. Committee on Nutritional Status During Pregnancy and Lactation, National Academy of Sciences. *Nutrition During Pregnancy*. Washington, DC: National Academy Press, 1990.

2. Smith, D.E., Lewis, J.L., Caveny, L.L., et al. Longitudinal changes in adiposity associated with pregnancy: the CARDIA study. J.A.M.A. 271:147–151, 1994.

3. Simpson, J.L. Are physical activity and employment related to preterm birth and low birth weight? Am. J. Obstet. Gynecol. 168:1231–1238, 1993.

4. Dewey, K.G. and McCrory, M.A. Effects of dieting and physical activity on pregnancy and lactation. Am. J. Clin. Nutr. 59(suppl):446S–453S, 1994.

5. American College of Sports Medicine. *ACSMs Guidelines for Exercise Testing and Prescription*, 5th ed. Baltimore: Williams & Wilkins, 1995.

6. Hollingsworth, D.R. *Pregnancy, Diabetes and Birth*, 2nd ed. Baltimore: Williams & Wilkins, 1992.

7. Belizan, J.M., Villar, J., Gonzalez, L., et al. Calcium supplementation to prevent hypertensive disorders of pregnancy. N. Engl. J. Med. 325:1399–1405, 1991.

8. Anonymous. Folate supplements prevent recurrence of neural tube defects. Nutr. Rev. 50:22–24, 1992.

9. Rothman, K.J., Moore, L.L., Singer, M.R., et al. Teratogenicity of high vitamin A intake. N. Engl. J. Med. 333:1369–1373, 1995.

10. Bendich, A. Lifestyle and environmental factors that can adversely affect maternal nutritional status and pregnancy outcomes. Ann. NY Acad. Sci. 678:255–265, 1993.

11. Worthington-Roberts, B. and Williams, S.R. *Nutrition in Pregnancy and Lactation*, 5th ed. St. Louis: Mosby, 1993.

12. Prentice, A. Maternal calcium requirements during pregnancy and lactation. Am. J. Clin. Nutr. 59(suppl):477S–482S, 1994.

13. Optimal Calcium Intake. NIH Consensus Statement. June 6–8, 12:1–31, 1994.

14. Specker, B.L. Do North American women need supplemental vitamin D during pregnancy or lactation? Am. J. Clin. Nutr. 59(suppl):484S–491S, 1994.

15. Bower, C. Folate and neural tube defects. Nutr. Rev. 53:S33–S38, 1995.

16. Czeizel, A.E. and Dudas, I. Prevention of the first occurrence of neural tube defects by periconceptional vitamin supplementation. N. Engl. J. Med. 327:1832–1835, 1992.

17. Werler, M., Shapiro, S., and Mitchell, A. Periconceptional folic acid and risk of occurrent neural tube defects. J.A.M.A. 269:1257–1261, 1993.

18. Centers for Disease Control. Recommendations for the use of folic acid to reduce the number of cases of spina bifida and other neural tube defects. Morb. Mortal. Wkly. Rep. 41:1–7, 1992.

19. Goldenberg, R.L., Tamura, T., Neggers, Y., et al. The effect of zinc supplementation on pregnancy outcome. J.A.M.A. 274:463–468, 1995.

20. Scholl, T.O. and Hediger, M.L. Anemia and iron-deficiency anemia: compilation of data on pregnancy outcome. Am. J. Clin. Nutr. 59(suppl):492S–500S, 1994.

21. Horner, R.D., Lackey, C.J., Kolasa, K., and Warren, K. Pica practices of pregnant women. J. Am. Diet. Assoc. 91:34–38, 1991.

22. Federal Provincial Subcommittee on Nutrition, 1986. Nutrition in Pregnancy National Guidelines. Ottawa: Minister of Health and Welfare, Health and Welfare Canada, 1987.

23. Centers for Disease Control: Infant mortality—United States, 1992. J.A.M.A. 273:101, 1995.

24. American Dietetic Association Position of the American Dietetic Association: Nutrition Care for Pregnant Adolescents. J. Am. Diet. Assoc. 94:449–450, 1994.

25. Rosenfield, A. and Maine, D. Maternal mortality: a neglected tragedy. Lancet 2:83, 1985.

26. Bleuscher, P., Larson, L., Nelson, M., and Lenihan, A. Prenatal WIC participation can reduce low birth weight and newborn medical costs: a cost benefit analysis of WIC participation in North Carolina. J. Am. Diet. Assoc. 93:163–166, 1993.

27. Lewis, D.D. and Woods, S.E. Fetal alcohol syndrome. Am. Fam. Physician 50:1025–1032, 1035–1036, 1994.

28. Abel, E.L. An update on incidence of FAS: FAS is not an equal opportunity birth defect. Neurotoxicol. Teratol. 17:437–443, 1995.

29. Streissguth, A.P. Fetal alcohol syndrome in older patients. Alcohol Alcohol Suppl. 2:209–212, 1993.

30. Levy, M. and Koren, G. Obstetric and neonatal effects of drugs of abuse. Emerg. Med. Clin. North Am. 8:633–652, 1990.

31. DiFranza, J.R. and Lew, R.A. Effect of maternal smoking on pregnancy complications and sudden infant death syndrome. J. Fam. Pract. 40:385–394, 1995.

32. Klonoff-Cohen, H.S., Edelstein, S.L., Lefkowitz, E.S., et al. The effect of passive smoking and tobacco exposure through breast milk on sudden infant death syndrome. J.A.M.A. 273:795–798, 1995.

33. American Heart Association. Active and passive tobacco exposure: a serious pediatric health problem. A statement from the Committee on Atherosclerosis and Hypertension in Children, Council on Cardiovascular Disease in the Young, American Heart Association. Circulation 90:2581–2590, 1994.

34. Nehlig, A. and Dedry, G. Potential teratogenic and neurodevelopmental consequences of coffee and caffeine exposure: a review on human and animal data. Neurotoxicol. Teratol. 16:531–543, 1994.

35. Sivak, A. Coteratogenic effects of caffeine. Regul. Toxicol. Pharmacol. 19:1–13, 1994.

36. Nehlig, A. and Debry, G. Consequences on the newborn of chronic maternal consumption of coffee during gestation and lactation. J. Am. Coll. Nutr. 13:6–21, 1994.

37. Van Dyke, D.C. and Fox, A.A. Fetal drug exposure and its possible implications for learning in the preschool and school-aged population. J. Learn. Disabil. 23:160–163, 1990.

38. Fox, C.H. Cocaine use in pregnancy. J. Am. Board Fam. Pract. 7:225–228, 1994.

39. Plessinger, M.A. and Woods, J.R., Jr. Maternal, placental, and fetal pathophysiology of cocaine exposure during pregnancy. Clin. Obstet. Gynocol. 36:267–278, 1994.

40. Witter, F.R. and Niebyl, J.R. Marijuana use in pregnancy and pregnancy outcome. Am. J. Perinatol. 7:36–38, 1990.

41. Potter, S., Hannum, S., McFarlin, B., et al. Does infant feeding method influence maternal postpartum weight loss? J. Am. Diet. Assoc. 91:441–446, 1991.

42. Kramer, E.M., Stunkard, A.J., Marshall, K.A., et al. Breast feeding reduces maternal lower body fat. J. Am. Diet. Assoc. 93:429–433, 1993.

43. Dewey, K.G., Heinig, M.J., and Nommsen, L.A. Maternal weight-loss patterns during prolonged lactation. Am. J. Clin. Nutr. 58:162–166, 1993.

44. Committee on Nutritional Status During Pregnancy and Lactation, National Academy of Sciences. *Nutrition During Lactation*. Washington, DC: National Academy Press, 1991.

45. Sowers, M., Corton, G., Shapiro, B., et al. Changes in bone density with lactation. J.A.M.A. 269:3130–3135, 1993.

46. Greer, F.R., Searcy, J.E., Levin, R.S., et al. Bone mineral content and serum 25-hydroxy vitamin D concentration in breast fed infants with and without supplemental vitamin D. J. Pediatr. 100:919–922, 1982.

47. American Dietetic Association. Position paper on promotion and support of breast-feeding. J. Am. Diet. Assoc. 93:467–469, 1993.

48. *Healthy People 2000: National Health Promotion and Disease Prevention Objectives*. Washington, DC: U.S. Department of Health and Human Services, 1991.

49. Williams, R.D. Breast-feeding best bet for babies. FDA Consumer, 28:19–23, Oct, 1995.

The Growing Years: Toddlers to Teens

CHAPTER CONCEPTS

1. Nutrient intake during childhood and adolescence can affect current and future health.

2. Normal growth is the best indication of adequate nutrient intake in children.

3. Nutrient intake throughout life can affect the risk of chronic disease. After age two, children's diets should be high in carbohydrate and low in fat and cholesterol.

4. Developing sound eating habits during childhood can promote healthful eating throughout life.

5. Nutrient intakes for children must meet the needs for growth and development as well as maintenance and activity.

6. Children's food choices are affected by their biological need for nutrients, their personal food preferences, and the environment in which they live.

7. The physiological changes that occur during sexual maturation cause differences in the nutrient requirements of males and females.

8. Nutrient intake in adolescence must continue to meet the needs for growth and development.

9. Meeting nutrient needs can be very difficult during adolescence because food choices are frequently influenced more by peer pressures than by physiological requirements.

10. Alcohol consumption can affect nutritional status, judgment, and health.

JUST A TASTE

Are high blood cholesterol and high blood pressure concerns in children?

Can fast food and sweetened cereals be part of a healthy diet?

Does watching television affect nutritional status?

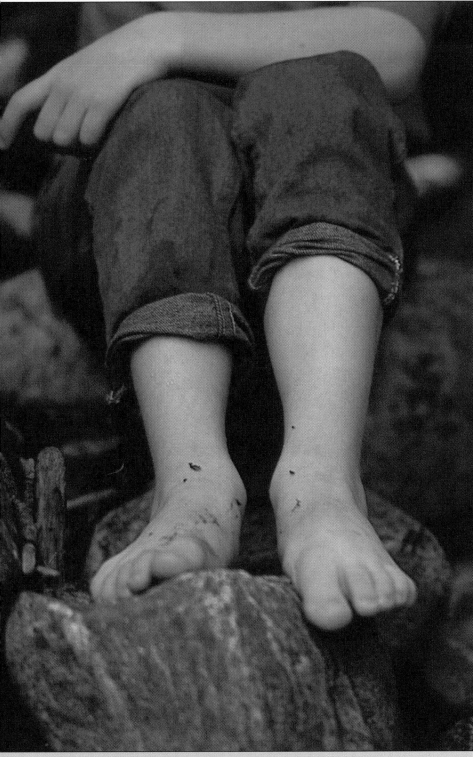

(Phillip Spears/Creative Sources/FPG International)

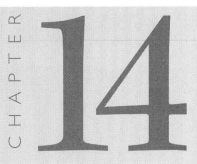

CHAPTER 14

Nutrient intake during childhood shapes the adult that the child will become. Thus, in the words of William Wordsworth, "the child is father of the man." Nutrition can affect health and the ability to achieve maximum growth potential as well as the propensity for developing chronic disease later in life. Eating habits developed during childhood and adolescence may last a lifetime.

Many physical changes occur between infancy and adulthood. During this period of rapid growth from birth to about 18 years of age, the diet must supply the nutrients needed for growth and development as well as maintenance and activity. However, many factors other than nutrient needs determine which foods are consumed. Taste always affects food choices, and as the child grows, influences from the outside world increase. When a child is enrolled in day-care, parents may no longer be in control or even aware of what the child is eating. When the child is in school, carefully packed lunches may be discarded or traded for more appealing foods. During adolescence a desire to be thin or to compete in athletics may dictate food choice. Sexual activity and alcohol use also have an impact on the nutritional status of some young adults.

In this chapter, we will discuss:

* How important is the development of sound nutritional habits early in life?
* What are the nutrient requirements from weaning through young adulthood?
* What social factors have an impact on food intake and nutrient needs?

NUTRITION AND THE HEALTH OF AMERICA'S YOUTH

Nutrient intake in children and adolescents can affect their health and longevity. In the United States, hunger and micronutrient deficiencies still exist in children, but the infant mortality rate and the incidence of malnutrition, as measured by low weight for age is decreasing.[1] Therefore the focus of public health nutrition for children, as with adults, is shifting away from concerns of underconsumption and dietary deficiencies toward the problems of overnutrition.

PROVIDING FOR OPTIMAL GROWTH AND DEVELOPMENT

The first goal of nutrition for children and adolescents is to meet the needs of growth and development. And, conversely, normal growth is the best indicator of adequate nourishment. Most children and adolescents follow standard patterns of growth. These patterns can be monitored using growth charts available for ages 0 to 36 months and 2 to 18 years of age (Appendix B). The rate of growth is slower in childhood than in infancy. In the second year of life, children generally grow about 5 inches, in the third year 4 inches, and thereafter about 2 to 3 inches per year. During adolescence, there is a period of growth that is almost as rapid as that of infancy.

Growth Patterns   Growth patterns are predictable, but growth occurs in spurts and plateaus. During a growth spurt, a child's or adolescent's appetite may seem insatiable, and between spurts they may seem to eat nothing. If the pattern of growth suddenly changes, the child should be evaluated by a physician to determine if there is a physiological reason for the sudden change in growth pat-

SUMMARY

1. Nutrition in childhood sets the stage for nutrition and health in the adult years. The diet must meet the needs for growth and development as well as reduce the risk of chronic disease later in life. Children with elevated blood pressure and blood cholesterol are more likely to have hypertension and heart disease as adults. Obese children are likely to become obese adults. Dental caries are more common when the diet is high in simple carbohydrates.

2. Energy and protein needs per kilogram of body weight decrease as children grow, but total needs increase because of the increase in total body weight and activity level. Fat intake should drop to 30% or less of energy beginning at two years of age. Dietary carbohydrates should come primarily from whole grains, vegetables, fruits, and milk.

3. Low dietary intakes of vitamin A, vitamin C, calcium, iron, and zinc put some American children at risk of deficiencies.

4. Children like to have control over what they eat. In order to meet nutrient needs and develop nutritious habits, a variety of healthy foods should be offered at meals and snacks throughout the day.

5. Once children reach school age, the outside world has more influence over their lives and food intake. Meals away from home at school or fast-food restaurants are common.

6. Occasionally, nutrition-related problems occur in childhood. Obesity among children is increasing in the United States. Lead poisoning is an environmental as well as nutritional concern. In some children, behavior may be affected by the types of food consumed.

7. The accelerated growth and sexual maturation that occur in adolescence have an impact on nutrient requirements.

The body composition and nutritional requirements of boys and girls diverge. Males gain more lean body tissue, while females have a greater increase in body fat.

8. During the adolescent growth spurt, total energy and protein requirements are higher than at any other time of life. Young men require more protein and energy than young women.

9. In adolescence, vitamin requirements increase to meet the needs of rapid growth. The minerals calcium, iron, and zinc are likely to be low in the adolescent diet. Iron deficiency anemia is common, especially in girls as they begin losing iron through menstruation.

10. In adolescence, food intake may be determined more by social activities and peer pressure than by nutrient needs. Since meals are frequently missed, healthy snacks should be included in the diet.

11. Psychosocial changes occur during the adolescent years. Obesity can be psychologically and socially devastating. Eating disorders are more common than at any other time. Adolescent athletes are susceptible to nutrition misinformation, and they may try dangerous practices such as anabolic steroids to increase muscle mass, or fad diets and fluid restriction to promote weight loss.

12. During the teen years, the use of oral contraceptives, pregnancy, and the consumption of alcohol may affect nutritional status.

13. Alcohol has short-term effects on the central nervous system, including the impairment of reasoning, judgment, and coordination, and eventually the loss of consciousness. Chronic alcohol use damages the liver and can cause malnutrition by decreasing nutrient intake and absorption and interfering with nutrient utilization.

SELF-TEST

1. What is the best way to determine if a child is eating enough?
2. How does nutrient intake during childhood affect health later in life?
3. What impact does parents' weight have on a child's weight?
4. What factors influence the maximum height a child will reach?
5. How do the recommendations for fat intake change when a child reaches the age of two years?
6. Why is anemia a problem in young children? In teenage girls?
7. Why are snacks an important part of children's diets?
8. Why is breakfast important?
9. What nutritional problems can be signaled by sudden changes in weight patterns?
10. How can fast foods be incorporated into a healthy diet?
11. What is the adolescent growth spurt? How does it affect nutrient requirements?
12. Describe two physiological differences between males and females after puberty that affect their nutrient needs.
13. Why are teenagers susceptible to eating disorders?
14. How can alcohol consumption affect nutritional status?

APPLICATIONS

These exercises are designed to help you apply your critical thinking skills to your own nutrition choices. Many are best performed using a diet analysis software program. If you do not have access to a computer program, these exercises can be hand calculated using the information in this text and its appendices.

1. Assume you had a Big Mac, fries, and a 12-ounce cola for lunch.
   a. How many servings from each food group of the Food Guide Pyramid does this represent?
   b. List the numbers of additional servings from each food

group that you would need to satisfy the daily recommendations of the Food Guide Pyramid.

c. Select foods from each group to complete your intake for the day.

d. Do the foods you selected meet the serving recommendations of the Food Guide Pyramid and your energy needs?

2. The table to the right gives a girl's heights and weights recorded from two to nine years of age.

a. Plot these values on the growth chart in Appendix B.

b. Is there anything unusual about her weight gain relative to her height?

c. If so, what should be done to correct the problem?

Age	Height (in.)	Weight (lb)
2	34	26
3	37	31
4	40	35
5	43	40
6	45	44
7	48	53
8	50	77
9	52	97

REFERENCES

1. Public Health Service. Mid-Term Review of Nutrition Objectives 2000. Washington, DC: U.S. Department of Health and Human Services, 1994.

2. Grantham-McGregor, S. A review of studies of the effect of severe malnutrition on mental development. J. Nutr. 125:2233S–2238S, 1995.

3. *Healthy People 2000: National Health Promotion and Disease Prevention Objectives*. Washington, DC: U.S. Department of Health and Human Services, 1990.

4. McDowell, M.A., Briefel, R.R., Alaimo, K., et al. Energy and macronutrient intakes of persons 2 months and over in the United States: Third National Health and Nutrition Examination Survey, Phase I, 1988–1991, Anvance data from Vital and Health Statistics: No. 255. Hyattsville, MD, NCHS, 1994.

5. Ernst, N. and Obarzanek, E. Child health and nutrition: obesity and high blood cholesterol. Prev. Med. 23:427–436, 1994.

6. Berensen, G.S., Wattigney, W.A., Srinivasan, S.R., and Radhakrishnamurthy, B. Rationale to study the early natural history of heart disease: the Bogalusa Heart Study. Am. J. Med. Sci. 310(suppl):22S–28S, 1995.

7. Snetselaar, L. and Lauer, R.M. Childhood, diet, and atherosclerotic process. Nutr. Today, 27:22–28, Jan/Feb 1992.

8. Lauer, R.M. and Clark, W.R. The use of cholesterol measurements in childhood for the prediction of adult hypercholesterolemia. The Muscatine Study. J.A.M.A. 264:3034–3038, 1990.

9. American Academy of Pediatrics. Committee on Nutrition. Statement on Cholesterol. Pediatrics 90:469–472, 1992.

10. Lauer, R.M., Clarke, W.R., Mahong, L.T., and Witt, J. Childhood predictors of high adult blood pressure. Pediatr. Clin. North Am. 40:23–39, 1993.

11. Shea, S., Basch, C.E., Gutin, B., et al. The rate of increase in blood pressure in children 5 years of age is related to changes in aerobic fitness and body mass index. Pediatrics 94:465–470, 1994.

12. Gillman, M.W. and Ellison, R.C. Childhood prevention of essential hypertension. Pediatr. Clin. North Am. 40:179–194, 1993.

13. Yip, R., Scanlon, D., and Trowbridge, F. Trends and patterns in height and weight status of low-income U.S. children. Crit. Rev. Food Sci. Nutr. 33:409–421, 1993.

14. Stunkard, A.J., Harris, J.R., Pedersen, N.L., and McClearen, G.E. The body-mass index of twins who have been reared apart. N. Engl. J. Med. 322:1483–1487, 1990.

15. Anonymous. Obesity: nature or nurture? Nutr. Rev. 49:21–22, 1990.

16. Gazzaniga, J. and Burns, R.L. Relationship between diet composition and body fatness with adjustment for resting energy expenditures and physical activity in preadolescent children. Am. J. Clin. Nutr. 58:21–28, 1993.

17. Nicklas, T.A., Webber, L.S., Srinivasan, S.R., and Berenson, G.S. Secular trends in dietary intakes and cardiovascular risk factors in 10 year old children: the Bogalusa Heart Study (1973–1988). Am. J. Clin. Nutr. 57:930–937, 1993.

18. Kennedy, E. and Goldberg, J. What are American children eating? Implications for public policy. Nutr. Rev. 53:111–126, 1995.

19. Nicklas, T.A., Bao, W., Srinivasan, S.R., and Berensen, G.S. Dietary intake patterns of infants and young children over a 12-year period: the Bogalusa Heart Study. J. Adv. Med. 5:89–103, 1992.

20. Fischer, J.O. and Birch, L.L. Fat preferences and fat consumption of 3 to 5 year old children are related to parental adiposity. J. Am. Diet. Assoc. 95:759–764, 1995.

21. Kleinman, R.E., Finberg, L.F., Klish, W.J., and Lauer, R.N. Dietary guidelines for children: U.S. recommendations. J. Nutr. 126:1028S–1030S, 1996.

22. Guthrie, H., Smiciklas-Wright, H., and Wang, W.Q. Characterizing nutrient intakes of children by socioeconomic factors. Public Health Reports 109:414–420, 1994.

23. Zive, M.M., Taras, H.L., Broyles, S.L., et al. Vitamin and mineral intakes of Anglo American and Mexican American preschoolers. J. Am. Diet. Assoc. 95:329–335, 1995.

24. National Consensus Conference. Optimum Calcium Intake. J.A.M.A. 272:1942–1948, 1994.

25. Centers for Disease Control, National Center for Health Statistics. The National Health and Examination Survey, 1988–1991, 1994.

26. Walter, T. Effect of iron deficiency anaemia on cognitive skills in infancy and childhood. Baillieres Clin. Haematol. 7:815–827, 1994.

27. Oski, F.A. Iron deficiency in infancy and childhood. N. Engl. J. Med. 329:190–193, 1993.

28. Hingley, A.T. Preventing childhood poisoning. FDA Consumer 30:7–11, March 1996.

29. Shannon, M.W. and Graef, J.W. Lead intoxication in infancy. Pediatrics 89:87–90, 1992.

30. Committee on Environmental Health, Lead Poisoning: from screening to primary prevention. Pediatrics 93:176–183, 1993.

31. Wender, E.H. and Solanto, M.V. Effects of sugar on aggressive and inattentive behavior in children with attention deficit disorder with hyperactivity and normal children. Pediatrics 88:960–966, 1991.

32. Boris, M. and Mandel, F.S. Foods and additives are common causes of attention deficit hyperactive disorder in children. Ann. Allergy 72:462–468, 1994.

33. Carter, C.M., Urbanowicz, M., Hemsley, R., et al. Effects of a few food diet in attention deficit disorder. Arch. Dis. Child. 69:564–568, 1993.

34. Birch, L.L., Johnson, S.L., Andresen, G., et al. The variability of young children's energy intake. N. Engl. J. Med. 324:232–235, 1991.

35. Nicklas, T., Weihang, B., Webber, L.S., and Berensen, G.S. Breakfast consumption affects adequacy of total daily intake in children. J. Am. Diet. Assoc. 93:886–891, 1993.

36. Pollitt, E. Does breakfast make a difference in school? J. Am. Diet. Assoc. 95:1134–1139, 1995.

37. ADA supports U.S.D.A. School Meals Initiative for Healthy Children but recommends more improvements for child nutrition. J. Am. Diet. Assoc. 94:841–842, 1994.

38. Gortmaker, S.L., Dietz, W.H., and Cheung, L.W. Inactivity, diet and the fattening of America. J. Am. Diet. Assoc. 90:1247–1252, 1990.

39. Sylvester, G.P., Achterberg, C., and Williams, J. Children's television and nutrition: friends or foes? Nutrition Today 30:6–15, Feb, 1995.

40. Klesges, R.C., Shelton, M.L., and Klesges, L.M. Effects of television on metabolic rate: potential implications for childhood obesity. Pediatrics 91:281–286, 1993.

41. Wong, N.D., Hei, T.K., Qaqundah, P.Y., et al. Television watching and pediatric hypercholesterolemia. Pediatrics 90:75–79, 1992.

42. Proos, L.A. Anthropometry in adolescence—secular trends, adoption, ethnic and environmental differences. Horm. Res. 39(suppl)3:18–24, 1993.

43. Carruth, B.R. Adolescence. In *Present Knowledge in Nutrition*. Brown, M.L., ed. Washington, DC: International Life Sciences Institute—Nutrition Foundation, 1990, pp. 325–332.

44. Calvo, M.S. The effects of high phosphorus intake on calcium homeostasis. Adv. Nutr. Res. 9:183–207, 1994.

45. U.S. Department of Agriculture, Human Nutrition Information Service. Food and nutrient intakes by individuals in the United States, 1 day, 1989. Nationwide Food Consumption Survey 1987088. NFCS Report No. 87-I-1, 1993.

46. Kaufman, L., Springen, K., Rogers, A., and Gordon, J. Children of the corn. Newsweek August 28:60–62, 1995.

47. Curcio, B.A. For college students, bulgur beats burgers. Eating Well, September/October:21, 1995.

48. Eichner, E.R. Sports anemia, iron supplements, and blood doping. Med. Sci. Sports Exerc. 24:315S–318S, 1992.

49. Sundjot-Borgen, J. Risks and trigger factors for the development of eating disorders in female elite athletes. Med. Sci. Sports Med. 26:414–419, 1994.

50. Horswill, C.A. Applied physiology of amateur wrestling. Sports Med. 14:114–143, 1992.

51. Roe, D.A. *Diet and Drug Interactions*. New York: Van Nostrand Reinhold, 1989.

52. National Research Council. *Diet and Health: Implications for Reducing Chronic Disease Risk*. Washington, DC: National Academy Press, 1989.

53. U.S. Department of Agriculture, U.S. Department of Health and Human Services. *Nutrition and Your Health: Dietary Guidelines for Americans*, 4th ed. Home and Garden Bulletin No. 232. Hyattsville, MD: U.S. Government Printing Office, 1995.

Nutrition and Aging: The Adult Years

CHAPTER CONCEPTS

1. With advances in medicine and technology, Americans are living longer than ever before—now the goal is to increase the number of healthy years.
2. A healthy lifestyle including exercise and a nutritious diet can postpone some of the degenerative changes and diseases that occur with aging.
3. Aging is the accumulation of changes that occur over a lifetime, resulting in an increasing susceptibility to disease and death.
4. With aging there are changes in sensory abilities, digestion and metabolism, hormonal balance, immune function, body composition, mobility, and mental capacity.
5. Older adults should consume nutrient-dense diets because their energy needs are decreased, whereas their other nutrient needs remain the same.
6. The risk of malnutrition increases with age because of physiological as well as socioeconomic changes that affect the ability to obtain, prepare, and consume an adequate diet.
7. Prescription drug use, which is higher in the elderly than in any other age group, can affect nutritional status.
8. Meeting the nutritional needs of older adults requires consideration of social, economic, and medical needs.

JUST A TASTE

Do specific foods, such as yogurt, increase longevity?

Does eating a healthy diet extend your healthy years?

Can antioxidant supplements increase longevity?

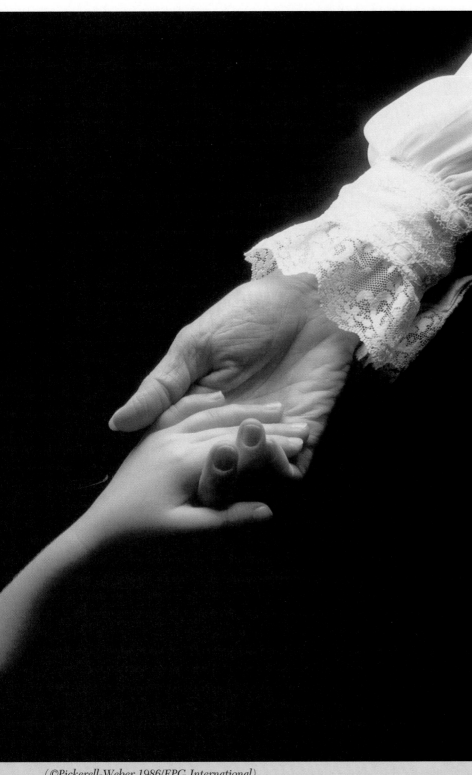

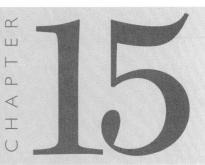

CHAPTER 15

W̲e are all getting older in a society obsessed with youth. Youth symbolizes beauty, fitness, and health. Aging is symbolized by gray hair, wrinkled skin, weak bodies, and forgetful minds. Are these unavoidable changes that occur with age, or can the diet and lifestyle choices we make slow or prevent these changes?

When trying to stop the physiological clock, nutrition is not always the first place people turn. They wash away gray hair in hair salons, and soften and fade wrinkles with creams, cleansers, and plastic surgery. These methods result only in cosmetic changes that help people look younger. They don't help maintain vitality at a youthful level. A healthy lifestyle on the other hand, may not remove the crow's feet, but can affect the health and vitality of one's later years.

The discovery of areas where inhabitants supposedly lived to a very old age generated hope that certain foods could extend life. Although the elderly in these regions are now believed to be no older than individuals throughout the rest of the world, they do remain healthier.[1] They are not overweight, hypertension is rare, and the incidence of heart disease and osteoporosis is low. No one food has been determined to be common among these people. But there are a number of lifestyle similarities. All are societies in which people engage in physical labor, consume largely vegetarian diets, and provide strong psychological support for the elderly. This suggests that although life is not extended, the physiological changes and chronic illness common in old age can be postponed by changes in lifestyle.

In this chapter we will discuss:

- What is aging?
- How can nutrition expand our healthy years?
- How can the nutritional health of the elderly be maintained?

WE ARE ALL GETTING OLDER

When does aging begin? At 21 we are no longer children, and at 45 we are considered middle aged, but when do we become old? The definition of "old" depends on who is defining the term. To a 5-year-old, anyone over 15 seems old. To the federal government, 62 is old enough to claim social security benefits, but to a healthy 80-year-old, "old" may mean 90.

Just as there are many definitions of old, there is great diversity among the elderly, and chronological age is not always the best indicator of aging. A person who is chronologically 75 may have the vigor and health of someone only 55, or vice versa. Individuals in their mid-sixties are strikingly different from those in their nineties, and the differences among 70-year-olds are greater than those among individuals in younger age groups. There are 70-year-olds riding bicycles and others in wheelchairs; some are healthy, independent, and active, while others are chronically ill, dependent, and institutionalized.

No matter how you define aging, as a population and as individuals we are getting older. Advances in technology and health care have allowed people to live longer lives. By the year 2000 there will be 35 million people in the United States over 65, and early in the next century one of five people will be over 65 (Figure 15-1). The fastest-growing segment of the population in industrialized nations is individuals over the age of 85.[2]

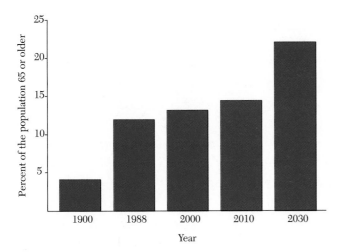

FIGURE 15-1

The percentage of people in the population over the age of 65 has been increasing over the last century. By early in the next century it is projected that one in every five individuals will be 65 or older. (Adapted from *Healthy People 2000: National Health Promotion and Disease Prevention Objectives.* Washington, DC: DHHS, 1991.)

HOW LONG CAN WE EXPECT TO LIVE?

Human **life span**, or the maximum age to which any human can live, is about 100 to 120 years. Most individuals don't live that long. **Life expectancy**, the average length of time that a person can be expected to live, varies between and within populations. It is affected by genetics, lifestyle, and environmental factors. In the United States in 1900, life expectancy was 50 years, but today the average is over 75 years. African Americans have a life expectancy of 69.4 years, whereas Caucasians have a life expectancy of 75.6 years.[2] In Zaire, life expectancy is currently only 47 years, whereas in Japan it is 79 years.[3] Women in the United States live an average of 79 years, seven years longer than the average man. How long an individual lives, or **longevity**, is affected by individual genetic makeup as well as by personal lifestyle and diet.

Life span—The maximum age to which a member of a species can live.

Life expectancy—The average length of life for a population of individuals.

Longevity—The duration of an individual's life.

HOW LONG CAN WE EXPECT TO BE HEALTHY?

Although average life expectancy in the United States has increased to over 75 years, the average healthy life span is only about 64 years. The last 11 years of life are restricted by disease and disability, which become more and more common with advancing age.[2] The goal of successful aging is to increase not only life expectancy but the number of years of healthy life that an individual can expect. This is achieved by slowing the changes that accumulate over time and postponing the diseases of aging long enough to approach or reach the limits of life span before any symptoms appear. This is referred to as **compression of morbidity**. For the population, this means that people are healthier and so more people live longer (Figure 15-2); for the individual, it means that he stays healthy until he reaches the limits of life span and dies. Compression of morbidity benefits not only aging individuals but also the family members who must find the time and resources to care for them and the public health programs that attempt to meet their needs.

Compression of morbidity—The postponement of the onset of chronic disease such that disability occupies a smaller and smaller proportion of the life span.

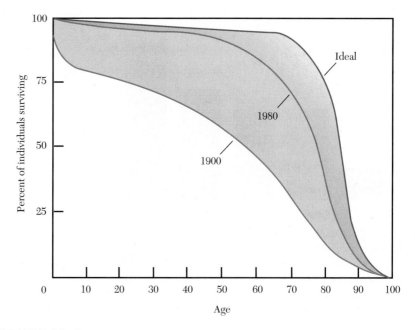

FIGURE 15-2
This graph illustrates the effect of compression of morbidity on survival in a population. The decline in deaths from infectious diseases between 1900 and 1980 allowed more people to survive into adulthood. Delaying the onset of chronic diseases will allow more people to remain healthy and survive into their seventies and eighties. (Adapted from Fries, J.F. Aging, natural death, and the compression of morbidity. N. Engl. J. Med. 303:130–135, 1980.)

CAN NUTRITION KEEP US YOUNG?

Is nutrition the key to immortality? Although the effects of diet and nutrition on the aging process itself are not fully understood, proper diet and exercise can help achieve compression of morbidity, that is, extend our healthy years.

The diseases that are the major causes of disability in older adults—cardiovascular disease, hypertension, diabetes, cancer, and osteoporosis—are all nutrition related. Exercise and a healthy diet will not necessarily prevent these diseases, but may slow the changes that accumulate over time, postponing the onset of disease symptoms. As discussed in Chapters 5 and 12, the risk of developing cardiovascular disease can be decreased by exercise and a diet low in total fat and saturated fat. As discussed in Chapter 10, the occurrence of hypertension may be reduced by consuming a diet low in sodium and adequate in potassium, calcium, and other minerals. As discussed in Chapters 4 and 7, the complications of diabetes are affected by carbohydrate and energy intake. As discussed in Chapter 10, osteoporosis may be slowed by adequate calcium and exercise throughout life. And as discussed throughout this text, the likelihood of getting cancer can be reduced by consuming a diet low in fat and high in fiber and grains, vegetables, and fruits containing antioxidant nutrients and phytochemicals. In addition to preventing chronic disease, consuming an adequate healthy diet can prevent malnutrition, which is a concern among the elderly.

CRITICAL THINKING
Can Your Diet Keep You Young?

Marilyn and Bob are a relatively healthy retired couple in their sixties. The only medication Bob is taking is Questran for high blood cholesterol. Marilyn is taking

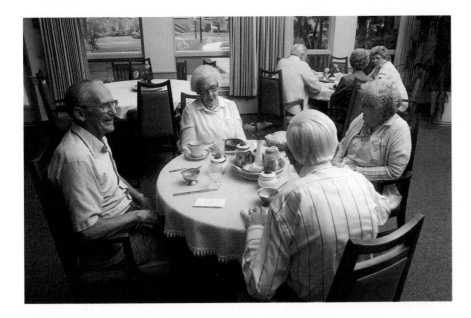

thinking and reasoning. In addition, the diets prescribed for some of these conditions may contribute to malnutrition.[63] This can occur when a diet restricts foods and those using the diet are not provided with enough information about how to substitute foods that will give them adequate energy, nutrients, and eating pleasure (see *Off the Label*: Using Food Labels to Follow Special Diets).

Drugs and Nutrition in the Elderly   Many older persons take 20 or more different drugs every day[64] (Figure 15-10). Medications commonly used by older individuals include aspirin, antacids, laxatives, diuretics (water pills), anticoagulants (blood thinners), anticonvulsives, heart stimulants, cholesterol-lowering medications, and pain medications. Both the effects of drugs on nutritional status and the effects of nutritional status on the effectiveness of the drugs must be considered in the elderly.

The Effect of Drugs on Nutritional Status   Drugs can affect nutrition by altering appetite, nutrient absorption, metabolism, or excretion (Table 15-3). These effects occur with both prescription and over-the-counter medications. In many situations, drugs do not significantly alter overall nutritional status, but they can have a significant impact for individuals who take medications for extended periods, those who take multiple medications, or those who already have marginal nutritional status.

Some medications directly affect the gastrointestinal tract. More than 250 drugs, including blood pressure medications, antidepressants, decongestants, and the pain reliever ibuprofen (found in Advil, Motrin, and Nuprin), can cause mouth dryness, which can decrease interest in eating by interfering with taste, chewing, and swallowing. People with such problems choose foods that are easy to chew and may therefore reduce their consumption of fresh fruits and vegetables, which are high in fiber, vitamins, and minerals. Aspirin is a stomach irritant and can cause small amounts of painless bleeding in the gastrointestinal tract, resulting in iron loss. Digoxin, which is a heart stimulant, can cause gastrointestinal upset, loss of appetite, and nausea. Narcotic pain medications, such as codeine, can lead to constipation, nausea, and vomiting.

Other drugs can decrease nutrient absorption. Cholestyramine (Questran), which is used to reduce blood cholesterol, can decrease the absorption of the fat soluble vitamins, vitamin B_{12}, iron, and folate. Antacids that contain aluminum or magnesium hydroxide (Rolaids or Maalox) combine with phosphorus and fluoride

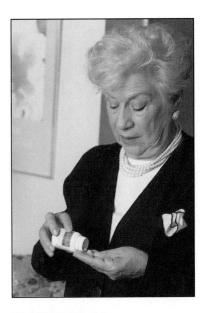

FIGURE 15-10
Most older adults take one or more medications every day. (© Michael Newman/Photo Edit)

TABLE 15-3	**Commonly Used Drugs That May Cause Nutritional Deficiencies**	
Drug Group	**Drug**	**Potential Deficiency**
Antacids	Sodium bicarbonate	Folate, phosphate, calcium, copper
	Aluminum hydroxide	
Anticonvulsants	Phenytoin, phenobarbital, primidone	Vitamins D and K
	Valproic acid	Carnitine
Antibiotics	Tetracycline	Calcium
	Gentamicin	Potassium, magnesium
Antibacterial agents	Neomycin	Fat, nitrogen
	Boric acid	Riboflavin
	Trimethoprim	Folate
	Isoniazid	Vitamins B_6, D, and niacin
Antiinflammatory agents	Sulfasalazine	Folate
	Aspirin	Vitamin C, folate, iron
Anticancer drugs	Colchine	Fat, vitamin B_{12}
	Prednisone	Calcium
	Methotrexate	Folate, calcium
Anticoagulant drugs	Warfarin	Vitamin K
Antihypertensive drugs	Hydralazine	Vitamin B_6
Diuretics	Thiazides	Potassium
	Furosemide	Potassium, calcium, magnesium
Hypocholesterolemic agents	Cholestyramine	Fat
	Colestipol	Vitamin K, vitamin A, folate, vitamin B_{12}
Laxatives	Mineral oil	Carotene, retinol, vitamin D, vitamin K
	Phenolphthalein	Potassium
	Senna	Fat, calcium, vitamin B_6, folate, vitamin C
Tranquilizers	Chlorpromazine	Riboflavin

Adapted from Roe, D.A. *Diet and Drug Interactions*, New York: Van Nostrand Reinhold, 1989.

in the gut to form compounds that cannot be absorbed. Chronic use can result in loss of phosphorus from bone and possibly accelerate osteoporosis. Repeated use of stimulant laxatives can deplete calcium and potassium. Mineral oil laxatives prevent the absorption of fat soluble vitamins. If it isn't possible to prevent constipation by consuming a diet high in fiber and fluid, bulk-forming laxatives are a safer choice.

The metabolism of drugs can also affect nutritional status. For example, anticonvulsive drugs taken by people prone to epileptic seizures increase the liver's capacity to metabolize and eliminate vitamin D and therefore increase the need for vitamin D.

Some drugs affect nutrient excretion. Diuretics, which are used to treat hypertension and edema, cause water loss; but some types (thiazides) also increase the excretion of potassium. People taking thiazide diuretics are advised to include several good sources of potassium in their diet each day or are prescribed supplements.

The Effect of Food and Nutritional Status on the Utilization of Drugs   Food components can either enhance or retard the absorption and metabolism of drugs. Some drugs, such as the pain medication Darvon, are absorbed better or faster if taken with food. Other drugs, such as aspirin and ibuprofen, should be taken with food because they are irritating to the gastrointestinal tract. Since food can delay how quickly drugs leave the stomach, some are best taken with just water. Other drugs interact with specific foods. For instance, the antibiotic tetracycline shouldn't be taken with milk because it binds with calcium, making both unavailable.

Nutritional status can also affect drug metabolism. If nutritional status is poor, the body's ability to detoxify drugs may be altered. For example, in a malnourished individual, theophylline, used to treat asthma, is metabolized slowly, resulting in high blood levels of the drug, which can cause loss of appetite, nausea, and vomiting.

Specific nutrients can also affect the metabolism of drugs. High-protein diets enhance drug metabolism in general, and low-protein diets slow it. Vitamin K hinders the action of anticoagulants, taken to reduce the risk of blood clots. On the other hand, omega-3 fatty acids, found in fish oils, inhibit blood clotting and may intensify the effect of an anticoagulant drug and cause bleeding. It is safe to eat fish while taking anticoagulant drugs; however, the use of fish oil supplements is not recommended.

Drugs can also interact with each other. For example, alcohol affects the metabolism of over a hundred medications. Drug interactions can exaggerate and, in some cases, diminish the effect of a medication. Mixing certain drugs can be fatal. Individuals taking any medication should consult their doctor, pharmacist, or dietitian regarding how the drug could affect their nutrition and how their nutrition could affect the action of the drug.

MEETING NUTRIENT NEEDS

Meeting the nutrient needs of older adults involves not only a consideration of nutrient requirements but also of how food intake and availability are affected by sensory changes, physical limitations, psychological needs, and socioeconomic factors. An understanding of the diversity in the elderly population as well as the factors that help maintain vitality and independence is key to meeting the needs of this segment of the population.

Nutritional Guidelines   A well-planned diet for older adults should follow the recommendations of the Food Guide Pyramid at the low end of the range of servings. Most of the nutritional recommendations that have been made for the general public also apply to elderly individuals. The *Dietary Guidelines* are designed for everyone over two years of age. The National Cholesterol Education Program, designed to reduce the risk of heart disease in the population, suggests that its guidelines be followed by older as well as younger adults. However, this program also cautions that, in the elderly, a very restrictive diet could lead to nutrient deficiencies.[65] Because of the decreased energy requirements of older adults, a nutrient-dense diet must be consumed to meet micronutrient needs. However, simply providing a nutrient-dense diet does not solve all of the nutritional problems that may accompany aging.

Food Choices   Often, food choices must be modified to meet needs. For instance, an individual with dental problems may not be able to chew fresh fruits and vegetables. Therefore, a texture modification is required. Canned and soft fruit or fruit juices can be substituted for hard-to-chew fruits, and cooked vege-

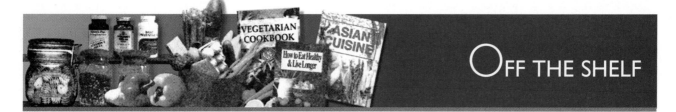

Are Frozen Meals a Healthy Option?

Shopping for and cooking meals that offer variety is difficult for many people who live alone. One choice that allows a different meal every night is frozen prepared meals. They are convenient, easy to prepare, and easy to clean up after, but are they healthy and economical?

Frozen dinners have come a long way. In the 1950s, frozen meals known as "TV dinners" were marketed as the meal of the future—convenient, fast, self-contained, a whole meal that Dad could cook by himself in 30 minutes without dirtying a pan. Selection was limited, however. If you weren't a fan of Salisbury steak, mashed potatoes, gravy, and mixed vegetables you were better off cooking for yourself. These original TV dinners were also high in fat, saturated fat, and sodium. Today the selection is extensive—the frozen meal section occupies a whole aisle of the grocery store. You can buy frozen breakfasts, lunches, entrées, or desserts. There are Hungry Man meals

that cater to big eaters, Lean Cuisine for those looking for a low-kcalorie option, and Kids Cuisine that target the food preferences of children. There are ethnic foods like burritos, egg rolls, and curries. Food technology has created complete microwaveable meals with heat susceptors to crisp the fries and protective coverings to only warm the pie.

Are these healthy options? It depends on the choices you make. There are meals that are low in energy, low in fat, and low in sodium. And, there are many that are very high in these nutrients. Check the labels to find the ones that suit your needs. A sodium content of 1000 mg may seem high, but if that meal is your entire dinner and you have limited your sodium intake for the rest of the day, it can be included in a healthy diet. Prepared meals can increase the nutrient content of the diet by adding variety. For example, a single-serving meal prepared at home

might be a potato or some pasta, but a frozen dinner provides sources of protein and complex carbohydrate, vegetables, and often fruit.

An important consideration with these meals is cost. The price of a frozen meal ranges from $1.50 for lunch to $4.50 for a large-serving-size dinner. This may seem expensive, but frozen meals don't need to be eaten at every meal every day. A breakfast of cereal or oatmeal and a lunch of a peanut butter sandwich are no more difficult to prepare than a frozen meal. It may be possible to budget the cost of a few frozen dinners a week. This cost must also be balanced against the cost of buying small amounts of fresh vegetables, fruits, and meats needed to prepare a single-serving meal at home. If cost is not prohibitive and choices are made wisely, frozen meals can be part of a diet that meets the recommendations of the *Dietary Guidelines* and the Food Guide Pyramid.

tables can replace raw ones. Meats can be stewed, providing an easier-to-chew protein source. To overcome changes in the sense of taste and smell, spicy or acidic foods may be limited or emphasized, depending on individual tastes. Constipation can be prevented by increasing the intake of cooked vegetables and fluid or by including a fiber supplement. In some cases, meeting nutrient needs involves providing assistance with shopping or meal preparation; in other cases, education about the requirements, economics, and preparation of foods may be beneficial.

Another problem that contributes to poor nutrient intake is loneliness. Living, cooking, and eating alone can decrease interest in food. This can be a problem not only for the elderly, but for anyone who typically eats alone. It is important for people of all ages to keep socially active and share and cook meals with others as often as possible. Even when eating alone, single people can eat convenient, nutritious, delicious foods (see *Off the Shelf*: Are Frozen Meals a Healthy Option?). To avoid spoilage of perishable items, grocers can be asked to break up packages of meat, eggs, fruits, and vegetables so small amounts can be purchased. Buying single servings of food is an option, although it can be expensive. Cooking larger portions and freezing foods in meal-size batches can be helpful not only with cost but also to relieve the boredom of eating the same leftovers several days in a row. Easy single meals can also be prepared by topping a potato with cooked

food does not mean that the food is hazardous. The potential of a substance to cause harm depends on how potent it is, the amount, or dose, that is consumed, how often it is consumed, and who consumes it. Some substances will cause no harm at any practical level of intake, but almost any substance can be toxic if a large enough amount is consumed. Many substances have a **threshold effect**; that is, they are harmless up to a certain dose or threshold, after which negative effects increase with increasing intake.

Body size, nutritional status, and how a substance is metabolized by the body can affect toxicity. Small doses are more dangerous in children and small adults because the amount of toxin per unit of body weight is greater. Poor nutritional or health status may decrease the body's natural ability to detoxify harmful substances. The way that a substance is stored or excreted also determines its potential for harm. Substances that are stored in the body are more likely to be toxic because they accumulate. Over time they are deposited in bone, adipose tissue, liver, or other organs until toxicity symptoms occur. For instance, vitamin A is stored in the liver and can be toxic if excess amounts are consumed over a long period. Substances that are easily excreted when consumed in excess, such as vitamin C, are less likely to cause toxicity. The interaction of toxins with one another and with other dietary factors also affects toxicity. For example, mercury, which is extremely toxic, is not absorbed well if the diet is high in selenium, and the absorption of cadmium and lead is decreased by the presence of iron and calcium in the diet.

WHO SAFEGUARDS THE FOOD SUPPLY?

The safety of the food supply is monitored by a number of different agencies at the international, federal, state, and local levels. Individual consumers must also share the responsibility for maintaining the safety of the foods they eat.

Federal Agencies   The Food and Drug Administration (FDA), the U.S. Department of Agriculture (USDA), the Environmental Protection Agency (EPA), and other agencies are all responsible for monitoring various segments of the food supply (see Table 16-1). They set standards and establish regulations on the safe and sanitary handling of food and water as well as the use of additives and packaging techniques. They also set standards for both the nutrition information and the safe handling information on food labels. They inspect food processing and storage facilities, monitor both domestic and imported foods for contamination, and investigate outbreaks of food-borne illness (see Figure 16-1).

These agencies work together to ensure a safe food supply. For instance, the EPA is responsible for determining allowable limits, or **tolerances**, for pesticide residues in raw foods. The tolerance limits set by the EPA are enforced by the FDA and the USDA. International cooperation on food inspection and regulatory standards helps to ensure the safety of imported foods. Approximately 40 different nations are now partners with the United States in ensuring food safety through agreements that regulate a variety of food products.

Traditional methods of monitoring the food industry depend on spot checking manufacturing conditions and randomly sampling final products. This is a daunting task, considering the variety of foods and the many processing methods used by the food industry. Many agencies are now switching to a system that focuses on preventing food-borne hazards rather than inspecting to see if they have occurred. This system, Hazard Analysis Critical Control Point, or HACCP, requires that the points in a food's production at which hazards can be prevented, controlled, or eliminated be identified.[1] Preventative measures are then established at each of these critical points, to avoid contamination or to limit it to an acceptable level. For example, to produce liquid and frozen eggs, the eggs are removed from the shells and then pasteurized to kill *Salmonella* and other microbial contaminants.

Threshold effect–When a substance can be ingested without effect up to a certain amount; after that, effects increase as the amount consumed increases.

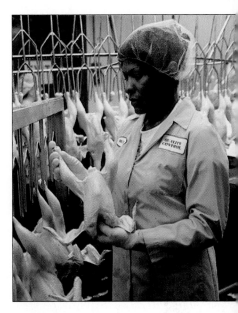

FIGURE 16-1
Inspecting food processing facilities is one way that food safety is monitored. (© Don Smetzer/Tony Stone Worldwide-Click/Chicago Ltd.)

Tolerances–Allowable levels of pesticide residues in foods, set by the EPA.

TABLE 16-1	Agencies Responsible for Food Safety
Agency	**Responsibility**
FDA (Food and Drug Administration)	Ensures the safety and wholesomeness of all foods sold in interstate commerce with the exception of red meat (beef, veal, pork and lamb), poultry, and eggs; inspects food plants and imported foods; sets standards for food composition; and enforces regulations for food labeling, food and color additives, and food sanitation.
USDA (U.S. Department of Agriculture)	Enforces standards for the wholesomeness and quality of red meat, poultry, and eggs.
EPA (Environmental Protection Agency)	Regulates pesticide levels and must approve all pesticides before they can be sold in the United States; establishes water quality standards.
National Marine Fishery Service (Department of Commerce)	Oversees the management of fisheries and fish harvesting. Provides a voluntary program of inspection and grading of fish products.
CDC (Centers for Disease Control and Prevention)	Monitors and investigates the incidence and causes of food-borne diseases.
Bureau of Alcohol, Tobacco, and Firearms	Enforces laws covering the production, distribution, and labeling of alcoholic beverages.

The critical control point for eliminating *Salmonella* is pasteurization. HACCP also involves establishing procedures for monitoring control points, taking corrective actions when a critical limit has not been met, and establishing effective record keeping and procedures to verify the system is working consistently. To monitor the effectiveness of pasteurization in the liquid and frozen egg industry, the pasteurized eggs are held refrigerated or frozen until the results of bacterial tests have been obtained. If the eggs are *Salmonella* free, they are released to the market. If they contain *Salmonella*, they cannot be sold and pasteurization conditions must be adjusted. The advantage of this system over standard inspections by the FDA is that the plan is preventative rather than punitive, oversight is easier, and the responsibility for food safety is placed on the manufacturer, not the regulatory agencies.

State and Local Governments   The FDA provides guidelines to state and local governments for regulating dairy products and food sold at restaurants. States then have the primary responsibility for milk safety and the inspection of restaurants, retail food stores, dairies, grain mills, and other food-related establishments within their borders (Figure 16-2). As a result, regulations vary from state to state.

Consumers   Consumers must also assume some of the responsibility for their food. They must decide what foods they will consume and evaluate the risks involved. They must also be actively involved in preventing food-borne illness. A food that has been manufactured, packaged, and transported with the greatest care can still cause food-borne illness if it is not carefully handled at home. Ways in which consumers can help to ensure the safety of their diets are included in the following discussions. Consumers can also protect themselves and others by reporting incidents involving unsanitary, unsafe, deceptive, or mislabeled food to the appropriate agencies (Table 16-2).

brings with it pesticides that are not used domestically. Domestic produce and imported produce do not differ in the amounts of pesticide residue, but they do differ in the types of pesticides they contain. Because of country-to-country differences in crops, pests, growing conditions, and pesticide regulations, imported foods may contain pesticides that are not used in the United States and for which the EPA has not set tolerance levels.[15]

To protect against the risk of pesticide exposure, the FDA not only regulates pesticide use but also measures the pesticide content of the total diet as well as of individual foods. In general, the amounts of pesticides to which people are exposed are small. According to the FDA's pesticide residue monitoring program, the levels of pesticides found in the American food supply are below tolerances. Of all FDA samples, domestic and imported, 60% contained no detectable pesticide residues and only 1% were above tolerance levels.[16] Since the foods we buy in the grocery store are shipped from many different locations, repeated exposure to large doses of any one pesticide is unlikely.

Reducing Pesticide Risks   Concern about the toxicity of pesticides has changed the pattern of pesticide use in the United States. New, more effective chemical pesticides are being developed, and the use of older, more toxic products is decreasing. One approach to the development of safer pesticides is genetic engineering. In 1991, the EPA approved the first genetically engineered pesticides. They are insect-killing proteins that are produced by bacteria. The bacteria containing the pesticides are killed and then sprayed on plants. Genetically engineered insect-killing viruses are also being tested.[17]

In addition to developing safer pesticides, production methods are being developed to make low-pesticide and pesticide-free produce available to the consumer. One such system is called **integrated pest management (IPM)**. IPM combines chemical and nonchemical methods of pest control and emphasizes the use of natural pesticides and more effective pesticide application.[15] Another system is organic farming, which does not use synthetic pesticides, herbicides, or fertilizers at all. These farming techniques reduce the exposure of farm workers to pesticides and decrease the quantity of pesticides introduced into the food supply and the environment.

Integrated pest management (IPM)–A method of agricultural pest control that integrates nonchemical and chemical techniques.

Exploiting Natural Toxins   Many toxins occur naturally in plants. They function as natural pesticides that offer protection from bacteria, molds, and insect pests. These naturally pest-resistant crops are advantageous in developing countries because they thrive without the use of expensive added pesticides. Plants high in natural pesticides are being produced through special breeding programs. Using these plants will reduce the need for added pesticides. The natural toxins in plants can also be isolated and applied to crops like synthetic pesticides. Unfortunately, these natural pesticides are not always safer than synthetic ones and they are not as extensively tested.[18]

As with all chemical toxins, natural toxins move through the food supply and the potential for toxicity depends on the dose of toxin and the health of the consumer. For example, a cow that has foraged on toxic plants can pass the toxin into her milk and poison the consumer of the milk. Abraham Lincoln's mother died from drinking milk from a cow that had eaten poisonous snakeroot plants. Most natural toxins in the food supply are consumed in doses that pose little risk to the consumer. For instance, solanine, a neurotoxin found in the green layer under potato skins is not toxic in amounts typically consumed. But consuming ten times the typical amount of potatoes could cause symptoms. Poisonous mushrooms contain toxins that can be fatal even in small amounts, but the varieties of mushrooms sold in grocery stores are safe and delicious. Natural toxins are also found in seafood and are responsible for about one third of reported cases of seafood-borne illness.[19]

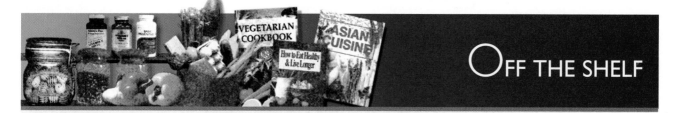

OFF THE SHELF

Herbal Teas or Herbal Hazards?

For thousands of years, herbs have been used medicinally, and today herbal teas are consumed for their aroma and flavor as well. While consuming herbal teas is thought to be a healthful alternative to caffeinated beverages, little is really known about the safety of some of the herbs.

Many of the herbal teas on the market have ingredient lists that look like a garden tour: lemon grass, rosebuds, spearmint, raspberry leaves, chamomile flowers. Most of these and other ingredients used in commercially prepared teas have been used for centuries with relative safety. However, problems arise when people consume herbal teas in excessive amounts or concoct their own brews. For example, comfrey tea has been implicated in liver disease. Comfrey roots and leaves contain chemicals that have been found to cause cancer in rats. Lobelia, also known as Indian tobacco, was used in the 19th century to treat asthma. When used in large amounts, lobelia tea can cause vomiting, breathing problems, convulsions, coma, and death. Sassafras tea, which

was once used as a stimulant, blood thinner, and reputed cure for rheumatism and syphilis, causes cancer in rats. Oil of sassafras and safrole from sassafras root bark were taken out of root beer over 30 years ago, and today sassafras bark is banned in all food products. There have been reports of illness caused by tea made from the leaves of foxglove plant, from which the heart drug digitalis is derived, and from oleander, which is poisonous. Abnormal menstrual bleeding was reported in a woman consuming a homemade brew that included, among others, tonka beans, melilot, and woodruff. These contain coumarin, an anticoagulant.

Currently, the regulation of herbal teas depends on the types of claims made about its use. If an herbal tea makes a claim to prevent or cure a disease, the FDA regulates it as a drug, and it must be approved as safe and effective for its intended use. For example, products claiming to help with smoking cessation, weight loss, constipation, or sore throats are considered drugs. Herb teas claiming

less dramatic effects, such as calming, relaxing, and soothing, are classified as dietary supplements by the FDA and therefore regulated like foods rather than drugs or additives.

Concern about the effects of herbs has prompted the FDA to collect samples of herbal products to determine health hazards and assess unsubstantiated claims. In Canada, an advisory committee was established to review information about herbs and make recommendations. The result was a ban on 57 herbs and warning labels on five others that may cause problems during pregnancy. The herb industry itself has also initiated a program to evaluate 200 or so commercially available herbs that are currently not approved for use as food flavorings. Their evaluations include factors such as the history of the herb in other countries, chemical composition, pharmacological properties, reports of adverse reactions, and toxicity studies. Advice for tea drinkers is to stick to commercial varieties and to avoid consuming any one variety in excess.

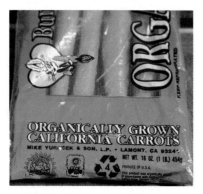

FIGURE 16-12

In many states, inspections ensure that foods labeled "organically grown" are produced using organic techniques. (Charles D. Winters)

Using Organic Techniques   Organically grown foods are grown without synthetic pesticides and are better for the environment, which is a benefit; but a food labeled organic is not always pesticide free, risk free, or the best choice for everyone. The National Organic Standards Law established national uniformity in the requirements for the certification and marketing of organically grown foods; however, currently only 16 states have inspections to ensure that foods labeled organic are really produced organically (Figure 16-12). Even if the food purchased is produced according to standards, it may not be pesticide free. Organically grown foods may contain traces of pesticides from irrigation water, rain, or a variety of other sources. An additional health concern when purchasing organically grown food is that it may have been fertilized with improperly treated compost or untreated animal manure that may contain harmful bacteria.[20] Consumers must also be aware that organically grown foods are not superior in quality, taste, or nutrient content to conventionally grown foods.[20] Economics and availability must also be factored into the risk-benefit analysis. Organic produce is usually more expensive and available in less variety than conventionally grown foods.

which may cause itching and hives in hypersensitive individuals, was not considered a great enough risk to be removed from the food supply.

PROCESSING AND PACKAGING

For thousands of years, humans have been treating foods in order to protect them from spoilage by microorganisms. Most of the oldest methods of food preservation—including drying, smoking, **fermentation**, and the addition of sugar or salt—are still used today. In more recent history, these techniques were supplemented with methods that rely on temperature to prevent microbial growth.

Using Temperature to Ensure Safety
Preservation techniques that rely on temperature include cooking, canning, **pasteurization**, sterilization, refrigeration, and freezing. These techniques benefit us by providing appealing safe food, but they are not risk free, particularly if used incorrectly. Techniques that heat food, such as canning and pasteurization, kill microorganisms and those that keep food cold, such as refrigeration and freezing, slow or stop microbial growth. If foods are not heated long enough or to a high enough temperature or if they are not kept cold enough, there is a risk of food-borne illness.

Cooking food is one of the oldest methods of ensuring food safety. It kills disease-causing organisms, destroys toxins, and increases flavor and digestibility. In addition to the risks posed by undercooking foods, cooking can generate a variety of mutagens and carcinogens (Figure 16-15). These are considered accidental contaminants, so they are not regulated by the FDA.

Fermentation—A process in which microorganisms metabolize components of a food and therefore change the composition, taste, and storage properties of the food.

Pasteurization—The process of heating food products to kill disease-causing organisms.

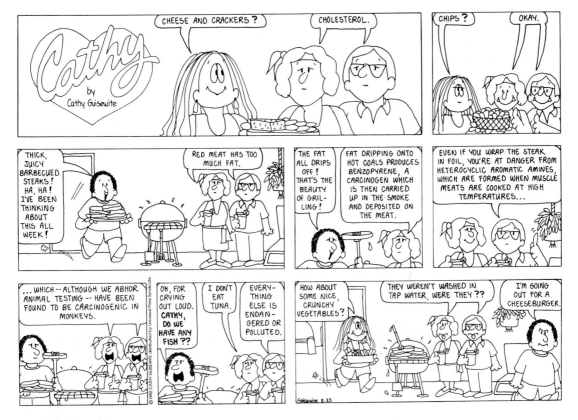

FIGURE 16-15
(© *Cathy Guisewite. Reprinted with permission of UNIVERSAL PRESS SYNDICATE. All rights reserved.*)

Polycyclic aromatic hydrocarbons (PAHs)–A class of mutagenic substances produced during cooking when there is incomplete combustion of organic materials, for example, when fat drips on a grill.

Heterocyclic amines (HAs)–A class of mutagenic substances produced when there is incomplete combustion of amino acids during the cooking of meats, for example, when meat is charred.

Aseptic processing–A method that places sterilized food in a sterilized package using a sterile process.

Modified atmosphere packaging (MAP)–A type of food packaging in which the gases inside the package are changed to control or retard chemical, physical, and microbiological changes.

Toxins Produced During Cooking The most familiar group of chemicals produced during food preparation is the **polycyclic aromatic hydrocarbons (PAHs)**. PAHs are formed when fat from beef, pork, lamb, poultry, or fish drips onto the flame of a grill. As early as 1775, PAH-containing soot was linked to cancer in chimney sweeps. Several of the PAHs found in food have been shown to cause cancer in laboratory animals. Eating grilled fatty meat every day is not recommended, but occasional grilling, particularly with lowfat meat, presents little risk.

Broiled foods, which are cooked with the heat source on the top, are low in PAHs. However, broiled and pan-fried meats contain another potential hazard—**heterocyclic amines**. Heterocyclic amines, such as benzopyrene, are formed from the burning of amino acids and other substances in meats. Well-done meat and meat cooked using hotter temperatures contain greater amounts. The cooking temperatures recommended by the FDA are designed to prevent microbial foodborne illness and minimize the production of heterocyclic amines. The levels of heterocyclic amines can be reduced by precooking meat in the microwave and discarding the juice.

Using Packaging to Ensure Safety Some of the newer methods of food preservation rely on modern packaging. In one type of preservation, referred to as **aseptic processing**, sterilized foods are placed in sterilized packages using sterilized packaging equipment.[5] Aseptic processing is currently used to produce boxes of sterile milk and juices. These can remain free of microbial growth at room temperature for years.

Consumer demand for fresh foods has led to a new generation of fresh refrigerated foods such as pasta, vegetables, fish, chicken, and beef. They are delicious, nutritious, and convenient, but are they safe? To make fresh refrigerated foods—for example, beef teriyaki—the raw ingredients are sealed in plastic pouches, the air is vacuumed out, and the pouch and its contents are partially precooked and immediately refrigerated.[32] This type of processing eliminates the need for the extreme cold of freezing or the extreme heat of canning, so flavor is better preserved. These vacuum-packed raw or partially cooked foods are known by the French words *sous vide*, meaning "under vacuum." In some products, the oxygen in the package is replaced with a gas such as carbon dioxide or nitrogen, in which microbes are unlikely to grow.[5] This is called **modified atmosphere packaging (MAP)**. These products must be kept refrigerated until use. Unlike canned foods, fresh refrigerated products are not heated to sufficient temperatures to kill all bacteria, and unlike frozen foods, they are not kept at temperatures low enough to prevent all bacteria from growing. Despite the modified atmosphere inside the package, some bacteria, such as *Listeria*, that can grow at temperatures of 33 to 39°F may still be a threat. These foods should be purchased only from reputable vendors, used by the expiration date printed on the package, refrigerated constantly until use, and heated according to the time and temperature on the package directions.

Contamination from Packaging Packaging can protect food from spoilage, but even the best packaging can introduce risk if it becomes a part of the food. A variety of substances leach into foods from the packaging in which they are contained. These substances come from plastics, paper, and even dishes. Components that are known to contaminate foods are indirect food additives and are regulated by EPA tolerance levels and FDA inspections. However, these regulations apply only to the intended use of the product. When used as intended, packaging enhances the safety of food, and the amounts and types of substances that enter food from it is regulated. However, when used improperly, packaging can migrate into food and become an accidental contaminant. For instance, some

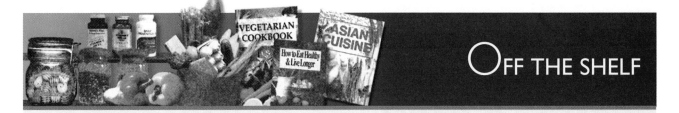

OFF THE SHELF

Food to Go . . .

Today, technology can process and package food to go to the bottom of the ocean or to orbit the globe. Many of the advances in processing technology have arisen from government and military needs, rather than consumer convenience. In fact, the packaging of food originated in response to military need.

In 1800, the battle of Marengo was nearly lost because Napoleon's men had to spend so much time foraging for food. While most of the soldiers were on a search for sustenance, the Austrians attacked and nearly won the battle. The French were not able to carry or keep enough fresh food for the months of battle, and they were not able to buy food because the Italians wouldn't accept their paper currency. Therefore, they were forced to trade or forage for food to feed the army. After this battle, Napoleon returned to France to create a gold-based monetary system and to offer a prize for the development of packaged, transportable food.

The first packaged food was prepared using the technology for bottling champagne. Nicholas Appert, who had worked in the champagne industry, placed foods in wine bottles

and sealed the bottles with corks held on by wire cages. The bottles were then bathed in boiling water. The first bottled foods were peas, beans, stew, and soup. Appert sold these to the French navy, who took them on a trial voyage to the Caribbean. When Appert's foods proved stable, he was awarded a prize by the French government for solving their need for portable food.

Military needs continue to promote the development of new processing and packaging techniques. Products must be developed that are stable in the jungle, the desert, in extreme cold, and at high altitudes. Special food engineering departments have been established expressly for the purpose of developing foods to meet military needs. If a branch of the military submits a request for a food with a specific shelf life, with specific preparation requirements, and to be used in a specific climate, a team of food scientists will go to work to develop the requested product.

Military rations range from frozen foods sent to military bases with full kitchens to MREs (Meal, Ready-to-Eat), that is, individually packaged meals including entrees, crackers,

fruit, dessert, candy, and beverage powders, which individual soldiers carry to the front lines. The latest developments include flameless heating units that heat MREs to 100°F above the ambient temperature in 12 minutes, and LLRPs (Long-Life Ration Packets), which are completely dehydrated, and therefore lightweight, meals. During the 1991 Gulf War the military's deployment capability often surpassed its logistic ability to feed the troops. As a result, the majority of meals were provided by MREs.[1]

Advances developed for the military soon find their way into the consumer market. T rations, which were developed as prepared meals in ready-to-cook and ready-to-eat serving trays, foreshadowed TV dinners. Lightweight, dehydrated beverages developed for astronauts are now common in most kitchen cabinets, and lightweight dehydrated meals now benefit the backpacker. The industry may have been born out of military need, but the result is technology that serves the everyday consumer.

[1] Feeney, R.E., Askew, E.E., and Jezior, D.A. The development and evolution of U.S. Army field rations. Nutr. Rev. 53:221–225, 1995.

---

plastics migrate into food when heated in a microwave oven. Only packages designated for microwave cooking should be used. The ink on plastic bags used to package foods is outside the bag and should not come in contact with food. If the bags are used improperly, food can be contaminated with lead from the ink. A survey on the use of empty bread bags found that some people are turning bread bags inside out and reusing them to store other foods or to pack lunches.[33] To avoid lead contamination from plastic bags, don't reuse them; if you do, don't let the inked side touch the food. (See *Off the Shelf*: Get the Lead Out, in Chapter 14.)

Lead can also contaminate food and water from the lead glaze used on some pottery, leaded crystal used in wine glasses, and lead solder used in water pipes. For information about lead contamination and kits for home use that test the amount of lead leaching from ceramic ware, call your local FDA office or FDA headquarters at (301)443-4667. The National Safety Council also maintains a National Lead Information Center, which supplies information in English and Spanish (1-(800)LEAD-FYI, or 1-(800)532-3394). In addition, most ceramic manufacturers in the United States maintain toll-free lines that can provide information about lead levels in their products.

IRRADIATED FOODS

Irradiation—A process of exposing foods to radiation to kill contaminating organisms and retard ripening and spoilage of fruits and vegetables.

Irradiation is a newer method of food preservation. The process exposes food to a high dose of x-rays, gamma radiation, or high-energy electrons, which kills microorganisms, destroys insects, and slows vital processes such as the germination and ripening of fruits and vegetables. It may, therefore, be used in place of chemicals to reduce insect and microbial contamination and to slow ripening during food storage.[34] Irradiation does produce some compounds that are unique to irradiated foods. As a result, irradiation is treated as a food additive, and the level of radiation that may be used is regulated by the FDA and USDA. At the allowed levels of irradiation, the amounts of these unique compounds produced are almost negligible and have not been found to be a risk to consumers. The effect of irradiation on texture, flavor, color, and nutrient composition varies with the food but is comparable to other methods of food processing and preservation.[34]

The FDA has approved irradiation to destroy contaminants in spices, prevent insect infestation in flour and spices, increase shelf life of potatoes, eliminate *Trichinella* in pork and bacteria in poultry, and slow the ripening and spoilage of some produce. Irradiated foods can be identified by the radura symbol shown in Figure 16-16 and the statement "treated with radiation" or "treated by irradiation." Products that contain irradiated spices do not need to display this symbol.

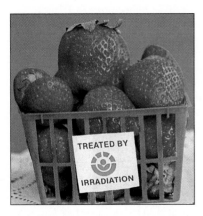

FIGURE 16-16
Foods that have been treated with irradiation can be identified by this symbol. (Courtesy of Nordion International, Inc.)

BIOTECHNOLOGY

Genetic modification or **genetic engineering—**A set of techniques used to manipulate DNA for the purpose of changing the characteristics of an organism or creating a new product.
Gene—A stretch of DNA that contains the instructions for making a protein.

In addition to the technological advances that have created new methods of processing and packaging foods, technology has also produced new foods and products. Some of these are produced using traditional food chemistry, but many are now being made using biotechnology. Biotechnology refers to the use of **genetic modification** or **genetic engineering** to alter the DNA of plants and animals to produce new traits or enhance desirable ones. The first step is to identify a stretch of DNA, or **gene**, for a given desirable trait, such as resistance to a particular disease. This gene could be in a plant, an animal, or a bacterial cell. The gene can be clipped out with specific DNA-cutting enzymes (Figure 16-17) and then pasted into or recombined with the DNA of a virus or bacteria. The virus or bacteria containing the gene for the desired trait then reproduces. Each reproduction produces **clones**, or copies of the gene. Each of the clones can now produce the protein that is coded for by that gene. For example, bovine somatotropin, used to increase milk production in cows, is produced by genetically engineered bacteria. Bacteria or viruses containing recombined genes can also be used to produce plants or animals with specific characteristics. To do this, the gene of interest must be inserted into a target plant or animal cell. For example, a gene for disease resistance might be introduced into the cells of wheat plants, making the wheat disease resistant. One way genes are inserted is by allowing a virus containing the desired gene to infect the target cell, hence introducing the recombinant DNA.

Clones—Copies of a gene that are identical to the original.

The Benefits of Biotechnology
The uses of biotechnology are as varied as the imagination. Crops being developed using biotechnology include fruits and vegetables that ripen more slowly so they will arrive at stores at their peak, virus-resistant vegetables, insect-resistant produce, vegetables with increased levels of

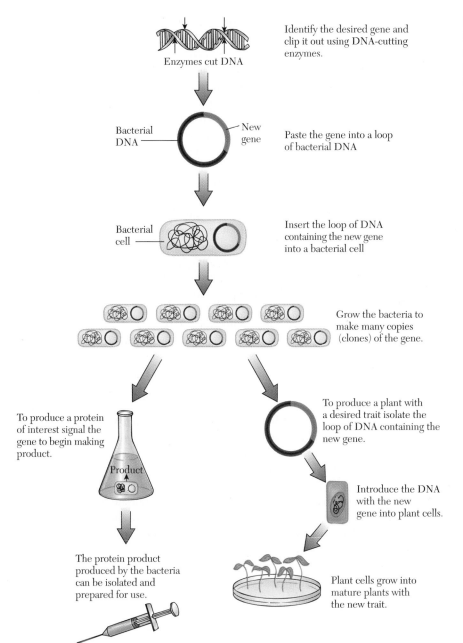

Identify the desired gene and clip it out using DNA-cutting enzymes.

Enzymes cut DNA

Paste the gene into a loop of bacterial DNA

Bacterial DNA — New gene

Insert the loop of DNA containing the new gene into a bacterial cell

Bacterial cell

Grow the bacteria to make many copies (clones) of the gene.

To produce a protein of interest signal the gene to begin making product.

To produce a plant with a desired trait isolate the loop of DNA containing the new gene.

Product

Introduce the DNA with the new gene into plant cells.

The protein product produced by the bacteria can be isolated and prepared for use.

Plant cells grow into mature plants with the new trait.

FIGURE 16-17
Genetic engineering involves inserting a gene for a desired trait into an organism to create a new strain of plant or animal or to produce large amounts of a desired gene product.

amino acids, low-caffeine coffee, long-lasting raspberries, and potatoes that absorb less fat when fried.[35,36] Vegetable crops can be developed that don't need as much cooking when they are canned or are more resistant to freezing. The first genetically engineered whole food to be approved by the FDA and marketed is the Flavr Savr tomato, a tomato that can be shipped vine ripened without rotting. To create this tomato, rather than inserting a gene that codes for slower rotting, researchers used a technique to inactivate the gene that causes tomato rotting (Figure 16-18).

Other advances in biotechnology that will have impact on the quantity, quality, safety, and shelf life of foods include environmentally friendly pesticides, and safer additives and preservatives. Genetically engineered enzymes are also used in food processing, and food colors and flavors are being produced from plant tissue grown in the laboratory in culture. Improvements in the treatment, prevention, and diagnosis of animal disease as well as developments that improve animal growth and fertility all can enhance food production.[37]

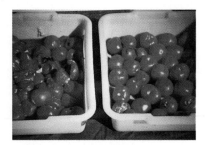

FIGURE 16-18
Tomatoes can be genetically engineered to delay ripening and extend shelf life. The genetically altered tomatoes on the right do not spoil as fast as those on the left. (Markel/Gamma Liaison, Inc.)

Does Biotechnology Carry Risks?   As with any new process or product, consumers may be reluctant to use genetically engineered foods. The FDA has ruled that there is no reason for extra regulations on most foods produced via genetic engineering.[35] No premarket approval will be required for genetically engineered foods unless the food contains substances not commonly found in foods, or the food contains a substance that does not have a history of safe use in foods. To help assure the public that this approach is appropriate for genetically engineered foods, the FDA plans to require that producers of these products notify the FDA before they are marketed so the FDA is kept aware of all new developments.

Because they are essentially no different from other foods, genetically engineered foods do not need special labeling. Exceptions are foods into which a potential allergen has been introduced. For example, if DNA from fish or peanuts, foods that commonly cause allergic reactions, is introduced into tomatoes or corn, these foods would have to be labeled in order to alert allergic consumers. Labeling would also be required if the nutrient content of a food were significantly altered. For example, tomatoes are an excellent source of vitamin C. If a tomato were developed that had no vitamin C, it would have be labeled to disclose this information.

The standard concerns about safety and labeling have been addressed, but genetic engineering has introduced some new concerns. One relates more to the environment than to the consumer. Because the chemical makeup of DNA is similar in all living things, genetic engineering can take traits from any living organism—plant, animal, or microbe—and incorporate them into another species. For example, one developer has explored the use of a gene isolated from a fish, the winter flounder, to impart freeze resistance into a tomato. If a trait introduced into a plant species could be passed on to one of its wild relatives, it might produce a plant that would become a fast-growing weed or that would be harmful to species that depend on it for food. Ethical and religious issues also need to be resolved. For example, can a tomato that contains some DNA from a fish be included in a vegan diet? Is corn that contains DNA from a pig appropriate for Jews and Moslems to eat? The FDA currently believes that the answer to these questions is yes, since plants and animals already share some of the same types of DNA, but this is an issue that will continue to be debated.[35]

CRITICAL THINKING
Individual Risk-Benefit Analysis

After reading a newspaper article about a child who died of food-borne illness contracted by eating an undercooked hamburger, Rex became concerned about the safety of the foods his family was eating. He thought more carefully about other food safety issues, such as eggs and poultry contaminated with *Salmonella*; pesticide residues on fruits and vegetables; and fish contaminated with industrial pollutants, bacteria, viruses, and parasites. He started to think it was too risky to eat at all but then decided to look at the foods his family eats and see if the benefits they provide are worth the risk.

In general his family eats a healthy diet and is rarely sick, but he knows that a few of the things they like carry risks. He enjoys his meat rare, his son is an athlete who drinks protein shakes containing raw eggs, his young daughter likes to lick the bowl where cookie dough containing raw eggs is mixed, and he and his wife enjoy eating sushi and raw oysters. He made the following list of foods and then recorded the risks and benefits of each:

Food	Risk	Benefit
Hamburger	Can be contaminated with dangerous strains of *E. coli*.	A good source of protein and iron in the diet.
Chicken	Raw chicken is often contaminated with *Salmonella*.	Chicken is an economical source of protein that is low in fat.
Eggs	Raw eggs can contain *Salmonella* inside the shell.	They are an inexpensive source of protein.
Fish	Large fish are often contaminated with environmental pollutants such as PCBs, and toxic metals.	Fish is a lowfat source of high-quality protein. Consumption has been associated with a reduced risk of cardiovascular disease.
Raw fish and shellfish	These are a source of bacterial, viral, and parasitic infections.	Fish is a lowfat source of high-quality protein.
Fruits and vegetables	Some may contain pesticide residues.	They are an excellent source of fiber and vitamins in the diet. They also contain health-promoting phytochemicals.

After reviewing the risks and benefits of his family's diet, Rex realizes he can minimize the risk of hamburger and chicken by thoroughly cooking them, since *E. coli* and its toxins and *Salmonella* are destroyed by heat.

What other changes can he make to minimize the risks associated with his family's typical diet while including foods that are beneficial?

Answer:

SUMMARY

1. The safety of the food supply is affected by biological contamination as well as chemical toxins. To determine the types and amounts of contaminants that will be tolerated in the food supply, regulatory agencies must weigh the risks against the benefits. The harm caused by toxins in the food supply depends on the type of toxin, the dose, the length of time over which the dose is consumed, and the health status of the consumer.

2. The food supply is monitored for safety at the federal level by the FDA, the USDA, and the EPA. State and local governments are also responsible for monitoring some aspects of food safety. In addition, consumers play an important role in limiting their risks of developing food-borne illness.

3. The most common cause of food-borne illness is microbial contamination, which often produces acute gastrointestinal symptoms. Some bacteria cause food infections because when ingested they are able to grow in the gastrointestinal tract. Others produce toxins in food and cause food intoxications when the food is consumed. Some may do both. Viruses that contaminate foods such as shellfish can also cause food-borne illness, as can toxins produced by molds that grow on foods, and parasites contracted by consuming contaminated water or raw or undercooked meat or fish.

4. The risk of food-borne illness can be decreased by proper food selection, preparation, and storage. Consumers should choose the freshest meats and produce, select frozen foods that have been kept at constant temperatures, and avoid packages with broken seals. Canned foods should be discarded if the can is bulging or the contents appear deteriorated or foul smelling. Once in the home, foods should be cooked thoroughly and leftovers stored properly. Kitchen surfaces, hands, and cooking utensils should be cleaned between different preparation steps.

5. Environmental contaminants such as pesticides applied to crops, drugs given to animals, and industrial wastes that leach into the water supply may find their way into the food supply.

6. To decrease the potential risk, safer pesticides are being developed and American farmers are reducing pesticide usage by using organic methods and integrated pest management.

7. Industrial pollutants such as PCBs, radioactive substances, and toxic metals have contaminated some waterways and the fish that live in them.

8. Consumers can reduce the amounts of pesticides and other environmental contaminants in food by careful selection and handling. Choose fruits and vegetables produced with fewer pesticides. Select lowfat saltwater varieties of fish caught well offshore in unpolluted waters. Wash produce and trim fat from meat, poultry, and fish before cooking.

9. Food additives include all substances that can reasonably be expected to find their way into a food during processing. This includes direct food additives, which are used to preserve or enhance the appeal of food, and indirect food additives, which are substances known to find their way into food during cooking, processing, and packaging. Direct and indirect food additives are regulated by the FDA. Accidental contaminants that enter food when it is used or prepared incorrectly are not regulated by the FDA.

10. Food additives are used only if their benefits outweigh their risks. Substances on the GRAS list are exempt from being defined as food additives and must be proved unsafe by the FDA before their usage can be banned. All new food additives must be demonstrated safe by the manufacturer before they are approved for addition to foods. If a substance is found to induce cancer in humans or animals at any level, the Delaney Clause prohibits its use as a food additive.

11. Processing and packaging techniques are used to prevent food spoilage. Some rely on high or low temperatures to kill microbes or prevent their growth. Cooking heats food to kill microorganisms but can also produce carcinogens that are considered accidental contaminants. Packaging also preserves foods. Aseptic packaging sterilizes the food and the package; modified atmosphere packaging reduces the oxygen available for microbial growth. Some substances may migrate from packaging into foods.

12. Irradiation is a newer method of food preservation. It kills microorganisms, destroys insects, and slows the germination and ripening of fruits and vegetables by exposing food to x-rays, gamma radiation, or high-energy electrons.

13. New foods and products can be produced using biotechnology. These techniques alter the DNA of plants or animals to produce new varieties with desired traits, such as disease resistance.

SELF-TEST

1. What is a risk-benefit analysis?
2. List three factors that affect the toxicity of a substance.
3. What is the most common cause of food-borne illness in the United States?
4. List three common bacterial food contaminants. What can be done to avoid the food-borne illnesses caused by these?
5. What temperature range allows the most rapid bacterial growth?
6. What is the difference between a food-borne infection and a food-borne intoxication?
7. Why do canned foods present a risk for botulism poisoning?
8. How do pesticides applied to agricultural crops find their way into animal products?
9. List some ways in which food processing reduces food-borne illnesses.
10. What is the GRAS list?
11. What is the Delaney Clause?
12. List four reasons for using food additives.
13. What is genetic engineering?

APPLICATIONS

These exercises are designed to help you apply your critical thinking skills to your own nutrition choices.

1. Read the labels from food products in your cupboard or the store.
   a. List ten additives and the food product in which they are contained.
   b. Describe why each additive is used and what might happen in each case if the additive were not used in the product.

2. After 67 people became ill from consuming food at a company picnic, investigators determined that the tossed salad, the egg salad, and the turkey slices were all contaminated with *Salmonella*. Invent a scenario that would explain how all three became contaminated.

REFERENCES

1. Kurtzweil, P. HACCP patrolling for food hazards. FDA Consumer 29:5–10, Jan/Feb, 1995.
2. Pariza, M.W. Risk assessment. Crit. Rev. Food Sci. Nutr. 31:205–209, 1992.
3. *Healthy People 2000: National Health Promotion and Disease Prevention Objectives.* Washington, DC: U.S. Department of Health and Human Services, 1990.
4. Knabel, S.J. Institute of Food Technologists Scientific Status Summary. Foodborne illness: role of home food handling practices. Food Technol. 49:119–131, 1995.
5. Jay, J.M. Microbiological food safety. Crit. Rev. Food Sci. Nutr. 31:177–190, 1992.
6. Miller, R.W. Get hooked on seafood safety. FDA Consumer 25:7–11, June, 1991.
7. Mims, C.A., Playfair, J.H.L., Roitl, I.M., et al. *Medical Microbiology.* London: Mosby Europe Limited, 1993.
8. Schmidt, R.D. and Schmidt, T.W. Infant botulism: a case series and review of the literature. J. Emerg. Med. 10:713–718, 1992.
9. Kohn, M.A., Farley, T.A., Ando, T., et al. An outbreak of Norwalk virus gastroenteritis associated with eating raw oysters. Implications for maintaining safe oyster beds. J.A.M.A. 273:466–471, 1995.
10. McKerrow, J.H. and Sakanari, J. Revenge of the sushi parasite. N. Engl. J. Med. 319:1228, 1988.
11. Kurtzweil, P. Can your kitchen pass the food safety test? FDA Consumer 28:14–18, Oct, 1994.
12. Marwick, C. Disease pattern changes with food system. J.A.M.A. 264:2858–2859, 1990.
13. Mehler, L.N., O'Malley, M.A., and Krieger, R.I. Acute pesticide morbidity and mortality. California Rev. Environ. Contam. Toxicol. 129:51–66, 1992.
14. Foulke, J.E. FDA reports on pesticides in foods. FDA Consumer 27:29–32, June, 1993.
15. Hotchkiss, J.H. Pesticide residue controls to ensure food safety. Crit. Rev. Food Sci. Nutr. 31:191–203, 1992.
16. The Food and Drug Administration. *Residues in Foods: 1989.* Washington, DC: U.S. Government Printing Office, 1990.
17. Adler, T. Mothra meets its match—Researchers engineer insect-killing viruses. Science News 146:154–155, 1994.
18. Ames, B.N., Profet, M., and Gold, L.S. Nature's chemicals and synthetic chemicals: comparative toxicology. Proc. Natl. Acad. Sci. USA 87:7782–7786, 1990.
19. Seafood safety. Highlights of the Executive Summary of the 1991 Report by the Committee on Evaluation of the Safety of Fishery Products of the Food and Nutrition Board, Institute of Medicine, National Academy of Sciences. Nutr. Rev. 49:357–363, 1991.
20. Organically grown foods. A Scientific Status Summary by the Institute of Food Technologists' Expert Panel on Food Safety and Nutrition. Food Technol. 44:123–130, 1990.
21. Russell, L. Consumers face little danger from residues in meat and poultry. Food News 6:10–11, 1990.
22. Wright, K. The policy response: in limbo. Science 249:24, 1990.
23. Ropp, K.L. New animal drug increases milk production. FDA Consumer 28:24–27, May, 1994.
24. Clarkson, T.W. Environmental contaminants in the food chain. Am. J. Clin. Nutr. 61(suppl):682S–686S, 1995.
25. Committee on Environmental Health. American Academy of Pediatrics. PCBs in Breast Milk. Pediatrics 84:122–123, 1994.
26. Foulke, J.E. Mercury in fish. Cause for concern? FDA Consumer 28:5–8, Sept, 1994.
27. Bradbard, L. Seafood hotline responds to consumer needs. FDA Consumer 27:9–11, Sept, 1993.
28. Segal, M. Ingredient labeling. What's in a food? FDA Consumer 27:14–18, April, 1993.
29. Walker, R. Nitrates, nitrites and N-nitrosocompounds: a review of the occurrence in food and diet and the toxicologic implications. Food Addit. Contam. 7:717–768, 1990.
30. Parke, D.V. and Lewis, D.F. Safety aspects of food preservatives. Food Addit. Contam. 9:561–577, 1992.
31. Henkel, J. From shampoo to cereal. FDA Consumer 27:14–21, Dec, 1993.
32. Foulke, J. What happens if the packaging gets into the food? FDA Consumer 25:9–11, Nov, 1991.
33. Taylor, R. A loaf of bread, a jug of wine, and lead. J. NIH Res. 3:36–38, May, 1991.
34. American Dietetic Association. Position of the American Dietetic Association: Irradiated Foods. J. Am. Diet. Assoc. 96:69–72, 1996.
35. Genetically engineered foods: fears and facts. FDA Consumer 27:11–14, Jan/Feb, 1993.
36. Henkel, J. Genetic engineering fast forwarding to future foods. FDA Consumer, 29:6–11, April, 1995.
37. Peters, A.R. Improving food quality through new technology. Vet. Rec. 126:543–546, 1990.

The Global View: Feeding the World

CHAPTER CONCEPTS

1. The overnutrition that is prevalent in developed countries contrasts sharply with the undernutrition that is a problem in much of the developing world.

2. The world population is currently growing faster than our ability to produce food.

3. In areas where food and nutrients are limited, a cycle of malnutrition produces poorly nourished infants who are at risk for infection, illness, and early death. Those who survive grow to be unhealthy adults who are unable to reach their full potential.

4. Food shortages are caused by overpopulation, inequitable distribution of resources, and agricultural practices that damage the environment, limiting future production.

5. Poor-quality diets and increased needs in certain groups cause malnutrition even in populations with adequate food supplies.

6. Solutions to the problem of worldwide undernutrition include short-term programs to feed the hungry and long-term programs to balance population with resources, foster economic self-sufficiency among households and nations, and encourage sustainable agricultural practices to preserve the environment for future use.

7. In the United States, the majority of the population is at risk for overnutrition; but poverty, particularly among women and children, the homeless, and the elderly, creates pockets of undernutrition.

8. Solutions to hunger at home involve providing food, education, and medical care as well as controlling food production and cost.

9. Overnutrition, with the resulting increase in the incidence of chronic disease, is a growing international problem.

JUST A TASTE

Is there enough food to feed the world?

Is hunger a problem in the United States?

Can the food choices you make affect the environment?

J.A., and Shike, M., eds. Philadelphia: Lea & Febiger, 1994, pp. 252–263.

14. Sommer, A. Vitamin A: its effect on childhood sight and life. Nutr. Rev. 52:S60–S66, 1994.

15. Sloham, J. Emergency feeding programmes. Still not delivering the goods. Br. J. Med. 305:596–597, 1992.

16. Bongaarts, J. Population policy options in the developing world. Science 263:771–776, 1994.

17. Ghebremeskel, K. The state of food production and nutrition in the developing countries. Nutr. Health 6:121–128, 1989.

18. Viteri, F.E., Alvarez, E., Batres, R., et al. Fortification of sugar with iron sodium ethylenediaminotetraacetate (FeNaEDTA) improves iron status in semirural Guatemalan populations. Am. J. Clin. Nutr. 61:1153–1163, 1995.

19. Waibel, H. Government intervention in crop protection in developing countries. Ciba Found. Symp. 177:76–90, 1993.

20. Henkel, J. Genetic engineering fast forwarding to future foods. FDA Consumer, 29:6–11, April, 1995.

21. National Center for Health Statistics. Health, United States, 1989 and Prevention Profile. Hyattsville, MD: U.S. Department of Health and Human Services, 1990.

22. Mayer, J. Hunger and undernutrition in the United States. J. Nutr. 120:919–923, 1990.

23. Wegman, M.E. Annual summary of vital statistics—1993. Pediatrics 94:792–803, 1994.

24. National Center for Health Statistics. Health, United States, 1990 and Prevention Profile. Hyattsville, MD: U.S. Department of Health and Human Services, 1991.

25. Hunger and Homelessness. Washington, DC: U.S. Conference of Mayors, 1990.

26. Wolgemuth, J., Myers-Williams, C., Johnson, P., and Henseler, C. Wasting, malnutrition and inadequate nutrient intakes in a multiethnic homeless population. J. Am. Diet. Assoc. 92:834–839, 1992.

27. Wiecha, J.L., Dwyer, J.T., Jacques, P.F., and Rand, W.M. Nutritional and economic advantages for homeless families in shelters providing kitchen facilities and food. J. Am. Diet. Assoc. 93:777–783, 1993.

28. Taylor, M.L. and Oblinsky, S.A. Food consumption and eating behavior of homeless preschool children. J. Nutr. Ed. 26:20–25, 1994.

29. Chernoff, R. Baby boomers come of age: nutrition in the 21st century. J. Am. Diet. Assoc. 95:650–654, 1995.

30. Pollitt, E. Poverty and child development: relevance of research in developing countries to the United States. Child Dev. 65:283–295, 1994.

31. Poppendieck, J. Hunger and public policy lessons from the Great Depression. J. Nutr. Ed. 24(Suppl):6S–10S, 1992.

32. Hughes, M.A. Poverty in cities: a research report of the National League of Cities. Washington, DC: National League of Cities, 1989.

33. Abrams, B. Preventing low birth weight: does WIC work? A review of evaluations of the special supplemental food program for women, infants, and children. Ann. N.Y. Acad. Sci. 678:306–316, 1993.

34. Bleuscher, P., Larson, L., Nelson, M., and Lenihan, A. Prenatal WIC participation can reduce low birth weight and newborn medical costs: a cost–benefit analysis of WIC participation in North Carolina. J. Am. Diet. Assoc. 93:163–166, 1993.

35. Friedman, B.J. Urban and rural food agencies provide adequate nutrition to the hungry. J. Am. Diet. Assoc. 91:1589–1590, 1991.

36. Posner, B.M., Franz, M., Quatromoni, P., and the INTERHEALTH steering committee. Nutrition and the global risk for chronic diseases: The INTERHEALTH Nutrition Initiative. Nutr. Rev. 52:201–207, 1994.

37. Posner, B.M., Quatromoni, P.A., and Franz, M. Nutrition policies and interventions for chronic disease risk reduction in international settings: The INTERHEALTH Nutrition Initiative. Nutr. Rev. 52:179–187, 1994.

APPENDICES

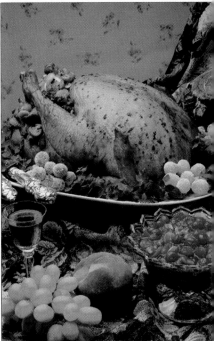

A
Nutrient Composition of Foods

B
Anthropometric Standards of Body Weight and Composition

C
Normal Blood Values of Nutritional Relevance

D
Sources of Information on Nutrition

E
Canadian Nutritional Recommendations and Guidelines

F
Nutrient Intake Recommendations
by the World Health Organization

G
Dietary Guidelines from Various Agencies and Countries

H
Healthy People 2000

I
Exchange Lists

J
Diet Planning Tools for Ethnic Diets

K
Food Labeling Information

L
Energy Expenditure for Various Activities

M
Answers to Critical Thinking Exercises

Appendix A
Nutrient Composition of Foods

EshaCode	Food Item	Qty	Meas	Wgt	Wtr	Cals	Prot	Carb	Fib	Fat	F_Sat
90095	Ac'cent flavor enhancer	.125	tsp	0	—	0	0	0	0	0	0
4639	Acorns, dried	2	oz.	57	5	289	5	30	1.9	18	2.3
5150	Alfalfa sprouts	1	cup	33	91	10	1	1	.8	0	0
57236	All Sport Drink, fruit punch	1.5	cup	360	—	933	53	67	5.3	51	26.7
26000	Allspice, ground	1	Tbs	6	8	16	0	4	1.3	1	.2
4567	Almond butter, honey and cinnamon	1	cup	250	2	1505	40	68	14.8	131	12.4
4572	Almond butter, plain, salted	1	cup	250	1	1582	38	53	14.8	148	14
4534	Almond butter, plain, unsalted	1	Tbs	16	1	101	2	3	.9	9	.9
15907	Almond chicken	1	cup	242	77	275	20	18	3.9	14	2
4657	Almond meal, partially defatted	2	oz.	57	7	231	22	16	5.6	10	1
4553	Almond paste, packed	.5	cup	114	16	508	14	50	16.9	31	2.9
4500	Almond, dried, unblanched, whole	1	cup	142	4	836	28	29	13.5	74	7.1
4549	Almond, dry roasted, unsalted, whole	1	cup	138	3	810	22	33	13.7	71	6.8
4548	Almonds, blanched, slices	1	cup	105	5	615	21	19	10.2	55	5.2
4547	Almonds, blanched, whole	1	cup	145	5	850	30	27	14.1	76	7.2
4727	Almonds, blanched, whole	1	cup	145	5	889	31	26	19	73	—
4501	Almonds, dried, unblanched, chopped	1	cup	130	4	766	26	26	12.4	68	6.5
4503	Almonds, dried, unblanched, slivered	1	cup	135	4	795	27	28	12.8	70	6.7
4571	Almonds, dry roasted, salted	1	cup	138	3	810	22	33	13.7	71	6.8
4730	Almonds, dry roasted, whole	1	cup	138	2	824	29	26	14.9	73	5.9
4732	Almonds, natural, whole	1	cup	142	4	851	29	28	17.5	72	5.1
4640	Almonds, oil roasted, blanched	1	cup	142	4	870	27	26	14.1	80	7.6
4620	Almonds, oil roasted, salted	1	cup	157	3	970	32	25	15.6	91	8.6
4505	Almonds, oil roasted, unsalted	1	cup	157	3	970	32	25	15.1	91	8.6
4729	Almonds, oil roasted, whole	1	cup	157	2	975	35	20	14.6	91	6.9
4566	Almonds, whole, toasted	1	oz.	28	3	167	6	6	2.8	14	1.4
5377	Amaranth leaves, cooked, drained	1	cup	132	92	28	3	5	2.3	0	.1
5375	Amaranth leaves, raw, chopped	1	cup	28	92	7	1	1	.4	0	0
38070	Amaranth, grain	1	cup	195	10	729	28	129	29.6	13	3.2
5376	Amaranth, raw leaf	1	each	14	92	4	0	1	.2	0	0
26106	Anise seed	1	Tbs	7	10	23	1	3	1	1	—
26484	Annatto seed	100	grams	100	10	360	13	68	36	4	—
49005	Apple brown betty	.75	cup	155	58	294	4	51	2.8	9	4.8
23000	Apple butter	2	Tbs	35	52	65	0	17	.5	0	0
49031	Apple crisp, recipe	.5	cup	141	62	230	3	46	—	5	1
45549	Apple dumpling	1	each	190	33	670	7	84	2.9	35	8.6
3008	Apple juice, canned/bottled	1	cup	248	88	117	0	29	.2	0	0
3010	Apple juice, prepared from frozen	1	cup	239	88	112	0	28	.2	0	0
3005	Apple rings, dried	10	each	64	32	156	1	42	5.6	0	0
3148	Apple slices, canned, sweetened	1	cup	204	82	137	0	34	3.5	1	.2

This table of food composition has been prepared for Saunders College Publishing and is copyrighted by ESHA Research in Salem, Oregon, developer and publisher of The Food Processor® and Genesis™ nutrition and labeling software systems. The table includes nutrient data for over 3900 foods, including brand-name items, ethnic foods, vegetarian products, nonfat and low-sodium alternatives, baby foods and formulas, and a large selection of common food items. The foods are presented alphabetically with corresponding units of measure. Over 1000 sources of scientific information are researched to provide the most accurate, reliable data available. Government sources of information are the base for all the data: the USDA Handbook series and its current supplemental data, as well as current data from both published and unpublished provisional data. Even with all the government data available, there are still missing values for some nutrients. Dashes in the table appear where there are no data available. Considerable effort has been made to report the most accurate data available and to eliminate missing values. The authors welcome any suggestions or comments for future editions.

Key: Esha Code = computer code for Esha Software; Wtr = water; Cals = kcalories; Prot = protein; Fib = fiber; F_Sat = saturated fat; FM_Un = monounsaturated fat; FP_Un = polyunsaturated fat; Choles = cholesterol; Calc = calcium; Phos = phosphorus; Pota = potassium; Magnes = magnesium; A_RE = vitamin A (RE); B1 = thiamin; B2 = riboflavin; B3 = niacin; Fola = folate.

FM_Un	FP_Un	Choles	Calc	Phos	Sodium	Pota	Zinc	Iron	Magnes	A_RE	Vit_C	B1	B2	B3	B6	Fola	B12
0	0	0	0	—	80	—	—	0	—	0	0	—	—	—	—	—	—
11.3	3.4	0	31	58	0	402	.4	.6	46	0	0	.08	.09	1.4	.39	65	0
0	.1	0	11	23	2	26	.3	.3	9	5	3	.02	.04	.2	.01	12	0
—	—	107	1066	—	1973	—	—	3.8	—	267	16	—	—	—	—	—	—
0	.1	0	40	7	5	63	.1	.4	8	3	2	.01	0	.2	—	—	0
84.8	27.5	0	668	1295	28	1875	7.5	9.2	750	0	2	.33	1.51	7.1	.19	161	0
96	31	0	68	1307	1125	1895	7.6	9.3	758	0	2	.33	1.53	7.2	.19	163	0
6.1	2	0	43	84	2	121	.5	.6	48	0	0	.02	.1	.5	.01	10	0
5.3	5.8	35	81	238	615	551	1.5	2	59	76	10	.08	.19	8.6	.42	32	.24
6.8	2.2	0	240	518	4	794	1.6	4.8	163	0	0	.18	.95	3.6	.06	32	0
20.2	6.5	0	262	508	10	738	3	3.6	295	0	1	.24	.84	3.3	.11	63	0
48.1	15.6	0	378	738	16	1039	4.2	5.2	420	0	1	.3	1.11	4.8	.16	83	0
46.2	14.9	0	389	756	15	1062	6.8	5.3	420	0	1	.18	.83	3.9	.1	88	0
35.8	11.6	0	259	559	10	788	3.3	3.8	300	0	1	.17	.71	3.3	.11	40	0
49.4	16	0	358	771	14	1087	4.6	5.3	415	0	1	.23	.98	4.6	.15	56	0
—	—	0	374	767	0	885	4.8	5.5	438	—	—	.22	.91	4.6	.16	55	—
44.1	14.3	0	346	676	14	952	3.8	4.8	385	0	1	.27	1.01	4.4	.15	76	0
45.8	14.9	0	359	702	15	988	4	5	400	0	1	.28	1.05	4.5	.15	79	0
46.2	14.9	0	389	756	1076	1062	6.8	5.3	420	0	1	.18	.83	3.9	.1	88	0
46.1	12.8	0	446	—	4	973	—	—	—	—	—	.06	1.97	3.1	—	61	—
44.9	16.5	0	—	—	—	—	—	—	—	—	—	.27	1.26	4.5	.16	62	—
52.1	16.9	0	275	819	17	984	2	7.5	412	0	1	.11	.4	5.5	.13	90	0
58.7	19	0	367	859	1223	1072	7.7	6	477	0	1	.2	1.55	5.5	.13	100	0
58.7	19	0	367	859	16	1072	7.7	6	477	0	1	.2	1.55	5.5	.13	100	0
52.6	21.5	0	482	785	0	929	4.9	6	403	—	—	.16	1.73	5.5	—	47	—
9.4	3	0	80	156	3	219	1.4	1.4	86	0	0	.04	.17	.8	.02	18	0
.1	.1	0	276	95	28	846	1.2	3	73	366	54	.03	.18	.7	.23	75	0
0	0	0	61	14	6	174	.3	.7	16	83	12	.01	.04	.2	.06	24	0
2.8	5.6	0	298	887	41	714	6.2	14.8	519	0	8	.16	.41	2.5	.44	96	0
0	0	0	30	7	3	86	.1	.3	8	41	6	0	.02	.1	.03	12	0
.7	.2	0	43	30	1	96	.4	2.5	11	—	—	—	—	—	—	—	0
—	—	—	180	—	15	—	—	32.5	—	—	3	—	—	—	—	—	—
2.6	.8	18	77	54	329	164	.4	2.1	17	68	0	.25	.15	2.1	.08	8	.02
0	.1	0	2	2	0	32	0	0	1	0	1	0	0	0	.01	0	0
2.2	1.5	0	40	35	257	137	.2	1.1	10	44	3	.12	.1	1.1	.06	7	—
15.2	9.2	0	14	75	607	129	.5	3.1	16	10	2	.39	.3	3.5	.05	11	0
0	.1	0	17	17	7	295	.1	.9	7	0	2	.05	.04	.2	.07	0	0
0	.1	0	14	17	17	301	.1	.6	12	0	1	.01	.04	.1	.08	1	0
0	.1	0	9	24	56	288	.1	.9	10	6	2	0	.1	.6	.08	0	0
0	.3	0	8	10	6	139	.1	.5	4	10	1	.02	.02	.1	.09	1	0

EshaCode	Food Item	Qty	Meas	Wgt	Wtr	Cals	Prot	Carb	Fib	Fat	F_Sat
3149	Apple slices, frozen, heated	1	cup	206	87	97	1	25	3.5	1	.1
3009	Apple slices, peeled, cooked	1	cup	170	85	95	0	24	4.8	1	.1
49015	Apple strudel	1	each	71	44	195	2	29	1.6	8	2.1
45550	Apple turnover	1	each	82	33	289	3	36	1.2	15	3.7
3308	Apple, baked, unsweetened	1	each	161	83	102	0	26	3.8	1	.1
3145	Apple, dried, cooked w/o sugar	.5	cup	128	84	73	0	20	2.6	0	0
3146	Apple, dried, cooked w/sugar	.5	cup	140	79	116	0	29	2.6	0	0
3003	Apple, no peel	1	each	128	84	73	0	19	2.4	0	.1
3004	Apple, peeled slices	1	cup	110	84	63	0	16	2.1	0	.1
3000	Apple, w/peel	1	each	138	84	81	0	21	2.7	0	.1
3002	Apple, w/peel, slices	1	cup	110	84	65	0	17	2.2	0	.1
3147	Applesauce, canned, sweetened	1	cup	255	80	194	0	51	3.1	0	.1
3006	Applesauce, unsweetened	1	cup	244	88	105	0	28	2.9	0	0
3332	Apricot halves w/skin, canned in water	3	each	84	92	23	1	5	1.1	0	0
3217	Apricot halves, dried, cooked	1	cup	250	76	213	3	55	8.5	0	0
3013	Apricot halves, dried, sulfured	10	each	35	31	83	1	22	2.7	0	0
3015	Apricot nectar, canned	1	cup	251	85	141	1	36	1.5	0	0
3218	Apricot nectar, canned, vitamin C added	1	cup	251	85	141	1	36	1.5	0	0
3157	Apricot, pitted, fresh	3	each	106	86	51	1	12	1.9	0	0
3011	Apricot, w/skin, canned in heavy syrup	1	cup	258	78	214	1	56	3	0	0
3153	Apricot, w/skin, canned in light syrup	1	cup	253	83	159	1	42	2.7	0	0
3151	Apricot, w/skin, canned w/juice	1	cup	248	87	119	2	30	2.9	0	0
3155	Apricots, frozen, sweetened	1	cup	242	73	237	2	61	4.1	0	0
3156	Apricots, halves, fresh	1	cup	155	86	74	2	17	2.8	1	0
3333	Apricots, peeled, canned in water	2	each	90	93	20	1	5	1.1	0	0
56335	Arby's Bac'n cheddar sandwich, deluxe	1	each	231	59	512	21	39	.3	32	8.7
69055	Arby's Philly beef'n swiss sandwich	1	each	197	53	467	24	38	—	25	9.7
69045	Arby's Q sandwich	1	each	190	55	190	18	48	—	15	5.5
69046	Arby's chicken sandwich, grilled, deluxe	1	each	230	62	430	24	42	—	20	3.5
56337	Arby's roast beef sandwich, Junior	1	each	89	48	233	12	23	.5	11	4.1
56336	Arby's roast beef sandwich, regular	1	each	155	47	383	22	35	1.1	18	7
69051	Arby's sandwich, light roast beef, deluxe	1	each	182	65	294	18	33	—	10	3.5
69052	Arby's sandwich, light roast chicken, deluxe	1	each	195	66	276	24	33	—	7	1.7
53256	Arby's sauce	.5	oz.	14	69	15	0	3	—	0	0
69048	Arby's sub sandwich, Italian	1	each	297	—	671	34	47	—	39	12.8
69049	Arby's sub sandwich, roast beef	1	each	305	60	623	38	47	—	32	11.5
69050	Arby's sub sandwich, tuna	1	each	284	42	663	74	50	—	37	8.2
69044	Arby's sub sandwich, turkey	1	each	277	62	486	33	46	—	19	5.3
57015	Arby's, Cheddar fries	5	oz.	142	45	399	6	46	—	22	9
69056	Arby's, Steak'n cheddar sandwich	1	each	194	34	508	25	43	—	26	7.7
6432	Arby's, curly fries	3.5	oz.	100	31	340	4	44	—	18	7.5
69042	Arby's, roast chicken club sandwich	1	each	238	60	503	30	37	—	27	6.9
5191	Artichoke heart, marinated	6	oz.	170	59	168	4	13	7.5	14	2
5360	Artichoke heart, raw	.5	cup	84	86	37	2	9	5	0	0
6493	Artichoke heart, raw	.595	cup	100	86	44	2	10	5.9	0	0
5077	Artichoke, Jerusalem, raw, freshly harvested	1	cup	150	78	114	3	26	2.4	0	0
5192	Artichoke, frozen, cooked	9	oz.	240	86	108	7	22	12.6	1	.3
5000	Artichoke, globe, cooked	1	each	120	84	60	4	13	6.5	0	0
6032	Arugula leaf, raw	5	each	10	92	2	0	0	—	0	—
6033	Arugula, chopped, raw	.5	cup	10	92	2	0	0	—	0	—
5362	Asparagus pieces, canned, w/liquid	.5	cup	122	95	17	2	3	2.1	0	.1
5645	Asparagus pieces, steamed	1	cup	180	92	41	4	8	3.8	0	.1
5646	Asparagus pieces, stir fried, no oil	1	cup	180	92	41	4	8	3.8	0	.1
5007	Asparagus spears, canned, drained	4	each	80	94	15	2	2	1.3	1	.1
5245	Asparagus spears, canned, not drained, low sodium	4	each	80	95	11	1	2	1.4	0	0
5363	Asparagus spears, canned, w/liquid	4	each	80	95	11	1	2	1.4	0	0
5004	Asparagus spears, cooked, unsalted	4	each	60	92	14	2	3	1.2	0	0
5006	Asparagus spears, frozen, cooked	4	each	60	91	17	2	3	1.2	0	.1
5842	Asparagus, canned w/liquid, low sodium	.5	cup	122	95	17	2	3	1.8	0	.1
5361	Asparagus, frozen, uncooked spears	4	each	58	92	14	2	2	1.2	0	0
5002	Asparagus, raw spears	4	each	58	92	13	1	3	1.2	0	0
42454	Aunt Anne's pretzel, original, soft	1	each	138	—	390	12	84	3	1	0
42456	Aunt Anne's pretzel, whole wheat, soft	1	each	140	—	390	13	82	8	2	0
3018	Avocado cubes	1	cup	150	74	242	3	11	6.2	23	3.7
3019	Avocado slices	1	piece	10	74	16	0	1	.4	2	.2

FM_Un	FP_Un	Choles	Calc	Phos	Sodium	Pota	Zinc	Iron	Magnes	A_RE	Vit_C	B1	B2	B3	B6	Fola	B12
0	.2	0	10	16	6	157	.1	.4	6	4	1	.03	.02	.1	.07	1	0
0	.2	0	8	14	2	158	.1	.3	5	7	1	.03	.02	.1	.08	1	0
4.4	1	20	11	23	191	69	.1	.3	6	6	1	.03	.02	.2	.02	4	.11
6.6	4	0	6	32	262	56	.2	1.3	7	4	1	.17	.13	1.5	.02	5	0
0	.2	0	12	12	0	179	.1	.3	9	7	8	.02	.02	.1	.08	3	0
0	0	0	4	12	26	134	.1	.4	5	2	1	.01	.02	.2	.06	0	0
0	0	0	4	11	27	137	.1	.4	4	2	1	.01	.02	.2	.07	0	0
0	.1	0	5	9	0	145	.1	.1	4	6	5	.02	.01	.1	.06	1	0
0	.1	0	4	8	0	124	0	.1	3	5	4	.02	.01	.1	.05	0	0
0	.1	0	10	10	0	159	.1	.2	7	7	8	.02	.02	.1	.07	4	0
0	.1	0	8	8	0	127	0	.2	6	6	6	.02	.02	.1	.05	3	0
0	.1	0	10	18	8	156	.1	.9	8	3	4	.03	.07	.5	.07	2	0
0	0	0	7	17	5	183	.1	.3	7	7	3	.03	.06	.5	.06	1	0
.1	0	0	7	11	3	161	.1	.3	6	108	3	.02	.02	.3	.04	1	0
.2	.1	0	40	103	8	1222	.6	4.2	42	590	4	.02	.08	2.4	.28	0	0
.1	0	0	16	41	4	482	.3	1.6	16	253	1	0	.05	1	.06	4	0
.1	0	0	18	23	8	286	.2	1	13	331	2	.02	.04	.7	.06	3	0
.1	0	0	18	23	8	286	.2	1	13	331	137	.02	.04	.7	.06	3	0
.2	.1	0	15	20	1	314	.3	.6	8	277	11	.03	.04	.6	.06	9	0
.1	0	0	23	31	10	361	.3	.8	18	317	8	.05	.06	1	.14	4	0
.1	0	0	28	33	10	349	.3	1	20	334	7	.04	.05	.8	.14	4	0
0	0	0	30	50	10	409	.3	.7	25	419	12	.04	.05	.9	.13	4	0
.1	0	0	24	46	10	554	.2	2.2	22	407	22	.05	.1	1.9	.14	4	0
.3	.1	0	22	30	2	459	.4	.8	12	405	16	.05	.06	.9	.08	13	0
0	0	0	7	14	10	139	.1	.5	8	163	2	.02	.02	.4	.05	2	0
12.7	10.1	38	110	—	1094	491	3	4.3	—	40	11	.34	.46	9.6	—	—	—
10.7	5.1	53	290	—	1144	409	3.8	4.1	—	100	19	.28	.46	8.8	—	—	—
6.4	3.5	29	70	—	1268	456	—	9.2	—	—	—	.27	.39	9.2	—	—	—
5.1	4.4	44	70	—	901	659	—	2.5	—	80	8	.32	.29	13.6	—	—	—
5.2	2.5	22	40	60	519	201	1.5	2.7	8	—	—	.18	.26	6.6	.1	7	—
8	3.5	43	60	120	936	422	3.8	4.9	16	1	1	.28	.48	11	.2	14	—
4.7	2.1	42	130	—	826	392	—	4.5	—	40	8	.27	.49	8.4	—	—	—
2.9	2.5	33	130	—	326	392	—	2.9	—	40	7	.44	.75	9.4	—	—	—
.1	.1	0	—	—	115	28	—	.4	—	—	—	—	—	—	—	—	—
15.7	8.5	69	410	—	2062	565	—	4.3	—	100	11	.92	.49	8.2	—	—	—
13	6.8	73	410	—	1847	708	—	7.7	—	100	9	.56	.71	10.1	—	—	—
11.8	17	43	410	—	1847	708	—	7.7	—	100	9	.56	.71	14.2	—	—	—
6	7	51	400	—	2033	500	—	4.7	—	—	—	13.2	.54	18.8	—	—	—
10	1.7	9	80	—	443	742	.9	1.4	—	—	—	.06	.14	2	—	—	—
12	6.8	52	150	—	1166	321	3	6.1	—	—	1	.42	.63	9.8	—	—	—
7.7	1.5	0	20	—	169	731	.6	1.4	—	—	—	.06	.07	2	—	—	—
9.8	10.4	46	180	—	1143	534	2.2	2.9	—	—	8	.51	.71	10.6	—	—	—
3	7.7	0	39	102	899	439	.5	1.6	48	28	52	.06	.17	1.4	.15	149	0
0	.1	0	33	50	55	221	.3	1.1	33	12	6	.05	.04	.5	.07	37	0
0	.1	0	39	60	66	263	.3	1.4	39	14	7	.06	.05	.6	.09	44	0
0	0	0	21	117	6	644	.2	5.1	26	3	6	.3	.09	2	.12	20	0
0	.5	0	50	146	127	634	.9	1.3	74	39	12	.15	.38	2.2	.21	286	0
0	.1	0	54	103	114	425	.6	1.6	72	21	12	.08	.08	1.2	.13	61	0
—	—	0	16	5	3	37	0	.1	5	24	2	0	.01	0	.01	10	0
—	—	0	16	5	3	37	0	.1	5	24	2	0	.01	0	.01	10	0
0	.1	0	17	46	425	187	.6	.7	11	58	20	.07	.11	1	.12	104	0
0	.2	0	38	101	4	491	.8	1.6	32	100	20	.23	.22	2	.21	194	0
0	.2	0	38	101	4	491	.8	1.6	32	94	20	.23	.22	2	.22	184	0
0	.2	0	13	34	312	138	.3	1.5	8	42	15	.05	.08	.8	.09	76	0
0	.1	0	11	30	3	122	.4	.5	7	38	13	.04	.07	.7	.08	68	0
0	.1	0	11	30	278	122	.4	.5	7	38	13	.04	.07	.7	.08	68	0
0	.1	0	12	32	7	96	.3	.4	6	32	6	.07	.08	.6	.07	88	0
0	.1	0	14	33	2	131	.3	.4	8	49	15	.04	.06	.6	.01	81	0
0	.1	0	17	46	5	187	.6	.7	11	58	20	.07	.11	1	.12	104	0
0	.1	0	14	37	5	147	.3	.4	8	55	18	.07	.08	.7	.06	111	0
0	.1	0	12	32	1	158	.3	.5	10	34	8	.08	.07	.7	.08	74	0
—	—	0	40	—	1100	—	—	2.7	—	0	—	—	—	—	—	—	—
—	—	0	40	—	1290	—	—	2.7	—	0	—	—	—	—	—	—	—
14.4	2.9	0	16	62	15	899	.6	1.6	58	92	12	.16	.18	2.9	.42	93	0
1	.2	0	1	4	1	60	0	.1	4	6	1	.01	.01	.2	.03	6	0

EshaCode	Food Item	Qty.	Meas	Wgt	Wtr	Cals	Prot	Carb	Fib	Fat	F_Sat
3210	Avocado, California	1	each	173	73	306	4	12	5.9	30	4.5
3211	Avocado, California, mashed	.5	cup	115	73	204	2	8	3.9	20	3
3212	Avocado, Florida	1	each	304	80	340	5	27	7.7	27	5.4
3213	Avocado, Florida, mashed	.5	cup	115	80	129	2	10	2.9	10	2
3016	Avocado, average	1	each	201	74	324	4	15	8.2	31	4.9
60754	Baby Food, bananas, strained, Heinz	1	Tbs	16	74	16	0	4	.3	0	0
60763	Baby Food, beef dinner supreme, stage 2, Beech-nut	1	each	128	83	147	2	9	1.1	10	—
60769	Baby Food, beef stew, toddler	1	Tbs	14	87	7	1	1	.2	0	.1
60765	Baby Food, carrots, stage 1, Beech-nut	1	oz.	28	91	12	0	2	1	0	0
60759	Baby Food, cereal, mixed, w/formula	1	Tbs	18	76	22	1	3	—	1	—
60761	Baby Food, cereal, rice w/fruit, Gerber	1	Tbs	14	80	11	0	3	.1	0	—
60757	Baby Food, chicken w/broth, stage 1, jar, Beech-nut	1	each	71	83	70	8	0	0	3	—
60758	Baby Food, chicken-rice dinner, stage 2, Beech-nut	4	oz.	113	88	80	1	9	1	3	—
60755	Baby Food, peaches, strained, Heinz	1	Tbs	16	80	12	0	3	.4	0	0
60762	Baby Food, pudding, cherry vanilla, Gerber	1	Tbs	14	83	10	0	2	0	0	—
60770	Baby Food, spaghetti w/meat sauce, toddler	1	Tbs	14	82	11	1	2	—	0	—
60766	Baby Food, sweet potatoes, stage 3, jar, Beech-nut	1	each	170	87	110	1	25	1	0	0
60756	Baby Food, tropical fruit medley, Gerber	1	Tbs	14	84	9	0	2	0	0	—
60764	Baby Food, turkey sticks, Gerber	1	each	10	76	13	1	0	0	1	.3
60760	Baby Formula, Enfamil w/iron, 24cal/oz, Mead Johnson	1	cup	247	86	192	4	20	—	11	5
60767	Baby Formula, Prosobee, RTS, 20cal/oz, Mead Johnson	1	cup	246	87	160	5	16	0	8	4.6
60768	Baby Formula, similac, liquid, 27cal/oz, Ross Labs	.46	cup	114	83	100	3	10	0	5	2.3
12002	Bacon, Canadian style, grilled	2	piece	47	62	87	11	1	0	4	1.3
12000	Bacon, cooked, regular	3	piece	19	13	109	6	0	0	9	3.3
44061	Bagel chips	5	piece	70	3	298	6	52	5.6	7	1.2
42092	Bagel, 100% whole wheat	1	each	55	28	145	6	31	5.4	1	.1
42100	Bagel, cinnamon raisin	1	each	71	32	195	7	39	1.9	1	.2
42101	Bagel, cinnamon raisin, toasted	1	each	66	27	194	7	39	1.9	1	.2
42041	Bagel, egg	1	each	71	33	197	8	38	1.6	1	.3
42102	Bagel, egg, toasted	1	each	66	28	197	8	38	1.5	1	.3
42103	Bagel, oat bran	1	each	71	33	181	8	38	8.1	1	.1
42104	Bagel, oat bran, toasted	1	each	66	28	181	8	38	8.1	1	.1
42000	Bagel, plain	1	each	68	33	187	7	36	1.5	1	.2
42099	Bagel, plain, toasted	1	each	66	28	195	7	38	1.6	1	.2
23119	Baking chips, butterscotch	1	cup	170	1	884	4	114	0	50	40.8
23120	Baking chips, peanut butter	1	cup	170	6	845	31	76	1.7	51	22.3
23121	Baking chips, white chocolate	1	cup	170	1	906	10	104	0	52	30.3
23180	Baking chocolate, bar, semi-sweet, Nestle	1	oz.	28	1	142	2	18	4	8	5.1
23179	Baking chocolate, bar, unsweetened	1	oz.	28	0	160	4	9	6	14	3.9
23179	Baking chocolate, bar, unsweetened, Nestle	1	oz.	28	0	162	4	9	6.1	14	4
28208	Baking chocolate, unsweetened, liquid, pkt	1	each	28	1	134	3	10	—	14	7.2
23178	Baking chocolate, unsweetened, premelted, ChocoBake	1	oz.	28	4	162	0	10	6.1	16	10.2
28059	Baking mix, reduced fat, Bisquick	.33	cup	40	—	150	3	28	.5	2	.5
28004	Baking powder, double acting, Calumet	1	tsp	5	5	2	0	1	0	0	0
28005	Baking powder, double acting, Rumford	1	tsp	5	4	2	0	1	0	0	0
28006	Baking powder, low sodium	1	tsp	4	6	4	0	2	0	0	0
28003	Baking soda/sodium bicarbonate	1	tsp	5	0	0	0	0	0	0	0
45516	Baklava	1	piece	78	25	333	5	29	1.6	23	9.3
5403	Balsam pear, leaftips, cooked	.5	cup	29	89	10	1	2	.6	0	—
5405	Balsam pear, pods, cooked	1	cup	124	94	24	1	5	2.5	0	—
5401	Bamboo shoot, sliced, canned	1	cup	131	94	25	2	4	3.5	1	.1
5230	Bamboo shoot, sliced, raw	1	cup	151	91	41	4	8	3.3	0	.1
5249	Bamboo shoots, cooked slices	1	cup	120	96	14	2	2	1.2	0	.1
5250	Bamboo shoots, cooked, whole	1	each	144	96	17	2	3	1.4	0	.1
3020	Banana	1	each	114	74	105	1	27	2.3	1	.2
3307	Banana chips, fried	1	cup	92	4	477	2	54	7.1	31	26.7
3325	Banana nectar	1	cup	250	81	177	1	46	1.4	0	.2
3021	Banana slices	1	cup	150	74	138	2	35	3	1	.3
2070	Banana split w/whipped cream	1	each	425	52	1076	15	120	1.2	66	37.9
23113	Banana, chocolate-covered, w/nuts	1	each	145	51	336	7	43	4.6	19	7
3023	Banana, dehydrated	1	cup	100	3	346	4	88	7.7	2	.7
3306	Banana, ripe, fried	1	each	91	60	184	1	24	1.6	11	2.2
38003	Barley, pearled, cooked	1	cup	157	69	193	4	44	7.8	1	.1
38002	Barley, pearled, dry	1	cup	200	10	704	20	155	27.4	2	.5
38001	Barley, whole, cooked	1	cup	200	65	270	7	59	13.6	2	.4

FM_Un	FP_Un	Choles	Calc	Phos	Sodium	Pota	Zinc	Iron	Magnes	A_RE	Vit_C	B1	B2	B3	B6	Fola	B12
19.4	3.5	0	19	73	21	1096	.7	2.1	71	106	14	.19	.21	3.3	.48	113	0
12.9	2.4	0	13	48	14	729	.5	1.4	47	70	9	.12	.14	2.2	.32	75	0
14.8	4.5	0	33	119	15	1483	1.3	1.6	103	185	24	.33	.37	5.8	.85	162	0
5.6	1.7	0	13	45	6	561	.5	.6	39	70	9	.12	.14	2.2	.32	61	0
19.3	3.9	0	22	82	20	1203	.8	2.1	78	123	16	.22	.24	3.9	.56	124	0
—	—	—	1	3	0	52	0	.1	—	2	6	0	.02	.1	.04	—	—
—	—	—	27	—	51	192	—	.3	—	813	0	.01	.06	1	—	—	—
.1	0	2	1	6	49	20	.1	.1	2	33	0	0	.01	.2	.01	1	.07
0	0	—	6	—	25	40	—	0	—	300	0	0	0	.1	—	—	—
—	—	—	7	—	3	—	—	.9	—	7	1	.02	.02	.3	.04	—	—
—	—	—	2	3	1	7	.1	.4	1	0	1	.02	.02	.3	.02	—	—
—	—	—	12	—	55	120	—	.6	—	—	0	.02	.08	1.2	—	—	—
—	—	—	36	—	70	115	—	.6	—	1260	0	.02	.03	.6	—	—	—
—	—	—	1	1	0	34	0	.1	—	16	10	0	.01	.2	0	—	—
—	—	—	1	1	1	6	—	0	0	0	0	0	0	0	0	—	—
—	—	—	3	6	51	23	.1	.1	2	12	1	.01	.01	.2	.01	1	.03
0	0	—	12	—	15	360	—	.3	—	855	0	.03	.04	.5	—	—	—
—	—	—	1	0	1	6	—	0	1	4	2	0	0	0	.01	—	—
—	—	9	10	13	43	12	.2	.1	1	0	0	0	.02	.2	.01	—	—
2.6	3.1	3	132	90	52	207	1.5	3.6	15	180	16	.15	.3	2.4	.12	30	.45
1.2	2.3	0	150	119	58	195	1.2	3	18	150	13	.12	.15	2	.1	25	.5
.9	1.9	2	90	70	34	132	.8	.2	7	60	9	.1	.15	1	.06	15	.25
1.9	.4	27	5	139	727	183	.8	.4	10	0	10	.39	.09	3.2	.21	2	.37
4.5	1.1	16	2	64	303	92	.6	.3	5	0	6	.13	.05	1.4	.05	1	.33
2	3.4	0	9	145	419	167	.9	1.4	41	0	0	.13	.12	1.6	.19	58	0
.1	.3	0	16	159	270	190	1.3	1.8	59	0	0	.17	.14	2.8	.18	40	0
.1	.5	0	14	55	229	108	.5	2.7	15	6	0	.27	.2	2	.04	15	0
.1	.5	0	13	55	228	108	.5	2.7	15	5	0	.22	.18	2	.04	11	0
.3	.5	17	9	60	359	48	.5	2.8	18	23	0	.38	.17	2.4	.06	16	.11
.3	.5	17	9	59	358	48	.5	2.8	18	21	0	.3	.15	2.2	.06	11	.11
.2	.3	0	9	117	360	145	1.5	2.2	40	0	0	.24	.24	2.1	.14	33	0
.2	.3	0	9	117	360	145	1.5	2.2	41	0	0	.19	.22	1.9	.13	23	0
.1	.5	0	50	65	363	69	.6	2.4	20	0	0	.37	.21	3.1	.04	15	0
.1	.5	0	53	68	379	72	.6	2.5	20	0	0	.31	.2	2.9	.03	11	0
5.8	.8	2	58	44	160	318	.2	.1	5	0	0	.14	0	.1	.02	3	.19
16.3	9.1	0	187	527	425	859	3.4	2.9	187	3	0	.08	.34	13.9	.38	162	.1
16.3	1.4	37	350	321	151	519	1.5	.3	7	109	1	.08	.48	.3	.09	26	1.28
—	—	0	0	—	0	109	—	.7	—	0	0	.02	0	.2	—	—	—
5.2	.7	0	0	—	0	236	—	0	—	0	0	.03	.04	.4	—	—	—
5.2	.7	0	0	—	0	239	—	0	—	0	0	.03	.04	.4	—	—	—
2.6	3	0	15	96	3	331	1	1.2	75	1	0	.01	.04	.6	.02	2	0
—	—	0	0	—	0	—	—	1.5	—	0	0	.04	.04	.4	—	—	—
—	—	0	40	—	460	30	—	1.4	—	—	—	.15	.1	1.6	—	—	—
0	0	0	270	101	488	1	0	.5	1	0	0	0	0	0	0	0	0
0	0	0	339	456	363	0	0	.5	2	0	0	0	0	0	0	0	0
0	0	0	186	295	4	434	0	.4	1	0	0	0	0	0	0	0	0
0	0	0	0	0	1258	0	0	0	0	0	0	0	0	0	0	0	0
8.5	3.8	36	34	88	291	139	.5	1.7	34	124	1	.17	.13	1.3	.05	9	.02
—	—	0	12	22	4	175	.1	.3	27	50	16	.04	.08	.3	.22	25	0
—	—	0	11	45	7	396	1	.5	20	14	41	.06	.07	.3	.05	63	0
.1	.2	0	10	33	9	105	.9	.4	5	1	1	.03	.03	.2	.18	4	0
0	.2	0	20	89	6	805	1.7	.8	5	3	6	.23	.11	.9	.36	11	0
0	.1	0	14	24	5	640	.6	.3	4	0	0	.02	.06	.4	.12	3	0
0	.1	0	17	29	6	768	.7	.3	4	0	0	.03	.07	.4	.14	3	0
0	.1	0	7	23	1	451	.2	.4	33	9	10	.05	.11	.6	.66	22	0
1.8	.6	0	17	52	6	493	.7	1.2	70	7	6	.08	.02	.7	.24	13	0
0	.1	0	8	18	5	347	.2	.3	27	7	8	.04	.09	.5	.5	17	0
.1	.1	0	9	30	2	594	.2	.5	44	12	14	.07	.15	.8	.87	29	0
18.8	5	209	468	477	354	779	2.7	1.5	89	545	2	.15	.9	.5	.17	19	1.41
7.5	3.2	0	28	153	7	596	1.8	1.4	93	8	9	.1	.19	3.3	.63	42	0
.2	.3	0	22	74	3	1491	.6	1.2	108	30	7	.18	.24	2.8	.54	40	0
4.6	3.3	0	10	23	120	366	.2	.3	30	142	6	.04	.1	.5	.53	10	.01
.1	.3	0	17	85	5	146	1.3	2.1	34	2	0	.13	.1	3.2	.18	25	0
.3	1.1	0	58	442	18	560	4.3	5	158	4	0	.38	.23	9.2	.52	46	0
.3	1.2	0	26	230	1	230	1.6	2.1	44	0	0	.16	.05	2.8	.19	16	0

EshaCode	Food Item	Qty.	Meas	Wgt	Wtr	Cals	Prot	Carb	Fib	Fat	F_Sat
38000	Barley, whole, dry	1	cup	184	9	651	23	135	31.8	4	.9
26001	Basil, dried	1	Tbs	4	6	11	1	3	.8	0	—
26046	Basil, fresh leaves	5	each	2	91	1	0	0	.1	0	0
26045	Basil, fresh, chopped	2	Tbs	5	91	1	0	0	.1	0	0
26107	Bay leaf, crumbled	1	Tbs	2	5	6	0	1	.5	0	0
7084	Bean cake, Japanese style	1	each	32	23	130	2	16	.9	7	1
7167	Bean paste, sweetened	100	grams	100	45	211	6	48	5.2	0	.1
5197	Bean sprouts, mung, canned, drained	1	cup	125	96	15	2	3	1	0	0
5021	Bean sprouts, mung, cooked, drained	1	cup	124	93	26	3	5	1	0	0
5020	Bean sprouts, mung, raw	1	cup	104	90	31	3	6	1.9	0	0
5246	Bean sprouts, mung, stir fried	1	cup	124	84	62	5	13	4.2	0	0
5240	Bean, Italian green, canned, drained, low sodium	1	cup	240	93	48	3	11	3.1	0	.1
7031	Bean, winged/goabean, dry, cooked	1	cup	172	67	253	18	26	4.2	10	1.4
7000	Beans Garbanzo/Chickpeas, dry	1	cup	200	12	728	39	121	24	12	1.2
7035	Beans, Adzuki, canned, sweetened	.5	cup	145	41	344	6	80	4.2	0	0
7034	Beans, Adzuki, cooked	.5	cup	115	66	147	9	28	1	0	0
57054	Beans, B & M baked, fat free	.5	cup	130	—	160	8	31	7	1	0
7001	Beans, Garbanzo/chickpea, cooked from dry	1	cup	164	60	269	14	45	8	4	.4
5232	Beans, Italian green, canned, not drained, low sodium	1	cup	240	94	36	2	8	1.9	0	.1
7022	Beans, Navy, dry, cooked	1	cup	182	63	258	16	48	16	1	.3
7038	Beans, baked, canned, vegetarian	.5	cup	127	73	118	6	26	6.4	1	.1
7040	Beans, baked, canned, w/pork	.5	cup	126	72	134	7	25	6.9	2	.8
7037	Beans, baked, home prepared	.5	cup	126	65	190	7	27	6.9	6	2.5
7085	Beans, baked, low sodium	1	cup	253	73	235	12	52	13.9	1	.3
7042	Beans, black turtle soup, canned w/liquid	.5	cup	120	76	109	7	20	4.3	0	.1
7041	Beans, black turtle soup, cooked	.5	cup	92	66	120	8	22	4.9	0	.1
7012	Beans, black, dry, cooked, no added salt	1	cup	172	66	227	15	41	15	1	.2
7027	Beans, broadbean/fava dry, cooked	1	cup	170	72	187	13	34	8.6	1	.1
7055	Beans, broadbean/fava, canned w/liquid	.5	cup	128	80	91	7	16	4.5	0	0
7043	Beans, cranberry, cooked	.5	cup	88	65	120	8	22	7.1	0	.1
7045	Beans, french, cooked	.5	cup	86	67	111	6	21	3.2	1	.1
7088	Beans, garbanzo/chickpeas, canned w/liquid	.5	cup	120	70	143	6	27	4.6	1	.1
7021	Beans, great northern, dry, cooked	1	cup	177	69	209	15	37	9.9	1	.2
5016	Beans, green, Italian, canned, drained	1	cup	135	93	27	2	6	2.6	0	0
5017	Beans, green, Italian, canned, not drained	1	cup	240	94	36	2	8	1.7	0	.1
5012	Beans, green, Italian, cooked	1	cup	125	89	44	2	10	4	0	.1
5014	Beans, green, Italian, frozen, cooked, drained	1	cup	135	92	35	2	8	4.5	0	0
5010	Beans, green, Italian, raw	1	cup	110	90	34	2	8	3.7	0	0
5239	Beans, green, canned, drained, low sodium	1	cup	135	93	27	2	6	1.8	0	0
5231	Beans, green, canned, not drained, low sodium	1	cup	240	94	36	2	8	1.9	0	.1
5571	Beans, green, seasoned, canned	.5	cup	114	94	18	1	4	—	0	.1
5015	Beans, green, snap/string, canned, drained	1	cup	135	93	27	2	6	2.6	0	0
5013	Beans, green, snap/string, frozen, cooked, drained	1	cup	135	92	35	2	8	4.5	0	0
5603	Beans, green, string, pickled	1	cup	135	91	38	2	9	2.1	0	0
5009	Beans, green/snap/string, raw	1	cup	110	90	34	2	8	3.7	0	0
5011	Beans, green/snap/string, raw, cooked	1	cup	125	89	44	2	10	4	0	.1
7029	Beans, hyacinth, dry, cooked	1	cup	194	69	227	16	40	1.6	1	.2
7046	Beans, kidney, California red, cooked	.5	cup	88	67	109	8	20	6.9	0	0
7087	Beans, kidney, all, canned w/liquid	.5	cup	128	78	104	7	19	8.9	0	.1
7048	Beans, kidney, red, canned w/liquid	1	cup	256	77	218	14	40	16.4	1	.1
7064	Beans, kidney, red, canned w/liquid, low sodium	1	cup	256	77	218	14	40	16.4	1	.1
7135	Beans, kidney, red, canned, drained	1	cup	256	69	302	19	55	22.8	1	—
7047	Beans, kidney, red, cooked	.5	cup	88	67	112	8	20	6.9	0	.1
7049	Beans, kidney, royal red, cooked	.5	cup	88	67	108	8	19	6.6	0	0
5527	Beans, lima, baby, canned, w/liquid, low sodium	1	cup	174	80	131	8	24	5.6	1	.1
7009	Beans, lima, baby, dry	1	cup	190	12	637	39	119	36.1	2	.5
7058	Beans, lima, baby, dry, cooked	.5	cup	91	67	115	7	21	7	0	.1
5019	Beans, lima, baby, frozen, cooked	.5	cup	90	72	94	6	18	6	0	.1
5193	Beans, lima, canned, drained	1	cup	170	67	164	9	31	7.3	1	.2
5247	Beans, lima, fordhook, frozen, cooked	1	cup	170	74	170	10	32	12.2	1	.1
5570	Beans, lima, immature, canned w/liquid	.5	cup	124	80	93	6	17	4	0	.1
5319	Beans, lima, immature, raw, cooked	.5	cup	85	67	105	6	20	4.5	0	.1
7011	Beans, lima, large, canned, not drained	1	cup	241	77	190	12	36	11.6	0	.1
7010	Beans, lima, large, dry, cooked	1	cup	188	70	216	15	39	13.2	1	.2
7059	Beans, mung, cooked, unsalted	.5	cup	101	73	106	7	19	3.7	0	.1

FM_Un	FP_Un	Choles	Calc	Phos	Sodium	Pota	Zinc	Iron	Magnes	A_RE	Vit_C	B1	B2	B3	B6	Fola	B12
.5	2	0	61	486	22	832	5.1	6.6	245	4	0	1.19	.52	8.5	.58	35	0
—	—	0	95	22	2	154	.3	1.9	19	42	3	.01	.01	.3	—	—	0
0	0	0	4	2	0	12	0	.1	2	10	0	0	0	0	0	2	0
0	0	0	8	4	0	24	0	.2	4	20	1	0	0	0	.01	3	0
0	0	0	15	2	0	10	.1	.8	2	11	1	0	.01	0	—	—	0
2.9	2.6	0	3	21	55	58	.2	.7	6	0	0	.07	.05	.5	.02	9	0
0	.1	0	13	81	107	370	.7	1.8	31	0	0	.12	.05	.3	.12	60	0
0	0	0	18	40	175	34	.4	.5	11	3	0	.04	.09	.3	.04	12	0
0	0	0	15	35	12	125	.6	.8	17	2	14	.06	.13	1	.07	36	0
0	.1	0	14	56	6	155	.4	.9	22	2	14	.09	.13	.8	.09	63	0
.1	.1	0	16	98	11	272	1.1	2.4	41	4	20	.17	.22	1.5	.16	86	0
0	.1	0	62	46	5	262	.7	2.2	31	84	12	.04	.13	.5	.09	76	0
3.7	2.7	0	244	263	22	482	2.5	7.4	93	0	0	.51	.22	1.4	.08	18	0
2.7	5.4	0	210	732	48	1750	6.9	12.5	230	13	8	.95	.42	3.1	1.07	1114	0
0	0	0	32	107	316	173	2.3	1.6	45	1	0	.15	.08	.9	.12	155	0
0	0	0	32	193	9	612	2	2.3	60	1	0	.13	.07	.8	.11	139	0
0	.5	0	60	—	220	—	—	3.6	—	0	0	—	—	—	—	—	—
1	1.9	0	80	276	12	477	2.5	4.8	79	4	2	.19	.1	.9	.23	282	0
0	.1	0	58	46	5	235	.5	2.1	31	78	10	.06	.12	.5	.07	44	0
.1	.4	0	127	286	2	670	2	4.5	107	0	2	.37	.11	1	.3	255	0
0	.2	0	64	132	504	376	1.8	.4	41	22	4	.19	.08	.5	.17	30	0
.8	.3	9	67	136	522	389	1.8	2.2	43	22	3	.07	.05	.6	.08	46	0
2.7	.9	6	77	137	532	451	.9	2.5	54	0	1	.17	.06	.5	.11	61	0
.1	.5	0	127	263	3	749	3.5	.7	81	43	8	.38	.15	1.1	.33	61	0
0	.2	0	42	130	461	370	.6	2.3	42	0	3	.17	.14	.7	.07	73	0
0	.1	0	51	140	3	398	.7	2.6	45	1	0	.21	.05	.5	.07	79	0
.1	.4	0	46	241	2	611	1.9	3.6	120	1	0	.42	.1	.9	.12	256	0
.1	.3	0	61	213	8	456	1.7	2.6	73	3	1	.16	.15	1.2	.12	177	0
.1	.1	0	33	101	580	310	.8	1.3	41	1	2	.03	.06	1.2	.06	42	0
0	.2	0	44	119	1	341	1	1.8	44	0	0	.18	.06	.5	.07	182	0
0	.4	0	54	88	5	318	.6	.9	48	0	1	.11	.05	.5	.09	64	0
.3	.6	0	38	108	359	206	1.3	1.6	35	3	5	.04	.04	.2	.57	80	0
0	.3	0	120	292	4	692	1.6	3.8	88	0	2	.28	.1	1.2	.21	181	0
0	.1	0	35	26	339	147	.4	1.2	18	47	6	.02	.08	.3	.05	43	0
0	.1	0	58	46	883	235	.5	2.1	31	78	10	.06	.12	.5	.07	44	0
0	.2	0	58	49	4	374	.4	1.6	31	83	12	.09	.12	.8	.07	42	0
0	.1	0	61	32	18	151	.8	1.1	28	71	11	.06	.1	.6	.08	11	0
0	.1	0	41	42	7	230	.3	1.1	28	74	18	.09	.12	.8	.08	40	0
.0	.1	0	35	26	3	147	.4	1.2	18	47	6	.02	.08	.3	.05	43	0
0	.1	0	58	46	5	235	.5	2.1	31	78	10	.06	.12	.5	.07	44	0
0	.1	0	25	18	425	106	.2	.5	15	60	4	.03	.06	.3	.05	20	0
0	.1	0	35	26	339	147	.4	1.2	18	47	6	.02	.08	.3	.05	43	0
0	.1	0	61	32	18	151	.8	1.1	28	71	11	.06	.1	.6	.08	11	0
0	.1	0	45	46	296	255	.3	1.3	31	75	16	.09	.12	.8	.08	37	0
0	.1	0	41	42	7	230	.3	1.1	28	74	18	.09	.12	.8	.08	40	0
0	.2	0	58	49	4	374	.4	1.6	31	83	12	.09	.12	.8	.07	42	0
.2	.6	0	78	233	14	654	5.6	8.9	159	0	0	.52	.07	.8	.07	7	0
0	0	0	58	121	4	369	.8	2.6	42	0	1	.11	.06	.5	.09	65	0
0	.2	0	35	134	444	329	.7	1.6	40	0	2	.14	.09	.6	.09	63	0
.1	.5	0	61	241	873	658	1.4	3.2	72	0	3	.27	.22	1.2	.06	130	0
.1	.5	0	61	241	5	658	1.4	3.2	72	0	3	.27	.22	1.2	.06	130	0
—	—	0	—	333	—	—	2	—	99	1	—	.37	.31	1.6	.08	179	0
0	.2	0	25	125	2	355	1	2.6	40	0	1	.14	.05	.5	.11	114	0
0	.1	0	39	125	4	333	.8	2.4	37	0	1	.08	.06	.5	.09	65	0
0	.3	0	49	124	7	468	1.1	2.8	59	30	15	.05	.08	.9	.11	28	0
.2	.8	0	154	703	25	2665	5	11.8	357	1	0	1.09	.41	3.2	.62	760	0
0	.2	0	26	116	3	365	.9	2.2	48	0	0	.15	.05	.6	.07	137	0
0	.1	0	25	101	26	370	.5	1.8	50	15	5	.06	.05	.7	.1	14	0
.1	.4	0	48	120	401	377	1.6	2.9	70	32	10	.06	.08	.8	.04	40	0
0	.3	0	37	107	90	694	.7	2.3	58	32	22	.13	.1	1.8	.21	36	0
0	.2	0	35	88	309	334	.8	2	42	21	11	.04	.05	.7	.08	20	0
0	.1	0	27	111	14	485	.7	2.1	63	32	9	.12	.08	.9	.16	22	0
0	.2	0	51	178	810	530	1.6	4.4	94	0	0	.13	.08	.6	.22	121	0
.1	.3	0	32	209	4	955	1.8	4.5	81	0	0	.3	.1	.8	.3	156	0
.1	.1	0	27	100	2	269	.8	1.4	48	2	1	.17	.06	.6	.07	161	0

EshaCode	Food Item	Qty.	Meas	Wgt	Wtr	Cals	Prot	Carb	Fib	Fat	F_Sat
7061	Beans, mungo, cooked	.5	cup	90	72	94	7	16	5.8	0	0
7050	Beans, pink, cooked	.5	cup	84	61	125	8	23	4.5	0	.1
7051	Beans, pinto, canned w/liquid	.5	cup	120	79	94	5	18	4.2	0	.1
7013	Beans, pinto, dry, cooked	1	cup	171	64	234	14	44	14.7	1	.2
7007	Beans, red kidney, dry	1	cup	184	12	620	41	113	35.1	2	.3
7008	Beans, red kidney, dry, cooked	1	cup	177	67	225	15	40	13.9	1	.1
7082	Beans, red mexican, dry, cooked	1	cup	224	70	252	16	47	18.1	1	.2
7024	Beans, refried/frijoles, canned	1	cup	253	72	271	16	47	13.4	3	1
7003	Beans, small white, dry, cooked	1	cup	179	63	254	16	46	14.1	1	.3
7054	Beans, white, canned w/liquid	.5	cup	131	70	153	10	29	6.3	0	.1
7053	Beans, white, dry, cooked, unsalted	.5	cup	90	63	125	9	23	5.7	0	.1
7030	Beans, winged/goabean, dry, mature	1	cup	182	8	744	54	76	12.5	30	9.5
7033	Beans, yardlong, dry, cooked	1	cup	171	69	202	14	36	2.8	1	.2
7032	Beans, yardlong, dry, mature	1	cup	167	8	579	41	103	6.5	2	.6
5438	Beans, yellow snap, canned, low sodium	1	cup	135	93	27	2	6	1.8	0	0
5196	Beans, yellow wax, canned, drained	1	cup	135	93	27	2	6	1.8	0	0
5194	Beans, yellow wax, cooked, drained	1	cup	125	89	44	2	10	1.6	0	.1
5195	Beans, yellow wax, frozen, cooked, drained	1	cup	135	92	35	2	8	4.2	0	0
7052	Beans, yellow, dry, cooked	.5	cup	88	63	127	8	22	1	1	.2
7036	Beans, yokan adzuki, confection, slices	3	piece	43	36	112	1	26	.9	0	0
4642	Beechnuts, dried	2	oz.	57	7	327	4	19	—	28	3.2
56153	Beef & noodles, w/tomato sauce, Hamburger Helper	1	cup	249	75	281	30	21	2.7	8	2.9
56150	Beef (roast) hash	1	cup	190	68	315	21	21	2.2	16	5
10073	Beef cube steak, fried, lean	3	oz.	85	55	196	29	0	0	8	2.9
10051	Beef jerky	1	each	20	25	67	8	3	0	3	1.2
16234	Beef pot pie, Banquet	1	each	198	68	330	9	38	3	15	7
70734	Beef pot pie, Swanson	1	each	198	—	380	12	39	3	19	8
10077	Beef round steak, fried, lean	3	oz.	85	55	196	29	0	0	8	2.9
10078	Beef sirloin steak, fried, lean	3	oz.	85	55	196	29	0	0	8	2.9
11008	Beef stroganoff	1	cup	256	71	405	25	16	1.4	27	10.6
10021	Beef, London Broil, broiled, lean	1	piece	21	61	44	6	0	0	2	.9
10035	Beef, bacon, Sizzlean	2	piece	22	26	99	7	0	0	8	3.2
10057	Beef, bottom round, pot roast, braised, lean	1	piece	42	58	88	13	0	0	3	1.2
10036	Beef, brisket, corned, cooked, lean	1	piece	42	60	105	8	0	0	8	2.7
10053	Beef, chuck, arm pot roast, braised, lean	1	piece	42	58	91	14	0	0	3	1.3
10008	Beef, corned, canned	1	cup	140	58	350	38	0	0	21	8.7
10081	Beef, cube steak, bread/flour fried, lean	3	oz.	85	48	235	23	9	.5	11	3.4
10009	Beef, dried, cured	6.75	piece	28	56	47	8	0	0	1	.5
10060	Beef, filet mignon steak, broiled, lean	3	oz.	85	60	179	24	0	0	8	3.2
10455	Beef, ground, baked, well done, extra lean	3	oz.	85	53	233	26	0	0	14	5.4
10722	Beef, ground, broiled, well done, extra lean	3	oz.	85	54	225	24	0	0	13	5.3
10032	Beef, ground, broiled, well done, lean	1	each	88	53	246	25	0	0	16	6.4
10724	Beef, ground, broiled, well done, lean	3	oz.	85	53	238	24	0	0	15	6.2
10463	Beef, ground, broiled, well done, regular	3	oz.	85	52	248	23	0	0	17	6.5
10030	Beef, ground, extra lean, broiled, well done	1	each	96	54	254	28	0	0	15	6
10461	Beef, ground, fried, well done, lean	3	oz.	85	54	235	24	0	0	15	5.9
10457	Beef, ground, fried, well, extra lean	3	oz.	85	54	224	24	0	0	14	5.3
10031	Beef, ground, patty, baked, well done, lean	1	each	88	51	257	26	0	0	16	6.4
10015	Beef, heart, simmered	3	oz.	85	64	149	24	0	0	5	1.4
10010	Beef, liver, fried	3	oz.	85	56	184	23	7	0	7	2.3
13000	Beef, lunchmeat, thin sliced	1	oz.	28	58	50	8	2	0	1	.5
10052	Beef, meat stick, smoked	1	each	20	19	109	4	1	—	10	4.1
11018	Beef, meatloaf	1	piece	108	62	230	18	7	.4	14	5
10028	Beef, porterhouse steak, choice, broiled, lean	1	each	170	60	371	48	0	0	18	7.4
10024	Beef, rib eye steak, broiled, lean	3	oz.	85	59	191	24	0	0	10	4
10056	Beef, rib steak, broiled, lean	3	oz.	85	58	188	24	0	0	10	3.8
10022	Beef, rib, whole, roasted, lean	1	piece	42	58	102	12	0	0	6	2.4
10002	Beef, rib, whole, roasted, lean & fat	1	piece	42	46	158	9	0	0	13	5.3
10004	Beef, roast, rump, braised, lean	1	piece	42	59	82	13	0	0	3	1
10003	Beef, roast, rump, braised, lean & fat	1	piece	42	53	109	12	0	0	6	2.4
10069	Beef, round steak, fried, lean & fat	3	oz.	85	51	245	26	0	0	15	5.6
10058	Beef, round tip, sirloin roast, roasted, lean	1	piece	42	65	78	12	0	0	3	1
10014	Beef, round, bottom, braised, lean	1	piece	42	57	92	13	0	0	4	1.3
10027	Beef, round, broiled, lean & fat	1	cup	140	55	384	36	0	0	26	10.2
10016	Beef, round, pot roasted, lean & fat	1	piece	42	52	116	12	0	0	7	2.7

FM_Un	FP_Un	Choles	Calc	Phos	Sodium	Pota	Zinc	Iron	Magnes	A_RE	Vit_C	B1	B2	B3	B6	Fola	B12
0	0	0	15	16	7	54	.1	.2	6	57	12	.02	.02	.1	.04	9	0
0	.3	0	72	100	41	491	.6	1.3	38	233	141	.1	.18	1	.24	107	0
2.2	4.9	16	67	71	62	242	.4	.9	20	102	53	.08	.13	.8	.11	43	.05
2.4	1	15	148	128	365	269	.7	.8	24	176	57	.06	.17	.5	.13	41	.18
0	.1	0	21	29	12	143	.2	.4	11	18	41	.03	.05	.3	.07	31	0
.1	0	0	2	8	864	14	0	.1	2	1	0	.01	.01	.1	.01	1	.04
0	0	0	0	—	130	—	—	0	—	0	4	—	—	—	—	—	—
.1	0	1	9	9	1152	18	0	.1	3	4	0	.01	.02	.2	0	2	.01
.4	.4	0	15	12	1483	24	0	.1	5	12	0	.01	.03	.2	0	2	.02
1	.2	0	3	11	21	69	0	.3	1	0	0	.02	.03	.2	0	0	0
2	2.8	9	6	26	83	61	.2	.6	11	4	0	.04	.05	.5	.01	3	.02
—	—	0	20	—	140	100	—	1.1	—	0	0	—	—	—	—	—	—
2.1	.6	4	7	25	78	37	.2	.6	8	5	0	.06	.05	.4	.01	3	.04
2.2	1.9	15	11	26	69	35	.2	.4	11	40	0	.03	.04	.2	.02	3	.03
0	.2	0	30	47	18	266	.3	1	17	60	52	.09	.07	.5	.15	50	0
.1	.4	0	56	87	33	495	.5	1.9	31	112	97	.17	.12	.9	.28	94	0
.1	.3	0	37	84	36	504	.6	1.2	37	91	71	.16	.18	.8	.45	157	0
0	.1	0	32	52	19	296	.3	1.1	18	67	65	.11	.07	.6	.17	46	0
0	.1	0	37	61	22	342	.4	1.2	20	78	75	.12	.08	.7	.19	54	0
.4	.4	0	14	139	8	174	1.2	1.6	101	0	0	.08	.08	1.9	.15	28	0
1.8	1.8	0	31	590	2	782	4.1	3.8	393	0	0	.17	.72	11.9	.36	51	0
.1	.2	0	18	73	9	124	1	1.8	58	0	0	.1	.05	1.8	.15	33	0
1.3	.4	0	63	40	252	64	.3	1.4	9	0	0	.22	.14	1.8	.02	12	.01
.2	.3	0	25	58	190	34	.4	1.3	12	0	0	.17	.08	2.1	.02	13	.11
1.3	.5	0	41	52	197	64	.5	1.7	21	0	0	.2	.13	1.9	.04	12	0
1.2	.4	0	56	35	224	56	.2	1.3	8	0	0	.19	.12	1.6	.02	11	.01
—	—	80	60	—	480	—	—	5.4	—	60	6	—	—	—	—	—	—
—	—	90	80	—	870	—	—	4.5	—	100	9	.33	.41	7	.35	—	—
—	—	115	250	—	1350	—	—	4.5	—	150	9	.34	.48	7	.33	—	—
—	—	137	203	—	1075	—	—	4.6	—	81	0	—	—	—	—	—	—
—	—	60	100	—	1400	—	—	3.6	—	0	0	—	—	—	—	—	—
—	—	90	60	—	980	—	—	2.7	—	20	1	—	—	—	—	—	—
—	—	76	153	—	783	—	—	3.7	—	81	5	—	—	—	—	—	—
—	—	62	62	—	543	—	—	3.7	—	41	5	—	—	—	—	—	—
7.2	2.2	8	33	31	443	219	.8	2.3	16	58	2	.36	.37	3.9	.16	8	1.07
2.5	1.8	28	214	180	1166	497	1.6	2.3	80	238	2	.22	.71	3.6	.24	82	.89
—	—	0	150	—	570	—	—	3.6	—	20	9	—	—	—	—	—	—
7.2	2.2	8	33	31	443	219	.8	2.3	16	134	2	.36	.37	3.9	.16	8	1.07
—	—	90	60	—	500	—	—	1.4	—	—	1	—	—	—	—	—	—
0	0	0	1	0	60	0	0	.1	0	0	0	0	0	0	0	0	0
24.4	3	219	24	23	747	26	0	.2	2	754	0	0	.03	0	0	3	.12
55.4	6.8	497	53	52	1877	59	.1	.4	5	1711	0	.01	.08	.1	.01	6	.28
1.2	.2	11	1	1	41	1	0	0	0	38	0	0	0	0	0	0	.01
55.4	6.8	497	53	52	25	59	.1	.4	5	1711	0	.01	.08	.1	.01	6	.28
18.4	2.3	166	18	17	625	20	0	.1	2	570	0	0	.03	0	0	2	.1
4.7	2.3	12	4	3	127	5	0	0	0	127	0	0	0	0	0	0	.01
—	—	0	42	5	5	15	.1	.8	2	0	15	.01	.01	.2	.04	3	0
—	—	0	97	11	7	616	.2	.1	13	5	30	.02	.02	.2	.09	10	0
—	—	0	27	3	2	159	0	0	4	1	9	0	0	0	.02	2	0
.6	.1	9	284	219	257	370	1	.1	27	20	2	.08	.38	.1	.08	12	.54
5.9	24.2	0	30	253	1	239	1.8	2.3	134	7	2	.22	.08	.6	.32	38	0
—	—	0	0	—	182	315	—	0	—	0	0	.12	.17	.1	—	—	—
0	.2	0	179	63	110	427	.3	1.4	32	15	5	.06	.11	.8	.3	95	0
0	.2	0	179	63	110	427	.3	1.4	32	458	65	.06	.11	.8	.31	89	0
0	.1	0	72	64	416	1279	.3	.7	18	28	1	0	.06	.3	.15	63	0
0	.1	0	158	49	58	631	.3	1.8	19	437	44	.05	.11	.7	.28	69	0
0	.1	0	74	26	46	176	.1	.6	13	6	2	.03	.05	.4	.14	46	0
0	.2	0	70	34	27	369	.3	.9	22	18	41	.07	.06	.4	.14	52	0
0	.2	0	70	34	27	369	.3	.9	22	19	41	.07	.06	.4	.13	55	0
.4	2.5	0	391	189	101	1224	1.1	2.2	101	167	254	.72	.69	3.6	1.43	252	0
.2	1.1	0	427	209	163	2233	1.6	5.4	136	121	292	.45	.36	2.7	.87	390	0
0	.1	0	145	59	995	375	.4	1.3	28	426	80	.07	.1	.8	.34	88	0
0	.1	0	86	35	918	315	.4	.9	19	124	0	.05	.12	.9	.38	92	0
0	.1	0	58	22	7	181	.2	.2	10	7	2	.03	.04	.3	.18	60	0
0	.1	0	38	46	11	268	.2	.4	12	11	4	.05	.05	.6	.21	64	0

EshaCode	Food Item	Qty.	Meas	Wgt	Wtr	Cals	Prot	Carb	Fib	Fat	F_Sat
5559	Cabbage, raw, fresh harvest	.5	cup	35	92	8	0	2	.6	0	0
5238	Cabbage, red, cooked, drained	.5	cup	75	94	16	1	3	2	0	0
5533	Cabbage, red, pickled	1	cup	150	60	220	1	57	1.2	0	0
5042	Cabbage, red, raw	1	cup	70	92	19	1	4	2.1	0	0
5534	Cabbage, red, sweet & sour	1	cup	150	60	220	1	57	1.2	0	0
5044	Cabbage, savoy, cooked, drained	1	cup	145	92	35	3	8	4.1	0	0
5043	Cabbage, savoy, raw	1	cup	70	91	19	1	4	2.4	0	0
5038	Cabbage, shredded, cooked, no added salt, drained	1	cup	150	94	33	2	7	4.2	1	.1
5036	Cabbage, shredded, raw	1	cup	70	92	18	1	4	1.4	0	0
5526	Cactus pad/nopales, cooked	1	each	29	87	12	0	3	1	0	0
5524	Cactus/nopales, raw	1	cup	118	88	48	1	11	4.2	1	.1
26100	Cajun seasoning	1	tsp	3	5	6	0	1	.2	0	—
46066	Cake, German chocolate, mix, prepared, w/frosting	1	piece	111	27	404	4	55	1.6	21	5.3
46004	Cake, angel food	1	piece	53	33	137	3	31	.8	0	.1
46050	Cake, angel food, mix, prepared	1	piece	50	33	129	3	29	.2	0	0
46051	Cake, angel food, recipe	1	piece	53	32	142	4	32	.2	0	0
46102	Cake, applesauce w/nuts & icing	1	piece	108	19	399	3	70	1.5	13	3.2
46098	Cake, applesauce, no icing	1	piece	87	22	313	3	52	1.7	11	2.9
46099	Cake, apricot, no icing	1	piece	87	22	313	3	52	1.7	11	2.9
46104	Cake, banana w/icing	1	piece	108	34	309	3	58	1.1	8	1.6
46103	Cake, banana, no icing	1	piece	87	37	245	3	43	1.1	7	1.6
46100	Cake, blackberry, no icing	1	piece	87	22	313	3	52	1.7	11	2.9
46010	Cake, carrot w/cream cheese frosting, recipe	1	piece	112	21	488	5	53	1.3	30	5.5
46054	Cake, carrot, mix, prepared, no frosting	1	piece	70	31	239	4	33	1	11	1.8
46055	Cake, cherry fudge, w/chocolate frosting	1	piece	71	46	187	2	27	—	9	3
46120	Cake, chocolate w/fluffy white icing	1	piece	91	33	262	4	48	1	8	1.8
46061	Cake, chocolate, mix, low sodium, prepared	1	piece	38	24	116	1	23	.6	3	1.4
46059	Cake, chocolate, mix, prepared	1	piece	65	32	198	4	32	1	8	1.8
46057	Cake, chocolate, mix, pudding type, prepared	1	piece	77	30	270	4	34	1.1	14	3
46062	Cake, chocolate, recipe, no frosting	1	piece	95	24	340	5	51	2.1	14	5.2
46013	Cake, chocolate, w/chocolate icing, commercial	1	piece	69	23	253	3	38	1.9	11	3.2
46117	Cake, chocolate, w/cream cheese icing	1	piece	103	26	355	4	57	1	14	3.7
46118	Cake, chocolate, w/vanilla icing	1	piece	103	25	358	4	58	1	14	3.6
46092	Cake, coffee, cheese	1	piece	76	32	258	5	34	.9	12	3.8
46263	Cake, coffee, cheese, Entenmann's	1	piece	54	32	190	4	24	0	8	3.5
46093	Cake, coffee, cinnamon, w/crumb topping	1	piece	63	22	263	4	29	2.1	15	3.6
46095	Cake, coffee, cinnamon, w/crumb topping, recipe	1	piece	60	21	240	4	30	.9	12	2.2
46096	Cake, coffee, creme filled, w/chocolate frosting	1	piece	90	29	298	4	48	1.8	10	2.5
46097	Cake, coffee, fruit	1	piece	50	32	156	3	26	1.2	5	1.2
46005	Cake, coffee, mix, prepared	1	piece	72	30	229	4	38	1.1	7	1.3
46106	Cake, date pudding	1	piece	42	35	131	2	19	.9	6	3
46063	Cake, fruit, recipe	1	piece	43	19	155	2	28	1.6	5	.6
45562	Cake, funnel, 6 inch diameter	1	each	90	41	285	7	29	.9	15	3.9
46006	Cake, gingerbread, mix, prepared	1	piece	63	33	195	3	32	2	6	1.6
46000	Cake, gingerbread, recipe	1	piece	110	28	392	4	54	.9	18	4.5
46108	Cake, graham cracker	1	piece	45	28	156	3	22	.4	7	1.7
46109	Cake, ice cream roll, chocolate	1	piece	34	39	102	1	14	.3	5	2.2
46110	Cake, ice cream roll, chocolate	1	each	340	39	1015	14	136	3.5	50	22
46111	Cake, lemon, w/icing, 2-layer	1	piece	109	21	388	3	70	.5	11	2.6
46119	Cake, marble w/chocolate icing	1	piece	111	25	404	3	59	.9	19	4.4
46068	Cake, marble, mix, pudding type, dry	1	oz.	28	3	118	1	22	.3	3	.7
46389	Cake, mix, Angle Food, prepared	.5	each	33	9	120	3	27	0	0	0
46387	Cake, mix, Devil's Food, prep w/oil & egg	1	piece	44	14	210	3	25	0	10	3
46112	Cake, oatmeal w/icing	1	piece	110	19	410	3	70	1.5	14	3.4
46070	Cake, pineapple upside-down cake, recipe	1	piece	115	32	367	4	58	.8	14	3.4
46107	Cake, plum pudding	1	piece	42	35	131	2	19	.9	6	3
46114	Cake, poppyseed, no icing	1	piece	90	24	354	7	43	1	18	6.5
46016	Cake, pound w/butter	1	piece	29	25	113	2	14	.2	6	3.2
46072	Cake, pound, commercial, not w/butter	1	piece	30	23	117	2	16	.3	6	1.3
46075	Cake, pound, old fashion, w/butter	1	piece	53	20	229	3	25	.4	13	7.6
46076	Cake, pound, old fashion, w/margarine	1	piece	53	20	230	3	25	.4	13	2.7
46074	Cake, pound, recipe, w/margarine	1	piece	54	23	206	3	28	.4	9	1.9
46101	Cake, rhubarb, no icing	1	piece	87	22	313	3	52	1.7	11	2.9
46077	Cake, shortcake, biscuit type, recipe	1	each	65	28	225	4	32	.8	9	2.4
46011	Cake, snack, chocolate, creme filled, w/icing	1	each	28	20	107	1	17	.1	4	.9

FM_Un	FP_Un	Choles	Calc	Phos	Sodium	Pota	Zinc	Iron	Magnes	A_RE	Vit_C	B1	B2	B3	B6	Fola	B12
0	0	0	16	8	6	86	.1	.2	5	4	18	.02	.01	.1	.03	20	0
0	.1	0	28	22	6	105	.1	.3	8	2	26	.03	.02	.2	.1	9	0
0	.1	0	71	33	27	307	.2	1.3	25	3	19	.03	.02	.2	.12	8	0
0	.1	0	36	29	8	144	.1	.3	10	3	40	.04	.02	.2	.15	14	0
0	.1	0	71	33	27	307	.2	1.3	25	2	19	.03	.02	.2	.12	8	0
0	.1	0	44	48	35	267	.3	.6	35	129	25	.07	.03	0	.22	67	0
0	0	0	24	29	20	161	.2	.3	20	70	22	.05	.02	.2	.13	56	0
0	.3	0	46	22	12	146	.1	.3	12	20	30	.09	.08	.4	.17	30	0
0	.1	0	33	16	13	172	.1	.4	10	9	22	.04	.03	.2	.07	30	0
0	.1	0	15	7	68	57	0	.1	24	1	3	0	.02	.1	.02	1	0
.1	.3	0	66	28	6	260	.1	.4	100	6	16	.02	.07	.5	.07	7	0
—	—	—	—	—	474	29	—	—	—	—	—	—	—	—	—	—	0
8.7	5.5	53	53	173	369	151	.5	1.2	19	24	0	.11	.14	1.1	.02	4	.1
0	.2	0	74	123	397	49	0	.3	6	0	0	.05	.26	.5	.02	2	0
0	.1	0	42	116	255	68	.1	.1	4	0	0	.05	.1	.1	0	2	.02
0	0	0	3	13	96	116	.1	.4	5	0	0	.05	.17	.4	0	2	.05
5.7	3.6	21	20	45	293	137	.2	1.3	10	49	1	.12	.12	1	.05	5	.05
4.9	2.9	22	17	46	285	145	.2	1.4	11	10	1	.14	.13	1.1	.06	6	.04
4.9	2.9	22	17	46	285	145	.2	1.4	11	10	1	.14	.13	1.1	.06	6	.04
3.2	2.3	31	28	48	292	198	.3	1	17	105	4	.13	.18	1.1	.25	12	.08
3.1	2.2	29	26	46	257	186	.3	1	16	100	3	.12	.16	1	.24	12	.07
4.9	2.9	22	17	46	285	145	.2	1.4	11	10	1	.14	.13	1.1	.06	6	.04
7.3	15.2	60	28	80	276	125	.5	1.4	20	430	1	.15	.18	1.1	.08	13	.11
3.4	5	51	77	123	249	84	.2	.9	5	173	2	.09	.12	.8	.06	8	.82
3.3	2	39	34	75	160	118	.4	.8	14	32	10	.02	.14	.5	—	6	.21
3.1	2.3	35	71	133	411	173	.5	2.1	22	16	0	.06	.11	.8	.02	8	.07
1.2	.2	0	11	102	130	82	.3	.8	14	0	0	.05	.06	.5	0	2	.01
3.1	2.3	35	70	132	370	153	.4	2.1	22	16	0	.06	.1	.6	.02	7	.06
4.7	5.9	53	64	146	402	161	.5	1.5	19	24	0	.08	.13	.9	.03	8	.32
5.7	2.6	55	57	101	299	133	.7	1.5	30	40	0	.13	.2	1.1	.04	10	.15
6.2	1.3	32	30	84	230	138	.5	1.5	24	19	0	.02	.09	.4	.03	6	.08
6.5	3.2	35	71	133	460	167	.4	2.2	22	60	0	.06	.1	.6	.02	7	.06
6.4	3.2	35	71	147	404	168	.4	2.1	22	102	0	.06	.1	.6	.02	7	.06
5.7	1.2	26	45	75	258	220	.4	.5	11	53	0	.08	.1	.5	.04	44	.11
—	—	30	40	—	160	55	—	0	—	20	0	—	—	—	—	—	—
8.3	1.8	20	34	68	221	78	.5	1.2	14	18	0	.13	.14	1.1	.02	20	.07
4.6	4.6	36	67	83	233	143	.5	1.3	24	99	0	.11	.12	.7	.06	9	.09
5.4	1.3	22	34	68	291	72	.4	.5	14	14	0	.07	.07	.8	.04	41	.05
2.9	.7	11	22	59	193	45	.3	1.2	8	10	0	.02	.1	1.3	.02	10	.02
2.8	2.3	35	98	155	303	81	.3	1	13	29	0	.12	.13	1.1	.04	9	.1
1.9	.3	16	40	35	56	196	.2	.8	23	8	0	.04	.06	.4	.08	3	.05
2	2	12	28	34	62	133	.3	.8	15	6	2	.07	.05	.5	.04	4	.02
4.5	5.9	66	115	128	236	153	.6	1.8	18	46	0	.24	.32	1.9	.05	14	.24
3.5	.8	22	44	106	289	152	.3	2.1	10	10	0	.12	.12	1	.02	6	.04
7.8	4.6	35	78	59	360	483	.4	3.2	77	15	0	.21	.18	1.9	.21	9	.07
3	1.8	34	44	52	176	78	.3	.7	8	80	0	.04	.14	.6	.02	5	.09
1.8	.7	16	43	38	69	57	.2	.5	9	22	0	.04	.07	.3	.01	2	.08
18.4	7	156	431	380	688	569	2.4	4.7	90	215	1	.4	.71	3	.14	23	.79
5.2	2.7	33	70	136	248	55	.2	.9	6	79	1	.1	.12	.8	.02	6	.07
7.4	6.2	53	43	172	311	143	.4	1.4	18	99	0	.07	.12	.7	.03	7	.1
1.4	1.1	0	22	78	147	35	.1	.5	5	0	0	.05	.04	.4	.01	3	0
0	0	0	15	—	200	35	—	0	—	0	0	0	0	0	—	—	—
3	3.5	25	20	—	270	170	—	1.1	—	0	0	.09	.1	.4	—	—	—
6.1	3.8	20	20	56	257	135	.3	1.8	14	57	1	.15	.11	1.1	.05	5	.05
6	3.8	25	138	94	367	129	.4	1.7	15	75	1	.18	.18	1.4	.04	8	.09
1.9	.3	16	40	35	56	196	.2	.8	23	8	0	.04	.06	.4	.08	3	.05
4.6	5.3	79	107	122	251	138	.7	1.7	20	94	1	.25	.29	1.7	.05	16	.18
1.6	.3	64	10	40	115	34	.1	.4	3	45	0	.04	.07	.4	.01	3	.05
3.8	.8	17	19	40	120	32	.1	.5	4	10	0	.04	.08	.4	.01	3	.04
3.9	.7	92	13	44	153	37	.3	.9	5	134	0	.1	.14	.8	.02	8	.13
5.6	3.9	60	13	44	169	39	.3	.9	5	147	0	.1	.14	.8	.02	8	.13
3.8	2.6	41	39	52	172	49	.3	.9	6	104	0	.11	.14	.9	.02	6	.1
4.9	2.9	22	17	46	285	145	.2	1.4	11	10	1	.14	.13	1.1	.06	6	.04
3.9	2.4	2	133	93	329	69	.3	1.7	10	12	0	.2	.18	1.7	.02	6	.05
1.5	1.2	5	21	26	121	35	.2	1	12	1	0	.06	.08	.7	.01	2	.03

EshaCode	Food Item	Qty.	Meas	Wgt	Wtr	Cals	Prot	Carb	Fib	Fat	F_Sat
46008	Cake, snack, cream filled, Twinkie	1	each	42	20	153	1	27	.5	5	1.2
46116	Cake, spice, w/icing	1	piece	109	24	374	4	65	1	11	3.8
46001	Cake, sponge, 1/12th	1	piece	65	30	188	4	40	.5	2	.5
46115	Cake, sponge, chocolate, no icing	1	piece	66	30	195	5	36	1	4	1.4
46105	Cake, sponge, fruit-cream filled, Twinkie	1	each	43	27	146	2	24	.4	5	1.4
46078	Cake, sponge, recipe	1	piece	63	29	187	5	36	.4	3	.8
46084	Cake, white, mix, low sodium, prepared	1	piece	38	26	118	1	23	.4	2	.4
46082	Cake, white, mix, prepared, pkg	1	each	739	31	2261	30	409	7.3	57	8.6
46080	Cake, white, mix, pudding type, prepared	1	each	826	28	2915	30	427	5.8	122	23
46007	Cake, white, no yolk, chocolate icing	1	piece	109	26	371	3	64	1.1	12	3.1
46003	Cake, white, w/coconut frosting, recipe	1	piece	70	21	249	3	44	.9	7	2.7
46017	Cake, white, w/white frosting	1	piece	71	20	266	2	45	.7	10	2.8
46090	Cake, yellow, mix, prepared	1	piece	69	30	221	3	38	.5	6	1.1
46012	Cake, yellow, w/chocolate frosting, commercial	1	piece	69	22	262	3	38	1.2	14	3.5
46015	Cake, yellow, w/vanilla frosting	1	piece	121	22	451	4	71	1.1	18	2.9
23021	Canduy, milk chocolate-covered peanuts	1	cup	170	2	882	22	84	7.1	57	24.8
23075	Candy, 3 Musketeers bar	1	each	60	6	251	2	46	1	8	3.9
23076	Candy, 3 Musketeers bar, snack size	1	each	18	6	75	1	14	.3	2	1.2
23125	Candy, 5th Avenue bar	1	each	56	2	261	4	38	—	12	—
23049	Candy, Almond Joy bar	1	each	49	8	227	2	29	4.3	14	8.1
23077	Candy, Alpine White bar, w/almonds	1	each	35	1	193	3	18	1.9	13	7
23110	Candy, Baby Ruth bar	1	each	60	5	281	5	38	1.7	13	6.4
23111	Candy, Bar None bar	1	each	42	4	219	3	22	1.4	14	—
23112	Candy, Bit-o-Honey chews	6	piece	48	7	186	1	39	—	4	—
23066	Candy, Butterfinger bar	1	each	61	2	286	4	43	1.5	11	5.6
23067	Candy, Butterfinger bar, snack size	1	each	21	2	98	1	15	.5	4	1.9
23116	Candy, Caramello bar	1	each	45	1	220	3	30	.7	11	—
23122	Candy, Chunky bar, small	1	each	35	3	179	3	20	1.7	10	5.3
23098	Candy, Crisped Rice bar, almond	1	each	28	7	130	2	18	1	6	1.1
23099	Candy, Crisped Rice bar, chocolate chip	1	each	28	7	115	1	21	.6	4	1.5
23123	Candy, Demet's Turtles	10	piece	170	6	825	11	99	—	47	18.4
23036	Candy, English toffee bar, Skor	1	each	39	4	206	2	22	.1	13	8.6
23130	Candy, Golden Almond Solitaires	1	each	85	1	455	10	40	8.5	32	—
23129	Candy, Golden Almond bar	1	each	85	1	466	9	41	8.8	32	—
23131	Candy, Golden III bar	1	each	91	3	471	6	51	5.3	30	—
23060	Candy, Kit Kat bar	1	each	42	2	214	3	26	.4	12	7
23061	Candy, Krackel bar	1	each	41	2	206	3	25	1	11	4.8
23048	Candy, M&M's, peanut, pieces	10	piece	20	2	99	2	12	.6	5	2.1
23047	Candy, M&M's, peanut, pkg	1	each	49	2	244	5	29	1.6	13	5.2
23046	Candy, M&M's, plain, pieces	10	piece	7	1	33	0	5	.2	2	.7
23045	Candy, M&M's, plain, pkg	1	each	48	1	228	3	33	1.5	11	5
23037	Candy, Mars almond bar	1	each	50	4	234	4	31	1	12	4.8
23038	Candy, Milky Way bar	1	each	61	6	256	3	44	1	9	4.8
23039	Candy, Milky Way bar, snack size	1	each	18	6	75	1	13	.3	3	1.4
23035	Candy, Mounds bar	1	each	53	15	191	2	31	1.7	11	6.1
23062	Candy, Mr. Goodbar bar	1	each	49	2	252	6	25	2.1	16	8.9
23136	Candy, Nestle 100 Grand bar	1	each	42	4	196	2	30	.6	8	4.3
23133	Candy, Nestle Crunch bar	1	each	40	1	198	2	26	1	10	6.1
23134	Candy, Nestle Crunch bar, snack size	1	each	10	1	49	1	6	.3	3	1.5
23135	Candy, Oh Henry! bar	1	each	57	6	246	6	37	2	10	3.8
23080	Candy, Planter's peanut bar	100	grams	100	2	522	16	47	3.3	34	4.3
23140	Candy, Reese's Pieces	10	piece	8	3	38	1	5	.3	2	—
23043	Candy, Reese's peanut butter cups	2	each	45	8	218	5	22	1.9	14	10.4
23141	Candy, Rolo chocolate-covered caramels	10	piece	55	2	260	3	38	.3	12	—
23143	Candy, Skittles, bite size	10	piece	11	1	43	0	11	0	0	—
23040	Candy, Snickers bar, 2.2oz	1	each	59	6	267	6	35	1.8	13	7
23057	Candy, Special Dark Sweet bar	1	each	41	1	195	2	25	2.3	12	8.5
23144	Candy, Starburst fruit chews	6	piece	59	7	232	0	50	0	5	—
23146	Candy, Symphony bar	1	each	42	1	219	3	24	1.1	14	—
23149	Candy, Twix Cookie bar, caramel	1	each	57	4	271	3	37	1	13	—
23150	Candy, Twix Cookie bar, peanut butter	1	each	48	1	245	5	28	1.6	14	—
23151	Candy, Whatchamacallit bar	1	each	48	2	241	4	28	1.4	12	—
23153	Candy, Y&S Nibs, cherry	2	oz.	57	1	212	2	52	0	1	—
23154	Candy, Y&S Twizzlers, strawberry	1	each	71	1	263	2	66	—	1	—
23152	Candy, York Peppermint Patty	1	each	42	9	145	1	33	—	4	—

FM_Un	FP_Un	Choles	Calc	Phos	Sodium	Pota	Zinc	Iron	Magnes	A_RE	Vit_C	B1	B2	B3	B6	Fola	B12
1.9	1.5	7	19	32	153	38	.1	.5	3	2	0	.06	.06	.5	.01	2	.05
5.1	1.4	48	77	201	271	150	.4	1.6	15	40	0	.13	.18	1.1	.04	9	.11
.6	.3	66	46	89	159	64	.3	1.8	7	30	0	.16	.18	1.2	.03	8	.16
1.5	.5	141	22	89	115	98	.6	1.6	20	63	1	.09	.21	.7	.05	14	.26
2.2	.8	23	46	92	132	34	.1	.6	4	11	0	.06	.08	.6	.01	5	.05
1	.4	107	26	63	144	89	.4	1	6	49	0	.1	.19	.8	.04	12	.23
1	.9	0	8	87	83	50	.1	.6	3	0	0	.07	.07	.6	0	2	.01
23.8	21.4	0	1019	1780	3591	702	2.5	7.3	66	1	1	.99	1.19	5.2	.13	37	.66
44.9	48.9	0	421	1470	3650	504	1.4	7.2	58	—	—	1.18	1.25	11.6	.11	33	.58
5.9	2.8	0	97	196	404	145	.4	1.3	15	82	0	.1	.12	.5	.01	3	.06
2.6	1.5	1	63	49	199	69	.2	.8	8	8	0	.09	.13	.7	.02	4	.04
4.2	2.5	6	34	46	166	41	.1	.6	4	23	0	.07	.09	.6	.01	4	.04
2.7	2.2	40	70	165	327	50	.2	.9	6	—	—	.08	.13	.8	.05	—	—
6.4	2.8	38	26	111	233	123	.4	1.4	21	19	0	.08	.11	.9	.02	6	.08
7.4	6.2	68	75	173	416	64	.3	1.3	7	23	0	.12	.08	.6	.04	11	.24
21.9	7.4	15	177	360	70	853	3.2	2.2	153	0	0	.2	.3	7.2	.36	14	.78
2.6	.3	7	51	55	117	80	.3	.4	18	16	0	.02	.08	.1	.01	0	.13
.8	.1	2	15	16	35	24	.1	.1	5	5	0	.01	.12	0	0	0	.04
—	—	2	39	84	104	184	.6	.6	35	4	0	.01	.12	1.8	.05	31	.1
2.6	1.2	1	39	69	66	182	.4	.6	32	2	0	.02	.07	.2	.03	4	.06
5	.9	4	81	82	26	146	.4	.2	13	9	0	.03	.15	.3	.03	5	.3
3.3	2.3	2	25	127	136	134	.5	.8	43	0	2	.02	.05	2.1	.06	31	.01
—	—	7	61	84	44	164	.5	.5	30	10	0	.02	.11	.7	.03	12	.18
—	—	0	27	32	124	60	.2	.1	10	0	0	0	.12	0	.01	2	0
2.7	1.6	1	18	58	121	145	.5	.7	32	12	2	.02	.03	2.1	.04	19	.09
.9	.6	0	6	20	42	50	.2	.2	11	4	1	.01	.01	.7	.01	7	.03
—	—	11	89	72	55	153	.4	.5	19	35	0	.02	.18	.5	.02	3	.28
3.9	1	4	50	73	18	202	.6	.4	26	4	0	.03	.14	.5	.04	8	.13
2.1	2.2	0	21	47	66	65	1.5	1.8	20	75	3	.37	.42	5	.5	0	0
1.1	1	0	6	38	79	48	.2	1.8	14	50	0	.15	.17	2	.2	40	0
18.9	7.9	37	269	335	160	524	2.5	2.3	89	58	1	.26	.41	.6	.09	17	.68
3	.4	24	44	58	90	93	.3	.2	13	27	0	.01	.13	0	.01	2	.11
—	—	10	305	255	46	428	1.6	1.2	100	8	0	.05	.42	.9	.04	18	.4
—	—	10	279	230	54	400	1.4	1.3	94	32	0	.05	.45	.9	.04	20	.37
—	—	17	275	200	79	413	1	.5	61	20	0	.06	.26	.1	.1	11	.41
3.3	.2	10	76	73	42	129	.4	.4	18	13	1	.02	.11	.2	.02	0	.29
2.9	2.3	8	73	91	56	140	.5	.3	23	5	0	.02	.12	.2	.01	3	.24
2.2	.8	3	27	55	19	78	.3	.3	16	2	0	.01	.04	.6	.04	11	.07
5.3	2.1	6	66	135	46	192	.8	.7	40	5	0	.03	.1	1.6	.09	28	.17
.4	0	0	12	14	7	27	.1	.1	5	2	0	0	.02	0	0	1	0
3	.3	0	81	93	49	187	.6	.7	32	12	0	.03	.12	.3	.03	4	0
4.4	.8	4	84	114	85	163	.6	.6	36	22	0	.02	.16	.5	.03	7	.16
3.3	.3	12	79	100	146	147	.4	.5	21	29	1	.02	.14	.2	.03	5	.31
1	.1	4	23	30	43	43	.1	.1	6	8	0	.01	.04	.1	.01	2	.09
3.5	.4	0	12	64	66	111	.6	2	36	0	0	.01	.03	0	.02	2	0
5.5	.7	10	54	137	17	221	.9	.6	47	5	0	.02	.13	2.3	.06	35	.22
2.6	.3	6	49	72	71	115	.3	.2	16	9	0	.02	.09	.1	.02	2	.16
3.8	.4	8	68	71	59	138	.4	.3	18	6	0	.02	.11	.2	.03	4	.15
1	.1	2	17	18	15	34	.1	.1	5	2	0	.01	.03	0	.01	1	.04
3.8	1.6	5	62	103	135	185	.7	.3	35	5	0	.01	.09	1.6	.04	19	.19
16.8	10.7	7	78	153	241	407	1.4	1	74	51	0	.1	.14	7.9	.11	60	.02
—	—	0	11	18	12	35	.1	.1	6	0	0	0	.02	.5	.01	4	.03
1	1	7	35	108	131	180	.6	.5	38	9	0	.02	.1	1.8	.04	13	.21
—	—	13	73	88	93	142	.4	.3	16	9	1	.03	.14	0	.04	4	.38
—	—	0	0	0	5	3	0	0	0	0	0	0	0	0	0	0	0
4	.5	7	68	124	157	191	.7	.5	35	18	0	.03	.11	1.8	.11	24	.24
4.8	.4	0	8	66	4	139	.6	.9	47	1	0	.01	.1	.3	.02	2	0
—	—	0	2	4	33	1	0	.1	1	0	31	0	0	0	0	0	0
—	—	12	99	105	36	162	.5	.4	23	5	0	.04	.16	.1	.02	3	.16
—	—	5	67	76	114	117	.4	.4	16	18	0	.03	.11	.2	.02	4	.22
—	—	6	57	98	143	153	.7	1	37	7	0	.05	.09	1.7	.05	11	.11
—	—	10	59	96	109	167	.5	.4	27	9	0	.29	.13	1	.03	5	.19
—	—	0	37	176	134	36	.1	.3	3	1	0	.01	.02	.1	.01	0	0
—	—	0	25	220	197	45	.1	.4	4	0	0	.01	.03	.1	.01	0	0
—	—	0	7	40	16	49	.3	.6	26	0	0	.01	.04	.4	0	2	.01

EshaCode	Food Item	Qty.	Meas	Wgt	Wtr	Cals	Prot	Carb	Fib	Fat	F_Sat
23020	Candy, almonds, chocolate-coated	1	cup	165	2	937	20	65	13.9	73	12.2
23115	Candy, butterscotch	5	piece	30	1	119	0	29	0	1	.3
23015	Candy, caramel, plain or chocolate	10	piece	80	8	306	4	62	1	6	5.3
23118	Candy, carob bar	1	each	87	1	464	11	43	5.6	29	7.4
23078	Candy, cherries, chocolate-covered	2	each	28	8	102	1	22	.3	3	1.5
23082	Candy, chewing gum	1	piece	4	3	14	0	4	0	0	0
23083	Candy, chewing gum, uncoated, sugarless	1	piece	4	4	11	0	4	0	0	0
23063	Candy, chocolate Kisses	6	piece	28	1	145	2	17	.8	9	5.2
23145	Candy, chocolate, sweet	1	each	41	0	207	2	24	2.3	14	8.2
23023	Candy, chocolate-covered mint patty	1	each	11	8	40	0	9	.1	1	.6
23053	Candy, divinity, no nuts	1	piece	20	9	70	0	18	.2	2	.2
23024	Candy, fondant/candy corn	1	cup	200	7	716	0	186	0	1	1
23124	Candy, fudge, brown sugar w/nuts, recipe	1	piece	14	8	55	0	11	—	1	.2
23126	Candy, fudge, chocolate marshmallow, recipe	1	piece	20	8	84	0	14	.4	3	2
23127	Candy, fudge, chocolate marshmallow, w/nuts, recipe	1	piece	22	7	96	1	15	.4	4	2.1
23026	Candy, fudge, chocolate w/nuts, recipe	1	piece	19	7	81	1	14	.2	3	1.1
23025	Candy, fudge, chocolate, recipe	1	piece	17	10	65	0	14	.1	1	.9
23128	Candy, fudge, peanut butter, recipe	1	piece	16	11	59	1	12	.1	1	.2
23027	Candy, fudge, vanilla, recipe	1	piece	16	11	59	0	13	0	1	.5
23028	Candy, fudge, vanilla, w/nuts, recipe	1	piece	15	8	62	0	11	.1	2	.6
23029	Candy, gumdrops	10	piece	35	1	135	0	35	0	0	0
23030	Candy, gummy bears	10	each	35	1	135	0	35	0	0	0
23031	Candy, hard, all flavor	1	oz.	28	1	106	0	28	0	0	0
23074	Candy, hard, dietetic	1	piece	3	1	11	0	3	0	0	0
23033	Candy, jellybeans	10	piece	11	6	40	0	10	0	0	0
23189	Candy, licorice	1	oz.	28	2	120	0	24	0	3	3.1
23087	Candy, licorice, Good & Plenty	1	oz.	28	6	104	0	26	0	0	.1
23032	Candy, lollipop	1	each	6	1	22	0	6	0	0	0
23084	Candy, malted milk balls, Whoppers	10	each	29	2	144	2	18	.8	8	4.6
23016	Candy, milk chocolate bar	1	each	44	1	226	3	26	1.5	14	8.1
23018	Candy, milk chocolate bar w/almonds	1	each	41	2	216	4	22	2.5	14	7
23019	Candy, milk chocolate w/peanuts	1	each	43	1	238	7	17	2.4	18	5.2
23058	Candy, milk chocolate w/rice cereal	1	each	40	2	198	3	25	1	11	6.4
23132	Candy, milk chocolate-covered peanuts, Goobers	10	piece	10	2	52	2	5	.8	3	1.3
23022	Candy, milk chocolate-covered raisins	1	cup	190	11	741	8	130	8	28	16.7
23214	Candy, milk chocolate-covered raisins, Raisinets	1	each	45	7	194	2	32	2.6	8	4.4
23081	Candy, peanut brittle, recipe	1	cup	147	2	666	11	102	2.9	28	7.4
23079	Candy, peanut butter cup, dietetic	2	each	16	4	88	2	7	1.1	6	5.1
23138	Candy, praline, recipe	1	piece	39	10	177	1	24	.7	9	.7
23142	Candy, sesame crunch	20	piece	35	2	181	4	18	2.7	12	1.6
23034	Candy, sugar-coated almonds, Jordan	7	each	28	2	129	2	20	1.3	5	.4
23147	Candy, taffy, recipe	1	piece	15	5	56	0	14	—	0	.3
23085	Candy, toffee, Almond Roca	1	piece	11	5	48	1	7	.3	2	1.1
23173	Candy, toffee, recipe	1	piece	12	1	65	0	8	0	4	2.4
23117	Candy, tootsie roll, bite size	7	each	35	7	126	1	31	.3	1	.2
23088	Candy, yogurt-covered peanuts	1	cup	170	4	774	15	64	7.1	52	10.1
23089	Candy, yogurt-covered raisins	1	cup	191	9	760	8	137	5.9	25	14.4
23148	Candym, truffle, recipe	1	piece	12	14	59	1	5	.2	4	2.6
3326	Cantaloupe Nectar	1	cup	250	84	151	1	38	.8	0	.2
5511	Capers	100	grams	100	86	4	4	2	3.7	0	—
3240	Carambola, raw (starfruit)	1	each	127	91	42	1	10	3.4	0	—
26018	Caraway seed	1	Tbs	7	10	22	1	3	2.6	1	0
26039	Cardamom, ground	1	Tbs	6	8	18	1	4	1.3	0	0
3241	Carissa, raw (natal plum)	1	each	20	84	12	0	3	—	0	—
44	Carob flavor mix, prepared w/milk	1	cup	256	84	195	8	22	1.7	8	5.1
5517	Carrot chips, dried	1	cup	74	4	272	7	54	14.7	1	.2
5226	Carrot juice, canned	.5	cup	123	89	49	1	11	1	0	0
5047	Carrot slices, cooked, no added salt, drained	.5	cup	78	87	35	1	8	2	0	0
5655	Carrot slices, steamed	1	cup	156	88	67	2	16	4.7	0	0
5656	Carrot slices, stir fried	1	cup	156	88	67	2	16	4.7	0	0
5439	Carrot, baby, raw (2.75inch)	1	each	10	90	4	0	1	.3	0	0
5633	Carrot, glazed	1	cup	161	70	234	2	34	4.2	11	2.2
5046	Carrot, raw, grated	.5	cup	55	88	24	1	6	1.4	0	0
5045	Carrot, whole, raw	1	each	72	88	31	1	7	1.9	0	0
5199	Carrots, canned, drained	.5	cup	73	93	17	0	4	1.4	0	0

FM_Un	FP_Un	Choles	Calc	Phos	Sodium	Pota	Zinc	Iron	Magnes	A_RE	Vit_C	B1	B2	B3	B6	Fola	B12
48	13	2	333	564	97	899	4.2	4.6	365	0	0	.2	.88	2.8	.12	128	0
.2	0	3	1	1	13	1	0	0	0	10	0	0	0	0	0	0	0
.7	.1	6	110	91	196	171	.4	.1	14	6	0	.01	.14	.2	.03	4	0
16.4	3.5	4	400	245	131	783	1.2	1.4	39	6	2	.02	.54	1	.16	28	.88
.9	.1	0	5	27	7	47	.1	.4	18	1	0	.01	.02	.2	0	0	0
0	0	0	0	0	0	0	0	0	0	0	0	0	0	0	0	0	0
0	0	0	1	0	0	0	0	0	0	0	0	0	0	0	0	0	0
2.8	.3	6	54	61	23	109	.4	.4	17	14	0	.02	.08	.1	.01	2	.11
4.6	.4	0	10	60	7	119	.6	1.1	46	1	0	.01	.1	.3	.02	1	0
.3	0	0	2	10	3	18	0	.2	7	0	0	0	.01	.1	0	0	0
.4	1.2	0	0	1	9	4	0	0	0	0	0	0	.01	0	0	0	0
0	0	0	4	4	80	32	.1	.1	2	0	0	0	.03	0	0	0	0
.3	.8	1	16	12	14	52	.1	.3	7	2	0	.01	.01	0	.02	2	0
1	.1	5	9	13	21	28	.1	.2	7	16	0	0	.02	0	0	0	.01
1.3	.7	5	11	18	21	37	.2	.2	10	16	0	.01	.02	0	.01	2	.01
.8	1	3	10	18	11	30	.1	.1	9	9	0	.01	.02	0	.02	2	.01
.4	.1	2	7	10	10	18	.1	.1	4	8	0	0	.01	0	0	0	.01
.5	.3	1	7	10	12	21	.1	0	4	2	0	0	.01	.2	.01	2	.01
.2	0	3	6	5	11	8	0	0	1	8	0	0	.01	0	0	0	.01
.5	.8	2	7	11	9	17	.1	.1	4	7	0	.01	.01	0	.01	2	.01
0	.1	0	1	0	15	2	0	.1	0	0	0	0	0	0	0	0	0
0	.1	0	1	0	15	2	0	.1	0	0	0	0	0	0	0	0	0
0	0	0	1	1	11	1	0	.1	1	0	0	0	0	0	0	0	0
0	0	0	0	0	0	0	0	0	0	0	0	0	0	0	0	0	0
0	0	0	0	0	3	4	0	.1	0	0	0	0	0	0	0	0	0
—	—	0	0	—	80	54	.1	0	3	0	0	—	—	—	—	—	—
0	0	0	1	1	7	10	0	.3	1	0	0	0	0	0	0	0	0
0	0	0	0	0	2	0	0	0	0	0	0	0	0	0	0	0	0
2.5	.2	6	50	56	42	100	.3	.2	14	3	0	.02	.08	.1	.02	3	.11
4.4	.4	10	84	95	36	169	.6	.6	26	21	0	.04	.13	.1	.02	3	.17
5.5	.9	8	92	108	30	182	.6	.7	37	6	0	.02	.18	.3	.02	5	.22
7.8	3.9	4	50	126	17	230	1	.8	53	9	0	.12	.08	3.2	.07	36	.08
3.5	.3	8	68	77	58	137	.5	.3	20	4	0	.02	.12	.2	.02	4	.15
1.5	.5	1	16	3	4	51	.1	.1	2	0	0	.01	.02	.6	.02	1	.03
9	1	6	163	272	68	977	1.5	3.3	86	13	0	.16	.31	.8	.22	10	.4
2.9	.3	3	49	65	15	245	.4	.6	20	5	0	.05	.07	.2	.05	2	.1
12.5	6.9	19	44	163	664	306	1.4	2	74	69	0	.28	.08	5.2	.15	103	.02
.7	.1	1	48	53	17	97	.4	.2	21	0	0	.03	.08	.4	.03	10	.12
5.9	2.4	0	12	42	24	82	.8	.5	20	2	0	.12	.02	.1	.03	5	0
4.4	5.1	0	247	155	8	154	1.3	1.5	88	0	0	.19	.07	1.3	.2	24	0
3.6	1.1	0	28	47	6	72	.5	.5	46	0	0	.01	.08	.3	.02	16	0
.1	0	1	0	0	13	1	0	0	0	5	0	0	0	0	0	0	0
.6	.2	1	16	19	20	34	.1	.1	5	2	0	.01	.02	.2	.01	3	.01
1.1	.1	13	4	4	22	6	0	0	0	38	0	0	.01	0	0	0	.01
.4	.3	0	8	14	9	35	.2	.1	11	1	0	0	.02	0	.01	0	.02
25.5	13.9	5	66	252	58	428	3.4	1.8	100	41	4	.19	.12	9.5	.19	192	.68
7.7	.8	18	219	259	85	1076	1	2.4	40	52	4	.21	.33	1	.32	16	.6
1.2	.1	6	19	21	9	37	.1	.1	6	17	0	.01	.03	0	0	0	.04
0	0	0	13	18	13	279	.2	.2	12	242	30	.03	.02	.5	.1	8	0
—	—	0	36	—	2108	—	—	1	—	24	0	—	—	—	—	—	—
—	—	0	5	20	3	207	.1	.3	11	62	27	.04	.03	.5	.09	12	0
.5	.2	0	46	38	1	90	.4	1.1	17	2	1	.03	.02	.2	—	—	0
0	0	0	22	10	1	65	.4	.8	13	0	—	.01	.01	.1	—	—	0
—	—	0	2	1	1	52	—	.3	3	1	8	.01	.01	0	—	—	0
2.4	.3	33	292	228	133	369	.9	.7	33	77	2	.1	.39	.3	.12	12	.87
.1	.5	0	162	251	222	1841	1.3	3	90	16042	41	.52	.36	5.3	.89	62	0
0	.1	0	30	52	36	359	.2	.6	17	3167	10	.11	.07	.5	.27	5	0
0	.1	0	24	23	52	177	.2	.5	10	1914	2	.03	.04	.4	.19	11	0
0	.1	0	42	69	55	504	.3	.8	23	3954	11	.14	.09	1.4	.22	21	0
0	.1	0	42	69	55	504	.3	.8	23	3954	12	.14	.09	1.4	.22	21	0
0	0	0	2	4	4	28	0	.1	1	20	1	0	0	.1	.01	3	0
4.9	3.6	0	63	48	263	379	.4	1.2	24	3435	3	.05	.08	.7	.34	19	.01
0	0	0	15	24	19	178	.1	.3	8	1547	5	.05	.03	.5	.08	8	0
0	.1	0	19	32	25	233	.1	.4	11	2025	7	.07	.04	.7	.11	10	0
0	.1	0	18	18	176	131	.2	.5	6	1005	2	.01	.02	.4	.08	7	0

EshaCode	Food Item	Qty.	Meas	Wgt	Wtr	Cals	Prot	Carb	Fib	Fat	F_Sat
5355	Carrots, canned, drained, low sodium	.5	cup	73	93	17	0	4	1.1	0	0
5198	Carrots, canned, not drained	.5	cup	123	93	28	1	6	1.1	0	0
5358	Carrots, frozen, cooked	.5	cup	73	90	26	1	6	2.6	0	0
6174	Carrots, julienne	1	cup	110	88	48	1	11	2.9	0	0
5048	Carrots, whole, cooked, no added salt, drained	1	each	46	87	21	1	5	1.2	0	0
4662	Cashew butter, salted	1	Tbs	16	3	94	3	4	.3	8	1.6
4537	Cashew butter, unsalted	1	Tbs	16	3	94	3	4	.5	8	1.6
15930	Cashew chicken	1	cup	162	56	409	27	11	2	29	4.8
4519	Cashew, dry roasted, salted	1	cup	137	2	786	21	45	4.4	64	12.5
4621	Cashews, dry roasted, unsalted	1	cup	137	2	786	21	45	4.1	64	12.5
4596	Cashews, oil roasted, salted	1	cup	130	4	749	21	37	4.1	63	12.4
4622	Cashews, oil roasted, unsalted	1	cup	130	4	749	21	37	4.1	63	12.4
5625	Cassava (yuca blanca), pieces, cooked	1	cup	137	68	165	4	37	.1	1	.1
5356	Cassava, raw	3.5	oz.	100	68	120	3	27	1.6	0	.1
27000	Catsup/ketchup	1	cup	245	67	255	4	67	3.2	1	.1
27032	Catsup/ketchup, low sodium	1	Tbs	15	67	16	0	4	.2	0	0
27001	Catsup/ketchup, packet	1	each	6	67	6	0	2	.1	0	0
5052	Cauliflower flowerets, cooked, drained	3	each	54	93	12	1	2	.9	0	0
5651	Cauliflower, chopped, steamed	1	cup	124	92	31	2	6	3	0	0
5652	Cauliflower, chopped, stir fried	1	cup	124	92	31	2	6	3	0	0
5051	Cauliflower, cooked, drained, cup measure	.5	cup	62	93	14	1	3	1.1	0	0
5539	Cauliflower, flowerets, batter-dipped, fried	5	piece	130	69	250	6	13	2.1	20	4.8
5607	Cauliflower, flowerets, pickled	1	each	27	88	11	0	3	.5	0	0
5053	Cauliflower, frozen, cooked, drained	1	cup	180	94	34	3	7	3.2	0	.1
5050	Cauliflower, raw flowerets	3	each	56	92	14	1	3	1.1	0	0
5049	Cauliflower, raw, cup measure	.5	cup	50	92	12	1	3	1	0	0
5641	Cauliflower, w/cheese sauce	1	cup	162	83	146	7	9	1.8	10	4.4
5200	Celeriac/celery root, cooked	3.5	oz.	100	92	25	1	6	3.9	0	0
5056	Celery pieces, cooked, no added salt	1	cup	150	94	27	1	6	2.4	0	.1
26040	Celery seed	1	tsp	2	6	8	0	1	.2	1	0
5054	Celery, chopped, raw	.5	cup	60	95	10	0	2	.9	0	0
5659	Celery, chopped, steamed	1	cup	150	95	24	1	5	2.6	0	.1
5660	Celery, chopped, stir fried	1	cup	150	95	24	1	5	2.6	0	.1
5606	Celery, pickled	1	cup	150	94	23	1	6	2.1	0	0
5055	Celery, raw, large outer stalk	1	each	40	95	6	0	1	.6	0	0
56320	Celery, stuffed w/cheesey	1	piece	32	78	44	2	1	.3	4	2.4
40059	Cereal, 100% Bran	1	cup	66	3	178	8	48	19.5	3	.6
40063	Cereal, 100% Natural	1	cup	104	2	489	12	65	8.8	22	15.1
40064	Cereal, 100% Natural w/apple cinnamon	1	cup	104	2	477	11	70	6.9	20	15.5
40065	Cereal, 100% Natural w/raisins & dates	1	cup	110	4	496	11	72	7.3	20	13.6
40003	Cereal, All Bran	.33	cup	28	3	71	4	21	10.1	1	.1
40027	Cereal, Alpha Bits	1	cup	28	1	111	2	25	1.2	1	.1
40123	Cereal, Amaranth flakes	1	cup	38	3	134	4	27	3.6	4	1
40028	Cereal, Apple Jacks	1	cup	28	2	110	2	26	.5	0	0
40029	Cereal, Bran Buds	.33	cup	28	3	73	4	22	10.6	1	.1
40025	Cereal, Bran Chex	1	cup	49	2	156	5	39	7.9	1	.2
40007	Cereal, Bran Flakes, Kellogg's	1	cup	39	3	127	5	30	5.5	1	.1
40090	Cereal, Bran Flakes, Post	1	cup	47	3	152	5	37	9.2	1	.2
40275	Cereal, Bran'ola raisin, Post	.5	cup	55	3	200	4	44	5	3	.5
40031	Cereal, C.W. Post w/raisins	1	cup	103	4	446	9	74	13.6	15	11
40030	Cereal, C.W. Post, plain	1	cup	97	2	432	9	70	7.2	15	11.3
40032	Cereal, Cap'n Crunch	1	cup	37	2	156	2	30	.7	3	2.2
40034	Cereal, Cap'n Crunch, peanut butter	1	cup	35	2	154	3	26	.5	5	1.9
40033	Cereal, Cap'n Crunchberries	1	cup	35	3	146	2	28	.7	3	1.9
40004	Cereal, Cheerios	1.25	cup	28	5	111	4	20	2	2	.3
40126	Cereal, Cinnamon Toast Crunch	1	cup	38	—	162	2	30	1.5	4	.8
40127	Cereal, Clusters	1	cup	57	2	221	7	39	5.8	7	.7
40035	Cereal, Cocoa Krispies	1	cup	36	2	139	2	32	.2	1	.2
40037	Cereal, Cocoa Pebbles	1	cup	32	2	131	2	28	.5	2	0
40215	Cereal, Common Sense Oat Bran w/raisins	.75	cup	37	—	130	4	29	3	1	0
40036	Cereal, Corn Bran	1	cup	36	2	125	2	30	6.8	1	.2
40038	Cereal, Corn Chex	1	cup	28	2	111	2	25	.5	0	.1
40005	Cereal, Corn Flakes, USDA	1	cup	25	3	97	2	22	.6	0	0
40067	Cereal, Corn Pops USDA	1	cup	28	3	108	1	26	.2	0	0
40039	Cereal, Cracklin' Oat Bran	1	cup	60	4	229	6	41	10	9	2.1

FM_Un	FP_Un	Choles	Calc	Phos	Sodium	Pota	Zinc	Iron	Magnes	A_RE	Vit_C	B1	B2	B3	B6	Fola	B12
0	.1	0	18	18	31	131	.2	.5	6	1005	2	.01	.02	.4	.08	7	0
0	.1	0	31	25	296	213	.4	.8	11	1619	3	.02	.03	.5	.14	10	0
0	0	0	20	19	43	115	.2	.3	7	1292	2	.02	.03	.3	.09	8	0
0	.1	0	30	49	39	357	.2	.6	17	3108	10	.11	.06	1	.16	16	0
0	0	0	14	14	30	104	.1	.3	6	1129	1	.02	.03	.2	.11	6	0
4.7	1.3	0	7	73	98	87	.8	.8	41	0	0	.05	.03	.3	.04	11	0
4.7	1.3	0	7	73	2	87	.8	.8	41	0	0	.05	.03	.3	.04	11	0
13	9.1	60	47	249	988	415	1.4	1.9	60	93	9	.14	.14	12.5	.56	40	.24
37.4	10.7	0	62	671	877	774	7.7	8.2	356	0	0	.27	.27	1.9	.35	95	0
37.4	10.7	0	62	671	22	774	7.7	8.2	356	0	0	.27	.27	1.9	.35	95	0
36.9	10.6	0	53	554	814	689	6.2	5.3	332	0	0	.55	.23	2.3	.32	88	0
36.9	10.6	0	53	554	22	689	6.2	5.3	332	0	0	.55	.23	2.3	.32	88	0
.1	.1	0	119	87	330	946	.3	4.7	86	1	43	.25	.12	1.7	.38	20	0
.1	.1	0	91	70	8	764	.2	3.6	66	1	48	.22	.1	1.4	.3	22	0
.1	.4	0	47	96	2905	1178	.6	1.7	54	249	37	.22	.18	3.4	.43	37	0
0	0	0	3	6	3	72	0	.1	3	15	2	.01	.01	.2	.03	2	0
0	0	0	1	2	71	29	0	0	1	6	1	0	0	.1	.01	1	0
0	.1	0	9	17	8	77	.1	.2	5	1	24	.02	.03	.2	.09	24	0
0	.1	0	27	55	37	376	.3	.5	19	2	49	.06	.07	.6	.25	60	0
0	.1	0	27	55	37	376	.3	.5	19	2	49	.06	.07	.6	.26	56	0
0	.1	0	10	20	9	88	.1	.2	6	1	28	.03	.03	.3	.11	27	0
5.2	9.1	30	167	173	239	332	.6	.9	19	45	47	.1	.16	.7	.19	40	.17
0	0	0	7	9	43	64	0	.1	3	10	12	.01	.01	.1	.04	8	0
0	.2	0	31	43	32	250	.2	.7	16	4	56	.07	.1	.6	.16	74	0
0	.1	0	12	25	17	170	.2	.2	8	1	26	.03	.04	.3	.12	32	0
0	.1	0	11	22	15	152	.1	.2	8	1	23	.03	.03	.3	.11	28	0
3.3	1.5	19	177	145	516	367	.7	.5	21	82	43	.08	.21	.6	.19	44	.33
0	.1	0	26	66	61	173	.2	.4	12	0	4	.03	.04	.4	.1	3	0
0	.1	0	63	38	137	426	.2	.6	18	20	9	.06	.07	.5	.13	33	0
.3	.1	0	35	11	3	28	.1	.9	9	0	0	.01	.01	.1	—	—	0
0	0	0	24	15	52	172	.1	.2	7	8	4	.03	.03	.2	.05	17	0
0	.1	0	60	38	131	432	.2	.6	16	19	9	.2	.06	.5	.12	36	0
0	.1	0	60	38	131	431	.2	.6	16	18	9	.2	.06	.5	.12	34	0
0	.1	0	51	31	366	354	.2	.6	17	16	7	.05	.05	.4	.1	24	0
0	0	0	16	10	35	115	.1	.2	4	5	3	.02	.02	.1	.04	11	0
1.1	.1	12	45	50	110	75	.2	.2	4	46	2	.01	.04	.1	.02	7	.06
.6	1.9	0	46	801	457	824	5.7	8.1	312	0	63	1.59	1.79	20.9	2.11	47	6.27
4.3	2	1	181	383	45	514	2.4	3.1	125	6	0	.31	.56	2.4	.19	31	.13
1.8	1.3	1	157	350	52	514	2	2.9	72	6	1	.33	.57	1.9	.11	17	.3
3.7	1.7	1	160	348	47	538	2.1	3.1	124	6	0	.31	.65	2.1	.16	45	.15
.1	.3	0	23	265	320	350	3.8	4.5	106	376	15	.37	.43	5	.51	100	0
.2	.3	0	8	51	180	110	1.5	2.7	17	376	0	.37	.43	5	.51	100	1.51
.9	1.8	0	6	126	13	134	.1	.7	10	3	1	.03	.04	1	.03	4	0
0	0	0	3	30	125	23	3.7	4.5	6	375	15	.37	.43	5	.51	100	0
.1	.4	0	19	246	174	474	3.7	4.5	90	375	15	.37	.43	5	.51	100	0
.2	.8	0	29	327	455	394	2.2	7.8	126	11	26	.64	.26	8.6	.88	173	2.6
.1	.4	0	19	192	303	248	5.2	24.8	71	516	0	.51	.59	6.9	.7	138	2.07
.2	.3	0	21	296	431	251	2.5	7.5	102	622	0	.62	.71	8.3	.85	166	2.49
—	—	0	0	100	220	220	1.5	4.5	40	250	0	.38	.42	5	.5	100	1.5
1.7	1.4	0	50	232	161	261	1.6	16.4	74	1363	0	1.35	1.56	18.1	1.85	364	5.46
1.7	1.4	0	47	224	167	198	1.6	15.4	67	1284	0	1.27	1.46	17.1	1.75	342	5.14
.4	.5	0	6	47	278	48	4	9.8	15	5	0	.66	.72	8.6	1	238	2.34
1.4	1	0	7	49	268	57	3.8	9.1	19	5	0	.61	.7	9	1.04	244	2.3
.4	.5	0	11	47	244	49	3.6	9	14	4	0	.6	.68	8.1	.93	128	2.51
.6	.7	0	48	134	307	101	.8	4.5	39	375	15	.37	.43	5	.51	6	1.5
—	—	0	50	76	262	54	.4	—	10	158	19	.48	.54	6.3	.64	0	—
2.9	2.8	0	103	212	270	273	.8	9	55	746	31	.78	.96	12	1.04	201	0
.2	.2	0	6	47	275	53	1.9	2.3	12	477	19	.47	.54	6.3	.65	127	.02
0	0	0	5	25	153	53	1.7	2	13	424	0	.42	.48	5.6	.58	113	1.7
—	—	0	20	146	250	180	3.8	8.1	48	225	—	.38	.43	5	.5	100	2
.3	.7	0	41	52	310	70	4	12.2	18	8	0	.38	.7	10.9	.86	232	1.39
.2	.6	0	3	11	271	23	.1	1.8	4	14	15	.37	.07	5	.51	100	1.5
0	0	0	1	16	256	23	.1	1.6	3	331	13	.33	.38	4.4	.45	88	0
0	.1	0	1	28	103	17	1.5	1.8	2	375	15	.37	.43	5	.51	100	0
2.3	3.5	0	40	241	487	355	3.2	3.8	116	794	32	.79	.91	10.6	1.08	212	0

EshaCode	Food Item	Qty.	Meas	Wgt	Wtr	Cals	Prot	Carb	Fib	Fat	F_Sat
40205	Cereal, Cracklin' Oat Bran, Kellogg's	.5	cup	28	—	110	3	21	4	3	1
40205	Cereal, Cracklin' Oat Bran	.5	cup	28	—	110	3	21	4	3	1
40040	Cereal, Crispy Wheat 'N Raisins	1	cup	43	7	150	3	35	2.8	1	.1
40006	Cereal, Farina, enriched, cooked	1	cup	233	88	117	3	25	3.3	0	0
40130	Cereal, Fiber One	1	cup	57	—	182	5	46	25.7	2	—
40042	Cereal, Froot Loops	1	cup	28	2	111	2	25	.6	1	.2
40198	Cereal, Frosted Bran, Kellogg's	.75	cup	30	—	102	2	26	3.3	0	.3
40020	Cereal, Frosted Flakes	.75	cup	28	2	108	1	26	.5	0	0
40085	Cereal, Fruit & Fibre, date-raisin-nut	.5	cup	28	9	96	2	22	3.8	1	.2
40086	Cereal, Fruitful Bran	.75	cup	34	1	144	4	37	6	0	.1
40046	Cereal, Fruity Pebbles	1	cup	32	3	130	1	28	.4	2	.4
40047	Cereal, Golden Grahams	1	cup	39	2	150	2	33	1.4	1	1
40197	Cereal, Granola, Kellogg's, low fat	.5	cup	55	—	209	4	42	3.3	4	0
40008	Cereal, Granola, Nature Valley	1	cup	113	4	503	12	76	6	20	13
40137	Cereal, Granola, low fat	.33	cup	31	3	120	3	25	2	2	0
40009	Cereal, Grape Nuts	1	cup	109	3	389	13	89	10.9	0	0
40049	Cereal, Grape Nuts Flakes	1	cup	39	3	140	4	32	3.9	0	.1
40129	Cereal, Heartwise, plain	1	cup	39	4	113	4	31	8.6	1	.2
40246	Cereal, Honey & Nut Corn Flakes	.667	cup	28	4	113	2	23	.3	2	.2
40052	Cereal, Honey Bran	1	cup	35	2	119	3	29	3.9	1	.1
40084	Cereal, Honey Buckwheat Crisp	.75	cup	28	5	110	3	23	2.5	1	.2
40125	Cereal, Honey Bunches of Oats	1	cup	43	2	173	3	36	2.1	2	.5
40053	Cereal, Honey Comb	1	cup	22	1	86	1	20	.6	0	.1
40051	Cereal, Honey Nut Cheerios	1	cup	33	3	125	4	26	1.4	1	.1
40068	Cereal, Honey Smacks	.75	cup	28	3	106	2	25	.4	1	.1
40134	Cereal, Just Right	1	cup	43	2	152	5	36	3	1	.2
40054	Cereal, King Vitaman	1	cup	21	2	85	1	18	.3	1	.7
40010	Cereal, Kix	1.5	cup	28	3	110	3	23	.5	1	.2
40011	Cereal, Life, plain/cinnamon	1	cup	44	4	162	8	32	2.6	1	.1
40055	Cereal, Lucky Charms	1	cup	32	3	125	3	26	1.4	1	.2
40015	Cereal, Maypo, cooked, no salt added	.75	cup	180	83	128	4	24	4.3	2	.3
40056	Cereal, Most	1	cup	52	5	175	7	40	7.3	1	.1
40124	Cereal, Mueslix Five Grain Muesli	1	cup	82	5	279	7	63	7.4	3	.5
40138	Cereal, Multi-grain, cooked	1	cup	246	78	200	7	40	3.9	2	.4
40057	Cereal, Nutri Grain Corn	1	cup	42	3	160	3	35	2.6	1	.1
40058	Cereal, Nutri Grain Wheat	1	cup	44	3	158	4	37	2.8	0	.1
40213	Cereal, Nutri Grain Wheat	.66	cup	28	—	90	3	23	3	0	0
40213	Cereal, Nutri Grain Wheat	.75	cup	30	—	95	3	24	3.2	0	0
40041	Cereal, Oat flakes, fortified	1	cup	48	3	177	9	35	1.4	1	.1
40072	Cereal, Oatmeal, instant, packet, prepared, plain	1	each	177	86	104	4	18	3	2	.3
40092	Cereal, Post Toasties	1	cup	24	3	93	2	21	.8	0	0
40012	Cereal, Product 19	1	cup	33	3	126	3	27	1.4	0	0
40066	Cereal, Quisp	1	cup	30	2	124	2	25	.5	2	1.5
40013	Cereal, Raisin Bran, Kellogg's	1	cup	56	8	175	6	42	6	1	.2
40091	Cereal, Raisin Bran, Post	1	cup	56	9	172	5	42	7.9	1	.2
40133	Cereal, Raisin Nut Bran	1	cup	57	5	221	4	42	5.6	6	1
40088	Cereal, Ralston, cooked	1	cup	253	86	134	6	28	6.1	1	.1
40026	Cereal, Rice Chex	1.13	cup	28	3	112	2	25	.5	0	.3
40017	Cereal, Rice Krispies	1	cup	28	2	111	2	25	.3	0	0
40210	Cereal, Rice Krispies	1	cup	28	—	110	2	25	0	0	0
40016	Cereal, Roman meal, cooked	.75	cup	181	83	110	5	25	1.1	1	.1
40062	Cereal, Shredded Wheat, large biscuit	1	each	24	6	83	3	19	2.3	0	.1
40022	Cereal, Shredded Wheat, small	.75	cup	32	5	115	4	26	3.1	1	.1
40019	Cereal, Special K	1	cup	28	2	111	6	21	.7	0	0
40211	Cereal, Special K	1	cup	28	—	100	6	20	1	0	0
40069	Cereal, Super Golden Crisp	1	cup	33	2	123	2	30	.5	0	0
40071	Cereal, Team Rice	1	cup	42	4	164	3	36	.5	1	.2
40131	Cereal, Total Corn Flakes	1	cup	33	3	126	3	28	2	1	.1
40021	Cereal, Total, wheat	1	cup	33	4	116	3	26	4.3	1	.1
40060	Cereal, Trix	1	cup	28	2	108	2	25	.3	0	.2
40128	Cereal, Uncle Sam's High Fiber	1	cup	110	6	427	17	79	29	5	.4
40061	Cereal, Wheat Chex	1	cup	46	2	169	5	38	4.1	1	.2
40080	Cereal, Wheatena, cooked, unsalted	1	cup	243	85	136	5	29	6.6	1	.2
40024	Cereal, Wheaties	1	cup	29	5	101	3	23	2.6	0	.1
38156	Cereal, cream of rye, cooked	1	cup	251	89	108	2	24	4.3	0	0

FM_Un	FP_Un	Choles	Calc	Phos	Sodium	Pota	Zinc	Iron	Magnes	A_RE	Vit_C	B1	B2	B3	B6	Fola	B12
2	0	0	15	123	140	160	1.5	1.8	45	225	15	.38	.43	5	.5	100	—
2	0	0	15	123	140	160	1.5	1.8	45	225	15	.38	.43	5	.5	100	—
.1	.4	0	71	117	204	174	.5	6.8	34	569	0	.56	.65	7.6	.77	15	2.28
0	.1	0	5	28	0	30	.2	1.2	5	0	0	.19	.12	1.3	.02	5	0
—	—	0	76	285	266	462	2.3	8.6	114	143	28	.71	.81	9.5	.95	0	—
.1	.1	0	3	24	145	26	3.7	4.5	7	375	15	.37	.43	5	.51	100	0
0	0	0	9	90	201	120	4	4.8	37	238	16	.4	.45	5.4	.53	105	1.59
0	0	0	1	21	230	18	0	1.8	2	375	15	.37	.43	5	.51	100	0
.6	.5	0	15	110	134	167	1.5	5.1	40	361	0	.38	.43	5	.5	100	1.5
.1	.2	0	23	152	264	276	1.3	5.4	67	270	0	.46	.52	6	.6	120	—
.3	.4	0	4	19	178	24	1.7	2	9	424	0	.42	.48	5.6	.58	113	1.7
.1	.2	0	24	56	385	86	.3	6.2	16	516	21	.51	.59	6.9	.7	6	2.07
—	—	0	23	127	55	160	6.4	7.7	45	384	—	.64	.73	8.8	.85	171	2.59
2.9	2.8	0	71	354	233	389	2.2	3.8	115	7	0	.4	.19	.8	.09	85	0
—	—	0	—	80	60	95	3.7	1.8	24	150	—	.37	.42	5	.5	100	1.5
0	.4	0	10	274	758	364	2.4	4.7	73	1443	0	1.43	1.65	19.2	1.96	385	5.78
0	.1	0	16	116	220	136	.8	11.2	43	516	0	.51	.59	6.9	.7	138	2.07
.3	.4	0	30	154	168	265	2.1	6.2	55	310	0	.52	.58	7	.69	137	1.95
.5	.7	0	3	13	225	36	.1	1.8	6	375	15	.37	.43	5	.51	100	0
.1	.4	0	16	132	202	151	.9	5.6	46	463	19	.46	.53	6.2	.63	24	1.86
.2	.4	0	40	80	269	106	.5	8.1	32	681	27	.68	.76	9	1.4	9	2.7
1.4	.3	0	8	66	272	77	.7	6	24	838	0	.55	.74	8.3	1.04	196	3.67
.1	.2	0	4	22	124	70	1.2	2.1	7	291	0	.29	.33	3.9	.4	78	1.17
.3	.3	0	23	122	299	115	.9	5.2	39	437	18	.43	.5	5.8	.59	22	1.75
.1	.2	0	3	31	75	42	.3	1.8	14	375	15	.37	.43	5	.51	100	0
.2	.4	0	11	94	288	98	22.8	27.3	29	341	0	2.27	2.58	30.3	3.03	607	9.1
.2	.2	0	2	27	161	26	.2	12.7	7	717	33	.93	1.06	12.9	1.18	286	4.12
.2	.2	0	35	39	290	44	.2	8.1	12	375	15	.37	.43	5	.51	100	1.5
.2	.4	0	154	238	229	197	1.5	11.6	14	9	0	.96	1	11.6	.08	37	0
.4	.5	0	36	89	227	66	.6	5.1	27	424	17	.42	.48	5.6	.58	6	1.7
.6	.8	0	94	185	7	158	1.1	6.3	38	527	22	.54	.54	7	.72	7	2.16
.2	.3	0	79	361	276	340	2.8	33	103	2753	110	2.76	3.13	36.7	3.69	734	11
1	1.2	0	38	215	107	369	7.5	8.9	82	747	1	.75	.84	9.8	.99	197	3.28
.9	.6	0	69	183	759	137	.9	5.4	66	0	0	.39	.46	4.4	.46	17	0
.2	.6	0	1	121	276	98	5.5	.9	27	556	22	.55	.63	7.4	.76	148	2.23
.1	.3	0	12	165	299	120	5.8	1.2	34	583	23	.58	.66	7.7	.79	155	2.33
0	0	0	9	92	170	90	3.8	.7	30	0	15	.38	.43	5	.5	100	2
0	0	0	10	97	180	95	4	.7	32	0	16	.4	.46	5.3	.53	106	2.12
.3	.3	0	68	176	429	343	1.5	13.7	58	636	0	.63	.72	8.4	.86	169	2.54
.6	.7	0	163	133	285	99	.9	6.3	42	453	0	.53	.28	5.5	.74	150	0
0	0	0	1	11	252	28	.1	.6	4	318	0	.31	.36	4.2	.43	85	1.27
0	.1	0	4	46	378	52	.5	21	12	1747	70	1.75	1.98	23.3	2.34	466	7
.3	.3	0	9	25	241	45	.2	6.3	12	5	0	.54	.76	5.8	.91	8	2.58
.2	.5	0	20	208	310	291	5.7	25.4	72	570	0	.57	.68	7.6	.78	152	2.3
.2	.4	0	26	235	365	345	3	8.9	95	741	0	.73	.85	9.9	1.01	198	2.97
1.6	2.9	0	80	201	302	302	1.7	9	64	753	0	.75	.86	10.1	1	201	0
.1	.4	0	13	147	5	154	1.4	1.6	58	0	0	.2	.18	2	.11	18	.11
.3	.4	0	4	28	237	33	.4	1.8	7	2	15	.37	.01	5	.51	100	1.51
0	.1	0	5	30	206	27	.5	.7	12	0	1	.11	.03	2	.04	3	.08
0	0	0	3	34	290	35	.4	1.8	11	225	15	.38	.43	5	.5	100	—
.1	.3	0	22	161	2	226	1.3	1.6	82	0	0	.18	.09	2.3	.08	18	0
.1	.2	0	10	86	0	77	.6	.7	40	0	0	.07	.07	1.1	.06	12	0
.1	.3	0	12	113	3	116	1.1	1.4	42	0	0	.08	.09	1.7	.08	16	0
0	0	0	8	55	265	49	3.7	4.5	16	375	15	.37	.43	5	.51	100	.02
0	0	0	10	57	230	55	3.8	4.5	18	225	15	.53	.6	7	.7	100	—
0	.1	0	7	60	29	123	1.8	2.1	20	437	0	.43	.5	5.8	.59	116	1.75
.2	.3	0	6	65	260	71	.6	2.6	18	556	22	.55	.63	7.4	.76	7	2.23
.2	.4	0	282	137	217	77	.1	21	37	1747	70	1.75	1.98	23.3	3.24	607	7
.1	.3	0	282	137	326	123	.8	21	37	1747	70	1.75	1.98	23.3	2.34	466	7
.1	.1	0	6	19	179	26	.1	4.4	6	371	15	.37	.42	4.9	.5	3	1.48
.9	3	0	77	417	251	518	2.9	4.1	134	0	0	2.62	2.77	23.1	.13	86	0
.2	.6	0	18	182	308	173	1.2	7.3	58	0	24	.6	.17	8.1	.83	162	2.44
.2	.5	0	10	146	5	187	1.7	1.4	49	0	0	.02	.05	1.3	.05	17	0
0	.2	0	44	100	276	108	.6	4.6	32	384	15	.38	.44	5.1	.52	102	1.54
0	.2	0	11	54	350	65	.6	.5	23	0	0	.08	.02	.2	.06	5	0

EshaCode	Food Item	Qty.	Meas	Wgt	Wtr	Cals	Prot	Carb	Fib	Fat	F_Sat
40078	Cereal, cream of wheat, cooked	1	cup	244	88	127	2	28	.2	0	.1
40244	Cereal, cream of wheat, cooked	1	cup	244	87	132	4	27	1.2	0	.1
40245	Cereal, cream of wheat, mix'n eat, prep, plain	1	each	142	82	102	3	21	.4	0	0
40077	Cereal, farina, unenriched, cooked w/o salt	1	cup	233	88	117	3	25	3.3	0	0
40043	Cereal, Frosted Mini Wheats, biscuits	4	each	31	5	111	3	26	2.4	0	.1
40045	Cereal, Frosted Rice Krispies	.75	cup	28	3	109	1	26	.2	0	0
40294	Cereal, honey cluster flake crunch, fat free	.75	cup	31	4	130	3	26	4	0	0
40014	Cereal, malt-o-meal, plain, cooked	1	cup	240	88	122	4	26	1	0	0
40136	Cereal, oat bran, cooked, Mother's brand	1	cup	242	90	63	4	17	4.1	2	.3
40000	Cereal, oatmeal, cooked	1	cup	234	85	145	6	25	4	2	.4
40073	Cereal, oatmeal, instant packet, prepared, apple-cinn	1	each	149	78	136	4	26	3.1	2	.3
40074	Cereal, oatmeal, instant packet, prepared, cinn-spice	1	each	161	73	177	5	35	2.6	2	.3
40075	Cereal, oatmeal, instant packet, prepared, maple	1	each	155	74	163	5	32	3.3	2	.3
40076	Cereal, oatmeal, instant, prepared, raisin-spice	1	each	158	75	161	4	32	2.2	2	.3
40018	Cereal, puffed rice, fortified 2% RDA	1	cup	14	3	56	1	13	.2	0	0
40023	Cereal, puffed wheat, fortified 2% RDA	1	cup	12	3	44	2	10	.5	0	0
40002	Cereal, rolled wheat, cooked	1	cup	240	84	149	5	33	3.8	1	.2
40070	Cereal, Tasteeos	1	cup	24	2	94	3	19	2.5	1	.2
22505	Champagne	.5	cup	119	86	91	0	2	0	0	0
5413	Chayote fruit, raw	1	each	203	93	49	2	11	6.1	1	—
5414	Chayote, cooked pieces	1	cup	160	93	38	1	8	.9	1	—
1001	Cheese food, American cold pack	1	piece	21	43	70	4	2	0	5	3.2
1071	Cheese food, swiss processed, slice	1	piece	21	44	68	5	1	0	5	3.3
1081	Cheese product, nonfat (Kraft Free Singles)	1	piece	19	61	30	4	3	0	0	0
44001	Cheese puffs (Cheetos)	1	cup	20	2	111	2	11	.2	7	1.3
1002	Cheese spread, American	1	cup	244	48	708	40	21	0	52	32.5
1094	Cheese spread, lowfat, low sodium (Velveeta)	1	piece	34	62	61	8	1	0	2	1.5
1072	Cheese, American food slice	1	piece	21	43	69	4	2	0	5	3.2
1000	Cheese, American processed	1	piece	21	39	79	5	0	0	7	4.1
1096	Cheese, American processed, lowfat	1	oz.	28	59	51	7	1	0	2	1.2
1132	Cheese, Gjetost	1	piece	28	13	132	3	12	0	8	5.4
1029	Cheese, asiago, shredded	1	cup	108	37	406	31	4	0	30	19.2
1039	Cheese, beer	1	oz.	28	41	105	7	1	0	8	5.3
1003	Cheese, blue	1	cup	135	42	477	29	3	0	39	25.2
1109	Cheese, brick w/salami	1	oz.	28	43	102	6	1	0	8	5
1037	Cheese, brick, shredded	1	cup	113	41	419	26	3	0	34	21.2
1004	Cheese, brie, sliced	1	cup	144	48	481	30	1	0	40	25.1
1006	Cheese, camembert	1	cup	246	52	738	49	1	0	60	37.6
1045	Cheese, caraway	1	piece	28	39	107	7	1	0	8	5.3
1423	Cheese, cheddar, low fat, Alpine Lace	.25	cup	31	48	89	10	1	0	5	3.3
1105	Cheese, cheddar, low sodim	1	oz.	28	39	113	7	1	0	9	5.9
1091	Cheese, cheddar, lowfat, low sodium	1	oz.	28	65	49	7	1	0	2	1.3
1008	Cheese, cheddar, shredded	1	cup	113	37	455	28	1	0	37	23.8
1046	Cheese, cheshire	1	piece	28	38	110	7	1	0	9	5.5
1011	Cheese, colby, cubed	1	cup	132	38	520	31	3	0	42	26.7
1107	Cheese, colby, low sodium	1	oz.	28	39	113	7	1	0	9	5.9
1089	Cheese, colby, lowfat, low sodium	1	oz.	28	65	49	7	1	0	2	1.3
1010	Cheese, colby, shredded	1	cup	113	38	445	27	3	0	36	22.8
1047	Cheese, cottage, 1% lowfat	1	cup	226	82	164	28	6	0	2	1.5
1014	Cheese, cottage, 2% lowfat	1	cup	226	79	203	31	8	0	4	2.8
1049	Cheese, cottage, creamed w/fruit	1	cup	226	72	280	22	30	0	8	4.9
1013	Cheese, cottage, creamed, large curd	1	cup	225	79	232	28	6	0	10	6.4
1099	Cheese, cottage, lowfat, low sodium	1	cup	225	84	162	28	6	0	2	1.4
1084	Cheese, cottage, nonfat (Knudsen)	.5	cup	122	84	80	15	4	0	0	0
1012	Cheese, cottage, small curd	1	cup	210	79	216	26	6	0	9	6
1015	Cheese, cream	1	cup	232	54	810	18	6	0	81	51
1098	Cheese, cream, lowfat	1	Tbs	15	64	35	2	1	0	3	1.7
1115	Cheese, cream, nonfat (Philadelphia Free)	2	Tbs	33	78	30	5	2	0	0	0
1083	Cheese, cream, soft (Philadelphia)	2	Tbs	30	56	100	2	1	0	10	7
1050	Cheese, edam	1	oz.	28	42	101	7	0	0	8	5
1016	Cheese, feta, shredded	1	cup	246	55	649	35	10	0	52	36.7
1052	Cheese, fontina	1	oz.	28	38	110	7	0	0	9	5.4
1078	Cheese, goat, hard	1	oz.	28	29	128	9	1	0	10	7
1080	Cheese, goat, soft	1	cup	246	61	659	46	2	0	52	35.9
1076	Cheese, gorgonzola	1	oz.	28	39	111	7	0	0	9	5.5

FM_Un	FP_Un	Choles	Calc	Phos	Sodium	Pota	Zinc	Iron	Magnes	A_RE	Vit_C	B1	B2	B3	B6	Fola	B12
.1	.1	0	7	42	2	49	.4	.5	7	0	0	0	0	1	.07	7	0
.1	.2	0	51	102	142	46	.3	10.5	12	0	0	.24	0	1.5	.03	10	0
0	.1	0	20	20	241	38	.2	8.1	7	376	0	.43	.28	5	.57	101	0
0	.1	0	5	28	0	30	.2	0	5	0	0	.02	.02	.2	.02	5	0
0	.2	0	10	81	9	106	1.6	2	25	410	16	.41	.47	5.5	.56	109	0
0	0	0	1	27	240	21	.3	1.8	5	375	15	.37	.43	5	.51	100	0
0	0	0	0	—	20	—	—	.4	—	20	1	—	—	—	—	—	—
0	.1	0	5	24	2	31	.2	9.6	5	0	0	.48	.24	5.8	.02	5	0
.6	.7	0	19	178	255	137	.9	1.3	62	0	0	.24	.05	.2	.04	9	0
.7	.9	0	19	178	2	131	1.2	1.6	56	4	0	.26	.05	.3	.05	9	0
.6	.7	0	158	118	222	107	.7	6.1	34	435	0	.48	.28	5.2	.7	137	0
.7	.8	0	172	145	280	105	1	6.6	52	473	0	.56	.34	5.7	.77	153	0
.7	.8	0	161	143	279	102	.9	6.4	42	451	0	.53	.33	5.4	.74	146	0
.6	.7	0	166	133	226	150	.7	6.6	36	441	0	.51	.36	5.5	.75	150	0
0	0	0	1	14	0	16	.1	.2	4	0	0	.02	.01	.4	.01	3	0
0	.1	0	3	43	0	42	.3	.6	17	0	0	.02	.03	1.3	.02	4	0
.2	.4	0	17	166	0	170	1.2	1.5	53	0	0	.17	.12	2.1	.18	26	0
.2	.3	0	11	96	183	71	.7	3.8	26	318	13	.31	.36	4.2	.43	9	1.27
0	0	0	6	8	7	95	.1	.4	10	0	0	0	.01	.1	.02	0	0
—	—	0	39	53	8	305	.7	.8	28	11	22	.06	.08	1	.27	56	0
—	—	0	21	46	2	277	.5	.4	19	8	13	.04	.06	.7	.19	29	0
1.5	.2	13	104	84	203	76	.6	.2	6	42	0	.01	.09	0	.03	1	.27
1.4	.1	17	152	110	326	60	.7	.1	6	51	0	0	.08	0	.01	1	.48
0	0	2	150	714	290	55	—	0	—	86	0	—	.07	—	—	—	—
4.1	1	1	12	22	210	33	.1	.5	4	7	0	.05	.07	.6	.03	24	.03
15.2	1.5	135	1371	1737	3281	590	6.3	.8	70	461	0	.12	1.05	.3	.28	17	.98
.7	.1	12	233	281	2	61	1.1	.1	8	22	0	.01	.13	0	.03	3	.26
1.5	.2	13	121	96	250	59	.6	.2	6	46	0	.01	.09	0	.03	2	.24
1.9	.2	20	129	156	300	34	.6	.1	5	61	0	.01	.07	0	.02	2	.15
.6	.1	10	194	234	405	51	.9	.1	7	18	0	.01	.11	0	.02	3	.22
2.2	.3	27	114	126	170	400	.3	.1	20	78	0	.09	.39	.2	.08	1	.69
7.8	1	99	1037	653	281	120	4.2	.2	39	273	0	.02	.39	.1	.09	7	1.81
2.4	.2	27	191	128	159	39	.7	.1	7	86	0	0	.1	0	.02	6	.36
10.5	1.1	102	713	522	1883	346	3.6	.4	31	308	0	.04	.52	1.4	.22	49	1.65
2.4	.3	26	172	118	173	40	.7	.2	7	77	0	.01	.1	.1	.02	5	.42
9.7	.9	107	762	510	633	154	3	.5	28	341	0	.02	.4	.1	.07	23	1.42
11.5	1.2	144	265	271	906	219	3.4	.7	29	262	0	.1	.75	.5	.34	94	2.38
17.3	1.8	177	954	854	2071	460	5.9	.8	49	620	0	.07	1.2	1.6	.56	153	3.2
2.4	.2	26	191	139	196	26	.8	.2	6	82	0	.01	.13	.1	.02	5	.08
—	—	17	277	—	105	—	—	.4	—	95	1	—	—	—	—	—	—
2.6	.3	28	199	137	6	32	.9	.2	8	82	0	.01	.11	0	.02	5	.24
.6	.1	6	199	137	6	32	.9	.2	8	18	0	.01	.01	0	.02	5	.24
10.6	1.1	119	815	579	702	111	3.5	.8	31	342	0	.03	.42	.1	.08	21	.94
2.5	.2	29	183	132	199	27	.8	.1	6	70	0	.01	.08	0	.02	5	.24
12.2	1.3	125	904	603	797	168	4.1	1	34	363	0	.02	.5	.1	.1	24	1.09
2.6	.3	28	199	137	6	32	.9	.2	8	82	0	.01	.11	0	.02	5	.24
.6	.1	6	199	137	6	32	.9	.2	8	18	0	.01	.01	0	.02	5	.24
10.5	1.1	107	774	516	683	144	3.5	.9	29	311	0	.02	.42	.1	.09	21	.93
.7	.1	10	138	303	918	193	.9	.3	12	25	0	.05	.37	.3	.15	28	1.43
1.2	.1	19	155	341	918	217	.9	.4	14	45	0	.05	.42	.3	.17	30	1.61
2.2	.2	25	108	237	915	151	.7	.2	9	81	0	.04	.29	.2	.12	22	1.12
2.9	.3	34	135	297	911	190	.8	.3	12	108	0	.05	.37	.3	.15	28	1.4
.7	.1	9	137	302	29	194	.9	.3	11	25	0	.04	.36	.3	.16	27	1.42
0	0	10	60	150	370	75	—	0	—	57	0	0	.17	—	.03	—	.6
2.7	.3	31	126	277	851	177	.8	.3	11	101	0	.04	.34	.3	.14	26	1.31
22.8	3	255	185	241	687	276	1.2	2.8	15	1013	0	.04	.46	.2	.11	31	.98
.8	.1	8	17	22	44	25	.1	.3	1	33	0	0	.04	0	.01	3	.09
0	0	2	100	150	160	65	.3	0	0	143	0	—	.34	—	—	—	.12
—	—	30	20	20	100	40	0	0	0	86	0	—	.03	—	—	—	0
2.3	.2	25	207	152	274	53	1.1	.1	8	72	0	.01	.11	0	.02	5	.44
11.4	1.4	219	1212	829	2745	152	7.1	1.6	47	315	0	.38	2.08	2.4	1.04	79	4.16
2.5	.5	33	156	98	227	18	1	.1	4	82	0	.01	.06	0	.02	2	.48
2.3	.2	30	254	207	98	14	.5	.5	15	156	0	.04	.34	.7	.02	1	.03
11.8	1.2	113	344	630	905	64	2.3	4.7	39	1131	0	.17	.94	1.1	.62	30	.47
2.4	.5	25	149	121	513	26	.6	.1	8	103	0	.01	.09	.2	.04	9	.26

EshaCode	Food Item	Qty	Meas	Wgt	Wtr	Cals	Prot	Carb	Fib	Fat	F_Sat
1054	Cheese, gouda	1	oz.	28	42	101	7	1	0	8	5
1074	Cheese, gruyere	1	oz.	28	33	117	8	0	0	9	5.4
1038	Cheese, havarti	1	oz.	28	41	105	7	1	0	8	5.3
1092	Cheese, imitation mozzarella, shredded	1	cup	113	61	202	18	14	0	8	5.2
1077	Cheese, liederkranz	1	oz.	28	53	87	5	0	0	8	5.3
1082	Cheese, light neufchatel (Kraft Philadelphia)	1	oz.	28	65	71	3	1	0	6	4
1055	Cheese, limburger	1	oz.	28	48	93	6	0	0	8	4.7
1018	Cheese, monterey jack, cubed	1	cup	132	41	492	32	1	0	40	25.2
1017	Cheese, monterey jack, shredded	1	cup	113	41	421	28	1	0	34	21.6
1059	Cheese, mozzarella sting/stick	1	each	28	54	72	7	1	0	5	2.9
1100	Cheese, mozzarella, low sodium	1	oz.	28	50	79	8	1	0	5	3.1
1101	Cheese, mozzarella, low sodium string/stick	1	each	28	50	79	8	1	0	5	3.1
1020	Cheese, mozzarella, lowfat, shredded	1	oz.	28	49	79	8	1	0	5	3.1
1019	Cheese, mozzarella, part skim, low moisture	1	cup	113	49	316	31	4	0	19	12.3
1058	Cheese, mozzarella, part skim, shredded	1	cup	113	54	287	28	3	0	18	11.4
1057	Cheese, mozzarella, whole milk, low moisture	1	cup	113	48	359	24	3	0	28	17.6
1056	Cheese, mozzarella, whole milk, shredded	1	cup	113	54	318	22	3	0	24	14.9
1021	Cheese, muenster	1	cup	113	42	416	26	1	0	34	21.6
1102	Cheese, muenster, low sodium	1	oz.	28	43	104	7	0	0	9	5.4
1060	Cheese, neufchatel	1	cup	235	62	611	23	7	0	55	34.8
1075	Cheese, parmesan, grated	1	cup	100	18	456	42	4	0	30	19.1
1061	Cheese, parmesan, hard, cubed	1	each	10	29	40	4	0	0	3	1.7
1103	Cheese, parmesan, low sodium, grated	1	cup	100	22	456	42	4	0	30	19.1
1112	Cheese, parmesan, shredded	2	oz.	57	25	235	22	2	0	16	9.9
1069	Cheese, pimento processed	1	oz.	28	39	106	6	0	0	9	5.6
1062	Cheese, port du salut	1	oz.	28	46	100	7	0	0	8	4.7
1023	Cheese, provolone	1	oz.	28	41	100	7	1	0	8	4.8
1024	Cheese, ricotta, part skim	1	cup	246	74	339	28	13	0	20	12.1
1064	Cheese, ricotta, whole milk	1	cup	246	72	428	28	8	0	32	20.4
1066	Cheese, romano, grated	1	cup	100	31	387	32	4	0	27	17.1
1026	Cheese, roquefort, crumbled	1	cup	135	39	498	29	3	0	41	26.1
1025	Cheese, roquefort, cubed	1	each	17	39	64	4	0	0	5	3.3
1035	Cheese, swiss	1	oz.	28	37	107	8	1	0	8	5
1428	Cheese, swiss, low fat, Alpine Lace	.25	cup	31	43	100	9	1	0	7	4.4
1104	Cheese, swiss, low sodium	1	oz.	28	38	107	8	1	0	8	5
1027	Cheese, swiss, shredded	1	cup	108	37	406	31	4	0	30	19.2
1067	Cheese, tilsit, whole milk	1	oz.	28	43	96	7	1	0	7	4.8
1114	Cheese, white cheddar	1	cup	113	37	455	28	1	0	37	23.8
1085	Cheese, yogurt	1	oz.	28	76	22	2	3	0	0	0
3242	Cherimoya, raw	1	each	547	74	514	7	131	13.1	2	—
3247	Cherries, ground, raw	1	cup	140	85	74	3	16	4.3	1	—
3459	Cherries, maraschino	1	cup	161	70	187	0	47	—	0	.1
3335	Cherries, sour, canned in extra heavy syrup	1	cup	261	70	298	2	76	3.4	0	.1
3035	Cherries, sour, canned in water	1	cup	244	90	88	2	22	2	0	.1
3159	Cherries, sour, frozen, unsweetened	1	cup	155	87	71	1	17	1.9	1	.2
3334	Cherries, sour, red, fresh, pitted	1	cup	155	86	78	2	19	1.9	0	.1
3038	Cherries, sweet, canned in heavy syrup	1	cup	257	78	213	2	55	1.8	0	.1
3336	Cherries, sweet, canned in juice	1	cup	250	85	135	2	34	1.8	0	0
3036	Cherries, sweet, fresh	10	each	68	81	49	1	11	1.2	1	.1
3037	Cherries, sweet, fresh, cup measure	1	cup	145	81	104	2	24	2.5	1	.3
3158	Cherries, sweet, frozen, sweetened	1	cup	259	76	231	3	58	2.6	0	.1
49023	Cherry crisp	1	cup	246	39	710	5	112	2.3	28	6.2
49007	Cherry crisp, piece, 3x3 in	1	piece	138	75	158	2	28	1.1	5	1
45552	Cherry turnover	1	each	78	41	238	3	31	.9	12	2.9
26108	Chervil, dried	1	Tbs	2	7	4	0	1	.2	0	—
4646	Chestnuts, Chinese, cooked	2	oz.	57	62	87	2	19	—	0	.1
4645	Chestnuts, Chinese, dried	2	oz.	57	9	206	4	45	—	1	.2
4644	Chestnuts, Chinese, raw	2	oz.	57	44	127	2	28	—	1	.1
4647	Chestnuts, Chinese, roasted	2	oz.	57	40	136	3	30	—	1	.1
4648	Chestnuts, European, cooked	2	oz.	57	68	74	1	16	3.8	1	.1
4530	Chestnuts, European, raw, peeled	1	oz.	28	52	56	0	12	1.4	0	.1
4538	Chestnuts, European, roasted, cup measure	1	cup	143	40	350	5	76	9	3	.6
4539	Chestnuts, European, roasted, whole	17	each	143	40	350	5	76	9	3	.6
25125	Chewing gum, Care Free sugarless	1	piece	2	—	5	0	2	—	0	—
44032	Chex party mix	.667	cup	28	4	120	3	18	—	5	—

FM_Un	FP_Un	Choles	Calc	Phos	Sodium	Pota	Zinc	Iron	Magnes	A_RE	Vit_C	B1	B2	B3	B6	Fola	B12
2.2	.2	32	198	155	232	34	1.1	.1	8	49	0	.01	.1	0	.02	6	.44
2.8	.5	31	287	172	95	23	1.1	0	10	85	0	.02	.08	0	.02	3	.45
2.4	.2	27	191	128	159	39	.7	.1	7	86	0	0	.1	0	.02	6	.36
2.4	.2	22	645	823	1296	261	2.9	.1	30	90	0	.04	.44	.2	.15	5	.51
2.2	.2	21	110	100	390	68	.7	.1	7	91	0	.01	.18	.1	.04	34	.26
—	—	20	20	40	122	30	0	0	0	58	0	—	.03	—	—	—	0
2.4	.1	26	141	111	227	36	.6	0	6	90	0	.02	.14	0	.02	16	.3
11.6	1.2	117	985	586	708	107	4	1	36	334	0	.02	.52	.1	.1	24	1.09
9.9	1	101	843	502	606	91	3.4	.8	30	286	0	.02	.44	.1	.09	21	.93
1.3	.1	16	183	131	132	24	.8	.1	7	50	0	0	.09	0	.02	2	.23
1.4	.1	15	207	149	5	27	.9	.1	7	54	0	.01	.1	0	.02	3	.26
1.4	.1	15	207	149	5	27	.9	.1	7	54	0	.01	.1	0	.02	3	.26
1.4	.1	15	207	149	150	27	.9	.1	7	54	0	.01	.1	0	.02	3	.26
5.5	.6	61	826	592	597	107	3.6	.3	30	216	0	.02	.39	.1	.09	11	1.05
5.1	.5	65	730	523	527	95	3.1	.2	26	200	0	.02	.34	.1	.08	10	.92
7.9	.9	101	650	466	469	84	2.8	.2	23	310	0	.02	.3	.1	.07	9	.82
7.4	.9	89	584	419	421	76	2.5	.2	21	272	0	.02	.28	.1	.06	8	.74
9.8	.7	108	810	529	710	151	3.2	.5	31	357	0	.02	.36	.1	.06	14	1.66
2.5	.2	27	203	133	5	38	.8	.1	8	90	0	0	.09	0	.02	3	.42
15.9	1.5	179	177	320	938	268	1.2	.7	18	620	0	.04	.46	.3	.1	27	.62
8.7	.7	79	1375	807	1861	107	3.2	1	51	173	0	.04	.39	.3	.1	8	1.4
.8	.1	7	122	72	165	10	.3	.1	4	15	0	0	.03	0	.01	1	.12
8.7	.7	79	1376	807	63	107	3.2	1	51	173	0	.04	.39	.3	.1	8	1.4
5	.4	41	710	417	962	55	1.8	.5	29	98	0	.02	.2	.2	.06	5	.79
2.5	.3	27	174	211	405	46	.8	.1	6	91	1	.01	.1	0	.02	2	.2
2.6	.2	35	184	102	151	39	.7	.1	7	105	0	0	.07	0	.02	5	.42
2.1	.2	20	214	141	248	39	.9	.1	8	75	0	0	.09	0	.02	3	.41
5.7	.6	76	669	450	308	308	3.3	1.1	36	278	0	.05	.46	.2	.05	32	.72
8.9	.9	124	509	389	207	258	2.9	.9	28	330	0	.03	.48	.3	.11	30	.83
7.8	.6	104	1063	760	1200	86	2.6	.8	41	141	0	.04	.37	.1	.08	7	1.12
11.4	1.8	122	894	529	2442	122	2.8	.8	40	404	0	.05	.79	1	.17	66	.87
1.5	.2	16	115	68	313	16	.4	.1	5	52	0	.01	.1	.1	.02	8	.11
2.1	.3	26	272	172	74	32	1.1	0	10	72	0	.01	.1	0	.02	2	.48
—	—	22	277	—	39	—	—	.4	—	95	1	—	—	—	—	—	—
2.1	.3	26	272	172	4	32	1.1	0	10	72	0	.01	.1	0	.02	2	.48
7.8	1	99	1037	653	281	120	4.2	.2	39	273	0	.02	.39	.1	.09	7	1.81
2	.2	29	198	142	213	18	1	.1	4	82	0	.02	.1	.1	.02	6	.6
10.6	1.1	119	815	579	702	111	3.5	.8	31	286	0	.03	.42	.1	.08	21	.94
0	0	1	56	44	22	72	.3	0	5	1	0	.01	.06	0	.01	3	.17
—	—	0	126	219	—	—	—	2.7	—	5	49	.55	.6	7.1	—	—	0
—	—	0	13	56	—	—	—	1.4	—	101	15	.15	.06	3.9	—	—	0
.1	.1	0	24	21	2	203	—	.5	—	0	0	0	0	0	—	—	0
.1	.1	0	26	24	18	238	.2	3.3	13	182	5	.04	.1	.4	.12	19	0
.1	.1	0	27	24	17	239	.2	3.4	15	184	5	.04	.1	.4	.11	20	0
.2	.2	0	20	25	2	192	.2	.8	14	135	3	.07	.05	.2	.1	7	0
.1	.1	0	25	23	5	268	.2	.5	14	198	16	.05	.06	.6	.07	12	0
.1	.1	0	23	46	8	373	.3	.9	23	40	9	.05	.1	1	.08	11	0
0	0	0	35	55	8	328	.2	1.4	30	31	6	.04	.06	1	.08	10	0
.2	.2	0	10	13	0	152	0	.3	7	15	5	.03	.04	.3	.02	3	0
.4	.4	0	22	28	0	325	.1	.6	16	31	10	.07	.09	.6	.05	6	0
.1	.1	0	31	41	3	515	.1	.9	26	49	3	.07	.12	.5	.09	11	0
13.2	7.3	0	157	284	592	223	.3	3.7	20	305	3	.27	.27	2.2	.09	16	.02
2.4	1.7	0	29	23	73	164	.2	2.2	12	145	3	.07	.08	.6	.06	10	.01
5.1	3.1	0	8	28	212	58	.2	1.6	7	27	1	.14	.11	1.2	.02	6	0
—	—	0	26	9	2	90	.2	.6	2	—	—	—	—	—	.02	—	0
.2	.1	0	7	37	1	174	.3	.6	33	8	14	.06	.07	.3	.16	26	0
.5	.3	0	16	88	3	412	.8	1.3	78	19	33	.15	.17	.7	.38	62	0
.3	.2	0	10	54	2	253	.5	.8	48	12	20	.09	.1	.5	.23	38	0
.4	.2	0	11	58	2	270	.5	.9	51	6	22	.08	.05	.9	.25	41	0
.3	.3	0	26	56	15	405	.1	1	31	1	15	.08	.06	.4	.13	22	0
.1	.1	0	5	11	1	137	.1	.3	9	1	11	.04	0	.3	.1	16	0
1.1	1.2	0	42	153	3	847	.8	1.3	47	3	37	.35	.25	1.9	.71	100	0
1.1	1.2	0	42	153	3	847	.8	1.3	47	3	37	.35	.25	1.9	.71	100	0
0	0	—	—	—	0	0	—	—	—	—	—	—	—	—	—	—	0
—	—	0	10	53	288	76	.6	7	18	4	14	.44	.14	4.8	.44	0	3.52

EshaCode	Food Item	Qty.	Meas	Wgt	Wtr	Cals	Prot	Carb	Fib	Fat	F_Sat
4610	Chia seeds, dried	1	oz.	28	5	134	5	14	7.2	7	3
56213	Chicken & dumplings, Chicken Helper	1	cup	244	71	373	27	20	.6	20	5.7
56090	Chicken & noodles, recipe	1	cup	240	71	367	22	26	1.8	18	5.9
15023	Chicken hearts, simmered	1	each	3	65	6	1	0	0	0	.1
15065	Chicken nuggets, fast food serving	1	each	102	49	290	17	16	.6	18	5.6
15927	Chicken parmigiana	1	piece	182	66	317	28	15	1.4	16	5.4
15902	Chicken patty, breaded, cooked	1	each	75	49	213	12	11	.3	13	4.1
16233	Chicken pot pie, Banquet	1	each	198	67	350	10	36	3	18	7
15037	Chicken roll, light meat	2	piece	57	69	91	11	1	0	4	1.2
56002	Chicken salad, w/celery	.5	cup	78	53	268	11	1	.2	25	4
15915	Chicken teriyaki, breast	1	each	128	67	176	26	7	.2	4	.9
15916	Chicken teriyaki, drumstick	1	each	68	67	93	14	4	.1	2	.5
15050	Chicken, back, skinless, fried	.5	each	58	48	167	17	3	.1	9	2.4
15051	Chicken, back, skinless, roasted	.5	each	40	59	96	11	0	0	5	1.4
15014	Chicken, back, w/skin, flour fried	1	each	72	44	238	20	5	.2	15	4
15015	Chicken, back, w/skin, roasted	1	each	53	54	159	14	0	0	11	3.1
15016	Chicken, boned, w/broth, can	1	each	142	69	234	31	0	0	11	3.1
15039	Chicken, breast meat, skinless, stewed	1	each	95	68	143	28	0	0	3	.8
15001	Chicken, breast w/skin, roasted	1	each	98	62	193	29	0	0	8	2.2
15057	Chicken, breast, skinless, fried	1	each	86	60	161	29	0	0	4	1.1
15004	Chicken, breast, skinless, roasted	1	each	86	65	142	27	0	0	3	.9
15003	Chicken, breast, w/skin, flour fried	1	each	98	57	218	31	2	.1	9	2.4
15038	Chicken, breast, w/skin, stewed	1	each	110	66	202	30	0	0	8	2.3
15208	Chicken, canned in water, Swanson	.25	cup	62	—	80	15	1	0	1	.5
15018	Chicken, canned, diced, dark meat	1	cup	205	69	338	45	0	0	16	4.5
15020	Chicken, canned, diced, light & dark meat	1	cup	205	69	338	45	0	0	16	4.5
15022	Chicken, canned, diced, light meat	1	cup	205	69	338	45	0	0	16	4.5
15026	Chicken, dark meat, skinless, fried	1	cup	140	56	335	41	4	.1	16	4.4
15027	Chicken, dark meat, skinless, roasted	1	cup	140	63	287	38	0	0	14	3.7
15030	Chicken, drumstick, batter fried	1	each	72	53	193	16	6	.2	11	3
15007	Chicken, drumstick, flour fried	1	each	49	57	120	13	1	0	7	1.8
15008	Chicken, drumstick, roasted	1	each	52	63	112	14	0	0	6	1.6
15042	Chicken, drumstick, skinless, fried	1	each	42	62	82	12	0	0	3	.9
15035	Chicken, drumstick, skinless, roasted	1	each	44	67	76	12	0	0	2	.7
15063	Chicken, fried, dark meat, 2 piece serving	1	each	148	49	431	30	16	.9	27	7
15064	Chicken, fried, white meat, 2 piece serving	1	each	163	46	494	36	20	1.1	30	7.8
15025	Chicken, gizzard, simmered	1	each	22	67	34	6	0	0	1	.2
15031	Chicken, light meat, skinless, fried	1	cup	140	60	269	46	1	0	8	2.1
15032	Chicken, light meat, skinless, roasted	1	cup	140	65	242	43	0	0	6	1.8
15092	Chicken, liver pate, canned	1	Tbs	13	66	26	2	1	0	2	.5
15005	Chicken, liver, simmered	7	each	140	68	220	34	1	0	8	2.6
15028	Chicken, meat, all types, skinless, fried	1	cup	140	58	307	43	2	.1	13	3.5
15000	Chicken, meat, all types, skinless, roasted	1	cup	140	64	266	40	0	0	10	2.9
15006	Chicken, meat, all types, skinless, stewed	1	cup	140	67	248	38	0	0	9	2.6
15131	Chicken, roaster, skinless, roasted	1	cup	140	67	234	35	0	0	9	2.6
15087	Chicken, skinless, stewed	1	cup	140	56	332	43	0	0	17	4.4
15088	Chicken, stewer w/giblets, cooked	1	each	593	54	1636	157	0	0	107	29.1
15011	Chicken, thigh, skinless, fried	1	each	52	59	113	15	1	0	5	1.4
15012	Chicken, thigh, skinless, roasted	1	each	52	63	109	14	0	0	6	1.6
15009	Chicken, thigh, w/skin, flour fried	1	each	62	54	162	17	2	.1	9	2.5
15010	Chicken, thigh, w/skin, roasted	1	each	62	59	153	16	0	0	10	2.7
15074	Chicken, whole, roasted	1	each	598	60	1429	163	0	0	81	22.7
15075	Chicken, whole, stewed	1	each	668	64	1462	165	0	0	84	23.4
15029	Chicken, wing, flour fried	1	each	32	49	103	8	1	0	7	1.9
15048	Chicken, wing, skinless, fried	1	each	20	60	42	6	0	0	2	.5
15059	Chicken, wing, skinless, roasted	1	each	21	63	43	6	0	0	2	.5
15002	Chicken, wing, w/skin, roasted	3	each	102	55	296	27	0	0	20	5.6
15903	Chicken, wings, buffalo type/spicy	1	piece	16	53	49	4	0	0	3	.9
6119	Chile, banana, cooked	100	grams	100	89	15	1	2	1.6	0	—
6118	Chile, banana, raw	100	grams	100	90	14	1	2	1.4	0	—
56112	Chiles rellenos	1	each	143	52	425	23	7	1	35	17
56001	Chili & beans, canned	1	cup	255	76	286	15	30	11.2	14	6
26072	Chili pepper, dried, Foran Spice	10	grams	10	6	42	1	6	1.6	1	—
26002	Chili powder	1	Tbs	8	8	24	1	4	2.6	1	.3
6532	Chilies, green, canned, Santiago	1	each	62	93	13	0	3	.7	0	0

A

FM_Un	FP_Un	Choles	Calc	Phos	Sodium	Pota	Zinc	Iron	Magnes	A_RE	Vit_C	B1	B2	B3	B6	Fola	B12
—	—	70	—	—	1280	—	—	—	—	—	—	—	—	—	—	—	—
2	—	10	123	—	120	180	—	2	—	—	—	—	—	—	—	—	—
—	—	25	—	—	290	—	—	—	—	—	—	—	—	—	—	—	—
—	—	—	—	—	12	—	—	—	—	0	120	—	—	—	—	—	0
9.2	6.2	0	17	95	0	124	1.2	.6	49	4	1	.25	.04	.3	.05	11	0
.4	1	0	16	69	292	16	1.7	1.5	28	0	0	0	0	0	.02	2	0
.4	.6	0	16	56	336	14	1.7	1	26	0	—	0	.01	.1	.01	2	0
.4	.6	0	16	56	336	14	1.7	1	26	18	0	0	.01	.1	.01	2	0
0	0	0	20	14	14	176	.7	1.4	7	0	8	0	.13	.4	.08	7	0
0	0	0	9	5	14	44	.2	.1	4	0	0	0	0	0	.01	2	0
2.6	.3	33	298	270	123	480	1.2	.8	56	85	2	.1	.44	.4	.11	12	.87
6.6	1.2	51	19	192	480	166	.8	3.3	10	6	3	.22	.4	3.8	.05	50	.3
7.8	.9	28	6	49	638	95	1	.7	6	0	15	.11	.07	1.5	.07	2	.75
7.8	.8	35	11	50	585	95	1.2	.8	2	0	14	.03	.06	1.4	.07	2	.88
3.8	1.8	46	43	48	617	38	.5	.9	4	17	0	.03	.05	1.4	.14	2	.11
2.5	2.2	48	48	60	642	81	1.4	.8	6	0	0	.02	.08	1.9	.1	4	.13
8.8	7.8	0	123	276	600	428	2.7	3.9	71	6	19	.23	.13	1	.98	146	0
—	—	60	300	—	2120	—	—	4.5	—	—	5	—	—	—	—	—	—
.7	1.6	10	61	42	147	32	.1	.7	5	9	0	.08	.07	.6	.02	4	.04
2.3	.8	20	207	228	182	395	.9	.6	33	57	2	.06	.3	1.1	.13	9	.65
2.7	1	21	161	155	92	271	.7	.3	24	58	2	.06	.28	.9	.08	18	.64
.6	.1	7	62	48	42	102	.4	.1	7	22	1	.02	.1	.1	.02	4	.24
3	1	21	72	86	48	151	.7	.4	21	55	0	.04	.14	.9	.04	7	.18
.1	0	1	129	99	55	173	.3	.1	14	2	0	.03	.18	.1	.05	1	.62
2.3	.4	24	70	62	43	126	.4	.2	11	63	0	.02	.13	.1	.03	3	.21
5.4	1.3	26	104	123	60	206	.9	.6	40	69	0	.05	.25	.6	.04	9	.23
2.6	.8	1	136	62	50	129	.3	.4	16	25	0	.02	.1	.5	.12	6	.2
.1	.1	0	1	4	6	4	0	.1	1	0	0	.01	.01	.2	0	0	0
2	.3	18	96	89	51	176	.4	.4	17	62	0	.04	.14	.3	.03	4	.27
.1	.1	0	4	10	32	14	.1	.4	3	0	0	.05	.04	.5	0	0	0
2.3	.4	32	102	88	72	158	.5	.2	11	84	0	.04	.2	.3	.04	4	.28
2.8	.4	29	95	89	66	169	.6	.4	18	77	0	.04	.19	.3	.04	4	.26
1.7	.4	20	60	64	36	122	.4	.3	13	53	0	.03	.12	.2	.03	5	.18
94.1	45.4	505	1733	2076	2765	3607	11.6	13.5	441	1377	7	.75	4.33	8.9	.75	94	4.98
1.7	.4	20	60	64	36	122	.4	.3	13	53	0	.03	.12	.2	.03	5	.18
.8	.2	10	30	31	18	60	.2	.1	6	26	0	.02	.06	.1	.01	2	.09
—	—	80	100	—	95	—	—	1.1	—	150	1	—	—	—	—	—	—
—	—	70	100	—	50	—	—	1.1	—	100	1	—	—	—	—	—	—
—	7	100	107	107	80	170	—	—	—	160	—	.16	.18	—	—	—	—
7.1	.7	38	74	139	56	260	1.1	1.1	63	95	0	.03	.21	.3	.04	2	.23
—	0	2	100	141	50	240	—	0	—	40	0	—	—	—	—	—	—
2	0	20	48	32	30	150	—	—	—	40	—	—	.1	—	—	—	.04
2.1	.3	22	72	71	50	164	.4	.6	19	78	0	.03	.13	.1	.04	11	.19
—	0	2	100	141	90	254	—	—	—	60	2	.03	.15	—	—	—	—
—	—	—	107	213	90	300	—	1.2	—	21	—	.1	.14	2.1	—	—	—
1	.3	0	179	162	96	357	1.6	.6	34	0	1	.06	.3	.2	.08	4	.75
.8	.2	0	180	142	97	287	1.4	.1	20	0	1	.05	.29	.1	.08	3	.77
.8	.2	0	180	142	97	287	1.4	.1	20	0	1	.05	.29	.1	.08	3	.77
—	—	60	64	64	30	114	—	0	—	85	6	.03	.11	.8	—	—	—
—	1.4	2	100	141	70	226	—	0	—	40	0	.03	.15	—	—	—	—
—	0	2	100	9	60	168	—	0	—	40	0	.03	.15	—	—	—	—
—	0	2	100	9	60	168	—	0	—	40	0	.03	.15	—	—	—	—
4.9	.6	43	206	184	89	384	1	.7	37	147	1	.07	.27	.2	.06	9	.64
3	.4	78	113	100	52	152	.4	.2	10	132	1	.04	.16	.1	.04	8	.43
1.6	.2	19	79	66	40	124	.2	.1	9	52	5	.03	.17	.1	.03	8	.2
—	—	2	100	—	50	—	—	0	—	8	0	—	—	—	—	—	—
2	0	20	64	48	40	125	—	—	—	40	—	.03	.14	—	—	—	.08
—	—	2	100	—	60	—	—	.4	—	8	0	—	—	—	—	—	—
2.1	.3	29	84	69	53	131	.5	.1	9	77	0	.03	.16	.1	.03	3	.26
2	.3	25	80	80	50	140	—	.1	—	60	—	.03	.15	—	—	—	.12
—	0	5	100	141	50	254	—	—	—	60	2	.05	.22	—	—	—	—
3.5	.4	45	87	70	41	118	.3	0	8	136	1	.03	.12	.1	.03	4	.27
1.2	.2	12	189	157	82	310	.8	.3	26	35	1	.06	.24	.2	.06	8	.59
2.4	.3	23	211	174	91	343	.8	.4	28	73	1	.07	.27	.2	.06	9	.66
1.7	.3	31	218	160	125	324	.7	.2	22	54	1	.1	.41	.2	.1	4	1.02

EshaCode	Food Item	Qty.	Meas	Wgt	Wtr	Cals	Prot	Carb	Fib	Fat	F_Sat
2059	Ice milk, strawberry, Breyer's Light	1	cup	136	61	245	6	37	0	8	5
2058	Ice milk, vanilla, Breyer's Light	1	cup	136	61	245	6	37	0	8	5
2009	Ice milk, vanilla, hard	.5	cup	66	68	92	3	15	.1	3	1.7
2010	Ice milk, vanilla, soft, 3% fat	.5	cup	88	70	111	4	19	.1	2	1.4
23051	Ice slushy	1	cup	193	67	151	1	63	0	0	0
23160	Ices, fruit flavor, sugar-free	1	each	51	93	12	0	3	—	0	—
23159	Ices, lime	.5	cup	96	67	75	0	31	0	0	0
42202	Injera (Ethiopian bread), 12 inch loaf	1	each	127	63	173	6	38	1.3	1	.3
62177	Instant breakfast, vanilla, Carnation	1	cup	281	12	975	56	167	0	0	0
101	Instant breakfast, w/1% milk	1	cup	281	79	233	15	36	.2	3	2
26	Instant breakfast, w/2% milk	1	cup	281	78	252	16	36	.2	5	3.3
27	Instant breakfast, w/nonfat milk	1	cup	282	80	216	16	36	.2	1	.6
25	Instant breakfast, w/whole milk	1	cup	281	77	280	15	36	.2	9	5.4
56430	Jack in the Box, BreakfastJack sandwich	1	each	121	49	300	18	30	0	12	5
56436	Jack in the Box, Jumbo Jack	1	each	229	55	560	26	41	0	32	10
56437	Jack in the Box, Jumbo Jack w/cheese	1	each	242	55	610	29	41	0	36	12
69032	Jack in the Box, bacon cheeseburger	1	each	242	49	710	35	41	0	45	15
69063	Jack in the Box, chicken caesar pita sandwich	1	each	237	59	520	27	44	4	26	6
69035	Jack in the Box, chicken sandwich	1	each	160	52	400	20	38	0	18	4
90094	Jack in the Box, cinnamon churritos, serving	1	each	75	21	330	3	34	3	21	5
56441	Jack in the Box, fajita, chicken pita	1	each	189	67	290	24	29	3	8	3
69036	Jack in the Box, fried steak sandwich	1	each	153	46	450	14	42	0	25	7
69033	Jack in the Box, hamburger, sourdough, grilled	1	each	223	48	670	32	39	0	43	16
69064	Jack in the Box, monterey roast beef sandwich	1	each	238	57	540	30	40	3	30	9
69040	Jack in the Box, sourdough breakfast sandwich	1	each	147	49	380	21	31	0	20	7
69065	Jack in the Box, ultimate breakfast sandwich	1	each	242	53	620	36	39	—	35	11
3248	Jackfruit, raw	2	oz.	57	73	53	1	14	.9	0	—
23175	Jam, cherry/strawberry	1	Tbs	20	29	54	0	14	—	0	0
23002	Jam, not cherry/strawberry	1	Tbs	20	29	54	0	14	.2	0	0
23166	Jam/marmalade, artificially sweetened	1	Tbs	20	46	2	0	11	.5	0	0
23054	Jam/preserves, 1 pkt	1	Tbs	20	34	48	0	13	.2	0	0
23167	Jam/preserves/marmalade, reduced sugar	1	Tbs	20	52	36	0	9	.6	0	0
3249	Java plum/jambolan, fresh	3	each	9	83	5	0	1	.1	0	—
23003	Jelly	1	Tbs	18	28	49	0	13	.2	0	0
23092	Jelly, dietetic	1	Tbs	19	42	6	0	11	.2	0	0
23004	Jelly, packet	1	each	14	28	38	0	10	.1	0	0
23165	Jelly, reduced sugar, all flavors	1	Tbs	19	53	34	0	9	.2	0	0
5224	Jicama, raw	1	cup	120	90	46	1	11	5.9	0	0
5436	Jicama/Yambean tuber, sliced, cooked	1	cup	100	90	38	1	9	1.1	0	0
5435	Jicama/Yambean tuber, sliced, raw	1	cup	120	90	46	1	11	3.7	0	0
3226	Juice drink, cranberry apricot, w/vitamin C	1	cup	253	83	170	0	43	.3	0	0
3225	Juice drink, cranberry blueberry, w/vitamin C	1	cup	253	83	170	0	43	.3	0	0
3227	Juice drink, cranberry grape, w/vitamin C	1	cup	253	83	170	0	43	.3	0	0
3224	Juice drink, cranberry raspberry, w/vitamin C	1	cup	253	83	170	0	43	.3	0	0
20280	Juice drink, orange, CapriSun Natural	1.2	cup	211	—	100	0	26	0	0	0
3238	Juice, acerola, fresh	1	cup	242	94	51	1	12	.7	1	—
3327	Juice, apple, frozen w/vit C, prepared	1	cup	239	88	112	0	28	.2	0	0
3328	Juice, apple, w/vit C, canned/bottled	1	cup	248	88	117	0	29	.2	0	0
3319	Juice, apple-cherry	1	cup	250	88	117	1	29	.8	0	.1
3321	Juice, apple-grape	1	cup	244	86	128	1	32	.2	0	.1
3320	Juice, apple-raspberry	1	cup	239	89	108	0	26	.2	0	0
20057	Juice, beef broth & tomato, canned	2	Tbs	30	90	11	0	3	.1	0	0
20042	Juice, clam and tomato	.69	cup	166	88	76	1	18	.2	0	0
3165	Juice, grapefruit, canned, sweetened	1	cup	250	87	115	1	28	.2	0	0
3092	Juice, orange, chilled	1	cup	249	88	110	2	25	.5	1	.1
3090	Juice, orange, fresh	1	cup	248	88	112	2	26	.5	0	.1
3091	Juice, orange, frozen concentrate, prepared	1	cup	249	88	112	2	27	.5	0	0
3093	Juice, orange, unsweetened, canned	1	cup	249	89	105	1	25	.5	0	0
3094	Juice, orange, unsweetened, frozen concentrate	.75	cup	213	58	339	5	81	1.7	0	.1
3200	Juice, passion fruit, purple, fresh	1	cup	247	86	126	1	34	.5	0	—
3201	Juice, passion fruit, yellow	1	cup	247	84	148	2	36	.5	0	—
3120	Juice, pineapple, canned, unsweetened	1	cup	250	86	140	1	34	.2	0	0
3119	Juice, pineapple, frozen concentrate, prepared	1	cup	250	86	130	1	32	.2	0	0
3323	Juice, pineapple, sweetened	1	cup	252	84	158	1	39	.2	0	0
3128	Juice, prune, bottled	1	cup	256	81	182	2	45	2.6	0	0

FM_Un	FP_Un	Choles	Calc	Phos	Sodium	Pota	Zinc	Iron	Magnes	A_RE	Vit_C	B1	B2	B3	B6	Fola	B12
3.8	1.1	42	134	178	768	282	2.6	2.7	27	—	2	.33	.31	3.8	.15	24	1.2
4.5	1.6	234	151	270	730	199	1.6	2.4	24	100	2	.49	.45	3.3	.15	33	.67
.2	0	3	132	101	84	175	—	.2	—	—	1	0	.02	.2	—	—	—
.1	.7	24	371	354	241	542	—	1	—	—	3	.12	.51	.4	.1	—	—
.1	.6	24	366	329	170	542	—	.3	—	—	3	.12	.51	.4	.11	—	—
.1	.6	24	360	327	194	534	—	.3	—	—	3	.12	.51	.3	—	—	—
2.3	1.9	0	7	51	332	213	.2	.3	11	0	3	.08	.02	.9	.08	8	—
4.6	5.8	11	108	503	746	285	.5	2	27	—	0	.24	.26	1.9	.09	0	.26
4.6	2.8	0	6	24	179	67	.2	1	6	10	1	.13	.09	1	.03	3	0
7.5	4.1	76	202	267	931	455	4.8	4.3	46	—	3	.49	.44	6.1	.25	49	2.25
3.7	2.4	42	9	199	353	210	.7	.6	17	0	0	.08	.11	5.2	.21	—	.21
—	—	35	80	—	310	—	—	.7	—	20	6	—	—	—	—	—	—
8.5	10.2	52	129	223	799	320	1.1	2.5	33	—	1	.91	.24	7.8	.39	37	.05
6.7	1.3	70	127	207	692	405	4.7	4.3	34	—	3	.39	.32	6.8	.24	27	2.58
8.7	1.6	97	143	—	1160	—	—	4.5	—	—	3	.39	.43	6.8	.26	33	2.89
3.7	.8	0	68	353	836	105	.3	1.8	9	0	0	.29	.23	2.2	.03	5	—
—	—	135	100	—	580	—	—	1.4	—	100	6	—	—	—	—	—	—
3.7	2.4	42	9	199	353	210	.7	.6	17	0	0	.08	.11	5.2	.21	—	.21
1.6	1	76	54	277	318	673	1.5	1.6	44	—	30	.51	.21	8.5	.52	83	.28
.5	1.1	47	117	327	506	433	.9	2.4	42	—	5	.43	.28	12.1	.55	38	.16
—	—	55	—	—	320	—	—	—	—	15	6	—	—	—	—	—	—
—	—	42	78	0	291	113	—	1	—	100	1	.3	.17	2	—	—	—
—	—	51	92	0	280	112	—	1.6	—	—	1	.3	.26	3	—	—	—
—	—	44	86	0	296	94	—	1	—	—	1	.3	.17	2	—	—	—
12	1.5	0	14	—	150	—	—	.7	—	0	12	.23	0	3	—	—	—
2.8	.9	28	126	113	533	261	2.3	2.7	24	—	2	.33	.26	3.8	.14	21	1.05
2.3	1.9	0	7	51	332	213	.2	.3	11	0	3	.08	.02	.9	.08	8	—
5.3	1.7	424	50	172	143	126	1.1	1.2	10	—	0	.07	.51	.1	.12	44	1.11
.1	.1	0	17	21	54	484	.3	.5	24	306	11	.29	.04	1.1	.18	44	0
.1	.1	0	18	27	14	494	.3	.3	18	515	68	.06	.03	.9	.18	27	0
.1	.2	0	29	45	24	825	.4	.6	29	860	113	.1	.06	1.5	.31	45	0
.3	.5	0	82	115	197	3444	1.2	6.6	131	49	262	.98	.33	6.6	.95	385	0
0	0	0	8	12	20	357	.1	.7	14	5	27	.1	.03	.7	.1	40	0
0	0	0	8	13	13	350	.1	.1	9	5	32	.1	.02	.8	.08	39	0
0	0	0	10	17	17	461	.1	.1	12	7	42	.13	.03	1	.1	51	0
2.6	.4	34	384	313	244	620	1.2	3.8	53	901	34	.73	1.26	10.9	1.02	32	.88
2.6	.4	34	305	265	172	498	1.1	.6	48	80	3	.13	.44	.6	.14	16	.93
2.5	.4	34	371	307	204	572	1.1	3.6	48	742	29	.71	1.14	10.4	.87	22	1.03
.8	.1	10	303	237	124	384	1	.1	34	145	2	.1	.41	.2	.11	12	.9
.8	.1	10	550	237	125	385	1	.1	34	146	2	.1	.41	.2	.11	13	.91
.7	.1	10	300	235	123	381	1	.1	34	144	2	.1	.41	.2	.1	12	.9
.8	.1	10	349	273	143	443	1.1	.1	39	145	3	.11	.47	.3	.12	14	1.05
1.4	.2	18	298	232	122	376	1	.1	33	139	2	.1	.4	.2	.1	12	.89
1.4	.2	19	352	276	145	448	1.1	.1	40	140	3	.11	.48	.2	.12	15	1.05
2.7	.4	28	327	271	122	498	.7	.1	34	137	3	.12	.34	.7	.11	1	.16
.8	.1	7	288	258	152	425	1	.6	33	148	2	.1	.42	.3	.1	12	.86
1.5	.2	17	285	255	151	423	1	.6	33	143	2	.09	.41	.3	.1	12	.85
.4	0	4	292	265	121	486	1.2	.7	46	142	2	.09	.34	.3	.1	14	.88
2.4	.3	34	292	229	147	460	.9	2.7	32	321	2	.1	.55	6.5	.1	12	.87
2.5	.3	30	280	253	149	418	1	.6	32	72	2	.09	.4	.3	.1	12	.84
7.4	1	104	869	774	389	1135	2.9	.6	79	248	8	.28	1.27	.6	.16	34	1.36
.1	0	12	836	670	373	1159	3	.2	80	483	4	.28	1.18	.6	.24	34	2.71
1.4	.2	20	717	483	285	821	2.2	.7	67	331	3	.11	.77	.4	.14	21	.59
.2	0	9	740	497	293	847	2.3	.7	69	298	3	.12	.79	.4	.14	22	.61
5.9	.6	74	658	512	267	764	1.9	.5	61	136	5	.12	.8	.5	.13	20	.41
4.1	1.2	34	79	34	42	126	.4	.1	8	157	12	.03	.09	.4	.03	13	.11
2.7	.9	0	200	244	134	366	.2	.2	2	149	0	0	0	.2	0	0	0
4.9	1.2	0	79	181	191	278	2.9	1	16	0	0	.03	.22	0	0	0	0
5.4	3.2	53	790	949	1306	2008	2.6	1.9	246	233	8	1.34	2.44	13.9	1.09	122	2.07
.1	0	4	301	247	126	407	1	.1	28	149	2	.09	.34	.2	.1	13	.93
0	0	4	284	224	131	388	1.1	.1	29	162	1	.09	.4	.2	.08	11	.91
.1	0	4	302	247	126	406	1	.1	28	149	2	.09	.34	.2	.1	13	.93
0	0	0	12	5	7	6	.1	.3	4	0	0	.02	.01	.1	.01	0	0
.2	0	5	350	274	144	446	1.1	.1	39	149	3	.11	.48	.2	.12	15	1.05
2.2	.3	30	275	215	120	348	.9	.2	30	70	2	.09	.4	.2	.1	12	.82

EshaCode	Food Item	Qty.	Meas	Wgt	Wtr	Cals	Prot	Carb	Fib	Fat	F_Sat
1	Milk, whole, 3.3% fat	1	cup	244	88	150	8	11	0	8	5.2
62	Milk, whole, extra rich, 3.7% fat	1	cup	244	88	157	8	11	0	9	5.6
52	Milk, whole, fluid, low sodium	1	cup	244	88	149	8	11	0	8	5.2
2020	Milkshake, chocolate	1.25	cup	283	72	359	10	58	.3	10	6.5
2022	Milkshake, strawberry	1.25	cup	283	74	320	10	54	.3	8	4.9
2024	Milkshake, vanilla	1.25	cup	283	75	314	10	51	.3	7	4.4
38052	Millet, cooked	.5	cup	120	71	143	4	28	1.6	1	.2
7503	Miso (soybean)	.5	cup	138	42	284	16	39	7.5	8	1.2
7563	Miso sauce	1	cup	248	57	383	13	72	5.9	7	1
3344	Mixed fruit canned in heavy syrup	1	cup	255	81	184	1	48	2.8	0	0
3168	Mixed fruit, dried	1	cup	136	31	330	3	87	5.8	1	.1
3169	Mixed fruit, frozen-sweetened-thawed	1	cup	250	74	245	4	60	4.8	0	.1
4595	Mixed nuts, no peanuts, oil roasted, salted	1	cup	144	3	886	22	32	7.9	81	13.1
4594	Mixed nuts, no peanuts, oil roasted, unsalted	1	cup	144	3	886	22	32	7.9	81	13.1
4592	Mixed nuts, w/peanuts, dry roasted, salted	1	cup	137	2	814	24	35	12.3	71	9.4
4591	Mixed nuts, w/peanuts, dry roasted, unsalted	1	cup	137	2	814	24	35	12.3	71	9.4
4593	Mixed nuts, w/peanuts, oil roasted, salted	1	cup	142	2	876	24	30	12.8	80	12.4
4533	Mixed nuts, w/peanuts, oil roasted, unsalted	1	cup	142	2	876	24	30	14.1	80	12.4
6462	Mixed vegetables, Chinese, LaChoy	100	grams	100	95	12	1	2	1.5	0	0
5305	Mixed vegetables, canned, drained	1	cup	163	87	77	4	15	6.3	0	.1
5516	Mixed vegetables, canned, low sodium	1	cup	182	90	66	3	13	5.6	0	.1
5548	Mixed vegetables, canned, w/liquid	1	cup	245	90	88	4	18	9.3	1	.1
5521	Mixed vegetables, dried-Salad Crunchies	1	Tbs	6	5	22	1	3	.8	1	.1
5549	Mixed vegetables, frozen	10	oz.	284	82	181	9	38	15.3	1	.3
5187	Mixed vegetables, frozen, cooked	1	cup	182	83	107	5	24	9.8	0	.1
70230	Mocha mix, vanilla	.75	cup	100	60	209	1	26	—	11	2.4
56323	Mock chicken leg, cooked	1	oz.	28	59	66	6	1	.1	4	1.2
25004	Molasses, blackstrap cane	1	cup	328	29	771	0	199	0	0	0
25003	Molasses, light cane	1	cup	328	26	872	0	226	0	0	0
56250	Moo goo gai pan	1	cup	216	77	281	15	12	2.7	20	4.7
7090	Mothbean, cooked, no salt	.5	cup	88	69	103	7	18	—	0	.1
56080	Moussaka, lamb & eggplant	1	cup	250	83	209	18	14	3.5	9	2.7
2667	Mousse, chocolate, recipe	.5	cup	202	62	446	9	33	—	33	18.6
44569	Muffin, blueberry, Weight Watchers	1	each	71	20	250	4	46	4	5	1
44516	Muffin, blueberry, commercial	1	each	57	38	158	3	27	2	4	.7
44505	Muffin, blueberry, mix, prepared	1	each	45	36	135	2	22	.9	4	.7
44520	Muffin, blueberry, recipe, w/2% milk	1	each	57	40	162	4	23	1.1	6	1.2
44501	Muffin, blueberry, recipe, w/whole milk	1	each	45	39	131	3	18	.8	5	1.1
44532	Muffin, buckwheat	1	each	47	34	144	4	20	1.4	6	1.7
44537	Muffin, carrot w/raisins & nuts	1	each	58	35	177	4	26	1	7	1.1
44534	Muffin, cheese	1	each	58	36	184	5	23	.7	8	3
44530	Muffin, chocolate chip	1	each	58	32	190	4	27	1	8	2.8
44521	Muffin, cornmeal, commercial	1	each	57	33	174	3	29	2.3	5	.9
44504	Muffin, cornmeal, mix, prepared	1	each	45	30	144	3	22	1.7	5	1.3
44524	Muffin, cornmeal, recipe w/2% milk	1	each	57	33	180	4	25	1.9	7	1.3
44503	Muffin, cornmeal, recipe, w/whole milk	1	each	45	32	144	3	20	1.5	6	1.2
44529	Muffin, cranberry nut	1	each	58	38	164	4	25	.8	5	1.5
70762	Muffin, egg-bacon-cheese, Great Starts	1	each	116	—	290	14	25	2	15	6
44514	Muffin, oat bran	1	each	57	35	154	4	28	4.3	4	.5
44533	Muffin, oatmeal	1	each	47	47	112	3	17	.7	3	1
44515	Muffin, plain, recipe, w/2% milk	1	each	57	38	169	4	24	1.5	6	1.2
44500	Muffin, plain, recipe, w/whole milk	1	each	45	37	135	3	19	1.2	5	1.1
44535	Muffin, pumpkin, w/raisins	1	each	58	28	181	3	34	1.1	4	.8
44518	Muffin, toaster type, blueberry	1	each	33	31	103	2	18	.8	3	.5
44519	Muffin, toaster type, blueberry, toasted	1	each	31	26	103	2	18	.7	3	.5
44522	Muffin, toaster type, corn	1	each	33	24	114	2	19	1.6	4	.6
44523	Muffin, toaster type, cornmeal, toasted	1	each	31	19	114	2	19	1.5	4	.6
44526	Muffin, toaster type, wheat bran-raisin	1	each	36	31	106	2	19	3.2	3	.5
44527	Muffin, toaster type, wheat bran-raisin, toasted	1	each	34	27	106	2	19	3.2	3	.5
44506	Muffin, wheat bran, mix, prepared	1	each	45	35	124	3	21	3.5	4	1.1
44528	Muffin, wheat bran, recipe, w/2% milk	1	each	57	35	161	4	24	4	7	1.3
44502	Muffin, wheat bran, recipe, w/whole milk	1	each	45	35	130	4	19	3.2	6	1.2
44531	Muffin, whole wheat	1	each	47	33	142	4	20	2.5	6	1.7
44536	Muffin, zucchini	1	each	58	30	210	3	26	.8	10	1.7
3309	Mulberries, raw	1	cup	140	88	60	2	14	2.4	1	0

FM_Un	FP_Un	Choles	Calc	Phos	Sodium	Pota	Zinc	Iron	Magnes	A_RE	Vit_C	B1	B2	B3	B6	Fola	B12
0	.3	0	43	48	3	324	.5	1.8	37	17	47	.05	.13	.7	.1	74	0
4.8	2	160	166	214	1541	400	1.4	3.1	32	245	9	.31	.42	2.9	.19	30	.38
2	.6	47	18	61	347	145	.9	1.1	11	53	6	.09	.12	1.6	.08	8	.46
2.6	.7	37	189	175	882	605	1.8	2.2	85	70	2	.13	.33	1.5	.2	112	.68
.6	.6	0	34	114	884	456	.6	1.4	47	146	66	.14	.11	2.4	.34	58	0
0	.1	0	30	22	88	105	0	.6	11	19	50	.08	.06	.3	.02	2	0
.1	0	0	4	3	81	31	0	.2	3	1	1	0	0	0	0	1	0
0	.6	0	49	34	1744	490	.2	2	12	24	15	0	.05	0	0	0	0
0	0	0	2	1	71	20	0	.1	0	1	1	0	0	0	0	0	0
.2	.1	0	28	34	657	259	.3	.7	20	27	11	.05	.04	.5	.09	19	0
.1	.3	0	151	143	7228	1269	.5	4.7	103	404	157	.23	.14	1.8	.46	40	0
.8	.1	10	171	133	71	248	.7	.4	27	60	1	.05	.21	.1	.06	7	.45
.7	.1	9	161	126	61	189	.5	.1	17	69	1	.05	.2	.1	.05	7	.44
1.3	.2	16	169	132	69	243	.7	.4	27	33	1	.05	.21	.1	.06	7	.44
1.2	.2	17	158	124	61	186	.5	.1	16	33	1	.05	.2	.1	.05	7	.44
6.9	5	0	294	46	193	289	.3	1.8	34	221	6	.15	.14	1.4	.05	14	.02
0	.5	0	348	19	2	230	.2	.5	29	17	8	.04	.06	.5	.05	13	0
0	1	0	105	17	5	351	.1	.3	15	12	10	.02	.04	.4	.03	9	0
6.3	6.2	0	47	1391	4	1232	5	15.4	648	0	0	2.28	.24	28.2	3.38	52	0
.2	.2	0	2	68	21	54	.5	.2	27	0	0	.01	.02	1.5	.02	4	0
.2	.2	0	2	58	52	50	.4	.2	20	0	0	.01	.02	1.2	.02	3	0
.2	.3	0	4	67	45	53	.5	.4	25	0	0	.01	.03	1.2	.02	4	0
.1	.1	0	1	32	29	26	.3	.1	12	0	0	0	.02	.7	.01	2	0
.2	.3	0	4	68	20	56	.5	.3	26	0	0	.02	.02	1.3	.03	1	0
.2	.2	0	2	68	41	52	.5	.3	24	0	1	.01	.02	1.3	.03	3	0
.2	.2	0	2	65	5	52	.5	.3	24	1	0	.01	.03	1.4	.03	4	0
1.2	.8	0	3	12	141	11	.2	.6	3	103	5	.11	.13	1.5	.16	30	0
0	0	0	9	26	1	60	.3	1	11	0	0	.01	.01	.8	.03	2	0
3	2.2	0	26	77	754	108	.8	2.4	19	86	1	.27	.03	2.6	.12	7	.01
5.1	4.7	0	72	1161	0	750	8.6	11.3	630	0	0	1.93	.19	29.6	.43	116	0
1.5	1.4	0	70	94	324	543	.8	2.4	40	115	39	.24	.08	3	.31	20	0
2.7	2.4	0	19	—	13	—	—	2.1	—	0	1	—	—	—	—	—	—
.6	.9	0	14	—	—	—	—	.9	—	0	1	—	—	—	—	—	—
—	—	—	39	450	20	533	—	6.3	—	0	—	.56	.22	9.2	—	—	—
.6	.6	0	20	162	10	84	1.2	.8	84	0	0	.19	.05	3	.28	8	0
.5	.5	0	14	120	7	62	.9	.6	62	0	0	.14	.04	2.2	.21	6	0
2	1.9	0	43	616	13	413	3.8	2.7	265	0	0	.74	.17	9.4	.94	37	0
.3	.3	0	10	76	1	77	.6	.5	43	0	0	.1	.01	1.3	.15	4	0
3	6.3	42	30	94	286	134	.9	1.8	24	21	4	.21	.11	2.2	.15	22	.11
—	—	0	14	—	16	—	—	1	—	0	3	—	—	—	—	—	—
2.3	2.4	0	17	—	14	—	—	3	—	0	2	—	—	—	—	—	—
.2	.2	0	20	88	2	72	1	2.5	25	0	0	.33	.03	3	.19	6	0
.4	.3	0	52	213	9	213	2	8	46	0	0	1.07	.09	7.8	.3	15	0
.2	.2	0	5	19	12	24	1	.3	12	0	0	.05	.03	.7	.06	2	0
.1	.1	0	10	18	4	5	.3	.8	6	0	0	.1	.06	1.1	.01	5	0
.1	.1	0	13	23	5	7	.4	1	8	0	0	.12	.08	1.4	.02	7	0
.1	.1	0	17	65	6	17	.9	4	11	0	0	.59	.06	5.2	.04	6	0
.1	.1	0	14	62	1	51	.7	1.8	17	0	0	.24	.02	2.2	.14	4	0
.1	.1	0	28	61	4	54	.4	1.6	17	0	0	.36	.03	2	.03	6	0
.1	.1	0	33	74	5	65	.5	2	21	0	0	.44	.03	2.4	.03	7	0
.3	.3	0	111	252	9	222	1.8	6.6	57	0	0	1.1	.13	6.7	.65	32	0
.1	.1	0	6	76	0	60	.9	3.1	27	0	0	.34	.03	3.8	.1	4	0
.1	.1	0	2	68	0	53	.8	3	16	0	0	.34	.03	3	.12	4	0
.1	.3	0	5	134	5	166	2.2	1	52	0	0	.08	.14	2.1	.22	43	0
.7	.9	66	18	340	115	775	.8	.8	51	98	0	.07	.12	5.8	.4	16	1.79
2.2	.5	0	10	104	250	19	.1	.8	4	0	0	.12	.07	1.1	.01	2	.02
2	.5	0	9	96	230	17	.1	.7	3	0	0	.14	.08	1.1	.01	2	.02
.7	.3	0	35	32	231	43	.3	1	8	0	0	.2	.11	1.6	.02	12	0
.2	.6	1	14	88	347	96	.8	3.7	22	4	0	.67	.45	6.3	.06	47	0
3.9	2.7	26	13	56	140	57	.4	1.8	10	88	0	.23	.21	2	.04	22	.06
2.6	.7	18	58	59	214	68	.3	1.2	10	12	0	.2	.18	1.2	.06	17	0
1.3	.4	2	54	44	210	39	.3	1.1	9	6	0	.16	.1	1.3	.02	15	.01
2.7	2.8	13	36	63	185	123	.4	1.5	16	60	0	.16	.16	1.3	.05	18	.06
.4	.7	0	34	33	148	38	.2	.9	7	0	0	.14	.09	1.1	.02	9	.01
.6	.6	0	6	54	126	53	.3	.9	15	0	0	.13	.1	1.1	.04	22	0

EshaCode	Food Item	Qty.	Meas	Wgt	Wtr	Cals	Prot	Carb	Fib	Fat	F_Sat
42170	Roll, dinner, bran, toasted	1	each	25	31	73	2	12	1.2	1	.2
42159	Roll, dinner, egg	1	each	35	30	107	3	18	1.3	2	.6
42018	Roll, dinner, enriched, brown+serve, browned	1	each	28	32	85	2	14	.9	2	.5
42158	Roll, dinner, homemade, w/2% milk	1	each	35	29	111	3	19	1.3	3	.6
42019	Roll, dinner, recipe, w/whole milk	1	each	35	29	112	3	19	1	3	.7
42160	Roll, dinner, wheat	1	each	28	37	77	2	13	—	2	.4
42057	Roll, dinner, whole wheat	1	each	35	33	93	3	18	2.4	2	.3
42184	Roll, garlic	1	each	35	32	104	3	18	.7	2	.5
42022	Roll, hard, white, enriched	1	each	50	31	147	5	26	1.5	2	.3
42188	Roll, jelly filled	1	each	55	30	173	4	28	.9	5	1.2
42070	Roll, oatmeal, toasted	1	each	33	44	78	3	13	1.4	2	.2
42058	Roll, rye, light	1	each	28	30	81	3	15	2	1	.2
42186	Roll, sourdough	1	each	45	31	131	4	25	1.2	1	.3
42034	Roll, submarine/hoagie	1	each	135	31	392	12	75	3.6	4	.9
42164	Roll, sweet, cheese	1	each	66	29	238	5	29	1.1	12	3.8
42033	Roll, sweet, cinnamon raisin, commercial	1	each	39	25	145	2	20	.8	7	1.7
3264	Rose apple, raw	2	oz.	57	93	14	0	3	.7	0	—
26030	Rosemary, dried	1	Tbs	3	9	11	0	2	1.2	1	—
5219	Rutabaga, cooked cubes	.5	cup	85	89	33	1	7	1.5	0	0
5220	Rutabaga, cooked, mashed	.5	cup	120	89	47	2	10	2.2	0	0
5218	Rutabaga, raw, cubes/pieces	1	cup	140	90	50	2	11	3.5	0	0
38084	Rye, whole grain	1	cup	158	11	529	23	110	23.1	4	.5
26111	Saffron	1	Tbs	2	12	7	0	1	.1	0	—
26306	Saffron safflower, flowers	100	grams	100	14	240	16	—	—	4	—
26311	Sage, fresh	1	Tbs	2	66	2	0	0	—	0	—
26031	Sage, ground	1	Tbs	2	8	6	0	1	.4	0	.1
8128	Salad dressing, Blue Cheese, low calorie	1	Tbs	15	80	15	1	0	0	1	.2
8017	Salad dressing, Dijon Vinegrarette Lite	1	Tbs	15	82	16	0	1	0	1	.2
8020	Salad dressing, Seven Seas Viva	1	Tbs	15	38	70	0	2	0	8	1.2
8147	Salad dressing, bacon & tomato, low calorie	1	Tbs	16	73	32	0	0	0	3	.6
8013	Salad dressing, blue cheese	1	cup	245	32	1234	12	18	0	128	24.3
8140	Salad dressing, buttermilk, light	1	Tbs	15	72	29	1	1	—	3	—
8066	Salad dressing, caesar's	.5	cup	92	36	418	11	2	.3	41	7.3
8138	Salad dressing, caesar, low calorie	1	Tbs	15	73	16	0	3	0	1	.1
8034	Salad dressing, cooked	1	Tbs	16	69	25	1	2	0	2	.5
8126	Salad dressing, creamy Italian	1	Tbs	15	39	71	0	1	0	8	1.1
8125	Salad dressing, creamy bacon	1	Tbs	15	39	71	0	1	0	8	1.1
8127	Salad dressing, creamy cucumber	1	Tbs	15	39	71	0	1	0	8	1.1
8152	Salad dressing, creamy cucumber, low calorie	1	Tbs	15	74	24	0	1	0	2	.3
8153	Salad dressing, creamy, oil free, low calorie	1	Tbs	15	74	24	0	1	0	2	.3
8015	Salad dressing, french	1	cup	250	38	1075	2	44	0	98	14.3
8146	Salad dressing, french, homemade	2	Tbs	28	24	177	0	1	0	20	3.5
8014	Salad dressing, french, low calorie	1	cup	260	69	348	1	56	.8	15	2.1
8124	Salad dressing, honey mustard	1	Tbs	16	35	50	0	7	.1	3	.4
8018	Salad dressing, italian	1	cup	235	38	1097	2	24	0	129	18.5
8016	Salad dressing, italian, low calorie	1	cup	240	82	252	0	12	.2	24	3.1
8149	Salad dressing, light, cholesterol free	1	Tbs	15	57	48	0	2	0	4	1.1
8122	Salad dressing, low calorie, Miracle Whip Light	1	Tbs	14	54	36	0	3	0	3	.4
8021	Salad dressing, mayonnaise type	1	cup	235	40	917	2	56	0	78	11.5
8141	Salad dressing, oil free, low calorie	1	Tbs	15	88	4	0	1	0	0	0
8030	Salad dressing, ranch	.5	cup	119	35	436	4	6	0	45	6.7
8129	Salad dressing, roquefort, low calorie	1	Tbs	15	80	15	1	0	0	1	.2
8022	Salad dressing, Russian	1	cup	245	34	1210	4	26	0	124	17.9
8139	Salad dressing, Russian, low calorie	2	Tbs	33	65	46	0	9	.1	1	.2
8144	Salad dressing, sesame seed	2	Tbs	31	39	136	1	3	—	14	1.9
8024	Salad dressing, thousand island	1	cup	250	46	943	2	38	5	89	15
8023	Salad dressing, thousand island, low calorie	1	cup	245	69	390	2	40	2.9	26	3.9
8019	Salad dressing, vinaigrette	1	Tbs	15	38	69	0	2	0	8	1.2
8035	Salad dressing, vinegar & oil	1	Tbs	16	47	72	0	0	0	8	1.5
8150	Salad dressing, vinegar & sugar & water	1	Tbs	16	84	8	0	2	0	0	0
8123	Salad dressing, yogurt	1	Tbs	15	85	11	0	1	0	1	.3
8151	Salad dressing/marinade, Korean	1	Tbs	15	90	5	0	1	.1	0	0
27050	Salad topping, Bac-O-Bits	1	Tbs	6	11	25	2	2	—	1	—
56109	Salad, carrot raisin	1	cup	175	58	404	3	42	5.3	28	4.1
56628	Salad, chef style w/turkey+ham+cheese	1.5	cup	326	82	267	26	5	—	16	8.2

FM_Un	FP_Un	Choles	Calc	Phos	Sodium	Pota	Zinc	Iron	Magnes	A_RE	Vit_C	B1	B2	B3	B6	Fola	B12
.5	.6	0	6	52	118	50	.3	.9	14	0	0	.1	.09	.9	.04	15	0
1.1	.4	18	21	35	191	37	.3	1.2	9	8	0	.18	.18	1.2	.03	19	.08
1	.3	0	34	33	148	38	.2	.9	7	0	0	.14	.09	1.1	.02	9	.01
1	.7	12	21	44	145	53	.2	1	7	32	0	.14	.14	1.2	.02	15	.05
1.1	.7	13	21	44	145	53	.2	1	7	28	0	.14	.14	1.2	.02	15	.05
.9	.3	0	50	34	96	38	.3	1	12	0	0	.12	.08	1.2	.02	4	0
.4	.8	0	37	78	167	95	.7	.9	30	0	0	.09	.05	1.3	.07	10	0
1	.3	0	35	30	176	34	.3	1	7	0	0	.14	.08	1.2	.02	13	0
.6	.9	0	48	50	272	54	.5	1.6	14	0	0	.24	.17	2.1	.03	8	0
2.4	.7	17	56	58	199	92	.3	1.2	10	11	0	.2	.17	1.2	.07	16	0
.5	.5	0	28	34	136	36	.3	1.4	10	0	0	.15	.1	1.6	.01	10	0
.4	.2	0	9	45	253	51	.3	.8	15	0	0	.11	.08	1.1	.02	6	0
.4	.5	0	40	38	261	40	.3	1.3	9	0	0	.18	.11	1.5	.02	14	0
1.3	1.4	0	122	115	783	122	.9	3.8	27	0	0	.54	.33	4.5	.05	40	0
6.1	1.4	37	78	65	236	87	.4	.5	12	41	0	.1	.09	.5	.04	20	.11
2.9	1.8	26	28	30	149	43	.2	.6	7	25	1	.13	.1	.9	.04	9	.05
—	—	0	16	5	0	70	0	0	3	19	13	.01	.02	.5	—	—	0
—	—	0	42	2	2	32	.1	1	7	10	2	.02	—	0	—	—	0
0	.1	0	41	48	17	277	.3	.5	20	48	16	.07	.04	.6	.09	13	0
0	.1	0	58	67	24	391	.4	.6	28	67	23	.1	.05	.9	.12	18	0
0	.1	0	66	81	28	472	.5	.7	32	81	35	.13	.06	1	.14	29	0
.5	1.8	0	52	591	9	417	5.9	4.2	191	0	0	.5	.4	6.8	.46	95	0
—	—	0	2	5	3	36		.2	—	—	—	—	—	—	—	—	0
—	—	—	619	256	—	—	—	20.2	—	—	21	.14	.38	8.6	—	—	—
—	—	—	12	1	0	8	0	—	3	4	—	0	—	—	—	—	0
0	0	0	33	2	0	21	.1	.6	9	12	1	.02	.01	.1	—	—	0
.5	.4	0	14	13	184	1	0	.1	1	0	0	0	.02	0	0	0	.04
.3	.9	1	0	1	118	2	0	0	0	0	0	0	0	0	0	0	0
1.8	4.8	0	2	1	118	2	0	0	0	4	0	0	0	0	0	1	.02
.9	1.8	1	1	4	176	18	0	0	1	4	1	.01	0	.1	.01	0	.02
30.1	68.1	42	198	181	2680	91	0	.5	0	162	5	.02	.24	.2	.09	20	.67
—	—	—	—	—	84	18	—	—	—	—	—	—	—	—	—	—	—
28.1	3.8	92	170	146	1552	154	.9	1.5	21	50	5	.03	.19	3.8	.09	12	.44
.3	.2	0	4	3	162	4	0	0	0	0	0	0	0	0	0	0	0
.6	.3	9	13	14	117	19	0	.1	0	20	0	.01	.02	0	0	0	0
1.9	4.4	1	2	2	173	4	0	0	1	3	0	0	0	0	0	0	0
1.9	4.4	1	2	2	173	4	0	0	1	3	0	0	0	0	0	0	0
1.9	4.4	1	2	2	173	4	0	0	1	3	0	0	0	0	0	0	0
.9	.8	0	1	1	153	5	0	0	0	1	0	0	0	0	0	2	.01
.9	.8	0	1	1	153	5	0	0	0	1	0	0	0	0	0	2	.01
21.8	57.2	145	28	35	3425	198	.2	1	0	50	0	.02	.04	0	.03	10	.35
5.8	9.4	0	2	1	184	7	0	.1	0	43	0	0	.01	0	0	0	0
3.7	8.8	16	29	36	2046	205	.5	1	0	0	0	0	0	0	0	0	0
.7	1.6	0	3	3	91	10	.1	.1	2	0	0	0	0	0	0	0	0
28.4	76	0	24	12	1849	35	.3	.5	2	55	0	.02	.04	0	.03	12	.38
4.8	14.4	14	5	12	1888	36	.3	.5	0	0	0	0	0	0	0	0	0
1.1	2.1	0	0	0	102	0	0	0	0	2	0	0	0	0	0	0	0
.7	1.4	4	2	4	99	1	0	0	0	9	0	0	0	0	0	1	.03
21.2	42.3	61	33	61	1670	21	.4	.5	5	197	0	.03	.06	0	.04	15	.49
0	0	0	1	1	256	7	0	0	2	0	0	0	0	0	0	0	0
19.4	17	47	119	100	522	158	.4	.3	12	86	1	.04	.17	.1	.05	6	.33
.5	.4	0	14	13	184	1	0	.1	1	0	0	0	.02	0	0	0	.04
28.9	72	44	47	91	2126	385	1	1.5	4	507	15	.12	.12	1.5	.07	26	.74
.3	.8	2	6	12	283	51	0	.2	0	5	2	0	0	0	0	1	.04
3.6	7.7	0	6	11	306	48	0	.2	0	63	0	0	0	0	0	0	0
20.8	49.5	65	28	42	1750	283	.4	1.5	5	240	0	.03	.06	0	.04	16	.52
5.9	15.2	37	27	42	2450	277	.4	1.5	2	235	0	.03	.05	0	.04	14	.45
1.8	4.8	0	1	1	116	2	0	0	0	3	0	0	0	0	0	1	.02
2.4	3.9	0	0	0	0	1	0	0	0	0	0	0	0	0	0	0	0
0	0	0	1	0	165	5	0	0	1	0	0	0	0	0	0	0	0
.2	.1	2	15	12	59	22	.1	0	2	4	0	0	.02	0	0	1	.05
0	0	0	4	4	39	15	0	.1	2	20	5	0	0	.1	.01	1	0
—	—	0	13	—	103	164	—	.4	—	—	—	.52	.02	.1	—	—	—
7.8	14.2	20	52	92	234	630	.4	1.5	28	2907	11	.16	.09	1.3	.44	18	.09
5.2	1.4	140	235	401	743	401	3.1	2	49	137	16	.39	.39	6	.42	101	.85

FM_Un	FP_Un	Choles	Calc	Phos	Sodium	Pota	Zinc	Iron	Magnes	A_RE	Vit_C	B1	B2	B3	B6	Fola	B12

EshaCode	Food Item	Qty.	Meas	Wgt	Wtr	Cals	Prot	Carb	Fib	Fat	F_Sat
19402	Salad, crab, w/imitation crab	1	cup	208	69	300	18	28	.7	13	1.8
44023	Salad, fruit, canned, juice pack	.5	cup	124	86	62	1	16	1.6	0	0
5637	Salad, mixed greens/lettuce	1	cup	55	94	9	1	2	.9	0	0
5537	Salad, spinach, no dressing	1	cup	74	74	89	4	10	1.6	4	.9
56643	Salad, taco	1.5	cup	198	72	279	13	24	—	15	6.8
56118	Salad, three bean	1	cup	150	82	139	4	14	2.9	8	1.2
5677	Salad, tossed green	.75	cup	104	95	19	1	4	1.2	0	0
56006	Salad, waldorf	1	cup	137	59	397	3	12	2.4	39	5.2
13023	Salami, beef, cooked	1	piece	23	58	60	3	1	0	5	2.1
13026	Salami, dry, beef & pork	2	piece	20	35	84	5	1	0	7	2.4
13025	Salami, turkey, cooked	2	piece	57	66	112	9	0	0	8	2.3
11063	Salisbury steak, 4-compartment, Swanson	1	each	298	72	390	17	42	5	18	7
27020	Salsa cruda (uncooked salsa)	1	cup	240	93	47	2	10	2.4	0	.1
5221	Salsify, cooked, drained	1	cup	135	81	92	4	21	4.2	0	0
26014	Salt	1	Tbs	16	0	0	0	0	0	0	0
26101	Salt Free 17	1	tsp	6	5	21	1	4	.7	0	—
26113	Salt blend, light, Papa Dash	35.7	tsp	100	0	55	0	14	—	0	0
26090	Salt substitute, Morton	1	tsp	6	2	0	0	0	0	0	0
26048	Salt, light, Morton	1	tsp	6	0	0	0	0	0	0	0
26089	Salt, light, Morton Lite	1	tsp	6	2	0	0	0	0	0	0
26091	Salt, seasoning, Morton	1	Tbs	5	2	2	0	0	0	0	—
8130	Sandwich spread w/chopped pickle	2	Tbs	31	41	119	0	7	.1	10	1.6
56008	Sandwich, BLT, on firm white	1	each	145	45	432	13	38	1.9	25	6
56022	Sandwich, avocado & cheese, on wheat	1	each	196	58	456	14	33	4.9	31	9
56281	Sandwich, bologna	1	each	83	42	257	7	26	1.2	14	4.2
13093	Sandwich, chicken frank on bun	1	each	85	45	235	9	24	.8	11	3
56016	Sandwich, chicken salad, on firm white	1	each	114	38	398	11	33	1.4	25	4
56020	Sandwich, corned beef & swiss, on rye	1	each	147	44	457	27	25	3.1	28	10
56024	Sandwich, egg salad, on firm white	1	each	121	41	411	10	33	1.3	27	4.7
66011	Sandwich, fish w/tartar sauce & cheese	1	each	183	45	523	21	48	.4	28	8.1
56268	Sandwich, french dip au jus	1	each	193	61	359	26	34	1.7	12	4.8
56012	Sandwich, grilled cheese, on firm white	1	each	127	36	426	18	34	1.3	24	12.4
69017	Sandwich, grilled chicken, Weight Watchers	1	each	113	58	210	18	24	2	5	2
56272	Sandwich, gyro	1	each	105	64	169	12	20	1.1	4	1.5
56033	Sandwich, ham & swiss, on rye	1	each	145	50	368	23	26	3.1	19	7.2
56066	Sandwich, ham salad, on wheat	1	each	126	46	363	10	32	2.4	22	5
56031	Sandwich, ham, on wheat	1	each	123	55	259	17	22	2	11	2.4
66004	Sandwich, hotdog, plain	1	each	98	54	242	10	18	—	14	5.1
56267	Sandwich, pastrami	1	each	134	53	334	14	27	1.7	18	6.3
56038	Sandwich, patty melt, on rye	1	each	177	42	600	35	24	3	40	14
56040	Sandwich, peanut butter & jam, on soft white	1	each	101	26	350	11	48	2.9	14	2.7
56266	Sandwich, reuben	1	each	181	51	496	23	31	4.1	31	10.6
56046	Sandwich, roast beef, on wheat	1	each	123	47	314	23	25	1.9	13	2.8
56671	Sandwich, submarine w/coldcuts	1	each	228	58	456	22	51	1.7	19	6.8
56047	Sandwich, tuna salad, on firm white	1	each	126	44	362	14	37	1.6	18	2.9
56059	Sandwich, turkey ham & cheese, on wheat	1	each	152	50	385	22	27	2.5	21	7.9
56103	Sandwich, turkey ham, on rye	1	each	116	57	239	16	19	2.5	10	2.2
56053	Sandwich, turkey, on whole wheat	1	each	136	53	294	21	26	3.9	12	2.2
3266	Sapodilla, raw	1	each	170	78	141	1	34	9	2	—
3267	Sapotes, raw	1	each	170	62	228	4	58	4.4	1	—
53388	Sauce, Alfredo, Di Girono	.25	cup	62	—	230	4	2	0	22	10
53396	Sauce, Alfredo, low fat, Di Girono	.25	cup	69	—	170	5	16	0	10	6
53085	Sauce, Tabasco brand pepper	1	Tbs	16	95	2	0	0	.1	0	0
57271	Sauce, alfredo, Progresso	.5	cup	124	66	310	10	5	0	27	15
53133	Sauce, armanino pesto	1	oz.	28	52	95	2	2	.5	9	1.5
53000	Sauce, barbecue	1	cup	250	81	188	5	32	3	5	.7
53018	Sauce, bechamel	.5	cup	145	84	142	2	7	.3	12	7.3
53100	Sauce, black bean	1	cup	275	79	257	7	28	3.9	12	2.2
53019	Sauce, bordelaise	.5	cup	233	86	197	3	10	.6	12	7.4
53015	Sauce, cheese	.5	cup	101	65	216	10	6	.1	17	8.3
53029	Sauce, cheese, dry mix w/milk	1	cup	279	77	307	16	23	.8	17	9.3
53097	Sauce, cheese, low fat	1	cup	243	73	338	23	16	.3	20	8.2
53227	Sauce, chili, hot green	1	cup	245	94	49	2	12	—	0	0
27003	Sauce, chili, tomato base	1	cup	273	68	284	7	68	3.6	1	.1
53226	Sauce, chili, unsalted, bottled	1	cup	273	68	284	7	68	—	1	0

FM_Un	FP_Un	Choles	Calc	Phos	Sodium	Pota	Zinc	Iron	Magnes	A_RE	Vit_C	B1	B2	B3	B6	Fola	B12
3.2	6.7	73	75	220	1784	421	.6	.7	66	43	2	.06	.19	3.1	.28	14	2.82
0	0	0	14	17	6	144	.2	.3	10	74	4	.01	.02	.4	.03	3	0
0	.1	0	30	18	14	174	.2	.7	13	150	9	.04	.05	.2	.04	64	0
1.4	.9	60	51	73	157	276	.5	1.6	33	240	10	.11	.26	1.4	.1	76	.16
5.2	1.8	44	192	143	762	416	2.7	2.3	52	77	4	.1	.36	2.5	.22	40	.63
1.9	4.9	0	35	65	514	224	.5	1.4	25	23	4	.07	.1	.4	.04	53	.03
0	.1	0	14	24	11	201	.2	.5	11	209	11	.05	.04	.4	.06	36	0
10.5	21.4	21	41	75	241	259	.6	.8	35	40	6	.09	.05	.3	.36	26	.09
2.2	.2	15	2	26	270	52	.5	.5	3	0	4	.02	.04	.7	.04	0	.71
3.4	.6	16	2	28	372	76	.6	.3	3	0	5	.12	.06	1	.1	0	.38
2.6	2	47	11	60	572	139	1	.9	9	0	0	.04	.1	2	.14	2	.12
—	—	50	40	—	880	523	—	2.7	—	30	1	.15	.19	4.7	—	—	—
.1	.2	0	22	50	936	388	.3	.9	23	354	86	.1	.08	1	.2	29	0
0	.1	0	64	76	22	382	.4	.7	24	0	6	.08	.23	.5	.29	20	0
0	0	0	4	0	6395	1	0	0	0	0	0	0	0	0	0	0	0
—	—	—	—	—	3	74	—	—	—	—	—	—	—	—	—	—	0
0	0	0	—	—	33028	2	—	—	—	0	0	0	0	0	0	0	0
0	0	0	30	28	0	2766	—	—	0	0	—	—	—	—	—	—	0
0	0	0	3	0	1099	1500	0	0	4	0	0	0	0	0	0	0	0
0	0	0	0	—	1150	1534	—	—	4	0	—	—	—	—	—	—	0
—	—	0	—	—	1	2078	—	—	—	0	—	—	—	—	—	—	0
2.3	6.1	23	4	8	306	11	.2	.1	1	26	0	0	.01	0	.01	2	.06
9.4	8.1	29	77	156	774	273	1.2	2.6	24	44	14	.45	.25	4.1	.2	35	.4
12.7	7.6	33	278	250	528	587	1.8	3	64	138	11	.33	.37	3.8	.36	76	.26
6.2	2.5	16	63	79	608	111	.8	1.9	16	54	6	.28	.21	2.7	.08	18	.38
5	2.2	45	83	82	819	76	.8	2	13	17	0	.19	.15	2.7	.16	17	.1
7.4	11.8	33	71	107	484	147	.8	2.1	19	34	1	.27	.19	3.7	.26	27	.12
9	6.4	79	307	290	1063	193	3.6	2.7	39	80	1	.22	.34	3.2	.21	32	1.36
8.2	11.9	150	81	126	550	125	.8	2.3	17	83	0	.27	.31	2.1	.21	38	.41
8.9	9.4	68	185	311	939	353	1.2	3.5	37	97	3	.46	.42	4.2	.11	31	1.08
5.2	.9	58	66	212	608	355	5.3	3.7	31	0	0	.3	.31	5.4	.24	26	2.11
7.8	2.4	56	411	489	1177	173	2.1	2.1	26	220	0	.28	.36	2.2	.06	28	.4
—	—	20	60	—	420	220	—	1.4	—	0	0	—	—	—	—	—	—
1.4	.4	34	44	117	212	209	2.3	2.2	20	11	4	.21	.25	3.5	.16	30	.9
6.2	4.6	56	309	353	1289	313	2.7	2	41	77	14	.73	.38	4.5	.37	29	.9
8.1	7.6	29	65	155	894	201	1.2	2.2	31	11	3	.48	.22	3.5	.22	24	.47
4.2	3.7	36	56	218	1285	332	1.8	2.1	34	6	17	.81	.27	5.1	.4	22	.52
6.8	1.7	44	24	97	670	143	2	2.3	13	0	0	.24	.27	3.7	.05	29	.51
8.9	1.2	53	71	142	1341	242	2.7	2.6	24	3	4	.29	.27	4.8	.13	21	.99
14.5	7.9	116	219	407	895	369	6.8	3.8	43	137	0	.28	.46	6.4	.35	38	2.1
6.5	4	2	61	133	293	258	1	2.2	51	0	0	.26	.17	5.2	.13	44	0
9.9	7.6	89	319	321	1308	247	4.2	2.9	36	101	11	.18	.32	3.1	.22	30	1.45
4.4	5	34	56	183	1264	381	3.2	3.4	34	9	10	.24	.25	5.4	.34	27	1.76
8.2	2.3	36	189	287	1650	394	2.6	2.5	68	80	12	1	.8	5.5	.14	55	1.09
5.4	8.1	17	72	156	587	169	.7	2.3	23	33	1	.27	.19	5.4	.14	27	.62
6.3	5.3	62	239	399	1349	345	3.1	3.6	43	88	0	.27	.39	4.2	.26	29	.35
3	4.3	41	40	178	1004	287	2.4	3	28	6	0	.2	.29	3.8	.23	24	.18
3.8	5.3	35	47	289	1339	336	1.9	2.2	62	9	0	.22	.19	7.9	.41	32	1.42
—	—	0	36	20	20	328	.2	1.4	20	10	25	0	.03	.3	.06	24	0
—	—	0	66	48	17	585	—	1.7	51	70	34	.02	.03	3.1	—	—	0
—	—	45	100	100	550	75	—	0	0	80	0	0	.1	0	—	—	—
—	—	30	150	100	600	80	—	0	8	80	0	0	.1	0	—	—	—
0	0	0	4	3	92	20	0	.4	1	65	0	.01	.01	.1	.03	0	9.36
7	1	75	300	—	670	—	—	0	—	150	0	—	—	—	—	—	—
—	—	5	82	—	182	—	—	.6	—	136	0	—	—	—	—	—	—
1.9	1.7	0	48	50	2037	435	.5	2.2	45	217	18	.08	.05	2.2	.19	10	0
3.5	.6	31	13	18	1125	28	.1	.5	5	113	0	.07	.06	.6	0	4	.03
5.4	4	0	64	105	2643	379	.8	1.7	44	19	5	.15	.1	1	.13	70	.02
3.5	.5	31	30	44	517	197	.2	1.5	17	119	7	.08	.09	1.5	.06	12	.11
5.9	2.1	38	279	207	539	127	1.1	.4	17	175	1	.06	.22	.3	.05	9	.46
5.3	1.6	53	569	438	1565	552	1	.3	47	117	2	.15	.56	.3	.14	13	1.12
7.5	3.6	44	661	724	1549	397	2.9	1	40	231	2	.14	.56	.6	.12	16	1.08
—	—	0	12	34	61	1381	—	1	—	149	167	.07	.07	1.7	—	—	—
.1	.3	0	55	141	3650	1010	.7	2.2	30	382	44	.25	.19	4.4	.32	20	0
—	—	0	55	142	55	1010	—	2.2	—	382	44	.25	.19	4.4	—	—	—

EshaCode	Food Item	Qty	Meas	Wgt	Wtr	Cals	Prot	Carb	Fib	Fat	F_Sat
53355	Sauce, creole	.25	cup	62	—	25	0	4	1	1	0
53016	Sauce, curry	.5	cup	115	89	74	3	3	.2	6	1.1
53103	Sauce, enchilada, green	1	cup	250	87	178	4	14	2.6	13	7.2
53102	Sauce, enchilada, red	1	cup	250	80	331	3	13	2.5	31	16.3
53104	Sauce, fish/bagoong	1	cup	272	64	283	57	1	0	3	.9
53351	Sauce, hoisin	2	Tbs	34	47	70	1	14	0	2	0
53110	Sauce, hollandaise, dry mix w/water	1	cup	259	84	238	5	14	.8	20	11.6
53098	Sauce, horseradish	1	Tbs	14	71	29	0	1	0	3	1.8
53408	Sauce, horseradish, Kraft	1	Tbs	5	—	0	0	0	0	0	0
27002	Sauce, hot chili/red pepper	2	Tbs	31	94	7	0	1	.1	0	0
50199	Sauce, lobster	1	cup	234	70	380	23	15	1.4	24	5
53120	Sauce, marinara tomato	1	cup	250	82	170	4	26	—	8	1.2
53125	Sauce, mole poblano	1	cup	265	76	315	11	28	5.4	21	4.8
53126	Sauce, mole verde	1	cup	265	86	157	9	16	4.4	8	1.5
53017	Sauce, mornay	.5	cup	172	61	429	17	11	.2	36	17.6
53106	Sauce, pesto	1	cup	232	21	1242	40	18	3.7	116	29
53032	Sauce, picante, Tostitos	6	Tbs	85	88	40	1	8	1.4	1	.1
53002	Sauce, soy (wheat & soy)	1	Tbs	18	71	10	1	2	.1	0	0
53267	Sauce, soy, lite, LaChoy	1	Tbs	18	67	15	1	2	0	0	0
53063	Sauce, soy, tamari	.25	cup	58	66	35	6	3	0	0	0
53010	Sauce, spaghetti w/meat, recipe	1	cup	248	76	289	16	22	4.2	17	4.6
53012	Sauce, spaghetti w/meatballs, canned	1	cup	250	75	255	12	28	1.8	10	2.6
53344	Sauce, spaghetti, Prego	.5	cup	125	—	150	2	22	2	6	2
53009	Sauce, spaghetti, canned	1	cup	249	75	271	5	40	8.5	12	1.7
53011	Sauce, spaghetti, meat flavor, canned	1	cup	250	74	300	8	37	8	14	2.8
53014	Sauce, spaghetti, w/mushrooms, canned	.75	cup	185	75	162	2	19	1.8	4	.6
53008	Sauce, spaghetti/marinara	1	cup	250	82	189	4	26	5.1	9	1.4
53058	Sauce, stroganoff w/milk & water	1.2	cup	296	78	272	12	34	.6	11	6.8
53001	Sauce, szechuan	1	cup	250	81	188	5	32	3	5	.7
53003	Sauce, tartar	1	Tbs	14	34	74	0	1	0	8	1.5
53415	Sauce, tartar, nonfat, Kraft	2	Tbs	30	—	23	0	5	.5	0	0
53004	Sauce, teriyaki	1	Tbs	18	68	15	1	3	0	0	0
53109	Sauce, teriyaki, dry w/water	1	cup	283	84	130	4	28	—	1	.1
5180	Sauce, tomato, canned, no added salt	1	cup	245	89	74	3	18	3.4	0	.1
53101	Sauce, white clam	1	cup	240	57	598	42	10	.2	43	5.6
53025	Sauce, white, dry mix, prep w/milk	1	cup	264	82	240	10	21	.3	14	6.4
53007	Sauce, white, recipe	1	cup	250	77	355	9	20	.4	27	7.8
53099	Sauce, worcestershire	1	cup	272	70	182	0	45	0	0	0
5531	Sauerkraut, canned, low sodium	1	cup	142	92	27	1	6	3.6	0	0
5145	Sauerkraut, canned, w/liquid	1	cup	236	92	45	2	10	5.9	0	.1
13022	Sausage, Polish, pork	1	oz.	28	53	93	4	0	0	8	2.9
13066	Sausage, braunschweiger	2	piece	57	48	205	8	2	0	18	6.2
13070	Sausage, chorizo, link	1	each	60	32	273	14	1	0	23	8.6
13043	Sausage, kielbasa	1	piece	26	54	81	3	1	0	7	2.6
13021	Sausage, pepperoni, pork/beef	4	piece	22	27	109	5	1	0	10	3.5
13015	Sausage, pork, Italian link, cooked	1	each	67	50	216	13	1	0	17	6.1
13030	Sausage, summer, thuringer, beef & pork	1	piece	23	51	77	4	0	0	7	2.8
13052	Sausage, turkey, breakfast type	1	piece	28	60	65	6	0	0	5	1.6
13053	Sausage, turkey, smoked	1	oz.	28	66	55	4	0	0	4	1.3
26112	Savory, ground	1	Tbs	4	9	12	0	3	1.3	0	—
42071	Scone	1	each	42	28	150	4	18	.6	7	2.1
42072	Scone, whole wheat	1	each	42	27	145	5	18	2.8	7	2.1
56257	Seafood salad	1	cup	208	73	331	25	5	.8	24	3.3
18816	Seafood souffle	1	cup	159	72	258	18	9	.2	17	4.7
5255	Seaweed, Irishmoss, raw	1	cup	80	81	39	1	10	1	0	0
5254	Seaweed, agar, dried	1	cup	15	9	46	1	12	1.2	0	0
5253	Seaweed, agar, raw	1	cup	80	91	21	0	5	.4	0	0
5256	Seaweed, kelp, raw	1	cup	80	82	34	1	8	1	0	.2
5257	Seaweed, laver, raw	1	cup	80	85	28	5	4	.2	0	0
5260	Seaweed, spirulina, dried	1	cup	15	5	44	9	4	.5	1	.4
7089	Seeds, lupin, cooked, no salt	.5	cup	83	71	99	13	8	2.3	2	.3
62000	Sego diet drink	1.25	cup	320	49	225	11	34	0	5	.1
62001	Sego lite diet drink	1.25	cup	320	49	150	11	20	0	3	.4
4655	Sesame butter, tahini, f/roasted/toasted kernels	1	Tbs	15	3	89	3	3	1.4	8	1.1
4619	Sesame meal, partially defatted	1	oz.	28	5	161	5	7	1.1	14	1.9

FM_Un	FP_Un	Choles	Calc	Phos	Sodium	Pota	Zinc	Iron	Magnes	A_RE	Vit_C	B1	B2	B3	B6	Fola	B12
—	—	0	20	—	340	—	—	0	—	40	0	—	—	—	—	—	—
2.6	1.7	0	9	38	392	103	.1	.5	3	61	0	.03	.05	1.6	.01	3	.11
3.5	1.1	39	78	118	368	584	.6	1.4	44	552	108	.11	.17	2.8	.2	18	.13
9.8	3	89	63	89	334	392	.5	1.1	31	779	20	.09	.2	1.3	.25	22	.11
.9	1.2	166	503	628	21760	1768	5.4	8.7	30	117	0	.08	.6	16.2	.35	49	21
—	—	0	0	—	500	—	—	0	—	0	0	—	—	—	—	—	—
5.9	.9	52	124	127	1565	124	.8	.9	8	220	0	.05	.18	.1	.52	21	.78
.8	.1	6	16	12	41	20	0	0	2	27	0	0	.02	0	0	1	.04
0	0	0	0	—	50	10	—	0	—	0	1	—	—	—	—	—	—
0	.1	0	3	5	8	174	.1	.2	3	297	9	0	.03	.2	.04	3	0
7.3	10	167	45	268	1934	456	2.3	1.9	33	50	2	.41	.39	4.7	.36	53	.81
4.3	2.3	0	45	88	1572	1060	.7	2	60	240	32	.11	.15	4	.62	34	0
9.2	5.4	2	88	261	626	671	1.9	3.7	120	1015	10	.15	.34	4.5	.41	32	.13
2.3	3.3	1	45	267	939	764	1.5	3.6	100	163	47	.12	.16	5.1	.22	35	.18
10.9	5	170	535	386	798	208	2	.8	31	367	1	.11	.38	.5	.11	18	1.16
72.6	8.4	71	1668	829	1688	826	4.1	9.7	134	346	21	.08	.41	1.8	.36	66	1.26
.4	.1	1	18	60	480	171	.9	.5	14	63	2	.03	.07	.5	.08	14	0
0	0	0	3	20	1028	32	.1	.4	6	0	0	.01	.02	.6	.03	3	0
—	—	0	3	—	505	—	—	.1	—	0	0	—	—	—	—	—	—
0	0	0	12	75	3238	123	.2	1.4	23	0	0	.04	.09	2.3	.12	11	0
5.6	4.7	46	58	172	1130	1084	3.4	3.9	62	229	35	.17	.25	5.8	.51	24	1.42
4.7	1.6	31	53	113	1105	245	2.2	3.3	28	220	5	.16	.19	2.4	.32	14	2.36
—	—	0	40	—	640	—	—	.7	—	—	15	—	—	—	—	—	—
6.1	3.3	0	70	90	1235	956	.5	1.6	60	306	28	.14	.15	3.8	.88	54	0
7	3.2	15	68	113	1179	952	1.4	1.9	60	289	26	.14	.17	4.5	.88	52	.49
2.3	1.2	0	22	45	744	500	.5	1.5	22	362	14	.12	.12	1.4	.24	19	0
2.1	5.3	0	63	102	1313	1129	.9	3.2	62	276	42	.19	.19	3.4	.46	23	0
3	.4	38	521	302	1829	672	1.1	1.3	38	127	1	.86	.77	.8	.12	9	.59
1.9	1.7	0	48	50	2037	435	.5	2.2	45	217	18	.08	.05	2.2	.19	10	0
2.6	4.1	7	3	4	99	11	0	.1	0	9	0	0	0	0	0	1	0
0	0	0	0	—	197	14	—	0	—	0	0	—	—	—	—	—	—
0	0	0	4	28	690	40	0	.3	11	0	0	0	.01	.2	.02	4	0
.2	.5	0	113	215	4791	215	.1	2.8	85	0	0	.03	.08	1.3	.14	28	0
.1	.2	0	34	78	1482	909	.6	1.9	47	240	32	.16	.14	2.8	.38	23	0
29.3	4.2	111	166	563	979	1060	4.6	46.7	33	288	38	.25	.71	5.6	.21	49	163
4.7	1.7	34	425	256	797	444	.5	.3	264	92	3	.08	.45	.5	.07	16	1.06
9.1	8.8	29	261	217	369	344	1	.7	32	310	2	.19	.42	1	.1	14	.78
0	0	0	291	163	2665	2176	.5	14.4	35	30	35	.19	.35	1.9	0	0	0
0	.1	0	43	28	437	241	.3	2.1	18	3	21	.03	.03	.2	.13	34	0
0	.1	0	71	47	1559	401	.4	3.5	31	4	35	.05	.05	.3	.31	56	0
3.8	.9	20	3	39	249	67	.6	.4	4	0	0	.14	.04	1	.05	1	.28
8.5	2.1	89	5	96	652	113	1.6	5.3	6	2405	6	.14	.87	4.8	.19	25	11.5
11	2.1	53	5	90	741	239	2	1	11	0	0	.38	.18	3.1	.32	1	1.21
3.4	.8	17	11	38	280	70	.5	.4	4	0	5	.06	.06	.7	.05	1	.42
4.6	1	17	2	26	449	76	.6	.3	4	0	0	.07	.06	1.1	.06	1	.55
8	2.2	52	16	114	618	204	1.6	1	12	0	1	.42	.16	2.8	.22	3	.88
3	.3	17	3	26	286	62	.6	.6	3	0	5	.04	.08	1	.06	0	1.27
1.8	1.2	23	5	52	191	76	1	.5	6	0	0	.03	.08	1.4	.08	1	.5
1.6	1	19	5	37	219	59	.7	.4	5	0	0	.02	.06	1.2	.06	1	.56
—	—	0	94	6	1	46	.2	1.7	17	23	—	.02	—	.2	—	—	0
2.5	1.4	51	62	61	246	50	.3	1.2	7	85	0	.14	.16	1.2	.03	8	.1
2.5	1.5	50	55	153	174	189	.8	1	32	84	0	.09	.11	1.3	.08	11	.1
16.6	2.4	127	90	275	548	498	3.2	2	53	53	13	.08	.1	2.3	.18	31	1.79
6.6	3.9	225	130	232	606	272	1.6	1.6	29	233	1	.1	.37	2.7	.16	26	1.07
0	0	0	58	126	54	50	1.6	7.1	115	9	8	.01	.37	.5	.06	146	0
0	0	0	94	8	15	169	.9	3.2	116	0	0	0	.03	0	.04	87	0
0	0	0	43	4	7	181	.5	1.5	54	0	0	0	.02	0	.03	68	0
.1	0	0	134	34	186	71	1	2.3	97	9	1	.04	.12	.4	0	144	0
0	.1	0	56	46	38	285	.8	1.4	2	416	31	.08	.36	1.2	.13	117	0
.1	.3	0	18	18	157	204	.3	4.3	29	9	2	.36	.55	1.9	.06	14	0
1	.6	0	42	106	3	203	1.2	1	45	1	1	.11	.04	.4	.01	49	0
2.2	1.9	4	250	250	362	602	3.7	4.5	100	374	15	.37	.43	5	.5	100	1.5
.5	1.1	4	250	250	362	602	3.7	4.5	100	374	15	.37	.43	5	.5	100	1.5
3	3.5	0	64	110	17	62	.7	1.3	14	1	0	.18	.07	.8	.02	15	0
5.1	6	0	43	219	11	115	2.9	4.1	98	2	0	.73	.08	3.6	.04	8	0

EshaCode	Food Item	Qty.	Meas	Wgt	Wtr	Cals	Prot	Carb	Fib	Fat	F_Sat
4524	Sesame seed kernels, dried	1	cup	150	5	882	40	14	13.6	82	11.5
4523	Sesame seed, whole, dried	1	cup	144	5	825	26	34	13.1	72	10
5428	Shallot, freeze dried, chopped	.25	cup	4	2	12	0	3	.2	0	0
5427	Shallot, raw, chopped	1	Tbs	10	80	7	0	2	.1	0	0
20186	Shasta Soda, cherry cola, diet	1.5	cup	360	100	0	0	0	0	0	0
20189	Shasta Soda, cream soda, diet	1.5	cup	360	100	0	0	0	0	0	0
20190	Shasta Soda, ginger ale, diet	1.5	cup	360	100	0	0	0	0	0	0
2011	Sherbet, orange	.5	cup	96	66	132	1	29	0	2	1.1
22506	Sherry, medium	.5	cup	120	86	168	0	10	0	0	0
8007	Shortening, vegetable (Crisco/Fluffo)	1	cup	205	0	1812	0	0	0	205	51.7
56239	Shrimp jambalaya	1	cup	243	73	306	28	26	1.7	10	1.9
19426	Shrimp marinara dinner, Healthy Choice	1	each	298	81	220	10	44	5	0	0
19418	Shrimp patty burger	1	each	120	60	248	18	15	1.3	13	3.4
56256	Shrimp salad	1	cup	182	72	282	27	6	.8	17	2.6
19410	Shrimp w/lobster sauce	1	cup	185	68	290	35	7	.6	12	2.5
19408	Shrimp, curried	1	cup	236	74	314	27	14	.4	16	5.1
23114	Snow cone	1	each	190	67	148	1	62	0	0	0
20208	Soda, 7-Up, Gold	.75	cup	180	89	78	0	19	—	0	0
20209	Soda, 7-Up, Gold, diet	.75	cup	180	99	2	0	1	—	0	0
20207	Soda, 7-Up, diet	1.5	cup	360	100	4	0	0	0	0	0
20055	Soda, 7-Up, regular	1.5	cup	360	89	151	0	37	0	0	0
20147	Soda, Coca Cola, can/bottle	1.5	cup	360	89	150	0	39	0	0	0
20148	Soda, Coca Cola, classic, can/bottle	1.5	cup	360	89	140	0	37	0	0	0
20150	Soda, Coca Cola, diet, can/bottle	1.5	cup	360	100	1	0	0	0	0	0
20027	Soda, Dr. Pepper type	1.5	cup	368	89	151	0	38	0	0	.3
20086	Soda, Dr. Pepper type, decaf, sugar free, 12 oz can	1	each	355	100	4	0	0	0	0	0
20167	Soda, Pepsi, diet	1	cup	240	100	0	0	0	0	0	0
20166	Soda, Pepsi, regular	1	cup	240	86	100	0	27	0	0	0
22508	Soda, Slice, apple, diet	1.5	cup	355	98	0	0	0	0	0	0
20068	Soda, Slice, lemon lime, diet	1	cup	240	97	0	0	1	0	0	0
57227	Soda, Slice, mandarin orange	1.5	cup	360	47	979	46	84	5.8	52	23
20125	Soda, Slice, mandarin orange, diet	1	cup	240	98	0	0	0	0	0	0
20125	Soda, Slice, mandarin orange, diet	1.5	cup	355	98	0	0	0	0	0	0
20125	Soda, Slice, mandarin orange, diet	1.5	cup	360	98	0	0	0	0	0	0
20163	Soda, Sprite, can/bottle	1.5	cup	360	90	137	0	35	0	0	0
20164	Soda, Sprite, diet, can/bottle	1.5	cup	360	100	4	0	0	0	0	0
20165	Soda, Tab, can/bottle	1.5	cup	360	100	1	0	0	0	0	0
20066	Soda, cherry cola, Slice	1.5	cup	372	88	179	0	46	0	0	0
20006	Soda, club	1.5	cup	355	100	0	0	0	0	0	0
20054	Soda, cola, caffeine-free, can/bottle	1.5	cup	365	89	162	0	41	0	0	0
20049	Soda, cola, diet, w/aspartame+saccharin	1.5	cup	355	100	4	0	0	0	0	0
20005	Soda, cola-type, regular	1.5	cup	370	89	152	0	38	0	0	0
20056	Soda, cola/coke, diet, caffeine-free	1.5	cup	360	100	0	0	0	0	0	0
20030	Soda, cola/coke, diet, w/aspartame, can/bottle	1.5	cup	355	100	4	0	0	0	0	0
20007	Soda, cola/pepper type, diet, w/saccharin	1.5	cup	355	100	0	0	0	0	0	0
20028	Soda, cream	1.5	cup	371	87	189	0	49	0	0	0
20085	Soda, cream, sugar-free, 12 fl oz can	1	each	355	100	0	0	0	0	0	0
20068	Soda, diet, lemon lime, Slice	1.5	cup	355	97	0	0	1	0	0	0
20008	Soda, ginger ale	1.5	cup	366	91	124	0	32	0	0	0
20084	Soda, ginger ale, sugar-free, 12 fl oz can	1	each	355	100	0	0	0	0	0	0
20031	Soda, grape, carbonated	1.5	cup	372	89	160	0	42	0	0	0
20032	Soda, lemon lime	1.5	cup	368	90	147	0	38	0	0	0
20271	Soda, mountain dew	1.5	cup	360	—	170	0	46	0	0	0
20160	Soda, orange, Minute Maid, can/bottle	1.5	cup	360	90	168	0	43	0	0	0
20269	Soda, pepsi, diet, caffeine free	1.5	cup	360	100	0	0	0	0	0	0
20009	Soda, root beer	1.5	cup	370	89	152	0	39	0	0	0
2066	Sorbet, fruit, citrus flavor	1	cup	200	76	184	1	46	.2	0	0
2065	Sorbet, fruit, non-citrus flavor	1	cup	200	82	140	2	33	0	0	.1
56075	Souffle, cheese	1	cup	112	71	195	11	5	.1	14	5.3
56076	Souffle, spinach	1	cup	136	74	219	11	3	3.8	18	7.2
50575	Soup, Home Cookin', hearty lentil, RTS	1	cup	245	—	150	7	26	5	2	.5
50124	Soup, Scotch broth, w/water	1	cup	241	92	80	5	10	1.2	3	1.1
50065	Soup, bean & ham, RTS, can	1	each	546	79	519	28	61	25.1	19	7.5
50064	Soup, bean & ham, chunky, RTS	1	cup	243	79	231	13	27	11.2	9	3.3
50063	Soup, bean and 'frank', w/water	1	cup	250	83	188	10	22	5.7	7	2.1

A

FM_Un	FP_Un	Choles	Calc	Phos	Sodium	Pota	Zinc	Iron	Magnes	A_RE	Vit_C	B1	B2	B3	B6	Fola	B12
31.1	36	0	197	1164	60	611	15.5	11.7	521	10	0	1.08	.13	7	.22	144	0
27.1	31.4	0	1404	906	16	674	11.2	21	505	1	0	1.14	.36	6.5	1.14	139	0
0	0	0	7	11	2	59	.1	.2	4	202	1	.01	0	0	.06	4	0
0	0	0	4	6	1	33	0	.1	2	0	1	.01	0	0	.04	3	0
0	0	0	—	73	66	0	—	—	—	—	—	—	—	—	—	—	0
0	0	0	—	0	65	0	—	—	—	—	—	—	—	—	—	—	0
0	0	0	—	—	65	0	—	—	—	—	—	—	—	—	—	—	0
.5	.1	5	52	38	44	92	.5	.1	8	13	4	.02	.06	.1	.03	4	.12
0	0	0	10	8	9	100	.1	.3	10	0	0	.01	.03	.1	.01	0	0
92.2	52.1	0	0	0	0	0	0	0	0	0	0	0	0	0	0	0	0
3.6	3.2	186	102	316	655	454	1.8	5.5	63	163	18	.18	.1	4.6	.24	11	1.21
—	—	50	60	—	220	—	—	1.8	—	60	27	—	—	—	—	—	—
5.4	3.5	143	58	197	299	328	1.1	2.3	39	29	5	.1	.1	2.7	.22	9	.78
4.5	8.4	205	87	280	391	366	1.5	3.4	52	42	6	.05	.06	3.2	.27	16	1.31
3.4	5	258	83	366	994	419	2.3	3.8	58	40	3	.2	.2	5	.27	24	1.56
5.9	3.9	183	226	363	632	436	1.8	3	60	188	4	.12	.3	3.2	.16	11	1.34
0	0	0	4	2	42	6	0	.3	2	0	2	0	0	0	0	0	0
0	0	—	—	34	35	—	—	—	—	0	—	—	—	—	—	—	0
0	0	—	—	34	35	—	—	—	—	0	—	—	—	—	—	—	0
0	0	0	7	—	10	27	—	.2	—	0	0	0	0	—	0	—	0
0	0	0	5	—	10	27	—	.2	—	0	0	0	0	—	0	—	0
0	0	0	11	53	8	4	0	.1	4	0	0	0	0	0	0	0	0
0	0	0	11	58	14	4	0	.1	4	0	0	0	0	0	0	0	0
0	0	0	14	28	8	18	.3	.1	4	0	0	.04	.07	0	0	0	0
0	0	0	11	40	37	4	.1	.1	0	0	0	0	0	0	0	0	0
0	0	0	14	32	21	0	.3	.1	4	0	0	.02	.08	0	0	0	0
0	0	0	0	27	23	5	—	0	—	0	0	—	—	—	—	—	—
0	0	0	0	35	23	—	—	0	—	0	0	—	—	—	—	—	—
0	0	0	0	0	49	—	—	0	—	0	0	—	—	—	—	—	—
0	0	0	0	0	23	—	—	0	—	0	0	—	—	—	—	—	—
—	—	101	720	—	2131	—	—	4.2	—	288	17	—	—	—	—	—	—
0	0	0	0	0	33	—	—	0	—	0	0	—	—	—	—	—	—
0	0	0	0	0	49	—	—	0	—	0	0	—	—	—	—	—	—
0	0	0	0	0	50	—	—	0	—	0	0	—	—	—	—	—	—
0	0	0	7	0	44	4	.2	.3	4	0	0	0	0	.1	0	0	0
0	0	0	14	1	9	99	.2	.1	—	0	0	0	0	0	0	0	0
0	0	0	12	47	8	18	—	.1	—	0	0	0	0	—	0	0	0
0	0	0	19	4	45	7	.4	.2	4	0	0	0	0	0	0	0	0
0	0	0	18	0	75	7	.4	0	4	0	0	0	0	0	0	0	0
0	0	0	—	50	24	0	—	—	—	—	—	—	—	—	—	—	0
0	0	0	14	32	32	0	.3	.1	4	0	0	.02	.08	0	0	0	0
0	.1	0	11	44	15	4	0	.1	4	0	0	0	0	0	0	0	0
0	0	0	—	49	51	54	—	—	—	—	—	—	—	—	—	—	0
0	0	0	14	32	21	0	.3	.1	4	0	0	.02	.08	0	0	0	0
0	0	0	14	39	57	7	.2	.1	4	0	0	0	0	0	0	0	0
0	0	0	19	0	44	4	.3	.2	4	0	0	0	0	0	0	0	0
0	0	0	14	39	57	7	.2	.1	4	0	0	0	0	0	0	0	0
0	0	0	0	0	34	—	—	0	—	0	0	—	—	—	—	—	—
0	0	0	11	0	26	4	.2	.7	4	0	0	—	—	—	—	—	—
0	0	0	14	39	57	7	.2	.1	4	0	0	0	0	0	0	0	0
0	0	0	11	0	56	4	.3	.3	4	0	0	0	0	0	0	0	0
0	0	0	7	0	40	4	.2	.3	4	0	0	0	0	.1	0	0	0
0	0	—	0	0	70	—	—	0	—	0	0	—	—	—	—	—	—
0	0	0	7	1	2	60	.2	.3	4	0	0	0	0	0	0	0	0
0	0	—	0	41	35	—	—	0	—	0	0	—	—	—	—	—	—
0	0	0	18	0	48	4	.3	.2	4	0	0	0	0	0	0	0	0
0	0	0	18	26	16	200	0	.9	16	54	51	.02	.06	.3	.04	44	0
0	0	0	4	0	92	4	.1	.1	2	0	0	0	0	0	0	0	0
4.8	2.7	207	202	200	291	145	1	.8	16	168	0	.08	.37	.3	.09	24	.8
6.8	3.1	184	230	231	763	201	1.3	1.4	38	675	3	.09	.3	.5	.12	62	1.37
—	—	0	40	—	860	—	—	3.6	—	—	2	—	—	—	—	—	—
.8	.6	5	14	55	1012	159	1.6	.8	5	218	1	.02	.05	1.2	.07	10	.26
8.6	2.1	49	175	322	2184	956	2.4	7.3	104	888	10	.33	.33	3.8	.27	66	.16
3.8	.9	22	78	143	972	425	1.1	3.3	46	395	4	.15	.15	1.7	.12	29	.07
2.7	1.6	12	88	165	1092	478	1.2	2.4	48	87	1	.11	.06	1	.13	30	.08

A

EshaCode	Food Item	Qty.	Meas	Wgt	Wtr	Cals	Prot	Carb	Fib	Fat	F_Sat
50151	Soup, bean w/bacon, dry, w/water	1	cup	265	90	106	6	16	9	2	1
50000	Soup, bean with bacon, prep w/water	1	cup	253	84	172	8	23	8.6	6	1.5
50198	Soup, beef and mushroom, w/water	1	cup	244	93	73	6	6	0	3	1.5
50001	Soup, beef broth/bouillon, condensed, prepared	1	cup	240	98	17	3	0	0	1	.3
50002	Soup, beef broth/bouillon, ready to serve can	1	each	397	98	28	5	0	0	1	.4
50153	Soup, beef noodle, dry, w/water	1	cup	251	95	40	2	6	.8	1	.3
50003	Soup, beef noodle, prep w/water	1	cup	244	92	83	5	9	.7	3	1.2
50206	Soup, beef stroganoff, chunky style	1	cup	240	80	235	12	22	1.4	11	5.1
50066	Soup, beef, chunky, RTS	1	cup	240	83	170	12	20	1.4	5	2.5
50067	Soup, beef, chunky, RTS, can	1	each	539	83	383	26	44	3.2	12	5.7
50134	Soup, bisque, tomato, prepared, w/milk	1	cup	251	82	198	6	29	.1	7	3.1
50135	Soup, bisque, tomato, w/water	1	cup	247	87	124	2	24	.1	3	.5
50060	Soup, black bean, w/water	1	cup	247	87	116	6	20	4.4	2	.4
50204	Soup, bouillabaisse	1	cup	227	78	242	34	5	.6	9	2
50035	Soup, broth, chicken, dry cube, prepared	1	cup	243	97	12	1	2	0	0	.1
50183	Soup, broth/bouillon, beef, canned, low sodium	1	cup	240	96	38	5	1	0	1	.4
50220	Soup, broth/bouillon, beef, condensed	1	each	298	96	36	7	2	0	0	0
50033	Soup, broth/bouillon, beef, dry cube, prepared	1	cup	241	98	7	1	1	0	0	.1
50032	Soup, broth/bouillon, beef, dry, w/water	1	cup	244	97	20	1	2	0	1	.3
50004	Soup, broth/bouillon, chicken, condensed, prepared	1	cup	244	96	39	5	1	0	1	.4
50155	Soup, cauliflower, dry, w/water	1	cup	256	93	69	3	11	.2	2	.3
50070	Soup, cheese, condensed, can	1	each	312	77	378	13	26	2.5	26	16.2
50071	Soup, cheese, prepared w/milk	1	cup	251	82	231	9	16	1	15	9.1
50072	Soup, cheese, prepared w/water	1	cup	247	88	156	5	10	0	10	6.7
50089	Soup, chicken & vegetable chunky, RTS	1	each	539	83	372	28	42	.5	11	3.2
50088	Soup, chicken & vegetable, chunky, RTS	1	each	298	83	206	15	24	.3	6	1.8
50074	Soup, chicken and dumpling, prep w/water	1	cup	241	92	96	6	6	.7	6	1.3
50077	Soup, chicken gumbo, prep w/water	1	cup	244	94	56	3	8	2	1	.3
50080	Soup, chicken mushroom, w/water	1	cup	244	90	132	4	9	0	9	2.4
50084	Soup, chicken noodle & meatballs, RTS	1	cup	248	91	99	8	8	.6	4	1.1
50081	Soup, chicken noodle, chunky, RTS	1	cup	240	84	175	13	17	3.8	6	1.4
50082	Soup, chicken noodle, chunky, RTS, can	1	each	539	84	393	29	38	8.6	14	3.1
50037	Soup, chicken noodle, dry, prep w/water	1	cup	252	94	53	3	7	.8	1	.3
50005	Soup, chicken noodle, prep w/water	1	cup	241	92	75	4	9	.7	2	.7
50085	Soup, chicken rice, chunky, RTS	1	cup	240	87	127	12	13	1	3	1
50086	Soup, chicken rice, chunky, RTS, can	1	each	539	87	286	28	29	2.2	7	2.2
50161	Soup, chicken rice, dry, w/water	1	cup	253	94	61	2	9	.8	1	.3
50020	Soup, chicken rice, w/water	1	cup	241	94	60	4	7	.7	2	.5
50038	Soup, chicken vegetable, dry, prep w/water	1	cup	251	95	50	3	8	.5	1	.2
50091	Soup, chicken vegetable, prep w/water	1	cup	241	93	75	4	9	1	3	.8
50052	Soup, chicken, chunky, ready to serve	1	cup	251	84	178	13	17	1.5	7	2
50053	Soup, chicken, chunky, ready to serve, can	1	each	305	84	217	16	21	1.8	8	2.4
50007	Soup, chili beef, w/water	1	cup	250	85	170	7	22	9.5	7	3.4
50166	Soup, consomme, w/gelatin, prepared mix	1	cup	249	95	17	2	2	0	0	0
50213	Soup, crab bisque	1	cup	248	81	254	20	12	.3	14	4.6
50099	Soup, crab, RTS	1	cup	244	92	76	6	10	.7	2	.4
50100	Soup, crab, RTS, can	1	each	369	92	114	8	16	1.1	2	.6
50056	Soup, cream of asparagus, condensed, can	1	each	305	84	210	6	26	1.2	10	2.5
50149	Soup, cream of asparagus, dry, w/water	1	cup	251	94	58	2	9	.4	2	0
50057	Soup, cream of asparagus, w/milk	1	cup	248	86	161	6	16	.7	8	3.3
50058	Soup, cream of asparagus, w/water	1	cup	244	92	85	2	11	.5	4	1
50188	Soup, cream of bacon, prepared w/water	1	cup	244	91	117	3	9	.2	7	2.1
50189	Soup, cream of broccoli	1	cup	237	81	234	9	16	1.8	16	6
50017	Soup, cream of celery, condensed, can	1	each	305	85	220	4	22	1.8	14	3.4
50157	Soup, cream of celery, dry, w/water	1	cup	254	94	64	3	10	.5	2	.3
50015	Soup, cream of celery, w/milk	1	cup	248	86	164	6	15	.7	10	3.9
50016	Soup, cream of celery, w/water	1	cup	244	92	90	2	9	.7	6	1.4
50019	Soup, cream of chicken, condensed, can	1	each	305	82	284	8	22	.6	18	5.1
50036	Soup, cream of chicken, dry, prep w/water	1	cup	261	91	107	2	13	.3	5	3.4
50006	Soup, cream of chicken, w/milk	1	cup	248	85	191	7	15	.2	12	4.6
50018	Soup, cream of chicken, w/water	1	cup	244	91	117	3	9	.2	7	2.1
50010	Soup, cream of mushroom, condensed, can	1	each	305	81	314	5	23	.9	23	6.2
50588	Soup, cream of mushroom, low sodium, RTS	1	each	298	87	174	3	14	2.9	14	5.1
50011	Soup, cream of mushroom, w/milk	1	cup	248	85	203	6	15	.5	14	5.1
50049	Soup, cream of mushroom, w/water	1	cup	244	90	129	2	9	.5	9	2.4

FM_Un	FP_Un	Choles	Calc	Phos	Sodium	Pota	Zinc	Iron	Magnes	A_RE	Vit_C	B1	B2	B3	B6	Fola	B12
1.6	1.4	0	55	72	1010	396	3.1	1.6	7	588	6	.07	.06	1.2	.19	17	0
3.6	3.1	0	124	162	2269	889	7	3.7	16	1320	14	.16	.15	2.7	.43	37	0
.3	.1	0	8	30	51	104	.2	.6	20	20	6	.05	.05	.8	.05	10	0
.8	.7	0	22	34	822	210	.5	1.1	7	301	1	.05	.05	.9	.06	11	0
1.7	.6	22	166	161	1061	322	.7	.5	17	67	1	.08	.24	.6	.09	9	.5
3	1	54	31	153	760	314	1.1	1.8	21	97	3	.42	.27	4.7	.19	19	.4
0	0	0	36	36	22	62	—	0	—	43	0	0	.06	—	—	—	.11
—	—	0	32	61	32	626	.2	1.4	47	0	46	.16	.11	2	.13	32	0
.5	1	0	257	—	94	322	.5	2.1	—	101	5	.16	.49	—	.16	26	.78
2	4.6	0	252	—	92	316	.5	2	—	100	5	.15	.48	—	.15	26	.76
.2	.5	0	212	593	18	2097	2.2	8.1	255	4	0	.61	.22	2.3	.5	268	0
.8	2	0	10	118	29	338	.6	1.4	46	8	0	.39	.17	.4	.1	4	0
0	0	0	90	—	14	4	—	.3	—	0	0	.02	.02	.7	—	—	0
4.7	10.7	0	116	305	3	1234	3	3.8	145	17	2	.08	.12	1.5	.25	190	0
.5	1.3	0	24	57	5	169	.4	.7	25	0	5	.12	.04	.4	.06	60	0
.9	2.4	0	56	127	9	334	1	1.2	56	1	8	.19	.05	1	.1	75	0
4.2	10.9	0	380	305	12	1275	5.3	15.1	201	0	23	.28	.33	0	.23	14	0
4.8	10.9	0	119	312	140	1264	3.1	3.8	149	17	2	.09	.12	1.5	.26	194	0
3.4	8.7	0	175	421	2	886	2	8.9	148	2	3	.27	.49	.7	.4	92	0
4.1	10.5	0	232	558	2	1173	4.1	3.4	196	2	4	.37	.65	.9	.19	176	0
1.1	2.7	0	131	142	13	485	.8	2.2	54	14	15	.23	.14	1.1	.05	100	0
4.8	10.9	0	119	312	3	1264	3.1	3.8	149	17	2	.09	.12	1.5	.26	194	0
3.9	3.9	22	52	113	1220	245	2.4	3.2	20	100	5	.15	.18	2.2	.12	5	.82
.4	.5	8	40	88	955	303	1.1	2.8	21	120	10	.35	.28	4.5	.13	6	0
13.1	2.2	49	83	323	436	513	2.8	22.6	39	128	16	.38	.45	4.8	.14	31	72.4
—	—	—	1660	—	349	—	—	192	—	—	1	—	—	—	—	—	—
0	.4	0	194	75	746	538	1	3.7	131	1505	32	.04	.25	.6	.19	136	0
0	.2	0	97	37	88	269	.5	1.8	66	753	16	.02	.12	.3	.09	68	0
0	.4	0	272	94	58	740	1	4.9	163	1878	31	.03	.3	.8	.21	209	0
0	.2	0	245	101	126	839	1.4	6.4	157	1474	18	.17	.42	.9	.44	263	0
0	.2	0	277	91	163	566	1.3	2.9	131	1478	23	.11	.32	.8	.28	205	0
0	.2	0	173	64	115	504	.7	3.2	90	1210	38	.13	.24	.7	.22	187	0
0	.1	0	55	27	44	312	.3	1.5	44	376	16	.04	.11	.4	.11	109	0
0	0	0	26	12	22	146	.1	.7	22	179	5	.02	.05	.2	.05	36	0
0	.3	0	178	88	142	1004	1	4.9	142	1089	43	.13	.32	1.2	.34	297	0
—	—	—	350	400	100	280	—	4.5	140	50	60	1.5	1.7	20	2	400	6
4.4	1.9	1	3	2	140	4	0	0	0	152	0	0	0	0	0	0	.01
2.7	1.6	37	13	58	304	124	.5	.8	10	14	2	.16	.13	1.3	.1	9	.12
0	.1	0	90	92	8	896	.3	1.9	88	88	22	.34	.03	1.8	.4	38	0
0	.1	0	108	110	10	1070	.4	2.3	105	105	26	.41	.03	2.2	.48	46	0
0	.1	0	64	66	7	644	.3	1.4	64	63	16	.24	.02	1.3	.29	28	0
0	.1	0	84	55	8	582	.3	1.2	60	1435	31	.15	.04	2	.25	39	0
0	.1	0	100	66	10	696	.3	1.5	71	1715	37	.18	.04	2.4	.3	47	0
0	.1	0	46	34	5	319	.3	1.4	22	801	8	.12	.09	1.1	.17	39	0
0	0	0	13	23	5	104	.3	.8	14	13	3	.02	.03	.5	.04	11	0
0	.2	0	49	70	2	346	.7	.6	43	52	10	.09	.09	.9	.17	36	0
.1	.6	0	41	55	19	859	.4	1.1	53	1448	23	.18	.11	1.3	.41	39	0
0	.1	0	18	34	1	168	.3	.4	23	10	13	.06	.03	.6	.1	25	0
0	.1	0	14	25	1	126	.2	.3	17	8	10	.05	.02	.4	.08	19	0
0	.2	0	33	22	28	181	.3	.5	17	17	5	.06	.03	1.3	.15	12	0
0	.2	0	49	70	2	346	.7	.6	43	52	10	.08	.07	.9	.12	36	0
0	.1	0	26	46	3	254	.3	.6	30	26	19	.08	.05	.7	.14	33	0
.1	.5	0	29	41	2	896	.5	.7	16	729	20	.17	.05	1.4	.15	57	0
.1	.6	0	34	48	557	1042	.6	.8	19	849	23	.2	.06	1.7	.17	67	0
0	.1	0	27	58	5	446	.4	.8	40	58	14	.11	.05	.7	.14	34	0
0	.1	0	38	56	4	433	.4	1.1	29	96	8	.09	.09	.9	.1	17	0
0	0	0	3	15	0	73	.1	.1	5	8	5	.01	.01	.1	.02	3	0
0	.1	0	39	66	849	622	.6	1.5	32	122	5	.1	.09	1.2	.34	69	0
0	0	0	23	72	5	455	.3	.6	40	43	8	.07	.07	.8	.14	30	0
0	.1	0	20	42	4	322	.3	.5	29	44	12	.09	.04	.5	.12	29	0
0	.1	0	27	58	5	446	.4	.8	40	55	14	.11	.05	.7	.14	32	0
3.1	.4	34	29	110	1006	426	4.2	2.2	39	262	7	.07	.12	2.4	.2	31	1.59
1.3	1	34	31	152	469	500	1.3	1.7	40	45	16	.1	.16	4.7	.28	47	.15
3.8	.7	52	36	200	1023	723	3.2	2.3	53	315	14	.24	.27	5.3	.41	34	1.49
2.1	.3	32	167	162	1041	235	10.3	1	20	44	4	.07	.23	.3	.06	10	2.65

EshaCode	Food Item	Qty.	Meas	Wgt	Wtr	Cals	Prot	Carb	Fib	Fat	F_Sat
50115	Stew, oyster, prep w/water	1	cup	241	95	58	2	4	0	4	2.5
50205	Stew, seafood, tomato base sauce	1	cup	252	83	169	20	15	2.4	3	.8
50201	Stew, veal, tomato base sauce	1	cup	252	83	190	16	16	2.6	7	2.8
50202	Stew, venison, tomato base sauce	1	cup	252	83	163	19	18	3	2	.7
3316	Strawberries, cooked, unsweetened	1	cup	242	94	49	1	11	4.2	1	0
3135	Strawberries, fresh	1	cup	166	92	50	1	12	2.5	1	0
3136	Strawberries, fresh slices	1	each	32	92	10	0	2	.5	0	0
3137	Strawberries, frozen, unsweetened	1	cup	149	90	52	1	14	2.4	0	0
3236	Strawberries, sliced, frozen, sweetened, thawed	1	cup	255	73	245	1	66	4.8	0	0
20212	Strawberry Julius	2	cup	430	85	340	1	82	.9	1	.2
49025	Strudel, berry	1	piece	64	44	159	2	29	1.4	4	.8
49027	Strudel, cheese	1	piece	64	38	195	6	24	.4	8	3.9
49026	Strudel, cherry	1	piece	64	39	179	3	29	1.1	6	.9
49028	Strudel, peach	1	piece	64	55	123	2	23	1.2	3	.6
42147	Stuffing mix, cornbread, prepared	.5	cup	100	65	179	3	22	—	9	1.8
5251	Succotash, cooked from fresh	1	cup	192	68	221	10	47	9.7	2	.3
5154	Succotash, frozen, cooked	1	cup	170	74	158	7	34	9.2	2	.3
5601	Succotash, whole corn & lima beans, canned	1	cup	255	82	161	7	36	13.8	1	.2
3270	Sugar apple (sweetsop), raw	1	each	155	73	146	3	37	6.8	0	—
25118	Sugar cane juice	100	grams	100	87	35	0	9	—	0	—
25040	Sugar, brown, Sugar Twin	1	tsp	0	0	1	0	0	0	0	0
25005	Sugar, brown, packed	1	cup	145	2	545	0	141	0	0	0
25043	Sugar, maple, piece	1	each	28	8	100	0	26	0	0	—
25006	Sugar, white, granulated	1	cup	200	0	774	0	200	0	0	0
25008	Sugar, white, powdered, sifted	1	cup	100	0	389	0	100	0	0	0
25009	Sugar, white, powdered, unsifted	1	cup	120	0	467	0	119	0	0	0
56244	Sukiyaki	1	cup	162	77	175	19	6	1.1	8	3
4661	Sunflower seed butter, salted	1	Tbs	16	1	93	3	4	2	8	.8
4550	Sunflower seed butter, unsalted	1	Tbs	16	1	93	3	4	1	8	.8
4545	Sunflower seed kernels, dry	.25	cup	36	5	205	8	7	2.2	18	1.9
4546	Sunflower seed kernels, oil roasted, unsalted	1	cup	135	3	830	29	20	8.4	78	8.1
4551	Sunflower seed, dry roasted	1	cup	128	1	745	25	31	8.1	64	6.7
4552	Sunflower seed, oil roasted, salted	1	cup	135	3	830	29	20	8.4	78	8.1
4597	Sunflower seeds, dry roasted, salted	1	cup	128	1	745	25	31	8.1	64	6.7
62150	Supplement, Osmolite, prepared, Ross Labs	1	cup	253	79	250	9	34	0	9	—
62214	Supplement, shake, vanilla, prepared, MenuMagic	.75	cup	195	66	300	9	47	0	9	1.5
56315	Sushi, w/egg, rolled in seaweed	1	cup	166	74	204	9	23	.4	8	2
56313	Sushi, w/vegetables & fish	1	cup	166	64	238	9	48	1.5	1	.2
56314	Sushi, w/vegetables, rolled in seaweed	1	cup	166	71	193	4	43	1	0	.1
5602	Swamp cabbage, chopped, cooked	1	cup	98	93	20	2	4	1.9	0	—
15921	Sweet & sour chicken breast	1	each	131	79	117	8	15	.8	3	.6
5429	Sweet potato leaves, raw	1	cup	35	88	12	1	2	.4	0	0
5430	Sweet potato leaves, steamed	1	cup	64	89	22	1	5	1.2	0	0
5155	Sweet potato, baked, then peeled	1	each	114	73	117	2	28	3.4	0	0
5158	Sweet potato, baked, then peeled	.5	cup	100	73	103	2	24	3	0	0
5166	Sweet potato, candied	1	piece	52	67	71	0	14	1	2	.7
5167	Sweet potato, candied, cup measure	1	cup	196	67	269	2	55	3.8	6	2.6
5554	Sweet potato, canned, w/syrup	1	cup	228	77	203	2	48	4.1	0	.1
5555	Sweet potato, canned, w/syrup, drained	1	cup	196	72	212	3	50	3.5	1	.2
5161	Sweet potato, peeled, boiled, mashed	1	cup	200	73	210	3	49	4.6	1	.2
5159	Sweet potato, peeled, boiled, medium size	1	each	156	73	164	3	38	3.6	0	.1
25045	Sweetener, Fruit Source, granular	100	grams	100	3	378	1	93	0	0	0
25036	Sweetener, NutraSweet, low calorie	5	grams	5	4	19	5	0	0	0	0
25041	Sweetener, saccharin, tablet	1	each	0	0	0	0	0	0	0	0
25070	Sweetener, sugar substitute, saccharin-based, liquid	1	tsp	5	98	0	0	0	0	0	0
5057	Swiss chard, chopped, raw	1	cup	36	93	7	1	1	.6	0	0
5059	Swiss chard, cooked, no added salt	1	cup	175	93	35	3	7	3.7	0	0
5058	Swiss chard, raw leaf	1	each	48	93	9	1	2	.8	0	0
23013	Syrup, chocolate, thin	1	cup	300	37	654	6	177	5.4	3	1.6
23056	Syrup, chocolate, thin	1	cup	300	29	735	5	197	5.4	4	2.3
25010	Syrup, corn, dark	1	cup	328	23	925	0	251	0	0	0
25000	Syrup, corn, light	1	cup	328	23	925	0	251	0	0	0
25002	Syrup, maple	1	Tbs	20	32	52	0	13	0	0	0
23042	Syrup, pancake	1	cup	314	24	901	0	238	0	0	0
23177	Syrup, pancake, Pillsbury Lite	2	Tbs	39	64	55	0	14	.5	0	0

FM_Un	FP_Un	Choles	Calc	Phos	Sodium	Pota	Zinc	Iron	Magnes	A_RE	Vit_C	B1	B2	B3	B6	Fola	B12
.9	.2	14	22	48	981	48	10.3	1	5	7	3	.02	.04	.2	.01	2	2.19
1	.6	96	80	221	985	811	1.8	9.4	45	532	31	.18	.21	3.5	.34	34	24.3
2.6	.6	56	37	193	607	547	2.1	1.4	36	615	12	.14	.23	6.9	.4	26	.55
.5	.4	58	31	208	679	765	2	3.5	45	534	27	.22	.4	5.6	.39	30	3.21
.1	.3	0	24	31	4	269	.2	.6	17	5	87	.03	.11	.4	.1	27	0
.1	.3	0	23	32	2	276	.2	.6	17	5	94	.03	.11	.4	.1	29	0
0	.1	0	4	6	0	53	0	.1	3	1	18	.01	.02	.1	.02	6	0
0	.1	0	24	19	3	221	.2	1.1	16	7	61	.03	.06	.7	.04	25	0
0	.2	0	28	33	8	250	.2	1.5	18	6	106	.04	.13	1	.08	38	0
.1	.2	0	54	—	15	165	—	.3	—	0	12	.02	.13	—	.02	—	0
1.7	1.2	11	15	26	103	55	.2	.8	6	53	5	.09	.09	.8	.02	6	.03
2.8	1.1	42	90	87	116	64	.6	.8	8	95	0	.08	.16	.7	.03	8	.12
2	2.9	9	19	40	88	100	.3	.8	15	79	3	.09	.08	.8	.05	8	.02
1.2	.9	8	12	22	75	102	.2	.6	7	59	3	.06	.07	1	.02	4	.02
3.9	2.7	0	26	34	455	62	.2	.9	13	85	1	.12	.09	1.2	.04	8	.01
.3	.7	0	33	225	33	787	1.2	2.9	102	56	16	.32	.18	2.6	.22	63	0
.3	.7	0	26	119	76	451	.8	1.5	39	39	10	.13	.12	2.2	.16	56	0
.3	.6	0	28	140	564	416	1.3	1.4	48	37	12	.07	.15	1.6	.12	81	0
—	—	0	37	50	14	383	.2	.9	33	2	56	.17	.18	1.4	.31	22	0
—	—	—	13	9	—	—	—	.1	—	—	—	.01	.01	.1	—	—	—
0	0	0	4	0	2	0	0	0	0	0	0	0	0	0	0	0	0
0	0	0	123	32	57	502	.3	2.8	42	0	0	.01	.01	.1	.04	1	0
—	—	0	26	1	3	78	1.7	.5	5	1	0	0	0	0	0	0	0
0	0	0	2	4	2	4	.1	.1	0	0	0	0	.04	0	0	0	0
0	0	0	1	2	1	2	0	.1	0	0	0	0	0	0	0	0	0
0	0	0	1	2	1	2	0	.1	0	0	0	0	0	0	0	0	0
3.2	.8	153	63	209	762	468	3.7	3.3	48	263	4	.13	.42	3.2	.36	62	1.56
1.5	5	0	20	118	83	12	.8	.8	59	1	0	.05	.04	.9	.13	38	0
1.5	5	0	20	118	0	12	.8	.8	59	1	0	.05	.04	.9	.13	38	0
3.4	11.8	0	42	254	1	248	1.8	2.4	127	2	1	.82	.09	1.6	.28	82	0
14.9	51.2	0	76	1537	4	652	7	9.1	171	7	2	.43	.38	5.6	1.07	316	0
12.2	42.1	0	90	1478	4	1088	6.8	4.9	165	6	2	.14	.32	9	1.03	303	0
14.9	51.2	0	76	1537	814	652	7	9.1	171	7	2	.43	.38	5.6	1.07	316	0
12.2	42.1	0	90	1478	998	1088	6.8	4.9	165	6	2	.14	.32	9	1.03	303	0
1.8	—	4	125	125	150	240	2.8	2.2	50	125	38	.38	.43	5	.5	100	1.5
—	—	4	300	200	200	350	3	3.6	120	200	12	.3	.34	4	.4	80	1.2
3.2	1.8	196	45	144	548	140	1.1	1.8	23	133	2	.14	.27	1.6	.14	28	.42
.2	.2	11	26	110	344	216	.8	2.4	27	172	4	.29	.07	3	.16	15	.33
.1	.1	0	23	68	151	111	.7	1.5	23	66	3	.21	.04	2	.15	11	0
—	—	0	53	41	120	278	.2	1.3	29	510	16	.05	.08	.5	.08	34	0
.8	1.5	23	16	75	732	187	.7	.8	21	20	12	.06	.08	3.1	.18	6	.08
0	0	0	13	33	3	181	.1	.4	21	36	4	.06	.12	.4	.07	28	0
0	.1	0	15	38	8	305	.2	.4	39	59	1	.07	.17	.6	.1	31	0
0	.1	0	32	63	11	397	.3	.5	23	2487	28	.08	.14	.7	.28	26	0
0	0	0	28	55	10	348	.3	.4	20	2182	25	.07	.13	.6	.24	23	0
.3	.1	4	14	14	36	98	.1	.6	6	218	3	.01	.02	.2	.02	6	0
1.2	.3	16	51	51	137	370	.3	2.2	22	821	13	.04	.08	.8	.08	22	0
0	.2	0	34	62	100	422	.4	1.8	30	1303	24	.06	.1	1	.12	15	0
0	.3	0	33	49	76	378	.3	1.9	24	1402	21	.05	.07	.7	.12	16	0
0	.3	0	42	54	26	368	.5	1.1	20	3410	34	.11	.28	1.3	.49	22	0
0	.2	0	33	42	20	287	.4	.9	16	2659	27	.08	.22	1	.38	17	0
0	0	0	33	49	49	297	—	.9	—	4	7	.02	.03	1.3	—	—	—
0	0	0	0	0	2	0	—	.1	—	0	0	0	0	0	—	—	0
0	0	0	0	0	0	1	0	0	0	0	0	0	0	0	0	0	0
0	0	0	0	0	1	5	0	0	0	0	0	0	0	0	0	0	0
0	0	0	18	17	77	136	.1	.6	29	119	11	.01	.03	.1	.04	5	0
0	.1	0	102	58	313	961	.6	4	151	550	32	.06	.15	.6	.15	15	0
0	.1	0	24	22	102	182	.2	.9	39	158	14	.02	.04	.2	.05	7	0
.9	.1	0	42	387	288	672	2.2	6.4	195	9	1	.03	.15	1	.02	12	0
1.3	.1	0	42	387	459	1443	2.2	40.8	195	3903	3	.01	2.48	101	.06	12	0
0	0	0	59	36	508	144	.1	1.2	26	0	0	.04	.03	.1	.03	0	0
0	0	0	10	7	397	13	.1	.2	7	0	0	.04	.03	.1	.03	0	0
0	0	0	13	0	2	41	.8	.2	3	0	0	0	0	0	0	0	0
0	0	0	3	28	261	6	.1	.3	6	0	0	.04	.03	.1	0	0	0
0	0	0	2	—	104	—	—	0	—	0	0	—	—	—	—	—	—

EshaCode	Food Item	Qty.	Meas	Wgt	Wtr	Cals	Prot	Carb	Fib	Fat	F_Sat
23176	Syrup, pancake, Pillsbury regular	2	Tbs	39	34	103	0	26	.1	0	0
23090	Syrup, pancake, buttery, Mrs. Butterworth's	1	cup	315	24	932	0	233	0	5	3.2
23091	Syrup, pancake, buttery, low cal, Butterworth's	1	Tbs	18	55	29	0	8	0	0	0
23172	Syrup, pancake, reduced-calorie	1	oz.	28	55	46	0	13	0	0	0
23161	Syrup, pancake, w/2% maple	1	cup	315	30	835	0	219	0	0	—
56916	Tabbouleh/tabbuli	1	cup	160	78	187	3	17	4.7	13	1.8
57062	Taco Bell, 7 Layer Burrito	1	each	276	—	440	19	67	10	9	3.5
57063	Taco Bell, Border Light taco	1	each	78	—	140	11	11	2	5	1.5
57065	Taco Bell, Border Light taco, soft	1	each	99	—	180	13	19	2	5	2.5
57067	Taco Bell, Border Light bean burrito	1	each	198	—	330	14	55	8	6	2
6490	Taco Bell, Border Light burrito supreme	1	each	248	—	350	20	50	4	8	3
56536	Taco Bell, Pintos & cheese	1	each	128	69	190	9	19	7	9	3.6
56690	Taco Bell, burrito, Big Beef Supreme	1	each	298	64	525	25	51	—	25	11
56688	Taco Bell, burrito, chicken	1	each	171	58	345	17	41	—	13	5
56691	Taco Bell, burrito, seven layer	1	each	234	60	458	14	55	8.5	20	5.9
45585	Taco Bell, cinnamon twist	1	each	35	5	139	1	20	.4	6	0
56531	Taco Bell, mexican pizza	1	each	223	55	574	19	40	2	38	12
56534	Taco Bell, nachos, bellgrande, svg	1	each	287	59	633	22	61	—	34	12.3
56684	Taco Bell, nachos, supreme, serving	1	each	145	52	364	12	39	—	18	5
56524	Taco Bell, taco	1	each	78	58	180	10	11	1	11	4.6
56689	Taco Bell, taco, soft, chicken	1	each	128	65	223	14	20	—	10	4
56693	Taco Bell, taco, soft, steak	1	each	100	56	217	12	21	—	9	4
56526	Taco Bell, taco, soft, supreme	1	each	124	60	262	13	20	1.9	14	7.3
56692	Taco Bell, taco, supreme	1	each	106	62	230	11	12	1	15	7.5
56553	Taco Time, Mexi-fries, svg	1	each	130	58	330	3	31	1	20	7
56540	Taco Time, burrito, bean, crispy	1	each	149	55	354	11	34	4	21	4
56541	Taco Time, burrito, beef, crispy	1	each	149	44	466	22	32	1	28	10
56544	Taco Time, burrito, combo, soft	1	each	255	60	520	27	48	4	25	10
56555	Taco Time, chicken fajita salad	1	each	297	66	541	28	39	2	31	7
56546	Taco Time, taco, natural super	1	each	283	61	575	28	49	4	31	13
42359	Taco shell, Ortega	2	each	30	—	140	2	20	2	7	1
42168	Taco shell, baked	1	each	13	6	61	1	8	1	3	.4
56061	Taco, chicken	1	each	78	56	175	15	10	.8	8	2.8
4532	Tahini (sesame butter)	1	Tbs	15	3	91	3	3	1.4	8	1.2
56113	Tamale, w/meat	1	each	70	51	183	7	16	2.9	10	3.7
82035	Tamales, Old El Paso	3	each	206	71	330	7	31	5	19	7
3269	Tamarind, raw	5	each	10	31	24	0	6	.5	0	0
3087	Tangelo, fresh	1	each	95	87	45	1	11	1.8	0	0
3237	Tangerine, canned in light syrup	1	cup	252	83	154	1	41	1.8	0	0
3138	Tangerine, fresh	1	each	84	88	37	1	9	1.3	0	0
44020	Taro chips	10	each	23	2	115	1	16	1.7	6	1.5
5543	Taro shoots, cooked slices	1	cup	140	95	20	1	4	—	0	0
5302	Taro slices, cooked	1	cup	132	64	187	1	46	6.7	0	0
5369	Taro, raw slices	1	cup	104	71	111	2	28	4.3	0	0
5544	Taro, tahitian, cooked slices	1	cup	137	86	60	6	9	—	1	.2
26032	Tarragon, ground	1	Tbs	5	8	14	1	2	.4	0	—
48057	Tart, lemon meringue	1	each	117	45	329	4	43	.6	16	4
20014	Tea, brewed	1	cup	240	100	2	0	1	0	0	0
20119	Tea, brewed, chamomile	.75	cup	178	100	2	0	0	0	0	0
20118	Tea, camomile	1	cup	240	100	2	0	0	0	0	0
20079	Tea, decaff, low calorie, frozen, prepared	1	cup	245	99	7	0	2	0	0	0
20022	Tea, from instant, sweetened, w/lemon	1	cup	262	91	89	0	22	0	0	0
20020	Tea, from instant, unsweetened	1	cup	237	100	2	0	0	0	0	0
20036	Tea, herbal, brewed	.75	cup	178	100	2	0	0	0	0	0
20040	Tea, instant, w/lemon, diet, dry, prepared	1	cup	238	99	5	0	1	0	0	0
20038	Tea, instant, w/lemon, prepared	1	cup	238	99	5	0	1	0	0	0
20078	Tea, presweetened, w/low calorie sweetener	1	cup	245	99	5	0	1	0	0	0
7564	Tempeh	1	cup	166	55	330	32	28	—	13	1.8
26312	Thyme, fresh	1	Tbs	4	69	4	0	1	—	0	—
26033	Thyme, ground	1	Tbs	4	8	12	0	3	.8	0	.1
45544	Toaster pastry, Pop Tarts, brown sugar cinnamon	1	each	50	—	220	3	32	1	9	1
45504	Toaster pastry, fruit filled, Poptart	1	each	52	12	204	2	37	.7	5	.8
7500	Tofu (soybean curd, reg)	.5	cup	124	85	94	10	2	1.5	6	.9
7546	Tofu yogurt	1	cup	262	78	254	9	43	.5	5	.7
7520	Tofu, fried, w/Nigari	1	piece	13	50	35	2	1	0	3	.4

FM_Un	FP_Un	Choles	Calc	Phos	Sodium	Pota	Zinc	Iron	Magnes	A_RE	Vit_C	B1	B2	B3	B6	Fola	B12
2.9	2.5	0	13	140	228	171	.4	1	7	0	0	.4	.27	2.7	.28	32	1.2
.8	1.2	0	70	286	694	478	1.7	5.6	47	102	21	.16	.09	1.6	.2	108	0
2.5	5.4	0	54	257	279	342	.8	1.1	13	0	0	.63	.51	6.8	.86	58	2.39
1.2	2.7	0	17	175	219	76	.6	.9	9	0	0	.56	.61	8.2	.5	40	1.22
2.6	5.6	0	28	296	576	188	1.1	1.5	15	0	0	.64	.37	7.4	.74	67	1.74
1.5	3.3	0	21	244	391	128	1.3	1.5	13	0	0	.64	.43	7.1	.85	55	1.7
1.5	3.3	0	20	241	385	126	1.3	1.5	13	0	0	.63	.42	7	.84	55	1.68
3.8	8.3	0	84	398	434	531	1.2	1.8	20	0	0	.97	.8	10.6	1.33	90	3.72
1.5	3.3	0	21	244	391	128	1.3	1.5	13	0	0	.64	.43	7.1	.85	55	1.7
4	3.7	13	146	372	931	211	2	2.7	26	45	1	.77	.55	8.1	.86	70	1.71
0	0	0	8	8	20	48	0	.4	6	0	0	.02	.02	0	.01	0	0
—	—	—	2	—	4	—	—	.2	—	0	0	—	—	—	—	—	—
0	0	0	14	22	2	240	0	1.4	53	0	0	0	0	0	0	0	0
—	—	—	9	6	—	—	—	3.1	—	—	—	.01	.01	.2	—	—	—
0	0	0	—	—	1	—	—	—	—	—	—	—	—	—	—	—	—
0	0	0	20	—	120	10	—	1.8	—	100	0	.15	.17	2	.2	40	—
1.6	.9	34	219	262	523	154	.5	1.2	16	29	2	.15	.23	1	.06	7	.2
4.2	2.4	90	584	699	1394	411	1.4	3.2	43	78	6	.39	.6	2.6	.16	20	.54
—	2`	15	20	—	250	40	—	1.8	—	100	0	.15	.17	2	.2	40	—
2.5	5.1	50	137	124	451	128	.6	1.6	14	26	0	.2	.27	1.6	.04	11	.16
2.2	3	75	110	108	312	124	.6	1.6	17	50	0	.21	.27	1.6	.08	16	.27
5.7	8.1	199	294	289	832	330	1.5	4.3	45	133	1	.55	.71	4.2	.22	43	.73
1.1	1.5	38	56	55	158	63	.3	.8	9	25	0	.1	.14	.8	.04	8	.14
1.1	1	8	81	147	275	45	.2	1.6	8	127	0	.14	.17	1.6	.31	12	.88
2.7	5.2	38	93	252	458	134	.4	1.2	15	20	0	.16	.19	1.2	.08	9	.2
1.2	2	28	83	104	146	123	.9	1.4	25	60	3	.14	.19	1.4	.11	23	.12
—	—	0	20	—	220	60	—	1.8	—	100	0	.15	.17	2	.2	40	—
1.1	2	0	8	131	214	189	.7	.7	38	57	0	.06	.06	.8	.03	15	.23
2.6	5.1	52	191	143	383	119	.5	1.7	14	49	0	.2	.26	1.6	.04	11	.19
1.9	1	39	84	83	150	91	.4	.7	16	25	0	.08	.13	.7	.04	7	.15
1.9	1	39	84	83	150	91	.4	.7	16	25	0	.08	.13	.7	.04	7	.15
17	46.9	0	113	380	12	602	3.3	2.9	203	15	4	.46	.18	1.2	.67	79	0
14.2	39.1	0	94	317	10	502	2.7	2.4	169	12	3	.38	.15	1	.56	66	0
10.2	30	0	46	371	1	419	2.7	2.5	162	24	3	.17	.09	.6	.44	52	0
15.9	46.9	0	72	580	1	655	4.3	3.8	253	37	4	.27	.14	.9	.69	82	0
0	0	0	5	0	7	0	.1	0	2	0	0	0	0	0	0	0	0
0	0	0	27	0	2	0	0	0	0	0	0	0	0	0	0	0	0
0	0	0	2	0	2	0	0	0	2	0	0	0	0	0	0	0	0
0	0	0	5	0	20	0	.5	0	0	0	0	0	0	0	0	0	0
0	0	0	14	39	57	7	.2	.1	4	0	0	0	0	0	0	0	0
0	0	0	4	0	15	0	.4	0	0	0	0	0	0	0	0	0	0
0	0	0	7	39	9	362	.3	0	14	0	2	.09	.12	.6	.2	10	0
0	0	0	3	13	6	83	.3	.6	4	0	1	.01	.02	.3	.11	4	0
0	0	0	1	5	2	34	.1	.2	1	0	0	0	.01	.1	.04	2	0
0	0	0	20	10	7	56	0	0	4	80	7	.02	.02	0	.02	2	0
0	0	0	30	15	10	82	0	0	5	118	11	.02	.03	0	.03	2	0
.1	.4	0	13	14	3	186	.1	.3	18	59	15	.13	.03	.3	.23	4	0
0	.1	0	16	15	93	4	.5	.3	9	0	9	.03	0	.3	.03	3	0
0	.1	0	25	25	147	8	.8	.5	13	0	17	.05	.14	.5	.05	7	0
9.6	3.4	22	137	103	818	131	1	1.2	10	14	10	.19	.16	2	.06	5	.59
—	—	55	400	356	260	776	1.4	1.1	65	100	0	.15	.67	.5	.17	25	1.2
—	—	45	150	—	840	—	—	3.6	—	100	6	—	—	—	—	—	—
—	—	60	150	342	910	384	5.9	3.6	39	80	9	.31	.32	6.6	.27	29	2.04
—	—	55	100	—	720	—	—	2.7	—	40	6	—	—	—	—	—	—
—	—	105	250	—	1510	578	—	6.3	—	200	15	.45	1.53	6	—	—	—
—	—	70	100	—	810	468	—	5.4	—	60	6	.43	.33	5.8	—	—	—
—	—	30	100	—	560	—	—	3.6	—	20	1	—	—	—	—	—	—
0	.1	0	3	26	0	33	.2	.3	12	0	0	.04	.01	.5	.03	4	0
.1	.4	0	13	182	0	213	1.3	1.9	110	0	0	.08	.09	2.2	.21	10	0
.2	.7	0	22	304	1	355	2.2	3.2	183	0	0	.16	.17	4.1	.39	24	0
1	4.5	0	29	632	9	669	9.2	4.7	179	0	0	1.13	.34	4.6	.88	148	0
1.4	6	0	39	842	12	892	12.3	6.3	239	0	0	1.88	.5	6.8	1.3	281	0
1.7	7.5	0	51	1294	5	1070	18.9	10.3	362	0	7	1.9	.93	6.3	1.11	398	0
1.3	5.5	0	37	971	3	802	14.1	7.7	271	0	14	1.42	.7	4.8	.83	298	0
.2	.7	0	29	294	4	344	2.5	3.3	117	0	0	.38	.18	5.4	.29	37	0

A

EshaCode	Food Item	Qty.	Meas	Wgt	Wtr	Cals	Prot	Carb	Fib	Fat	F_Sat
38068	Wheat sprouts	1	cup	108	48	214	8	46	1.2	1	.2
22540	Whiskey sour mix, packet	1	each	17	1	64	0	16	0	0	0
22541	Whiskey sour, canned	2	Tbs	31	77	37	0	4	0	0	0
22518	Wine, dessert, dry	.5	cup	118	80	149	0	5	0	0	0
22507	Wine, dessert, sweet	.5	cup	118	72	181	0	14	0	0	0
20076	Wine, non-alcoholic	1	cup	232	98	14	1	3	0	0	0
20077	Wine, non-alcoholic, light	1	cup	251	98	15	1	3	0	0	0
22501	Wine, red	.5	cup	118	88	85	0	2	0	0	0
22600	Wine, rice	100	grams	100	78	134	0	5	0	0	0
22502	Wine, rose'	.5	cup	118	89	84	0	2	0	0	0
22601	Wine, sangria	100	grams	100	83	82	0	11	0	0	0
22509	Wine, sherry, dry	.5	cup	117	89	82	0	2	0	0	0
22511	Wine, sweet vermouth	.5	cup	120	72	184	0	14	0	0	0
22503	Wine, white, dry	.5	cup	119	90	79	0	1	0	0	0
22504	Wine, white, medium	.5	cup	118	90	80	0	1	0	0	0
5433	Winged bean/goabean leaves, raw	1	cup	100	77	74	6	14	2.5	1	.3
5434	Winged bean/goabean tuber, raw	1	cup	100	57	159	12	28	7.4	1	.2
56111	Wonton, fried, meat filled	3	piece	57	43	183	8	12	.6	11	2.2
49016	Wonton/eggroll wrapper	1	each	8	29	23	1	5	—	0	0
5370	Yam, Hawaii Mountain, steamed	1	cup	145	77	119	3	29	4.4	0	0
5553	Yam, orange, canned in syrup	1	cup	228	77	203	2	48	4.1	0	.1
5168	Yam, white, cooked	1	cup	136	70	158	2	38	5.3	0	0
5156	Yams, orange, baked, then peeled, mashed	.5	cup	100	73	103	2	24	3	0	0
5163	Yams, orange, canned, mashed	.5	cup	128	74	129	3	30	1.9	0	.1
5160	Yams, orange, peeled, boiled, mashed	1	cup	200	73	210	3	49	4.6	1	.2
28007	Yeast, baker's, compressed cake	1	each	17	69	18	1	3	1.6	0	0
28000	Yeast, baker's, dry active	4	Tbs	30	8	88	12	12	8.3	1	.2
28002	Yeast, brewer's	1	Tbs	8	5	23	3	3	2.5	0	0
44068	Yogurt chips	1	oz.	28	5	146	3	16	.5	8	2.1
2002	Yogurt, custard fruit, lowfat	1	cup	245	74	250	11	47	.2	3	1.7
70637	Yogurt, frozen, banana-strawberry, HaagenDaz	.5	cup	98	—	170	6	27	—	4	2
70633	Yogurt, frozen, peach, HaagenDaz	.5	cup	98	—	170	6	26	—	4	2
2001	Yogurt, fruit, lowfat	1	cup	245	74	250	11	47	.2	3	1.7
2034	Yogurt, fruit, nonfat, low cal sweetener	1	cup	241	86	122	11	19	1.3	0	.2
2101	Yogurt, lowfat, fruit & nuts	1	cup	245	72	290	11	47	.5	7	2
2015	Yogurt, lowfat, maple	1	cup	245	79	209	12	34	0	3	2
2014	Yogurt, lowfat, vanilla/lemon	1	cup	245	79	209	12	34	0	3	2
2096	Yogurt, nonfat, lemon	1	cup	245	76	223	12	43	0	0	.3
2099	Yogurt, nonfat, lemon	1	cup	245	76	223	12	43	0	0	.3
2098	Yogurt, nonfat, vanilla	1	each	227	76	207	12	40	0	0	.2
2000	Yogurt, plain, lowfat	1	cup	245	85	155	13	17	0	4	2.3
2012	Yogurt, plain, nonfat	1	cup	245	85	137	14	19	0	0	.3
2013	Yogurt, plain, whole milk	1	cup	245	88	150	9	11	0	8	5.2

A

FM_Un	FP_Un	Choles	Calc	Phos	Sodium	Pota	Zinc	Iron	Magnes	A_RE	Vit_C	B1	B2	B3	B6	Fola	B12
.2	.6	0	30	216	17	183	1.8	2.3	89	0	3	.24	.17	3.3	.29	41	0
0	0	0	45	2	46	3	0	.1	3	1	0	0	0	0	0	0	0
0	0	0	0	2	14	3	0	0	0	0	0	0	0	0	0	0	0
0	0	0	9	11	11	109	.1	.3	11	0	0	.02	.02	.3	0	0	0
0	0	0	9	11	11	109	.1	.3	11	0	0	.02	.02	.3	0	0	0
0	0	0	21	35	16	204	.2	.9	23	0	0	0	.02	.2	.05	2	0
0	0	0	23	38	18	221	.2	1	25	0	0	0	.02	.3	.05	3	0
0	0	0	9	16	6	132	.1	.5	15	0	0	.01	.03	.1	.04	2	.01
0	0	0	5	6	2	25	0	.1	6	0	0	0	0	0	0	0	0
0	0	0	9	18	6	117	.1	.4	12	0	0	0	.02	.1	.03	1	.01
0	0	0	4	5	7	35	.1	.1	3	1	4	.01	.01	0	.01	2	0
0	0	0	9	16	9	104	.1	.5	12	0	0	0	.02	.1	.03	1	.01
0	0	0	10	11	11	110	.1	.3	11	0	0	.02	.02	.3	0	0	0
0	0	0	11	7	5	73	.1	.4	11	0	0	0	.01	.1	.02	0	0
0	0	0	11	16	6	94	.1	.4	12	0	0	0	.01	.1	.02	0	0
.3	.2	0	224	63	9	176	1.3	4	8	809	45	.83	.6	3.5	.23	16	0
.2	.2	0	30	45	35	586	1.4	2	24	0	0	.38	.15	1.6	.08	19	0
4.9	3.6	39	17	72	250	114	.7	1.2	13	65	1	.24	.17	1.8	.1	10	.17
0	0	1	4	6	46	7	.1	.3	2	0	0	.04	.03	.4	0	1	0
0	.1	0	12	58	17	718	.5	.6	14	0	0	.12	.02	.2	.3	18	0
0	.2	0	34	62	100	422	.4	1.8	30	1303	24	.06	.1	1	.12	15	0
0	.1	0	19	67	11	911	.3	.7	24	0	16	.13	.04	.8	.31	22	0
0	0	0	28	55	10	348	.3	.4	20	2182	25	.07	.13	.6	.24	23	0
0	.1	0	38	67	96	269	.3	1.7	31	1936	7	.04	.12	1.2	.3	14	0
0	.3	0	42	54	26	368	.5	1.1	20	3410	34	.11	.28	1.3	.49	22	0
.2	0	0	3	57	5	102	1.7	.6	7	0	0	.32	.19	2.1	.07	133	0
.8	0	0	19	387	15	600	1.9	5	29	0	0	.71	1.64	11.9	.46	702	.01
0	0	0	17	140	10	151	.6	1.4	18	0	0	1.25	.34	3	.4	313	0
3.5	2.1	1	37	47	13	63	.3	.9	7	3	0	.12	.12	1	.02	5	.08
.7	.1	10	372	292	143	478	1.8	.2	36	27	2	.09	.44	.2	.1	23	1.14
2	0	60	146	195	50	170	—	.4	—	—	4	—	.17	—	—	—	—
2	0	40	146	146	45	160	—	.4	—	—	—	—	.17	—	—	—	—
.7	.1	10	372	292	143	478	1.8	.2	36	27	2	.09	.44	.2	.1	23	1.14
.1	0	3	369	291	139	550	1.8	.6	41	6	26	.1	.45	.5	.11	32	1.11
3.7	1.3	10	364	305	139	490	2.2	.3	44	27	2	.15	.43	.3	.11	25	1.11
.8	.1	12	419	331	161	537	2	.2	40	32	2	.1	.49	.3	.11	26	1.29
.8	.1	12	419	331	161	537	2	.2	40	32	2	.1	.49	.3	.11	26	1.29
.1	0	4	436	343	168	559	2.1	.2	42	4	2	.1	.52	.3	.12	27	1.34
.1	0	4	436	343	168	559	2.1	.2	42	4	2	.1	.52	.3	.12	27	1.34
.1	0	4	404	318	155	518	2	.2	39	4	2	.1	.48	.3	.11	25	1.24
.9	.1	15	448	353	172	573	2.2	.2	43	39	2	.11	.52	.3	.12	27	1.38
.1	0	4	488	385	187	625	2.4	.2	47	5	2	.12	.57	.3	.13	30	1.5
2.2	.2	31	296	233	114	380	1.4	.1	28	74	1	.07	.35	.2	.08	18	.91

Anthropometric Standards of Body Weight and Composition

B

1983 Metropolitan Life Insurance Co. Height and Weight Tables			
Height	**Small Frame**	**Medium Frame**	**Large Frame**
		lb	
Men°			
5'2"	128–134	131–141	138–150
5'3"	130–136	133–143	140–153
5'4"	132–138	135–145	142–156
5'5"	134–140	137–148	144–160
5'6"	136–142	139–151	146–164
5'7"	138–145	142–154	149–168
5'8"	140–148	145–157	152–172
5'9"	142–151	148–160	155–176
5'10"	144–154	151–163	158–180
5'11"	146–157	154–166	161–184
6'0"	149–160	157–170	164–188
6'1"	152–164	160–174	168–192
6'2"	155–168	164–178	172–197
6'3"	158–172	167–182	176–202
6'4"	162–176	171–187	181–207
Women†			
4'10"	102–111	109–121	118–131
4'11"	103–113	111–123	120–134
5'0"	104–115	113–126	122–137
5'1"	106–118	115–129	125–140
5'2"	108–121	118–132	128–143
5'3"	111–124	121–135	131–147
5'4"	114–127	124–138	134–151
5'5"	117–130	127–141	137–155
5'6"	120–133	130–144	140–159
5'7"	123–136	133–147	143–163
5'8"	126–139	136–150	146–167
5'9"	129–142	139–153	149–170
5'10"	132–145	142–156	152–173
5'11"	135–148	145–159	155–176
6'0"	138–151	148–162	158–179

°Weights at ages 25 to 59 based on lowest mortality. Weight in pounds according to frame (in indoor clothing weighing 5 lb, shoes with 1" heels).

†Weights at ages 25 to 59 based on lowest mortality. Weight in pounds according to frame (in indoor clothing weighting 3 lb, shoes with 1" heels).

Courtesy of Metropolitan Life Insurance Company.

Weight-for-Height Tables for Adults—Gerontology Center Recommendations

Height (ft and in)	Gerontology Research Center* (Age-specific weight range in pounds for men and women)				
	20–29 yr	30–39 yr	40–49 yr	50–59 yr	60–69 yr
4'10"	84–111	92–119	99–127	107–135	115–142
4'11"	87–115	95–123	103–131	111–139	119–147
5'0"	90–119	98–127	106–135	114–143	123–152
5'1"	93–123	101–131	110–140	118–148	127–157
5'2"	96–127	105–136	113–144	122–153	131–163
5'3"	99–131	108–140	117–149	126–158	135–168
5'4"	102–135	112–145	121–154	130–163	140–173
5'5"	106–140	115–149	125–159	134–168	144–179
5'6"	109–144	119–154	129–164	138–174	148–184
5'7"	112–148	122–159	133–169	143–179	153–190
5'8"	116–153	126–163	137–174	147–184	158–196
5'9"	119–157	130–168	141–179	151–190	162–201
5'10"	122–162	134–173	145–184	156–195	167–207
5'11"	126–167	137–178	149–190	160–201	172–213
6'0"	129–171	141–183	153–195	165–207	177–219
6'1"	133–176	145–188	157–200	169–213	182–225
6'2"	137–181	149–194	162–206	174–219	187–232
6'3"	141–186	153–199	166–212	179–225	192–238
6'4"	144–191	157–205	171–218	184–231	197–244

*Values in this table are for height without shoes and weight without clothes.

Healthy Weight Ranges for Men and Women

Height*	Weight (in Pounds)[†]
4'10"	91–119
4'11"	94–124
5'0"	97–128
5'1"	101–132
5'2"	104–137
5'3"	107–141
5'4"	111–146
5'5"	114–150
5'6"	118–155
5'7"	121–160
5'8"	125–164
5'9"	129–169
5'10"	132–174
5'11"	136–179
6'0"	140–184
6'1"	144–189
6'2"	148–195
6'3"	152–200
6'4"	156–205
6'5"	160–211
6'6"	164–216

*Without shoes.
[†]Without clothes.
Source: Dietary Guidelines for Americans, USDA, DHHS, 1995. Derived from National Research Council, 1989, for adults, p. 564.

B

B

GIRLS: BIRTH TO 36 MONTHS
PHYSICAL GROWTH
NCHS PERCENTILES*

NAME _____   RECORD # _____

AGE (MONTHS)

LENGTH

WEIGHT

AGE (MONTHS)

MOTHER'S STATURE _____   GESTATIONAL
FATHER'S STATURE _____   AGE _____ WEEKS

DATE	AGE	LENGTH	WEIGHT	HEAD CIRC.	COMMENT
	BIRTH				

*Adapted from: Hamill PVV, Drizd TA, Johnson CL, Reed RB, Roche AF, Moore WM: Physical growth: National Center for Health Statistics percentiles. AM J CLIN NUTR 32: 607-629, 1979. Data from the Fels Research Institute, Wright State University School of Medicine, Yellow Springs, Ohio.
© 1982 ROSS LABORATORIES

GIRLS: 2 TO 18 YEARS
PHYSICAL GROWTH
NCHS PERCENTILES*

NAME _____   RECORD # _____

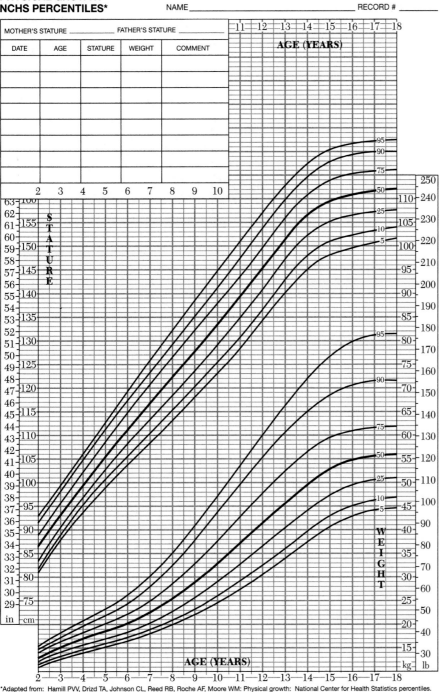

MOTHER'S STATURE _____   FATHER'S STATURE _____

DATE	AGE	STATURE	WEIGHT	COMMENT

*Adapted from: Hamill PVV, Drizd TA, Johnson CL, Reed RB, Roche AF, Moore WM: Physical growth: National Center for Health Statistics percentiles.
AM J CLIN NUTR 32: 607-629, 1979. Data from the Fels Research Institute, Wright State University School of Medicine, Yellow Springs, Ohio.
© 1982 ROSS LABORATORIES

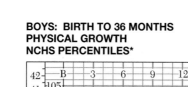

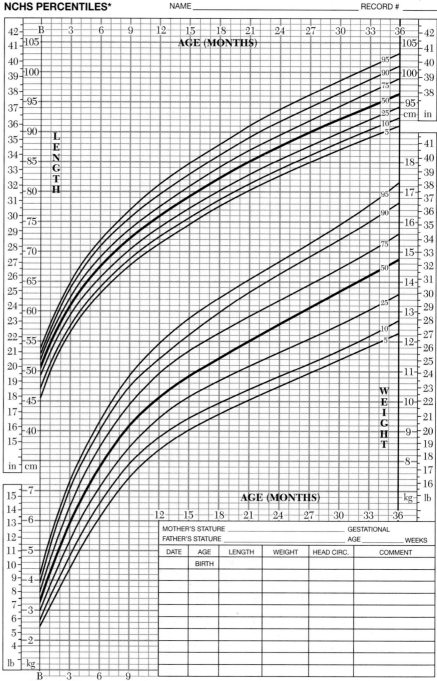

3) vitamin and mineral content per serving
    "contains" or "source"—at least 5% RDI
    "high" or "good source" at least 15% (vitamin C—30%) RDI
    "very high" or "excellent source"—at least 25% (vitamin C—50%) RDI

h) Biological role claims may include generally accepted functions of nutrients associated with maintaining normal metabolism and good health, with the precise wording at the discretion of the manufacturer. Drug-like claims or claims pertaining to the prevention, treatment or cure of a disease are to be avoided.

i) It is the responsibility of the manufacturers to ensure that information concerning nutrient levels in their products is valid.

THE CANADIAN EXCHANGE SYSTEM

The Canadian exchange system of meal planning is called the *Good Health Eating Guide*. Foods are divided into lists according to carbohydrate, fat, and protein content. An energy value is given for each food group and foods are interchangeable within a group. Most foods are eaten in measured amounts. The Canadian exchange system tables are adapted from the Good Health Eating Guide Resource, copyright 1994, with permission of the Canadian Diabetes Association.

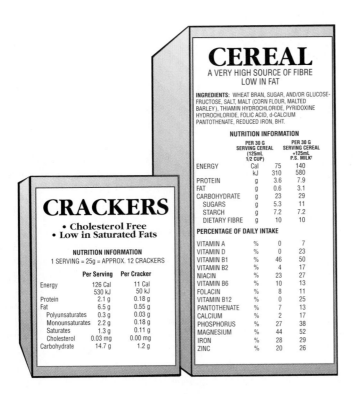

(Canadian Dietetic Association Fact Sheet)

Canadian Exchange System: Starch Foods

1 starch choice = 15 g carbohydrate (starch), 2 g protein, 290 kJ (68 kcal)

Food	Measure	Mass (Weight)
Breads		
Bagels	½	30 g
Bread crumbs	50 mL (¼ c)	30 g
Bread cubes	250 mL (1 c)	30 g
Bread sticks	2	20 g
Brewis, cooked	50 mL (¼ c)	45 g
Chapati	1	20 g
Cookies, plain	2	20 g
English muffins, crumpets	½	30 g
Flour	40 mL (2½ tbs)	20 g
Hamburger buns	½	30 g
Hot dog buns	½	30 g
Kaiser rolls	½	30 g
Matzo, 15 cm	1	20 g
Melba toast, rectangular	4	15 g
Melba toast, rounds	7	15 g
Pita, 20-cm (8″) diameter	¼	30 g
Pita, 15-cm (6″) diameter	½	30 g
Plain rolls	1 small	30 g
Pretzels	7	20 g
Raisin bread	1 slice	30 g
Rice cakes	2	30 g
Roti	1	20 g
Rusks	2	20 g
Rye, coarse or pumpernickel	½ slice	30 g
Soda crackers	6	20 g
Tortillas, corn (taco shell)	1	30 g
Tortilla, flour	1	30 g
White (French and Italian)	1 slice	25 g
Whole-wheat, cracked-wheat, rye, white enriched	1 slice	30 g
Cereals		
Bran flakes, 100% bran	125 mL (½ c)	30 g
Cooked cereals, cooked	125 mL (½ c)	125 g
Dry	30 mL (2 tbs)	20 g
Cornmeal, cooked	125 mL (½ c)	125 g
Dry	30 mL (2 tbs)	20 g
Ready-to-eat unsweetened cereals	125 mL (½ c)	20 g
Shredded wheat biscuits, rectangular or round	1	20 g
Shredded wheat, bite size	125 mL (½ c)	20 g
Wheat germ	75 mL (⅓ c)	30 g
Cornflakes	175 mL (⅔ c)	20 g
Rice Krispies	175 mL (⅔ c)	20 g
Cheerios	200 mL (¾ c)	20 g
Muffets	1	20 g
Puffed rice	300 mL (1¼ c)	15 g
Puffed wheat	425 mL (1⅔ c)	20 g

Canadian Exchange System: Starch Foods *Continued*

1 starch choice = 15 g carbohydrate (starch), 2 g protein, 290 kJ (68 kcal)

Food	Measure	Mass (Weight)
Grains		
Barley, cooked	125 mL (½ c)	120 g
Dry	30 mL (2 tbs)	20 g
Bulgur, kasha, cooked, moist	125 mL (½ c)	70 g
Cooked, crumbly	75 mL (⅓ c)	40 g
Dry	30 mL (2 tbs)	20 g
Rice, cooked, brown & white (short & long grain)	125 mL (½ c)	70 g
Rice, cooked, wild	75 mL (⅓ c)	70 g
Tapioca, pearl and granulated, quick cooking, dry	30 mL (2 tbs)	15 g
Couscous, cooked moist	125 mL (½ c)	70 g
Dry	30 mL (tbs)	20 g
Quinoa, cooked moist	125 mL (½ c)	70 g
Dry	30 mL (2 tbs)	20 g
Pastas		
Macaroni, cooked	125 mL (½ c)	70 g
Noodles, cooked	125 mL (½ c)	80 g
Spaghetti, cooked	125 mL (½ c)	70 g
Starchy Vegetables		
Beans and peas, dried, cooked	125 mL (½ c)	80 g
Breadfruit	1 slice	75 g
Corn, canned, whole kernel	125 mL (½ c)	85 g
Corn on the cob	½ medium cob	140 g
Cornstarch	30 mL (2 tbs)	15 g
Plantains	⅓ small	50 g
Popcorn, air-popped, unbuttered	750 mL (3 c)	20 g
Potatoes, whole (with or without skin)	½ medium	95 g
Yams, sweet potatoes (with or without skin)	½	75 g

Food	Exchanges per Serving	Measure	Mass (Weight)
Note: Food items found in this category provide more than 1 starch exchange:			
Bran flakes	1 starch + ½ sugar	150 mL (⅔ c)	24 g
Croissant, small	1 starch + 1½ fats	1 small	35 g
Large	1 starch + 1½ fats	½ large	30 g
Corn, canned creamed	1 starch + ½ fruits and vegetables	12 mL (½ c)	113 g
Potato chips	1 starch + 2 fats	15 chips	30 g
Tortilla chips (nachos)	1 starch + 1½ fats	13 chips	20 g
Corn chips	1 starch + 2 fats	30 chips	30 g
Cheese twists	1 starch + 1½ fats	30 chips	30 g
Cheese puffs	1 starch + 2 fats	27 chips	30 g
Tea biscuit	1 starch + 2 fats	1	30 g
Pancakes, homemade using 50 mL (¼ c) batter (6″ diameter)	1½ starches + 1 fat	1 medium	50 g
Potatoes, french fried (homemade or frozen)	1 starch + 1 fat	10 regular size	35 g
Soup, canned° (prepared with equal volume of water)	1 starch	250 mL (1 c)	260 g
Waffles, packaged	1 starch + 1 fat	1	35 g

°Soup can vary according to brand and type. Check the label for Food Choice Values and Symbols or the core nutrient listing.

Canadian Exchange System: Fruits and Vegetables

1 fruits and vegetables choice = 10 g carbohydrate, 1 g protein, 190 kJ (44 kcal)

Food	Measure	Mass (Weight)
Fruits (fresh, frozen, without sugar, canned in water)		
Apples, raw (with or without skin)	½ medium	75 g
Sauce unsweetened	125 mL (½ c)	120 g
Sweetened	see *Combined Food Choices*	
Apple butter	20 mL (4 tsp)	20 g
Apricots, raw	2 medium	115 g
Canned, in water	4 halves, plus 30 mL (2 tbs) liquid	110 g
Bake-apples (cloudberries), raw	125 mL (½ c)	120 g
Bananas, with peel	½ small	75 g
Peeled	½ small	50 g
Berries (blackberries, blueberries, boysenberries, huckleberries, loganberries, raspberries)		
Raw	125 mL (½ c)	70 g
Canned, in water	125 mL (½ c), plus 30 mL (2 tbs) liquid	100 g
Cantaloupe, wedge with rind	¼	240 g
Cubed or diced	250 mL (1 c)	160 g
Cherries, raw, with pits	10	75 g
Raw, without pits	10	70 g
Canned, in water with pits	75 mL (⅓ c), plus 30 mL (2 tbs) liquid	90 g
Canned, in water, without pits	75 mL (⅓ c), plus 30 mL (2 tbs) liquid	85 g
Crabapples, raw	1 small	55 g
Cranberries, raw	250 mL (1 c)	100 g
Figs, raw	1 medium	50 g
Canned, in water	3 medium, plus 30 mL (2 tbs) liquid	100 g
Foxberries, raw	250 mL (1 c)	100 g
Fruit cocktail, canned, in water	125 mL (½ c), plus 30 mL (2 tbs) liquid	120 g
Fruit, mixed, cut-up	125 mL (½ c)	120 g
Gooseberries, raw	250 mL (1 c)	150 g
Canned, in water	250 mL (1 c), plus 30 mL (2 tbs) liquid	230 g
Grapefruit, raw, with rind	½ small	185 g
Raw, sectioned	125 mL (½ c)	100 g
Canned, in water	125 mL (½ c), plus 30 mL (2 tbs) liquid	120 g
Grapes, raw, slip skin	125 mL (½ c)	75 g
Raw, seedless	125 mL (½ c)	75 g
Canned, in water	75 mL (⅓ c), plus 30 mL (2 tbs) liquid	115 g
Guavas, raw	½	50 g
Honeydew melon, raw, with rind	½	225 g
Cubed or diced	250 mL (1 c)	170 g
Kiwis, raw, with skin	2	155 g
Kumquats, raw	3	60 g
Loquats, raw	8	130 g
Lychee fruit, raw	8	120 g
Mandarin oranges, raw, with rind	1	135 g
Raw, sectioned	125 mL (½ c)	100 g
Canned, in water	125 mL (½ c), plus 30 mL (2 tbs) liquid	100 g
Mangoes, raw, without skin and seed	⅓	65 g
Diced	75 mL (⅓ c)	65 g

Canadian Exchange System: Protein Foods *Continued*

1 protein choice = 7 g protein, 3 g fat, 230 kJ (55 kcal)

Food	Exchanges per Serving	Measures	Mass (Weight)
Note: The following choices provide more than 1 protein exchange:			
Cheese			
Cheeses	1 protein + 1 fat	1 piece	25 g
Cheese, coarsely grated (e.g., Cheddar)	1 protein + 1 fat	50 mL (¼ c)	25 g
Cheese, dry, finely grated (e.g., parmesan)	1 protein + 1 fat	45 mL	15 g
Cheese, ricotta, high fat	1 protein + 1 fat	50 mL (¼ c)	55 g
Fish			
Eel	1 protein + 1 fat	1 slice	50 g
Meat			
Bologna	1 protein + 1 fat	1 slice	20 g
Canned lunch meats	1 protein + 1 fat	1 slice	20 g
Corned beef, canned	1 protein + 1 fat	1 slice	25 g
Corned beef, fresh	1 protein + 1 fat	1 slice	25 g
Ground beef, medium-fat	1 protein + 1 fat	30 mL (2 tbs)	25 g
Meat spreads, canned	1 protein + 1 fat	45 mL	35 g
Mutton chop	1 protein + 1 fat	½ chop, with bone	35 g
Paté (see *Fats and Oils* group, p. A-150)			
Sausages, garlic, Polish or knockwurst	1 protein + 1 fat	1 slice	50 g
Sausages, pork, links	1 protein + 1 fat	1 link	25 g
Spareribs or shortribs, with bone	1 protein + 1 fat	1 large	65 g
Stewing beef	1 protein + 1 fat	1 cube	25 g
Summer sausage or salami	1 protein + 1 fat	1 slice	40 g
Wiener, hot dog	1 protein + 1 fat	½ medium	25 g
Miscellaneous			
Blood pudding	1 protein + 1 fat	1 slice	25 g
Peanut butter	1 protein + 1 fat	15 mL (1 tbs)	15 g

E

Canadian Exchange System: Fats and Oils

1 fat choice = 5 g fat, 190 kJ (45 kcal)

Food	Measure	Mass (Weight)	Food	Measure	Mass (Weight)
Avocado°	⅛	30 g	Nuts (*continued*):		
Bacon, side, crisp°	1 slice	5 g	Seasame seeds	15 mL (1 tbs)	10 g
Butter°	5 mL (1 tsp)	5 g	Sunflower seeds		
Cheese spread	15 mL (1 tbs)	15 g	Shelled	15 mL (1 tbs)	10 g
Coconut, fresh°	45 mL (3 tbs)	15 g	In shell	45 mL (3 tbs)	15 g
Coconut, dried°	15 mL (1 tbs)	10 g	Walnuts	4 halves	10 g
Cream, half and half			Oil, cooking and salad	5 mL (1 tsp)	5 g
(cereal), 10%°	30 mL (2 tbs)	30 g	Olives, green	10	45 g
Light (coffee), 20%°	15 mL (1 tbs)	15 g	Ripe black	7	57 g
Whipping, 32 to 37%°	15 mL (1 tbs)	15 g	Pâté, liverwurst, meat spread	15 mL (1 tbs)	15 g
Cream cheese°	15 mL (1 tbs)	15 g	Salad dresssing: blue cheese, French, Italian,	10 mL (2 tsp)	10 g
Gravy°	30 mL (2 tbs)	30 g	mayonnaise,	5 mL (1 tsp)	
Lard°	5 mL (1 tsp)	5 g	Thousand Island	30 mL (2 tbs)	5 g
Margarine	5 mL (1 tsp)	5 g	Salad dressing, low-calorie		30 g
Nuts, shelled:			Salt pork, raw or cooked°	5 mL (1 tsp)	5 g
Almonds	8	5 g	Sesame oil	5 mL (1 tsp)	5 g
Brazil nuts	2	10 g	Sour cream		
Cashews	5	10 g	12% milkfat	30 mL (2 tbs)	30 g
Filberts, hazelnuts	5	10 g	7% milkfat	60 mL (4 tbs)	60 g
Macadamia	3	5 g	Shortening°	5 mL (1 tsp)	
Peanuts	10	10 g			
Pecans	5 halves	5 g			
Pignolias, pine nuts	25 mL (5 tsp)	10 g			
Pistachios, shelled	20	10 g			
Pistachios, in shell	20	20 g			
Pumpkin and squash seeds	20 mL (4 tsp)	10 g			

°These items contain higher amounts of saturated fat.

Canadian Exchange System: Extras

Extras have no more than 2.5 g carbohydrate, 60 kJ (14 kcal)

Vegetables 125 mL (½ c)

Artichokes
Asparagus
Bamboo shoots
Bean sprouts, mung or soya
Beans, string, green, or yellow
Bitter melon (balsam pear)
Bok choy
Broccoli
Brussels sprouts
Cabbage
Cauliflower
Celery
Chard
Cucumbers
Eggplant
Endive
Fiddleheads
Greens: beet, collard, dandelion, mustard, turnip, etc.
Kale
Kohlrabi
Leeks
Lettuce
Mushrooms
Okra
Onions, green or mature
Parsley
Peppers, green, yellow or red
Radishes
Rapini
Rhubarb
Sauerkraut
Shallots
Spinach
Sprouts: alfalfa, radish, etc.
Tomato wedges
Watercress
Zucchini

Free Foods (may be used without measuring)

Artificial sweetener, such as cyclamate or aspartame
Baking powder, baking soda
Bouillon from cube powder, or liquid
Bouillon or clear broth
Chowchow, unsweetened
Coffee, clear
Consommé
Dulse
Flavorings and extracts
Garlic
Gelatin, unsweetened
Ginger root
Herbal teas, unsweetened
Horseradish, uncreamed
Lemon juice or lemon wedges

Lime juice or lime wedges
Marjoram, cinnamon, etc.
Mineral water
Mustard
Parsley
Pimentos
Salt, pepper, thyme
Soda water, club soda
Soya sauce
Sugar-free Crystal Drink
Sugar-free Jelly Powder
Sugar-free soft drinks
Tea, clear
Vinegar
Water
Worcestershire sauce

Condiments

Food	Measure
Anchovies	2 fillets
Barbecue sauce	15 mL (1 tbs)
Bran, natural	30 mL (2 tbs)
Brewer's yeast	5 mL (1 tsp)
Carob powder	5 mL (1 tsp)
Catsup	5 mL (1 tsp)
Chili sauce	5 mL (1 tsp)
Cocoa powder	5 mL (1 tsp)
Cranberry sauce, unsweetened	15 mL (1 tbs)
Dietetic fruit spreads	5 mL (1 tsp)
Maraschino cherries	1
Nondairy coffee whitener	5 mL (1 tsp)
Nuts, chopped pieces	5 mL (1 tsp)
Pickles	
Unsweetened dill	2
Sour mixed	11
Sugar substitutes, granular	5 mL (1 tsp)
Whipped toppings	15 mL (1 tbs)

E

Canadian Exchange System: Combined Food Choices

Food	Exchanges per Serving	Measures	Mass (Weight)
Angel food cake	½ starch + 2½ sugars	1/12 cake	50 g
Apple crisp	½ starch + 1½ fruits & vegetables + 1 sugar + 1–2 fats	125 mL (½ c)	
Applesauce, sweetened	1 fruits & vegetables + 1 sugar	125 mL (½ c)	
Beans and pork in tomato sauce	1 starch + ½ fruits & vegetables + ½ sugar + 1 protein	125 mL (½ c)	135 g
Beef burrito	2 starches + 3 proteins + 3 fats		110 g
Brownie	1 sugar + 1 fat	1	20 g
Cabbage rolls°	1 starch + 2 proteins	3	310 g
Caesar salad	2–4 fats	20 mL dressing (4 tsp)	
Cheesecake	½ starch + 2 sugars + ½ protein + 5 fats	1 piece	80 g
Chicken fingers	1 starch + 2 proteins + 2 fats	6 small	100 g
Chicken and snow pea Oriental	2 starches + ½ fruits & vegetables + 3 proteins + 1 fat	500 mL (2 c)	
Chili	1½ starches + ½ fruits & vegetables + 3½ protein	300 mL (1¼ c)	325 g
Chips			
Potato chips	1 starch + 2 fats	15 chips	30 g
Corn chips	1 starch + 2 fats	30 chips	30 g
Tortilla chips	1 starch + 1½ fats	13 chips	
Cheese twist	1 starch + 1½ fats	30 chips	30 g
Chocolate bar			
Aero®	2½ sugars + 2½ fats	bar	43 g
Smarties®	4½ sugars + 2 fats	package	60 g
Chocolate cake (without icing)	1 starch + 2 sugars + 3 fats	1/10 of a 8″ pan	
Chocolate devil's food cake (without icing)	2 starches + 2 sugars + 3 fats	9″ pan	
Chocolate milk	2 milks 2% + 1 sugar	250 mL (1 c)	300 g
Clubhouse (triple-decker) sandwich	3 starches + 3 proteins + 4 fats		
Cookies			
Chocolate chip	½ starch + ½ sugar + 1½ fats	2	22 g
Oatmeal	1 starch + 1 sugar + 1 fat	2	40 g
Donut (chocolate glazed)	1 starch + 1½ sugars + 2 fats	1	65 g
Egg roll	1 starch + ½ protein + 1 fat		75 g
Four bean salad	1 starch + ½ protein + 1 fat	125 mL (½ c)	
French toast	1 starch + ½ protein + 2 fats	1 slice	65 g
Fruit in heavy syrup	1 fruits & vegetables + 1½ sugars	125 mL (½ c)	
Granola bar	½ starch + 1 sugar + 1–2 fats		30 g
Granola cereal	1 starch + 1 sugar + 2 fats	125 mL (½ c)	45 g
Hamburger	2 starches + 3 proteins + 2 fats	junior size	
Ice cream and cone, plain flavour			
Ice cream	½ milk + 2–3 sugars + 1–2 fats		100 g
Cone	½ sugar		4 g
Lasagna			
Regular cheese	1 starch + 1 fruits & vegetables + 3 proteins + 2 fats	3″ × 4″ piece	
Low-fat cheese	1 starch + 1 fruits & vegetables + 3 proteins	3″ × 4″ piece	
Legumes			
Dried beans (kidney, navy, pinto, fava, chick peas)	2 starches + 1 protein	250 mL (1 c)	180 g

Canadian Exchange System: Combined Food Choices *Continued*

Food	Exchanges per Serving	Measures	Mass (Weight)
Dried peas	2 starches + 1 protein	250 mL (1 c)	210 g
Lentils	2 starches + 1 protein	250 mL (1 c)	210 g
Macaroni and cheese	2 starches + 2 proteins + 2 fats	250 mL (1 c)	210 g
Minestrone soup	1½ starches + ½ fruits & vegetables + ½ fat	250 mL (1 c)	
Muffin	1 starch + ½ sugar + 1 fat	1 small	45 g
Nuts (dry or roasted without any oil added)			
almonds, dried slicd	½ protein + 2 fats	50 mL (¼ c)	22 g
Brazil nuts, dried unblanched	½ protein + 2½ fats	5 large	23 g
Cashew nuts, dry roasted	½ starch + ½ protein + 2 fats	50 mL (¼ c)	28 g
Filbert hazelnuts, dry	½ protein + 3½ fats	50 mL (¼ c)	30 g
Macadamia nuts, dried	½ protein + 4 fats	50 mL (¼ c)	28 g
Peanuts, raw	1 protein + 2 fats	50 mL (¼ c)	30 g
Pecans, dry roasted	½ fruits & vegetables + 3 fats	50 mL (¼ c)	22 g
Pine nuts, pignolia dried	1 protein + 3 fats	50 mL (¼ c)	34 g
Pistachio nuts, dried	½ fruits & vegetables + ½ protein + 2½ fats	50 mL (¼ c)	27 g
Pumpkin seeds, roasted	2 proteins + 2½ fats	50 mL (¼ c)	47 g
Sesame seeds, whole dried	½ fruits & vegetables + ½ protein + 2½ fats	50 mL (¼ c)	30 g
Sunflower kernel, dried	½ protein + 1½ fats	50 mL (¼ c)	17 g
Walnuts, dried choppd	½ protein + 3 fats	50 mL (¼ c)	26 g
Perogies	2 starches + 1 protein + 1 fat	3	
Pie, fruit	1 starch + 1 fruits & vegetables + 2 sugars + 3 fats	1 piece	120 g
Pizza, cheese	1 starch + 1 protein + 1 fat	1 slice (⅛ of a 12″)	50 g
Pork stir fry	½ to 1 fruits & vegetables + 3 proteins	200 mL (¾ c)	
Potato salad	1 starch + 1 fat	125 mL (½ c)	130 g
Potatoes, scalloped	2 starches + 1 milk + 1–2 fats	200 mL (¾ c)	210 g
Pudding, bread or rice	1 starch + 1 sugar + 1 fat	125 mL (½ c)	
Pudding, vanilla	1 milk + 2 sugars	125 mL (½ c)	
Raisin bran cereal	1 starch + ½ fruits & vegetables + ½ sugar	175 mL (⅔ c)	40 g
Rice krispie squares	½ starch + 1½ sugars + ½ fat	1 square	30 g
Shepherd's pie	2 starches + 1 fruits & vegetables + 3 proteins	325 mL (1⅓ c)	
Sherbet, orange	3 sugars + ½ fat	125 mL (½ c)	
Spaghetti and meat sauce	2 starches + 1 fruits & vegetables + 2 proteins + 3 fats	250 mL (1 c)	
Stew	2 starches + 2 fruit & vegetables + 3 proteins + ½ fat	200 mL (¾ c)	
Sundae	4 sugars + 3 fats	125 mL (½ c)	
Tuna casserole	1 starch + 2 proteins + ½ fat	125 mL (½ c)	
Yogurt, fruit bottom	1 fruits & vegetables + 1 milk + 1 sugar	125 mL (½ c)	125 g
Yogurt, frozen	1 milk + 1 sugar	125 mL (½ c)	125 g

° If eaten with sauce, add ½ fruits & vegetables exchange.

APPENDIX F

Nutrient Intake Recommendations by the World Health Organization

F

Recommended Intakes of Nutrients—WHO—1974*

Age	Body Weight (kg)	Energy[1] (kcal)	Energy[1] (MJ)	Protein[1,2] (gm)	Vitamin A[3,4] (μg)	Vitamin D[5,6] (μg)
Children						
<1	7.3	820	3.4	14	300	10.0
1–3	13.4	1360	5.7	16	250	10.0
4–6	20.2	1830	7.6	20	300	10.0
7–9	28.1	2190	9.2	25	400	2.5
Male adolescents						
10–12	36.9	2600	10.9	30	575	2.5
13–15	51.3	2900	12.1	37	725	2.5
16–19	62.9	3070	12.8	38	750	2.5
Female adolescents						
10–12	38.0	2350	9.8	29	575	2.5
13–15	49.9	2490	10.4	31	725	2.5
16–19	54.4	2310	9.7	30	750	2.5
Adult man (moderately active)	65.0	3000	12.6	37	750	2.5
Adult woman (moderately active)	55.0	2200	9.2	29	750	2.5
Pregnancy (later half)		+350	+1.5	38	750	10.0
Lactation (first 6 months)		+550	+2.3	46	1200	10.0

[1]Energy and Protein Requirements. Report of a Joint FAO/WHO Expert Group, FAO, Rome, 1972. [2]As egg or milk protein. [3]Requirements of vitamin A, thiamin, riboflavin and niacin. Report of a Joint FAO/WHO Expert Group, FAO, Rome, 1965. [4]As retinol. [5]Requirements of ascorbic acid, vitamin D, vitamin B_{12}, folate and iron. Report of a Joint applied FAO/WHO Expert Group, FAO, Rome, 1970. [6]As cholecalciferol. [7]Calcium requirements. Report of a FAO/WHO Expert Group, FAO, Rome, 1961. [8]On each line the lower value applies when over 25 per cent of calories in the diet come from animal foods, and the higher value when animal foods represent less than 10 per cent of calories. [9]For women whose iron intake throughout life has been at the level recommended in this table, the daily intake of iron during pregnancy and lactation should be the same as that recommended for nonpregnant, nonlactating women of childbearing age. For women whose iron status is not satisfactory at the beginning of pregnancy, the requirement is increased, and in the extreme situation of women with no iron stores, the requirement can probably not be met without supplementation.
*From Passmore, Nicol and Rao: *Handbook on Human Nutritional Requirements.* Geneva, WHO Monogr. Ser. No. 61, 1974, Table 1.
ADDENDUM: Dietary allowances, official or unofficial for many European countries, as of 1976 or earlier, appear in the Proceedings of the Second European Nutrition Conference, Munich, 1976. (Nutr. Metab. 21:210, 1977.)

Thiamin[3] (mg)	Riboflavin[3] (mg)	Niacin[3] (μg)	Folic Acid[5] (μg)	Vitamin B$_{12}$[5] (μg)	Ascorbic Acid[5] (mg)	Calcium[7] (gm)	Iron[5,8] (mg)
0.3	0.5	5.4	60	0.3	20	0.5–0.6	5–10
0.5	0.8	9.0	100	0.9	20	0.4–0.5	5–10
0.7	1.1	12.1	100	1.5	20	0.4–0.5	5–10
0.9	1.3	14.5	100	1.5	20	0.4–0.5	5–10
1.0	1.6	17.2	100	2.0	20	0.6–0.7	5–10
1.2	1.7	19.1	200	2.0	30	0.6–0.7	9–18
1.2	1.8	20.3	200	2.0	30	0.5–0.6	5–9
0.9	1.4	15.5	100	2.0	20	0.6–0.7	5–10
1.0	1.5	16.4	200	2.0	30	0.6–0.7	12–24
0.9	1.4	15.2	200	2.0	30	0.5–0.6	14–28
1.2	1.8	19.8	200	2.0	30	0.4–0.5	5–9
0.9	1.3	14.5	200	2.0	30	0.4–0.5	14–28
+0.1	+0.2	+2.3	400	3.0	50	1.0–1.2	(9)
+0.2	+0.4	+3.7	300	2.5	50	1.0–1.2	(9)

F

The Population Nutrient Goals From WHO

| | Limits for Population Average Intakes | |
	Lower limit	Upper limit
Total fat	15% of energy	30% of energy[a]
Saturated fatty acids	0% energy	10% of energy
Polyunsaturated fatty acids	3% of energy	7% of energy
Dietary cholesterol	0% mg/day	300 mg/day
Total carbohydrate	55% of energy	75% of energy
Complex carbohydrates[b]	50% of energy	75% of energy
Dietary fibre[c]		
As non-starch polysaccharides (NSP)	16 g/day	24 g/day
As total dietary fibre	27 g/day	40 g/day
Free sugars[d]	0% of energy	10% of energy
Protein	10% of energy	15% of energy[e]
Salt	—[e]	6 g/day

Total energy
Energy intake needs to be sufficient to allow for normal childhood growth, for the needs of pregnancy and lactation, and for work and desirable physical activities, and to maintain appropriate body reserves of energy in children and adults. Adult populations on average should have a body-mass index (BMI) of 20–22
(BMI = body mass in kg/[height in metres]^2).

The lower limit defines the minimum intake needed to prevent deficiency diseases, while the upper limit expressed the maximum intake compatible with the prevention of chronic diseases.

[a]An interim goal for nations with high fat intakes; further benefits would be expected by reducing fat intake towards 15% of total energy.
[b]A daily minimum intake of 400 g vegetables and fruits, including at least 30 g of pulses, nuts, and seeds, should contribute to this component.
[c]Dietary fibre includes the non-starch polysaccharides (NSP), the goals for which are based on NSP obtained from mixed food sources. Since the definition and measurement of dietary fibre remain uncertain, the goals for total dietary fibre have been estimated from the NSP values.
[d]These sugars include monosaccharides, disaccharides, and other short-chain sugars extracted from carbohydrates by refining. These refined, or purified sugars do not include the natural sugars consumed when eating fruits and vegetabls or drinking milk.
[e]Not defined.
Source: Diet, Nutrition and the Prevention of chronic diseases. A report of the WHO Study Group on Diet, Nutrition and Prevention of Noncommunicable Diseases. Nutr. Rev. 49:291–301, 1991.

Cholesterol (mg/day)	Complex Carbohydrates and Fiber	Simple Sugars	Sodium Chloride	Alcohol Intake	Other Recommendations
Reduce	NC	NC	Reduce for HR <5 g/day	Moderation	Avoid trace element deficiencies; food labeling; focus on HR groups
Restrict through less organ meats and egg yolks; for HR <300 mg	Increase	NC	Limit	Limit	Focus on HR groups; limit protein
<300	Increase to derive ≥50% kcal from total carbohydrates	NS	≤3 g/day of sodium	1–2 oz ethanol/day	Protein to make up remainder of calories; wide variety of foods

Restrict Sodium Chloride	Food Preparation Methods	Food Additives and Contaminants	Alcohol Intake	Other Recommendations
Indirectly	Minimize cured, pickled, and smoked foods	Monitor, test, and reduce exposure	Drink less, if at all	Monitor and test mutagens and carcinogens; recommendations made to government, scientists, and industry
Yes	Avoid hot drinks and burned food	NC	Same as NRC (1982)	Varied diet; chew food well
NS	Same as NRC (1982)	NS	Same as NRC (1982)	NC
NS	Same as NRC (1982)	Same as NRC (1982)	Two of fewer drinks	NC
To <5 g/day	Same as NRC (1982) and NCI (1987)	Same as NRC (1982) and NCI (1987)	Same as NRC (1982)	Varied diet; recommendations made to government, scientists, and industry
NS	Same as NRC (1982); avoid frying and high-temperature cooking	NC	Same as NRC (1982)	Balanced diet; read labels; follow USDA/DHHS (1985) guidelines

G

APPENDIX H
Healthy People 2000

Priority Areas for Healthy People 2000

Health Promotion

1. Physical Activity and Fitness
2. Nutrition
3. Tobacco
4. Alcohol and Other Drugs
5. Family Planning
6. Mental Health and Mental Disorders
7. Violent and Abusive Behavior
8. Educational and Community-Based Programs

Health Protection

9. Unintentional Injuries
10. Occupational Safety and Health
11. Environmental Health
12. Food and Drug Safety
13. Oral Health

Preventive Services

14. Maternal and Infant Health
15. Heart Disease and Stroke
16. Cancer
17. Diabetes and Chronic Disabling Conditions
18. HIV Infection
19. Sexually Transmitted Diseases
20. Immunization and Infectious Diseases
21. Clinical Preventive Services

Surveillance and Data Objectives

22. Surveillance and Data Systems

H

YEAR 2000 NATIONAL NUTRITION OBJECTIVES

2.1° Reduce coronary heart disease deaths to no more than 100 per 100,000 people. (Age-adjusted baseline: 135 per 100,000 in 1987)

2.2° Reverse the rise in cancer deaths to achieve a rate of no more than 130 per 100,000 people. (Age-adjusted baseline: 133 per 100,000 in 1987)

2.3° Reduce overweight to a prevalence of no more than 20% among people aged 20 years and older and maintain prevalence at no more than 15% among adolescents aged 12 through 19 years. (Baseline: 26% for people aged 20 through 74 years in 1976–1980, 24% for men and 27% for women; 15% for adolescents aged 12 through 19 years in 1976–1980)

Special Population Targets

Overweight prevalence	1976–1980 baseline	2000 target
Low-income women ≥ age 20	37%	25%
Black women ≥ age 20	44%	30%
Hispanic women ≥ age 20		25%
Mexican-American women	39%	
Cuban women	34%	
Puerto Rican women	37%	
American Indians/Alaska Natives	29%–75%	30%
People with disabilities	36%	25%
Women with high blood pressure	50%	41%
Men with high blood pressure	39%	35%

2.4 Reduce growth retardation among low-income children aged 5 years and younger to less than 10%. (Baseline: Up to 16% among low-income children in 1988, depending on age and race/ethnicity)

Special Population Targets

Prevalence of short stature	1988 baseline	2000 target
Low-income black children < age 1	15%	10%
Low-income Hispanic children < age 1	13%	10%
Low-income Hispanic children age 1	16%	10%
Low-income Asian/Pacific Islander children age 1	14%	10%
Low-income Asian/Pacific Islander children age 2 to 4	16%	10%

2.5° Reduce dietary fat intake to an average of 30% of energy or less and average saturated fat intake to less than 10% of energy among people aged 2 years and older. (Baseline: 36% of energy from total fat and 13% from saturated fat for people aged 20 through 74 in 1976–1980; 36% and 13% for women aged 19 through 50 in 1985)

2.6° Increase complex carbohydrate and fiber-containing foods in the diets of adults to five or more daily servings for vegetables (including legumes) and fruits, and to six or more daily servings for grain products. (Baseline: two and a half servings of vegetables and fruits and three servings for grain products for women aged 19 through 50 in 1985)

2.7° Increase to at least 50% the proportion of overweight people aged 12 years and older who have adopted sound dietary practices combined with regular physical activity to attain an appropriate body weight. (Baseline: 30% of overweight women and 25% of overweight men for people aged 18 and older in 1985)

°Objectives jointly shared between the nutrition priority areas and other priority areas

A-166

2.8 Increase calcium intake so at least 50% of youth aged 12 through 24 years and at least 50% of pregnant and lactating women consume three or more servings daily of foods rich in calcium, and at least 50% of people aged 25 years and older consume two or more servings daily. (Baseline: 7% of women and 14% of men aged 19 through 24 and 24% of pregnant and lactating women consumed three or more servings, and 15% of women and 23% of men aged 25 through 50 consumed two or more servings in 1985–1986)

2.9 Decrease salt and sodium intake so at least 65% of home meal preparers prepare foods without adding salt, at least 80% of people avoid using salt at the table, and at least 40% of adults regularly purchase foods modified or lower in sodium. (Baseline: 54% of women aged 19 through 50 years who served as the main meal preparer did not use salt in food preparation, and 68% of women aged 19 through 50 did not use salt at the table in 1985; 20% of all people aged 18 and older regularly purchased foods with reduced salt and sodium content in 1988)

2.10 Reduce iron deficiency to less than 3% among children aged 1 through 4 years and among women of childbearing age. (Baseline: 9% for children aged 1 through 2 years, and 4% for children aged 3 through 4 years, and 5% for women aged 20 through 44 years in 1976–1980)

Special Population Targets

Iron deficiency prevalence	1976–80 baseline	2000 target
Low-income children age 1 to 2	21%	10%
Low-income children age 3 to 4	10%	5%
Low-income women for childbearing age	8%	4%

Anemia prevalence	1983–85 baseline	2000 target
Alaska Native children age 1 to 5	22%–28%	10%
Black, low-income pregnant women (third trimester)	41%	20%

2.11° Increase to at least 75% the proportion of mothers who breast-feed their babies in the early postpartum period, and to at least 50% the proportion who continue breast-feeding until their babies are 5 to 6 months old. (Baseline: 54% at discharge from birth site and 21% at 5 to 6 months in 1988)

Special Populaton Targets

Mothers breast-feeding their babies:	1988 baseline	2000 target
during early postpartum period		
Low-income mothers	32%	75%
Black mothers	25%	75%
Hispanic mothers	51%	75%
American Indian/Alaska Native mothers	47%	75%
at age 5 to 6 months		
Low-income mothers	9%	50%
Black mothers	8%	50%
Hispanic mothers	16%	50%
American Indian/Alaska Native mothers	28%	50%

2.12° Increase to at least 75% the proportion of parents and caregivers who use feeding practices that prevent baby bottle tooth decay. For parents and caregivers with less than a high school education and for American Indian/Alaska native parents and caregivers, there is a special population target of 65%. (Baseline data available in 1991)

2.13 Increase to at least 85% the proportion of people aged 18 and older who use food labels to make nutritious food selections. (Baseline: 74% used labels to make food selections in 1988)

2.14 Achieve useful and informative nutrition labeling for virtually all processed foods and at least 40% of fresh meats, poultry, fish, fruits, vegetables, baked goods, and ready-to-eat carry-away foods. (Baseline: 60% of sales of processed foods regulated by FDA had nutrition labeling in 1988; baseline data on fresh and carry-away foods unavailable)

2.15 Increase to at least 5,000 brand items the availability of processed food products that are reduced in fat and saturated fat. (Baseline: 2,500 items reduced in fat in 1986)

2.16 Increase to at least 90% the proportion of restaurants and institutional food service operations that offer identifiable low-fat, low-calorie food choices, consistent with the *Dietary Guidelines for Americans*. (Baseline: About 70% of fast food and family restaurant chains with 350 or more units had at least one low-fat, low-calorie item on their menu in 1989)

2.17 Increase to at least 90% the proportion of school lunch and breakfast services and at least 50% of child care food services with menus that are consistent with the nutrition principles in the *Dietary Guidelines for Americans*. (Baseline data available in 1993)

2.18 Increase to at least 80% the receipt of home foodservices by people aged 65 and older who have difficulty in preparing their own meals or are otherwise in need of home-delivered meals. (Baseline data available in 1991)

2.19 Increase to at least 75% the proportion of the nation's schools that provide nutrition education from preschool through grade 12, preferably as part of quality school health education. (Baseline data available in 1991)

2.20 Increase to at least 50% the proportion of work sites with 50 or more employees that offer nutrition education and/or weight management programs for employees. (Baseline: 17% offered nutrition education activities in 15% offered weight control activities in 1985)

2.21 Increase to at least 75% the proportion or primary care providers who provide nutriton assessment and counseling and/or referral to qualified nutritionists or dietitians. (Baseline: Physicians provided diet counseling for an estimated 40% to 50% of patients in 1988)

H

APPENDIX I
Exchange Lists

Foods are listed with their serving sizes, which are usually measured after cooking. When you begin, you should measure the size of each serving. This may help you learn to "eyeball" correct serving sizes.

The following chart shows the amount of nutrients in one serving from each list.

The exchange lists provide you with a lot of food choices (foods from the basic food groups, foods with added sugars, free foods, combination foods, and fast foods). This gives you variety in your meals. Several foods, such as dried beans and peas, bacon, and peanut butter, are on two lists. This gives you flexibility in putting your meals together. Whenever you choose new foods or vary your meal plan, monitor your blood glucose to see how these different foods affect your blood glucose level.

Groups/Lists	Carbohydrate (grams)	Protein (grams)	Fat (grams)	Calories
Carbohydrate Group				
Starch	15	3	1 or less	80
Fruit	15	—	—	60
Milk				
Skim	12	8	0–3	90
Low-fat	12	8	5	120
Whole	12	8	8	150
Other carbohydrates	15	Varies	Varies	Varies
Vegetables	5	2	—	25
Meat and Meat Substitute Group				
Very lean	—	7	0–1	35
Lean	—	7	3	55
Medium-fat	—	7	5	75
High-fat	—	7	8	100
Fat Group	—	—	5	45

©1995 by the American Diabetes Association, Inc., and The American Dietetic Association.

STARCH LIST

One starch exchange equals 15 grams carbohydrate, 3 grams protein, 0–1 grams fat, and 80 calories.

Bread
Bagel.. ½ (1 oz)
Bread, reduced-calorie .... 2 slices (1½ oz)
Bread, white, whole-wheat, pumpernickel, rye .... 1 slice (1 oz)
Bread sticks, crisp, 4 in. long × ½ in. .... 2 (⅔ oz)
English muffin .... ½
Hot dog or hamburger bun......................... ½ (1 oz)
Pita, 6 in. across .... ½
Roll, plain, small .... 1 (1 oz)
Raisin bread, unfrosted .... 1 slice (1 oz)
Tortilla, corn, 6 in. across................................ 1
Tortilla, flour, 7–8 in. across 1
Waffle, 4½ in. square, reduced-fat........................ 1

Cereals and Grains
Bran cereals .... ½ cup
Bulgur... ½ cup
Cereals.. ½ cup
Cereals, unsweetened, ready-to-eat .... ¾ cup
Cornmeal (dry) .... 3 Tbsp
Couscous .... ⅓ cup
Flour (dry)... 3 Tbsp
Granola, low-fat .... ¼ cup
Grape-Nuts .... ¼ cup
Grits .... ½ cup
Kasha .... ½ cup
Millet .... ¼ cup
Muesli .... ¼ cup
Oats .... ½ cup
Pasta .... ½ cup
Puffed cereal .... 1½ cups
Rice milk .... ½ cup
Rice, white or brown .... ⅓ cup
Shredded Wheat .... ½ cup
Sugar-frosted cereal...................................... ½ cup
Wheat germ .... 3 Tbsp

Dried Beans, Peas, and Lentils
(Count as 1 starch exchange, plus 1 very lean meat exchange.)
Beans and peas (garbanzo, pinto, kidney, white, split, black-eyed) .... ½ cup
Lima beans.. ⅔ cup
Lentils... ½ cup
Miso ⬛ .... 3 Tbsp
⬛ = 400 mg or more of sodium per serving.

Starchy Vegetables
Baked beans .... ⅓ cup
Corn.. ½ cup
Corn on cob, medium .... 1 (5 oz)
Mixed vegetables with corn, peas, or pasta............... 1 cup
Peas, green .... ½ cup
Plantain... ½ cup
Potato, baked or boiled .... 1 small (3 oz)
Potato, mashed .... ½ cup

continued

Starchy Vegetables

Squash, winter (acorn, butternut)................................. 1 cup
Yam, sweet potato, plain .... ½ cup

Crackers and Snacks

Animal crackers 8
Graham crackers, 2½ in. square 3
Matzoh .... ¾ oz
Melba toast.. 4 slices
Oyster crackers 24
Popcorn (popped, no fat added or low-fat microwave)................ 3 cups
Pretzels .... ¾ oz
Rice cakes, 4 in. across.. 2
Saltine-type crackers.. 6
Snack chips, fat-free (tortilla, potato)............... 15–20 (¾ oz)
Whole-wheat crackers, no fat added .... 2–5 (¾ oz)

Starchy Foods Prepared with Fat
(Count as 1 starch exchange, plus 1 fat exchange.)

Biscuit, 2½ in. across.. 1
Chow mein noodles... ½ cup
Cron bread, 2 in. cube .... 1 (2 oz)
Crackers, round butter type.. 6
Croutons... 1 cup
French-fried potatoes .... 16–25 (3 oz)
Granola.. ¼ cup
Muffin, small .... 1 (1½ oz)
Pancake, 4 in. across... 2
Popcorn, microwave .... 3 cups
Sandwich crackers, cheese or peanut butter filling 3
Stuffing, bread (prepared)..................................... ⅓ cup
Taco shell, 6 in. across 2
Waffle, 4½ in. square 1
Whole-wheat crackers, fat added........................ 4–6 (1 oz)

FRUIT LIST

One fruit exchange equals 15 grams carbohydrate and 60 calories. The weight includes skin, core, seeds, and rind.

Fruit

Apple, unpeeled, small .... 1 (4 oz)
Applesauce, unsweetened .... ½ cup
Apples, dried .... 4 rings
Apricots, fresh .... 4 whole (5½ oz)
Apricots, dried .... 8 halves
Apricots, canned .... ½ cup
Banana, small .... 1 (4 oz)
Blackberries .... ¾ cup
Blueberries .... ¾ cup
Cantaloupe, small .... ⅓ melon (11 oz) or 1 cup cubes
Cherries, sweet, fresh .... 12 (3 oz)
Cherries, sweet, canned .... ½ cup
Dates 3
Figs, fresh........................ 1½ large or 2 medium (3½ oz)
Figs, dried 1½
Fruit cocktail.. ½ cup
Grapefruit, large .... ½ (11 oz)
Grapefruit sections, canned .... ¾ cup
Grapes, small .... 17 (3 oz)
Honeydew melon................ 1 slice (10 oz) or 1 cup cubes

Kiwi .... 1 (3½ oz)
Mandarin oranges, canned................................... ¾ cup
Mango, small .... ½ fruit (5½ oz) or ½ cup
Nectarine, small .... 1 (5 oz)
Orange, small.. 1 (6½ oz)
Papaya .... ½ fruit (8 oz) or 1 cup cubes
Peach, medium, fresh... 1 (6 oz)
Peaches, canned.. ½ cup
Pear, large, fresh... ½ (4 oz)
Pears, canned.. ½ cup
Pineapple, fresh.. ¾ cup
Pineapple, canned... ½ cup
Plums, small .... 2 (5 oz)
Plums, canned.. ½ cup
Prunes, dried.. 3
Raisins .... 2 Tbsp
Raspberries.. 1 cup
Strawberries .... 1¼ cup whole berries
Tangerines, small...................................... 2 (8 oz)
Watermelon .... 1 slice (13½ oz) or 1¼ cup cubes

Fruit Juice

Apple juice/cider.. ½ cup
Cranberry juice cocktail .... ⅓ cup
Cranberry juice cocktail, reduced-calorie .... 1 cup
Fruit juice blends, 100% juice................................. ⅓ cup
Grape juice.. ⅓ cup
Grapefruit juice... ½ cup
Orange juice.. ½ cup
Pineapple juice.. ½ cup
Prune juice.. ⅓ cup

MILK LIST

One milk exchange equals 12 grams carbohydrate and 8 grams protein.

Skim and Very Low-fat Milk
(0–3 grams fat per serving)

Skim milk .... 1 cup
½% milk .... 1 cup
1% milk .... 1 cup
Nonfat or low-fat buttermilk.................................. 1 cup
Evaporated skim milk... ½ cup
Nonfat dry milk .... ⅓ cup dry
Plain nonfat yogurt .... ¾ cup
Nonfat or low-fat fruit-flavored yogurt sweetened with aspartame
    or with a nonnutritive sweetener .... 1 cup

Low-fat
(5 grams fat per serving)

2% milk .... 1 cup
Plain low-fat yogurt .... ¾ cup
Sweet acidophilus milk.. 1 cup

Whole Milk
(8 grams fat per serving)

Whole milk.. 1 cup
Evaporated whole milk.. ½ cup
Goat's milk .... 1 cup
Kefir.. 1 cup

OTHER CARBOHYDRATES LIST

One exchange equals 15 grams carbohydrate, or 1 starch, or 1 fruit, or 1 milk.

Food	Serving Size	Exchanges Per Serving
Angel food cake, unfrosted	¹⁄₁₂th cake	2 carbohydrates
Brownie, small, unfrosted	2 in. square	1 carbohydrate, 1 fat
Cake, unfrosted	2 in. square	1 carbohydrate, 1 fat
Cake, frosted	2 in. square	2 carbohydrates, 1 fat
Cookie, fat-free	2 small	1 carbohydrate
Cookie or sandwich cookie with creme filling	2 small	1 carbohydrate, 1 fat
Cupcake, frosted	1 small	2 carbohydrates, 1 fat
Cranberry sauce, jellied	¼ cup	2 carbohydrates
Doughnut, plain cake	1 medium (1½ oz)	1½ carbohydrates, 2 fats
Doughnut, glazed	3¾ in. across (2 oz)	2 carbohydrates, 2 fats
Fruit juice bars, frozen, 100% juice	1 bar (3 oz)	1 carbohydrate
Fruit snacks, chewy (pureed fruit concentrate)	1 roll (¾ oz)	1 carbohydrate
Fruit spreads, 100% fruit	1 Tbsp	1 carbohydrate
Gelatin, regular	½ cup	1 carbohydrate
Gingersnaps	3	1 carbohydrate
Granola bar	1 bar	1 carbohydrate, 1 fat
Granola bar, fat-free	1 bar	2 carbohydrates
Hummus	⅓ cup	1 carbohydrate, 1 fat
Ice cream	½ cup	1 carbohydrate, 2 fats
Ice cream, light	½ cup	1 carbohydrate, 1 fat
Ice cream, fat-free, no sugar added	½ cup	1 carbohydrate
Jam or jelly, regular	1 Tbsp	1 carbohydrate
Milk, chocolate, whole	1 cup	2 carbohydrates, 1 fat
Pie, fruit, 2 crusts	⅙ pie	3 carbohydrates, 2 fats
Pie, pumpkin or custard	⅛ pie	1 carbohydrate, 2 fats
Potato chips	12–18 (1 oz)	1 carbohydrate, 2 fats
Pudding, regular (made with low-fat milk)	½ cup	2 carbohydrates
Pudding, sugar-free (made with low-fat milk)	½ cup	1 carbohydrate
Salad dressing, fat-free 🥄*	¼ cup	1 carbohydrate
Sherbet, sorbet	½ cup	2 carbohydrates
Spaghetti or pasta sauce, canned 🥄*	½ cup	1 carbohydrate, 1 fat
Sweet roll or Danish	1 (2½ oz)	2½ carbohydrates, 2 fats
Syrup, light	2 Tbsp	1 carbohydrate
Syrup, regular	1 Tbsp	1 carbohydrate
Syrup, regular	¼ cup	4 carbohydrates
Tortilla chips	6–12 (1 oz)	1 carbohydrate, 2 fats
Yogurt, frozen, low-fat, fat-free	⅓ cup	1 carbohydrate, 0–1 fat
Yogurt, frozen, fat-free, no sugar added	½ cup	1 carbohydrate
Yogurt, low-fat with fruit	1 cup	3 carbohydrates, 0–1 fat
Vanilla wafers	5	1 carbohydrate, 1 fat

🥄* = 400 mg or more of sodium per serving.

VEGETABLE LIST

Vegetables that contain small amounts of carbohydrates and calories are on this list. Vegetables contain important nutrients. Try to eat at least 2 or 3 vegetables choices each day. In general, one vegetable exchange is:

   ½ cup of cooked vegetable or vegetable juice, or
   1 cup of raw vegetables.

If you eat 1 to 2 vegetable choices at a meal or snack, you do not have to count the calories or carbohydrates because they contain small amounts of these nutrients.

One vegetable exchange equals 5 grams carbohydrate, 2 grams protein, 0 grams fat, and 25 calories.

Artichoke
Artichoke hearts
Asparagus
Beans (green, wax, Italian)
Bean sprouts
Beets
Broccoli
Brussels sprouts
Cabbage
Carrots
Cauliflower
Celery
Cucumber
Eggplant
Green onions or scallions

Greens (collard, kale, mustard, turnip)
Kohlrabi
Leeks
Mixed vegetables (without corn, peas, or pasta)
Mushrooms
Okra
Onions
Pea pods
Peppers (all varieties)
Radishes
Salad greens (endive, escarole, lettuce, romaine, spinach)

continued

VEGETABLE LIST

Sauerkraut 🥢
Spinach
Summer squash
Tomato
Tomatoes, canned
Tomato sauce 🥢

Tomato/vegetable juice 🥢
Turnips
Water chestnuts
Watercress
Zucchini

🥢 = 400 mg or more sodium per exchange.

VERY LEAN MEAT AND SUBSTITUTES LIST

One exchange equals 0 grams carbohydrate, 7 grams protein, 0–1 grams fat, and 35 calories.

One very lean meat exchange is equal to any one of the following items.

Poultry: Chicken or turkey (white meat, no skin), Cornish hen (no skin) .... 1 oz
Fish: Fresh or frozen cod, flounder, haddock, halibut, trout; tuna fresh or canned in water .... 1 oz
Shellfish: Clams, crab, lobster, scallops, shrimp, imitation shellfish .... 1 oz
Game: Duck or pheasant (no skin), venison, buffalo, ostrich .... 1 oz
Cheese with 1 gram or less fat per ounce:
Nonfat or low-fat cottage cheese .... ¼ cup
Fat-free cheese .... 1 oz
Other: Processed sandwich meats with 1 gram or less fat per ounce, such as deli thin, shaved meats, chipped beef 🥢, turkey ham .... 1 oz
Egg whites 2
Egg substitutes, plain .... ¼ cup
Hot dogs with 1 gram or less fat per ounce 🥢 .... 1 oz
Kidney (high in cholesterol) .... 1 oz
Sausage with 1 gram or less fat per ounce .... 1 oz

Count as one very lean meat and one starch exchange.

Dried beans, peas, lentils (cooked) .... ½ cup

🥢 = 400 mg or more sodium per exchange.

LEAN MEAT AND SUBSTITUTES LIST

One exchange equals 0 grams carbohydrate, 7 grams protein, 3 grams fat, and 55 calories.

One lean meat exchange is equal to any one of the following items.

Beef: USDA Select or Choice grades of lean beef trimmed of fat, such as round, sirloin, and flank steak; tenderloin; roast (rib, chuck, rump); steak (T-bone, porterhouse, cubed), ground round .... 1 oz
Pork: Lean pork, such as fresh ham; canned, cured, or boiled ham; Canadian bacon 🥢; tenderloin, center loin chop .... 1 oz
Lamb: Roast, chop, leg .... 1 oz
Veal: Lean chop, roast .... 1 oz
Poultry: Chicken, turkey (dark meat, no skin), chicken white meat (with skin), domestic duck or goose (well-drained of fat, no skin) .... 1 oz

Fish:
Herring (uncreamed or smoked) .... 1 oz
Oysters .... 6 medium
Salmon (fresh or canned), catfish .... 1 oz
Sardines (canned) .... 2 medium
Tuna (canned in oil, drained) .... 1 oz
Game: Goose (no skin), rabbit .... 1 oz
Cheese:
4.5%-fat cottage cheese .... ¼ cup
Grated Parmesan .... 2 Tbsp
Cheeses with 3 grams or less fat per ounce .... 1 oz
Other:
Hot dogs with 3 grams or less fat per ounce 🥢 .... 1½ oz
Processed sandwich meat with 3 grams or less fat per ounce, such as turkey pastrami or kielbasa .... 1 oz
Liver, heart (high in cholesterol) .... 1 oz

🥢 = 400 mg or more sodium per exchange.

MEDIUM-FAT MEAT AND SUBSTITUTES LIST

One exchange equals 0 grams carbohydrate, 7 grams protein, 5 grams fat, and 75 calories.

One medium-fat meat exchange is equal to any one of the following items.

Beef: Most beef products fall into this category (ground beef, meatloaf, corned beef, short ribs, Prime grades of meat trimmed of fat, such as prime rib) .... 1 oz
Pork: Top loin, chop, Boston butt, cutlet .... 1 oz
Lamb: Rib roast, ground .... 1 oz
Veal: Cutlet (ground or cubed, unbreaded) .... 1 oz
Poultry: Chicken dark meat (with skin), ground turkey or ground chicken, fried chicken (with skin) .... 1 oz
Fish: Any fried fish product .... 1 oz
Cheese: With 5 grams or less fat per ounce
Feta .... 1 oz
Mozzarella .... 1 oz
Ricotta .... ¼ cup (2 oz)
Other:
Egg (high in cholesterol, limit to 3 per week) 1
Sausage with 5 grams or less fat per ounce .... 1 oz
Soy milk .... 1 cup
Tempeh .... ¼ cup
Tofu .... 4 oz or ½ cup

HIGH-FAT MEAT AND SUBSTITUTES LIST

One exchange equals 0 grams carbohydrate, 7 grams protein, 8 grams fat, and 100 calories.

Remember these items are high in saturated fat, cholesterol, and calories and may raise blood cholesterol levels if eaten on a regular basis. One high-fat meat exchange is equal to any one of the following items.

Pork: Spareribs, ground pork, pork sausage .... 1 oz
Cheese: All regular cheeses, such as American 🥢, cheddar, Monterey Jack, Swiss .... 1 oz
continued

HIGH-FAT MEAT AND SUBSTITUTES LIST

Other: Processed sandwich meats with 8 grams or less fat per ounce, such as bologna, pimento loaf, salami .... 1 oz

Sausage, such as bratwurst, Italian, knockwurst, Polish, smoked .... 1 oz

Hot dog (turkey or chicken) 🔖 1 (10/lb)

Bacon.. 3 slices (20 slices/lb)

Count as one high-fat meat plus one fat exchange.

Hot dog (beef, pork, or combination) 🔖 1 (10/lb)

Peanut butter (contains unsaturated fat)........................... 2 Tbsp

🔖 = 400 mg or more sodium per exchange.

FATS LIST

MONOUNSATURATED FATS

One fat exchange equals 5 grams fat and 45 calories.

Avocado, medium .... ⅛ (1 oz)

Oil (canola, olive, peanut) .... 1 tsp

Olives: ripe (black).. 8 large

Green, stuffed 🔖 .... 10 large

Nuts

Almonds, cashews .... 6 nuts

Mixed (50% peanuts) .... 6 nuts

Peanuts .... 10 nuts

Pecans.. 4 halves

Peanut butter, smooth or crunchy....................................... 2 tsp

Sesame seeds.. 1 Tbsp

Tahini paste... 2 tsp

POLYUNSATURATED FATS

One fat exchange equals 5 grams fat and 45 calories.

Margarine: stick, tub, or squeeze .... 1 tsp

Lower-fat (30% to 50% vegetable oil).......................... 1 Tbsp

Mayonnaise: regular .... 1 tsp

Reduced-fat.. 1 Tbsp

Nuts, walnuts, English... 4 halves

Oil (corn, safflower, soybean) .... 1 tsp

Salad dressing: regular 🔖 .... 1 Tbsp

Reduced-fat... 2 Tbsp

Miracle Whip Salad Dressing®: regular .... 2 tsp

Reduced-fat.. 1 Tbsp

Seeds: pumpkin, sunflower .... 1 Tbsp

🔖 = 400 mg or more sodium per exchange.

SATURATED FATS*

One fat exchange equals 5 grams of fat and 45 calories.

Bacon, cooked...................................... 1 slice (20 slices/lb)

Bacon, grease .... 1 tsp

Butter: stick.. 1 tsp

Whipped.. 2 tsp

Reduced-fat.. 1 Tbsp

Chitterlings, boiled .... 2 Tbsp (½ oz)

Coconut, sweetened, shredded.. 2 Tbsp

Cream, half and half.. 2 Tbsp

Cream cheese: regular.................................... 1 Tbsp (½ oz)

Reduced-fat... 2 Tbsp (1 oz)

Fatback or salt pork, see below†

Shortening or lard... 1 tsp

Sour cream: regular .... 2 Tbsp

Reduced-fat.. 3 Tbsp

*Saturated fats can raise blood cholesterol levels

†Use a piece 1 in. × 1 in. × ¼ in. if you plan to eat the fatback cooked with vegetables. Use a piece 2 in. × 1 in. × ½ in. when eating only the vegetables with the fatback removed.

FREE FOODS LIST

A *free food* is any food or drink that contains less than 20 calories or less than 5 grams of carbohydrate per serving. Foods with a serving size listed should be limited to three servings per day. Be sure to spread them out throughout the day. If you eat all three servings at one time, it could affect your blood glucose level. Foods listed without a serving size can be eaten as often as you like.

Fat-free or Reduced-fat Foods

Cream cheese, fat-free .... 1 Tbsp

Creamers, nondairy, liquid.. 1 Tbsp

Creamers, nondairy, powdered... 2 tsp

Mayonnaise, fat-free .... 1 Tbsp

Mayonnaise, reduced-fat .... 1 tsp

Margarine, fat-free .... 4 Tbsp

Margarine, reduced-fat.. 1 tsp

Miracle Whip®, nonfat.. 1 Tbsp

Miracle Whip®, reduced-fat .... 1 tsp

Nonstick cooking spray

Salad dressing, fat-free .... 1 Tbsp

Salad dressing, fat-free, Italian .... 2 Tbsp

Salsa.. ¼ cup

Sour cream, fat-free, reduced-fat .... 1 Tbsp

Whipped topping, regular or light...................................... 2 Tbsp

Sugar-free or Low-sugar Foods

Candy, hard, sugar-free... 1 candy

Gelatin dessert, sugar-free

Gelatin, unflavored

Gum, sugar-free

Jam or jelly, low-sugar or light... 2 tsp

Sugar substitutes°

Syrup, sugar-free.. 2 Tbsp

°Sugar substitutes, alternatives, or replacements that are approved by the Food and Drug Administration (FDA) are safe to use. Common brand names include: Equal® (aspartame), Sprinkle Sweet® (saccharin), Sweet One® (acesulfame K), Sweet-10® (saccharin), Sugar Twin® (saccharin), Sweet 'n Low® (saccharin)

Drinks

Bouillon, broth, consommé 🔖

Bouillon or broth, low-sodium

Carbonated or mineral water

Cocoa powder, unsweetened .... 1 Tbsp

Coffee

Club soda

Diet soft drinks, sugar-free

continued

Drinks
Drink mixes, sugar-free
Tea
Tonic water, sugar-free

Condiments
Catsup .... 1 Tbsp
Horseradish
Lemon juice
Lime juice
Mustard
Pickles, dill ➤₊ .... 1½ large
Soy sauce, regular or light ➤₊
Taco sauce .... 1 Tbsp
Vinegar

Seasonings
Be careful with seasonings that contain sodium or are salts, such as garlic or celery salt, and lemon pepper.

Flavoring extracts
Garlic
Herbs, fresh or dried
Pimento
Spices
Tabasco® or hot pepper sauce
Wine, used in cooking
Worcestershire sauce

➤₊ = 400 mg or more of sodium per choice.

COMBINATION FOOD LIST

Many of the foods we eat are mixed together in various combinations. These combination foods do not fit into any one exchange list. Often it is hard to tell what is in a casserole dish or prepared food item. This is a list of exchanges for some typical combination foods. This list will help you fit these foods into your meal plan. Ask your dietitian for information about any other combination foods you would like to eat.

Food	Serving Size	Exchanges Per Serving
Entrees		
Tuna noodle casserole, lasagna, spaghetti with meatballs, chile with beans, macaroni and cheese ➤₊	1 cup (8 oz)	2 carbohydrates, 2 medium-fat meats
Chow mein (without noodles or rice)	2 cups (16 oz)	1 carbohydrate, 2 lean meats
Pizza, cheese, thin crust ➤₊	¼ of 10 in. (5 oz)	2 carbohydrates, 2 medium-fat meats, 1 fat
Pizza, meat topping, thin crust ➤₊	¼ of 10 in. (5 oz)	2 carbohydrates, 2 medium-fat meats, 2 fats
Pot pie ➤₊	1 (7 oz)	2 carbohydrates, 1 medium-fat meat, 4 fats
Frozen entrees		
Salisbury steak with gravy, mashed potato ➤₊	1 (11 oz)	2 carbohydrates, 3 medium-fat meats, 3–4 fats
Turkey with gravy, mashed potato, dressing ➤₊	1 (11 oz)	2 carbohydrates, 3 lean meats
Entree with less than 300 calories ➤₊	1 (8 oz)	2 carbohydrates, 3 lean meats
Soups		
Bean ➤₊	1 cup	1 carbohydrate, 1 very lean meat
Cream (made with water) ➤₊	1 cup (8 oz)	1 carbohydrate, 1 fat
Split pea (made with water) ➤₊	½ cup (4 oz)	1 carbohydrate
Tomato (made with water) ➤₊	1 cup (8 oz)	1 carbohydrate
Vegetable beef, chicken noodle, or other broth-type ➤₊	1 cup (8 oz)	1 carbohydrate

➤₊ = 400 mg or more sodium per exchange.

FAST FOODS LIST*

Food	Serving Size	Exchanges Per Serving
Burritos with beef ➤₊	2	4 carbohydrates, 2 medium-fat meats, 2 fats
Chicken nuggets ➤₊	6	1 carbohydrate, 2 medium-fat meats, 1 fat
Chicken breast and wing, breaded and fried ➤₊	1 each	1 carbohydrate, 4 medium-fat meats, 2 fats
Fish sandwich/tartar sauce ➤₊	1	3 carbohydrates, 1 medium-fat meat, 3 fats
French fries, thin	20–25	2 carbohydrates, 2 fats
Hamburger, regular	1	2 carbohydrates, 2 medium-fat meats
Hamburger, large ➤₊	1	2 carbohydrates, 3 medium-fat meats, 1 fat
Hot dog with bun ➤₊	1	1 carbohydrate, 1 high-fat meat, 1 fat
Individual pan pizza ➤₊	1	5 carbohydrates, 3 medium-fat meats, 3 fats
Soft-serve cone ➤₊	1 medium	2 carbohydrates, 1 fat
Submarine sandwich ➤₊	1 sub (6 in.)	3 carbohydrates, 1 vegetable, 2 medium-fat meats, 1 fat
Taco, hard shell ➤₊	1 (6 oz)	2 carbohydrates, 2 medium-fat meats, 2 fats
Taco, soft shell ➤₊	1 (3 oz)	1 carbohydrate, 1 medium-fat meat, 1 fat

➤₊ = 400 mg or more of sodium per serving.
*Ask at your fast-food restaurant for nutrition information about your favorite fast foods.

**Mexican American Foods
and the Food Guide Pyramid**

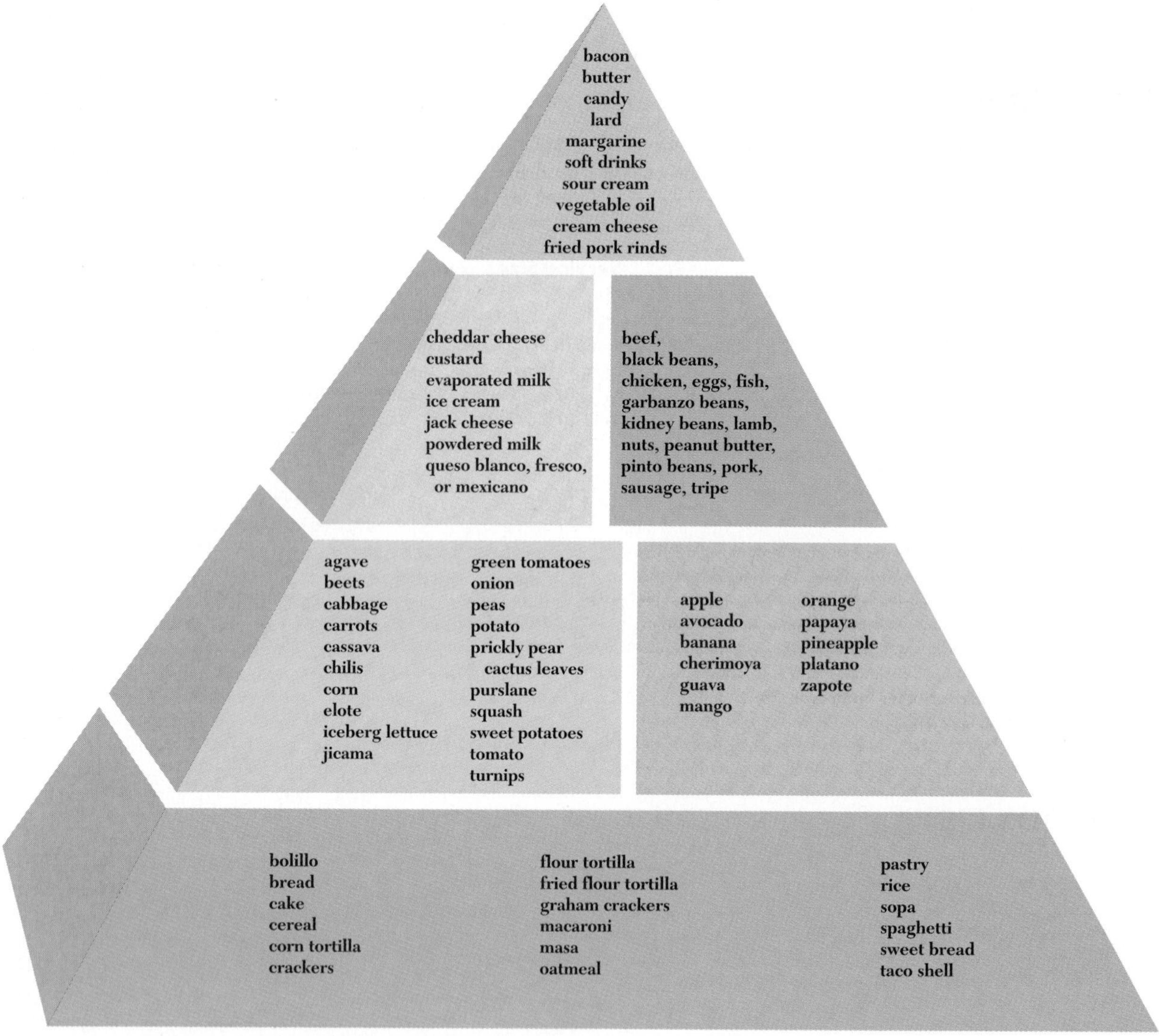

bacon
butter
candy
lard
margarine
soft drinks
sour cream
vegetable oil
cream cheese
fried pork rinds

cheddar cheese
custard
evaporated milk
ice cream
jack cheese
powdered milk
queso blanco, fresco,
or mexicano

beef,
black beans,
chicken, eggs, fish,
garbanzo beans,
kidney beans, lamb,
nuts, peanut butter,
pinto beans, pork,
sausage, tripe

agave
beets
cabbage
carrots
cassava
chilis
corn
elote
iceberg lettuce
jicama

green tomatoes
onion
peas
potato
prickly pear
  cactus leaves
purslane
squash
sweet potatoes
tomato
turnips

apple
avocado
banana
cherimoya
guava
mango

orange
papaya
pineapple
platano
zapote

bolillo
bread
cake
cereal
corn tortilla
crackers

flour tortilla
fried flour tortilla
graham crackers
macaroni
masa
oatmeal

pastry
rice
sopa
spaghetti
sweet bread
taco shell

© 1993 *Pyramid Packet*, Penn State Nutrition Center, 417 East Calder Way, University Park, PA 16801-5663; (814)865-6323

Sources: Ethnic and Regional Food Practices—A Series: Mexican American Food Practices, Customs, and Holidays; Diabetes Care and Education
Practice Group of the American Dietetic Association; contributors, Susan J. Algert, MS, RD, and Teri Hall Ellison, MPH, RD. 1989.

Comidas Hispana en Dietas Diabetica. Spanish Foods in Diabetic Diets. Visiting Nurse Association of Milwaukee. 1975.

J

The Mediterranean Diet Pyramid

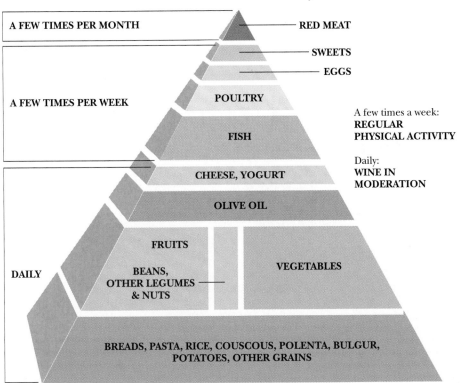

A FEW TIMES PER MONTH — RED MEAT

— SWEETS

— EGGS

A FEW TIMES PER WEEK

POULTRY

FISH

A few times a week:
REGULAR PHYSICAL ACTIVITY

CHEESE, YOGURT

Daily:
WINE IN MODERATION

OLIVE OIL

FRUITS

BEANS, OTHER LEGUMES & NUTS

VEGETABLES

DAILY

BREADS, PASTA, RICE, COUSCOUS, POLENTA, BULGUR, POTATOES, OTHER GRAINS

HEALTH HINTS FROM THE MEDITERRANEAN DIET PYRAMID

• Eat most food from plant sources including fruits, vegetables, potatoes, breads, beans, nuts and seeds.

• Use seasonally fresh, locally grown food with a minimum of processing.

• Let olive oil be your principal fat, replacing other fats, oils, butter and margarine.

• Eat red meat only a few times per month and favor the lean cuts.

• If you drink wine, enjoy only 1 or 2 glasses a day, preferably with meals.

• Engage in regular exercise to promote a healthy weight, fitness and well-being.

J

Chinese American Foods
and the Food Guide Pyramid

bacon fat,
butter,
coconut milk,
corn oil,
duck sauce, honey, lard,
maltose syrup, peanut oil,
sesame oil, sesame paste,
soybean oil, suet, sugar

buffalo milk

cow's milk

fish bones

soybean milk

yogurt

bean paste, beef,
chestnuts, chicken,
duck, eggs,
fish (e.g., carp, catfish),
lamb,
legumes (e.g., mung
   beans, soy beans),
pork, quail, rice birds,
shellfish and other seafood
(e.g., shrimp, squid), squab

amaranth, arrowheads, bamboo shoots,
bitter gourd, black mushroom, bok choy,
cabbage, celery, chayote, chilis,
Chinese broccoli, choy sum, dried wood ear,
eggplant, garland chrysanthemum, garlic,
ginger, green beans, hairy cucumber, leek,
lotus root, mustard greens, okra, onions,
Oriental radish, peas, pickled cucumber, potatoes,
scallion, spinach, sprouts, straw mushrooms, taro,
tomatoes, turnip, water chestnut, watercress,
winter melon, yard-long beans

carambola, Chinese banana,

Chinese pear, guava, jujube,

kumquats, litchi, longan, mango,

orange, papaya, persimmon,

pummelo, watermelon

barley	glutinous rice	nin goh		rice flour
bing	hua juan	noodles, including—celophane noodles		steamed rice
		—rice sticks		sorghum
dumplings	mianbao	—rice vermicelli		Wonton wrappers
fried rice	mantou	rice congee		zong-zi

J

GUÍA PARA LA
BUENA
ALIMENTACÍON
GUIDE TO GOOD EATING

Cómo alimentarse para mantener buena salud:
1. *Coma alimentos de los cinco grupos alimenticios todos los días.*
2. *Coma diferentes alimentos de cada grupo cada día.*

To eat for good health:
1. *Eat foods from all Five Food Groups every day.*
2. *Eat different foods from each food group every day.*

Todos los días coma:
Every day eat:

Las porciones que se recomiendan
Suggested Serving Sizes

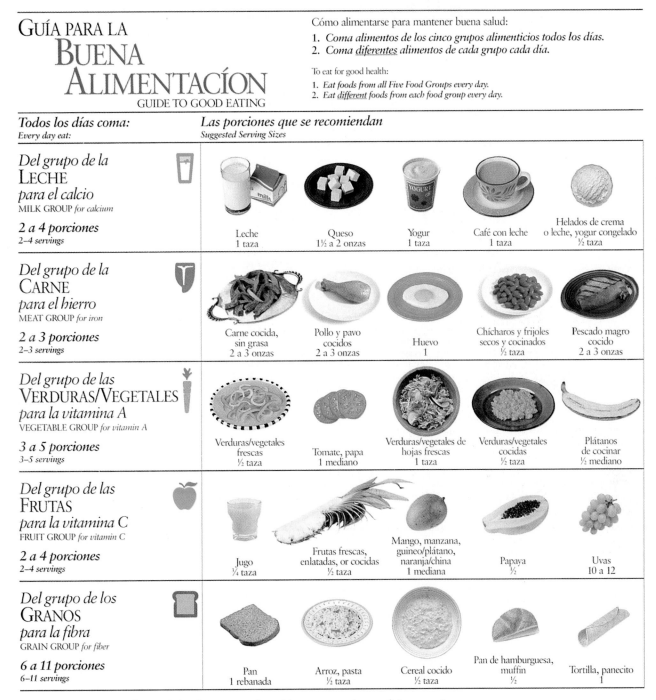

Del grupo de la
LECHE
para el calcio
MILK GROUP *for calcium*

2 a 4 porciones
2–4 servings

Leche
1 taza

Queso
1½ a 2 onzas

Yogur
1 taza

Café con leche
1 taza

Helados de crema
o leche, yogur congelado
½ taza

Del grupo de la
CARNE
para el hierro
MEAT GROUP *for iron*

2 a 3 porciones
2–3 servings

Carne cocida,
sin grasa
2 a 3 onzas

Pollo y pavo
cocidos
2 a 3 onzas

Huevo
1

Chícharos y frijoles
secos y cocinados
½ taza

Pescado magro
cocido
2 a 3 onzas

Del grupo de las
VERDURAS/VEGETALES
para la vitamina A
VEGETABLE GROUP *for vitamin A*

3 a 5 porciones
3–5 servings

Verduras/vegetales
frescas
½ taza

Tomate, papa
1 mediano

Verduras/vegetales de
hojas frescas
1 taza

Verduras/vegetales
cocidas
½ taza

Plátanos
de cocinar
½ mediano

Del grupo de las
FRUTAS
para la vitamina C
FRUIT GROUP *for vitamin C*

2 a 4 porciones
2–4 servings

Jugo
¼ taza

Frutas frescas,
enlatadas, or cocidas
½ taza

Mango, manzana,
guineo/plátano,
naranja/china
1 mediana

Papaya
½

Uvas
10 a 12

Del grupo de los
GRANOS
para la fibra
GRAIN GROUP *for fiber*

6 a 11 porciones
6–11 servings

Pan
1 rebanada

Arroz, pasta
½ taza

Cereal cocido
½ taza

Pan de hamburguesa,
muffin
½

Tortilla, panecito
1

"Los otros" no entran en ninguno de los cinco grupos alimenticios porque no tienen suficientes nutrientes.
Se pueden comer pero con moderación.
"Others" don't have enough nutrients to fit in any of the Five Food Groups. These foods are okay to eat in moderation.

Categoría de
"LOS OTROS"
"OTHERS" CATEGORY
Grasas y aceites, dulces, meriendas
saladas, bebidas alcohólicas, otras
bebidas, condimentos
Fats and oils, sweets, salty snacks, alcohol,
other beverages, and condiments

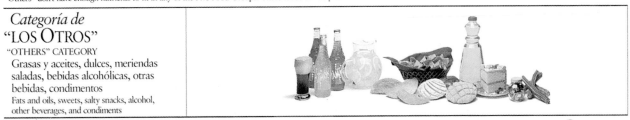

001NS 1 1993, Copyright © 1993, 6th Edition, NATIONAL DAIRY COUNCIL, Rosemont, IL 60018-5516. All rights reserved. Printed in U.S.A.

Samoan Foods in the Exchange Lists

Calcium/Milk exchanges—one serving contains approximately 90 kcal, 12 g carbohydrate, 8 g protein, and a trace of fat

Dark, green, leafy vegetables (calcium may not be readily absorbed)	3 c
Tofu, prepared with calcium (omit 1 fat group)	½ c
Fish, sardines, mackerel	3 oz
Salmon, canned with bones (omit 1 fat group)	3 oz

Starch exchanges—one serving contains approximately 80 kcal, 15 g carbohydrate, and 3 g protein

Banana, plantain (cooking banana)	1 medium (2″ × 1⅞″)
Cassava	⅓ c
Breadfruit	¼ c
Taro	½ c
O'o (sprouting coconut meat; omit 1 fat)	1¾ c

Fruit exchanges—one serving contains approximately 60 kcal and 15 g carbohydrate

Guava (good source of vitamin C)	1 medium
Soursop, pulp	⅓ c
Lychees	10 fruits
Passion fruit juice (good source of vitamin C)	½ c
Star fruit	1½ c, cubed

Vegetable exchanges—one serving contains approximately 25 kcal, 5 g carbohydrate, and 2 g protein

Bamboo shoot	½ c
Papaya, green	½ c
Banana bud	½ c
Squash, leaf tips (Good source of vitamin A)	½ c
Bittermelon, fruit	½ c
Sweet potato leaves (Good source of vitamin A)	½ c
Bittermelon, leaves (Good source of vitamin A)	½ c
Taro leaves (Good source of vitamin A)	½ c

Meat exchanges—meat exchanges are divided into three groups (A, B, and C) on the basis of fat content

Meat A Group—one serving contains approximately 55 kcal, 7 g protein, and 3 g fat

Clams, crab, lobster, prawns	1 oz
Fish (eg, aku, opakapaka, mahimahi, tuna)	1 oz or 1 slice (3″ × 1″ × ¾″)
Cuttlefish, squid, octopus	1 oz
Sea slug	1 c

Meat B Group—one serving contains approximately 75 kcal, 7 g protein, and 5 g fat

Chicken wing	1 wing
Tofu	⅓ c
Corned beef	1 oz

Meat C Group—one serving contains approximately 100 kcal, 7 g protein, and 8 g fat

Canned luncheon meat	1 oz
Turkey tails	½ oz
Mutton flaps (flank of mature sheep)	1 oz
Turkey wings	½ wing

Fat exchanges—one serving contains approximately 45 kcal and 5 g fat

Coconut, mature meat	1 piece (1″ × 1″ × ⅜″)
Coconut, cream (no water added)	1 tbsp
Coconut, milk (1 c water, 1 c cream)	2 tbsp
Coconut, grated	2 tbsp

J

Daily Reference Values

Food Component	Daily Reference Value (2000 kcal)
Total fat	Less than 65 g (30% of energy)
Saturated fat	Less than 20 g (10% of energy)
Cholesterol	Less than 300 mg
Total carbohydrate	300 g (60% of energy)
Dietary fiber	25 g (11.5 g/1000 kcal)
Sodium	Less than 2400 mg
Potassium	3500 mg
Protein	50 g (10% of energy)

Health Claims Allowed on Food Labels

Calcium and osteoporosis	Adequate calcium intake throughout life helps maintain bone health and reduce the risk of osteoporosis.
Sodium and hypertension (high blood pressure)	Diets high in sodium may increase the risk of high blood pressure.
Dietary fat and cancer	Diets high in fat increase the risk of some types of cancer.
Saturated fat and cholesterol and cardiovascular disease	Diets high in saturated fat and cholesterol increase blood cholesterol and, thus, the risk of heart disease.
Foods high in fiber and cancer	Diets low in fat and rich in fiber-containing grain products, fruits, and vegetables may reduce the risk of some types of cancer.
Foods high in fiber and risk of cardiovascular disease	Diets low in saturated fat and cholesterol and rich in fruits, vegetables, and grain products that contain fiber, particularly soluble fiber, may reduce the risk of coronary heart disease.
Fruits and vegetables and cancer	Diets low in fat and rich in fruits and vegetables may reduce the risk of some types of cancer.
Folic acid and neural tube defect–affected pregnancy	Adequate folic acid intake by the mother reduces the risk of birth defects of the brain or spinal cord in their babies.

K

Nutrient Content Descriptors Commonly Used on Food Labels

Free	Means that a product contains no amount of, or a trivial amount of, fat, saturated fat, cholesterol, sodium, sugars, or kcalories. For example, "sugar-free" and "fat-free" both mean less than 0.5 g per serving. Synonyms for "free" include "without," "no," and "zero."
Low	Used for foods that can be eaten frequently without exceeding the Daily Value for fat, saturated fat, cholesterol, sodium, or kcalories. Specific definitions have been established for each of these nutrients. For example, "low fat" means that the food contains 3 g or less per serving, and "low cholesterol" means that the food contains less than 20 mg of cholesterol per serving. Synonyms for "low" include "little," "few," and "low source of."
Lean and extra lean	Used to describe the fat content of meat, poultry, seafood, and game meats. "Lean" means that the food contains less than 10 g fat, less than 4.5 g saturated fat, and less than 95 mg of cholesterol per serving and per 100 g. "Extra lean" means that the food contains less than 5 g fat, less than 2 g saturated fat, and less than 95 mg of cholesterol per serving and per 100 g.
High	Can be used if a food contains 20% or more of the Daily Value for a particular nutrient. Synonyms for "high" include "rich in" and "excellent source of."
Good source	Means that a food contains 10 to 19% of the Daily Value for a particular nutrient per serving.
Reduced	Means that a nutritionally altered product contains 25% less of a nutrient or of energy than the regular or reference product.
Less	Means that a food, whether altered or not, contains 25% less of a nutrient or of energy than the reference food. For example, pretzels may claim to have "less fat" than potato chips. "Fewer" may be used as a synonym for "less."
Light	May be used in different ways. First, it can be used on a nutritionally altered product that contains one-third fewer kcalories or half the fat of a reference food. Second, it can be used when the sodium content of a low-calorie, lowfat food has been reduced by 50%. The term "light" can be used to describe properties such as texture and color as long as the label explains the intent, for example, "light and fluffy."
More	Means that a serving of food, whether altered or not, contains a nutrient that is at least 10% of the Daily Value more than the reference food. This definition also applies to foods using the terms "fortified," "enriched," or "added."
Healthy	May be used to describe foods that are low in fat and saturated fat and contain no more than 480 mg of sodium and no more than 60 mg of cholesterol per serving and provide at least 10% of the Daily Value for vitamins A or C, or iron, calcium, protein, or fiber.
Fresh	May be used on foods that are raw and have never been frozen or heated and contain no preservatives.

Federal Register 58, 1993, Jan. 6. U.S. Government Printing Office, Superintendent of Documents, Washington, DC.

Recommended Dietary Intakes*

Vitamins and Minerals	Units of Measurement	Adults and Children 4 or More Years of Age	Infants	Children Under 4 Years of Age	Pregnant or Lactating Women
Vitamin A	International Units (micrograms)[†]	5000 (1000 µg)	1,500	2,500	8,000
Vitamin D	International Units (micrograms)[†]	400 (10 µg)	400	400	400
Vitamin E	International Units (micrograms)[†]	30 (10 µg)	5	10	30
Vitamin C	Milligrams	60	35	40	60
Folic Acid	Micrograms	400	0.1	0.2	0.8
Thiamin	Milligrams	1.5	0.5	0.7	1.7
Riboflavin	Milligrams	1.7	0.6	0.8	2.0
Niacin	Milligrams	20	8	9	20
Vitamin B_6	Milligrams	2.0	0.4	0.7	2.5
Vitamin B_{12}	Micrograms	6.0	2	3	8
Biotin	Micrograms	300	0.05	0.15	0.30
Pantothenic acid	Milligrams	10	3	5	10
Calcium	Milligrams	1000	0.6	0.8	1.3
Phosphorus	Milligrams	1000	0.5	0.8	1.3
Iodine	Micrograms	150	45	70	150
Iron	Milligrams	18	15	10	18
Magnesium	Milligrams	400	70	200	450
Copper	Milligrams	20	0.6	1.0	2.0
Zinc	Milligrams	15	5	8	15
Vitamin K	Micrograms	80	—[‡]	—[‡]	—[‡]
Chromium	Micrograms	120	—	—	—
Selenium	Micrograms	70	—	—	—
Molybdenum	Micrograms	75	—	—	—
Manganese	Milligrams	2	—	—	—
Chloride	Milligrams	3400	—	—	—

* Based on National Academy of Sciences' 1968 Recommended Dietary Allowances.
[†] The RDIs for fat soluble vitamins are expressed in International Units (IU). The current RDAs use a newer system of measurement. Values that are approximately equivalent are given in parentheses.
[‡] No values yet established for vitamin K, chromium, selenium, molybdenum, manganese, or chloride for this population.

**SAMPLE LABEL
FOR A GRANOLA BAR**

Granola bars

Nutrition Facts

Serving Size 1 bar (24g)
Servings Per Container 12

Amount Per Serving

Calories 120   Calories from Fat 45

% Daily Value*

Total Fat 5g	8%
Saturated Fat 1g	5%
Cholesterol 0mg	0%
Sodium 65mg	3%
Total Carbohydrate 17g	6%
Dietary Fiber 1g	4%
Sugars 6g	
Protein 2g	

Vitamin A 0%	•	Vitamin C 0%	
Calcium 0%	•	Iron 4%	

* Percent Daily Values are based on a 2,000 calorie diet. Your daily values may be higher or lower depending on your calorie needs:

		Calories:	2,000	2,500
Total Fat	Less than		65g	80g
Sat Fat	Less than		20g	25g
Cholesterol	Less than		300mg	300mg
Sodium	Less than		2,400mg	2,400mg
Total Carbohydrate			300g	375g
Dietary Fiber			25g	30g

Calories per gram:
Fat 9 • Carbohydrate 4 • Protein 4

Ingredients: Rolled oats, sugar, sunflower oil, brown sugar syrup, honey, salt, soy lecithin

Type of Activity	Kcalories per Hour				
	100 lb	120 lb	150 lb	180 lb	200 lb
Aerobics (heavy)	363	435	544	653	726
Aerobics (light)	136	163	204	245	272
Aerobics (medium)	227	272	340	408	454
Archery	159	190	238	286	317
Back-packing	408	490	612	735	816
Badminton (doubles)	181	218	272	327	363
Badminton (singles)	231	278	347	416	463
Basketball (nonvigorous)	431	517	646	776	862
Basketball (vigorous)	499	599	748	898	998
Bicycling (10 mph)	249	299	374	449	499
Bicycling (11 mph)	295	354	442	531	590
Bicycling (12 mph)	340	408	510	612	680
Bicycling (13 mph)	385	463	578	694	771
Bicycling (6 mph)	159	190	238	286	317
Billiards	91	109	136	163	181
Bowling	177	212	265	318	354
Boxing—competition	603	724	905	1086	1206
Boxing—sparring	376	452	565	678	753
Calisthenics (heavy)	363	435	544	653	726
Calisthenics (light)	181	218	272	327	363
Canoeing (2.5 mph)	150	180	224	269	299
Canoeing (5 mph)	340	408	510	612	680
Carpentry	227	272	340	408	454
Climbing (mountain)	454	544	680	816	907
Disco dancing	272	327	408	490	544
Ditch digging (hand)	263	316	395	473	526
Fencing	340	408	510	612	680
Fishing (bank/boat)	159	190	238	286	317
Fishing (in waders)	249	299	374	449	499
Football (touch)	340	408	510	612	680
Gardening	145	174	218	261	290
Golf (carry clubs)	227	272	340	408	454
Golf (pull cart)	163	196	245	294	327
Golf (ride in cart)	113	136	170	204	227
Handball (vigorous)	454	544	680	816	907
Hiking (X-country)	249	299	374	449	499
Hiking (mountain)	340	408	510	612	680
Horseback trotting	231	278	347	416	463
Housework	181	218	272	327	363
Hunting (carry load)	272	327	408	490	544
Ice hockey (vigorous)	454	544	680	816	907

L

Type of Activity	Kcalories per Hour				
	100 lb	120 lb	150 lb	180 lb	200 lb
Ice skating (10 mph)	263	316	395	473	526
Jazzercize (heavy)	363	435	544	653	726
Jazzercize (light)	136	163	204	245	272
Jazzercize (medium)	227	272	340	408	454
Jog (10 min/mile)	454	544	680	816	907
Jog (12 min/mile)	385	463	578	694	771
Jog (13 min/mile)	317	381	476	571	635
Jog (14 min/mile)	272	327	408	490	544
Jog (15 min/mile)	227	272	340	408	454
Jog (17 min/mile)	181	218	272	327	363
Jog (9 min/mile)	499	599	748	898	998
Lawn mowing (hand)	295	354	442	531	590
Lawn mowing (power)	163	196	245	294	327
Music playing	113	136	170	204	227
Racquetball (social)	385	463	578	694	771
Racquetball (vigorous)	454	544	680	816	907
Roller skating	231	278	347	416	463
Rowboating (2.5 mph)	200	239	299	359	399
Rowing (11 mph)	590	707	884	1061	1179
Run (5 min/mile)	816	980	1224	1469	1633
Run (6 min/mile)	703	844	1054	1265	1406
Run (7 min/mile)	612	735	918	1102	1224
Run (8 min/mile)	544	653	816	980	1088
Sailing	159	190	238	286	317
Shuffleboard/skeet	136	163	204	245	272
Skiing (X-country)	454	544	680	816	907
Skiing (downhill)	363	435	544	653	726
Square dancing	272	327	407	490	544
Swimming (compete)	680	816	1020	1224	1361
Swimming (fast)	426	512	639	767	853
Swimming (slow)	349	419	524	629	698
Table tennis	236	283	354	424	472
Tennis (doubles)	227	272	340	408	454
Tennis (singles)	295	354	442	531	590
Tennis (vigorous)	385	463	578	694	771
Volleyball	231	278	347	416	463
Walking (20 min/mile)	159	190	238	286	317
Walking (26 min/mile)	136	163	204	245	272
Water skiing	317	381	476	571	635
Weightlifting (heavy)	408	490	612	735	816
Weightlifting (light)	181	218	272	327	363
Wood chopping (sawing)	295	354	442	531	590

Data reprinted with permission from N-Squared Computing, First Databank Division of the Hearst Corporation.

L

The answers given below are some of the possible answers. For many of these questions, many more answers are possible.

CHAPTER 1: CRITICAL THINKING: NUTRITIONAL ASSESSMENT

Start your own nutritional assessment. Is your weight within the normal range? Have you lost or gained weight recently? Weight tables are included in Appendix B.

CHAPTER 2: CRITICAL THINKING: WHAT IS WRONG WITH THIS EXPERIMENT?

Was the study well controlled? No, the groups were not evaluated before and after taking the supplement.

Was the proper number of experimental subjects tested? There was no mention of the statistics used to determine the correct number, but 50 in each group may be enough.

Were the experimental data objective? Yes, grades are an objective measure.

Is the conclusion valid? No, there are many variables other than Brain Power that could have had an impact on the students' grades. The students may have been taking more difficult courses during the semester that they were not taking Brain Power. In addition, the difference in grade point was only 3.0 to 3.1, a difference that is unlikely to be meaningful when analyzed statistically.

CHAPTER 2: CRITICAL THINKING: HOW TO APPLY THE FOOD GUIDE PYRAMID TO YOUR DIET

Does Naomi's diet meet the minimum number of servings recommended by the Food Guide Pyramid? No, her diet needs more grains and vegetables. It provides 3 breads, and the recommendation is 6 to 11; 3 milks, and the recommendation is 2 to 3; 3 fruits, and the recommendation is 2 to 5; 2 vegetables, and the recommendation is 3 to 5; 2 meats, and the recommendation is 2 to 3; and she consumes many fats and sweets, whereas the recommendation is to consume these in moderation.

What snacks could she choose to decrease the number of servings of fats and sweets and increase grains and vegetables? She could take a sandwich for lunch and have carrots for a snack. She could replace the soda with water or milk. And she could eliminate the ice cream; it counts as a serving of milk but is also high in fat.

CHAPTER 3: CRITICAL THINKING: GI PROBLEMS CAN AFFECT NUTRITION

What nutrient should this person avoid? Fat, because the gallbladder contracts to secrete bile when fat is consumed, causing the pain associated with gallbladder problems.

CHAPTER 4: CRITICAL THINKING: WHAT HAPPENS IF YOU CONSUME TOO LITTLE CARBOHYDRATE?

Why can insulin-dependent diabetics develop ketosis even when consuming plenty of carbohydrate? Individuals with insulin-dependent diabetes do not produce enough insulin to allow glucose uptake by the body cells. Therefore, even though glucose is available in the blood, it cannot enter cells. The cells respond as they do in starvation and begin using fatty acids for fuel. Without glucose the fatty acids cannot be completely metabolized and ketones are produced. When diabetics inject insulin, glucose can enter cells.

CHAPTER 4: CRITICAL THINKING: CHOOSING A DIET HIGH IN COMPLEX CARBOHYDRATE

Calculate the percent carbohydrate in Mercedes' modified diet: 247 g carbohydrate × 4 kcal/g = 988 kcal of carbohydrate divided by 1700 total kcalories × 100 = 58%.

Suggest some other modifications to Mercedes' diet so that it provides at least 17 grams of fiber. The beans she adds to her burrito increase her fiber intake; she could eat the potatoes in their skins; she could eat fruits instead of fruit juices; she could have a high-fiber cereal for breakfast instead of the chorizo; she could have whole wheat rather than white toast.

CHAPTER 5: CRITICAL THINKING: DIETARY FAT AND HEART DISEASE RISK

What risk factors does Rafael have for developing cardiovascular disease? He has a moderately stressful lifestyle; his total cholesterol is over 200 and HDL cholesterol is less than a fourth of his total cholesterol; his intake of fat, saturated fat, and cholesterol exceeds the recommendations for a healthy diet; he consumes more servings of meat and fewer servings of vegetables and fruits than is recommended by the Food Guide Pyramid.

What dietary and lifestyle changes would you recommend to reduce his risks? He could begin an exercise program

M

after consulting with his physician; he could reduce his intake of fat, saturated fat, and cholesterol and increase his intake of vegetables and fruits.

If Rafael were to replace all of the fat in his diet with olive oil, would he reduce his risk of cardiovascular disease to the level found in Mediterranean countries? No. The low risk of cardiovascular disease in Mediterranean countries is a result not only of olive oil consumption but also of the total diet being high in vegetables and fruits and carbohydrates and other lifestyle factors. Even if he added olive oil to his diet, it would still be low in fruits and vegetables, his lifestyle would still be stressful, and he still wouldn't be getting enough exercise.

CHAPTER 5: CRITICAL THINKING: HOW TO REDUCE YOUR FAT INTAKE

Her total energy intake is 2100 kcalories. What is the percent of kcalories from fat in her original diet? To determine the percent of energy from fat in her diet, Menchu multiplies the total grams of fat by 9 kcalories per gram (82.7 g × 9 kcal/g = 744.3 kcal from fat) and divides this by her total intake of 2100 kcalories (744.3 kcal from fat / 2100 kcal = 0.35). Multiplying this by 100 (0.35 × 100 = 35%) gives her the percent of her energy intake that is fat.

Does her modified diet contain less than 30% energy from fat and meet the recommendations of the Food Guide Pyramid? 34.2 g fat × 9 kcal/g = 307.8 kcal from fat. 307.8 kcal divided by 2100 total kcal × 100 = 14.7% energy as fat. Her diet meets all of the recommendations of the Food Guide Pyramid except for the milk, yogurt, and cheese group. The only dairy products she consumes is the ¾ cup of frozen yogurt, which is equal to less than 1 serving from this food group.

CHAPTER 6: CRITICAL THINKING: WHAT DOES NITROGEN BALANCE TELL US?

What is his nitrogen balance? Subject B consumes 11.2 grams and excretes 11.2 grams of nitrogen, 11.2 − 11.2 = 0. Therefore he is in neutral nitrogen balance.

What is her nitrogen balance? Subject C consumes 12.8 grams and excretes 10.4 grams of nitrogen, 12.8 − 10.4 = 2.4 g. She is in positive nitrogen balance, retaining more nitrogen in her body than she consumes.

Does her nitrogen balance make sense metabolically? Yes, this makes sense because she is pregnant and therefore gaining protein. The protein that is retained in her body is used to make proteins for maternal and fetal tissues.

CHAPTER 6: CRITICAL THINKING: MEETING PROTEIN NEEDS WITH A VEGETARIAN DIET

How much protein would his diet provide if he eliminated dairy products from his diet? It would provide 46.2 grams.

What substitutions could he make to meet his needs with a vegan diet? He would need to add about 10 grams of protein. He could have a cup of cooked cereal at breakfast, adding about 3 grams. He could increase his portion of the curry,

adding another 3 grams. He could add another vegetable to dinner, supplying 2 more grams. He could add bread or cookies to lunch or dinner to make up the last 2 grams.

CHAPTER 7: CRITICAL THINKING: IS SHE DESTINED TO BE OBESE?

What is her energy expenditure? April estimates her RMR using Table 7-2. At 23 years of age and 140 pounds, her RMR is 1437 kcal/24 hours or 59.9 kcal/hr. The energy required for April's activities can be estimated as a factor of her resting metabolic rate shown (Table 7-3):

8 hrs of resting requires 8 hr × (1 × RMR in kcal/hr) = 8 hr × 1 × 59.9 kcal/hr = 479 kcal

14 hr of very light activity requires 14 hr × (1.5 × 59.9 kcal/hr) = 1258 kcal

2 hr of light activity requires 2 hr × (2.5 × 59.9 kcal/hr) = 300 kcal

Total for RMR and activity = 2037 kcalories

The Thermic Effect of Food: The thermic effect of food is about 10% of daily energy intake.

Since she consumes 2650 kcalories, her TEF is 2650 kcalories × 10% = 265 kcalories.

Total energy expenditure = RMR + activity + TEF = 2037 + 265 = 2302 kcalories.

How much additional energy will this burn? 2 hours of moderate activity would add: 2 hr × 5 × 59.9 kcal/hr = 599 kcalories, replacing 180 kcalories of very light activity (2 hr × 1.5 × 59.9 kcal/hr = 180 kcal) for a net increase of 599 kcal − 180 kcal = 419 kcalories.

What other substitutions could she make to decrease her intake? She could have broiled chicken breast instead of the chicken nuggets and save about 150 kcalories, she could have pretzels instead of the candy bar and save 200 kcalories, and she could have macaroni with tomato sauce instead of macaroni and cheese and save about 100 kcalories.

CHAPTER 7: CRITICAL THINKING: DO YOU THINK THIS DIET WILL WORK?

Does the program promote changes in eating habits and lifestyle that will encourage weight maintenance? No. The formula will promote weight loss in the short term, but this weight loss is unlikely to be maintained. Replacing meals with a liquid meal substitute doesn't help promote healthy food choices. In addition, there is no behavior modification component to promote a permanent change in eating patterns, and there is no exercise component to increase energy expenditure.

CHAPTER 8: CRITICAL THINKING: SHOULD FOODS BE FORTIFIED WITH FOLATE?

What are the risk, benefits, and costs of this alternate approach? The risks are that despite public education programs, many people may not change their diets to increase the consumption of foods high in folate, and therefore the incidence of neural tube defects would not decline significantly. The benefits are that people who do change their diets are getting more than just additional folate. Foods high in folate are also good sources of other nutrients and phytochemicals. In terms of cost, producing an educational program is probably less expensive than altering grain processing to add folate and modifying food labels to reflect this. Who will bear the cost is also an issue. The cost of educational programs will be borne by public health agencies, while the costs of fortifying foods would go to manufacturers. If educational programs are not effective, the financial and emotional cost of caring for neural tube defect–affected children must be considered.

CHAPTER 9: CRITICAL THINKING: EVALUATING VITAMIN SUPPLEMENTS

What are the risks and benefits of taking these supplements? Vitamin B$_6$ and niacin are taken at doses known to cause symptoms in some individuals. Supplements are expensive and because he is taking supplements, Miquel may pay less attention to his food choices. If Miquel's diet is deficient in any of these nutrients, he could benefit from taking a supplement in the amount of the RDA. There are potential benefits to increasing one's intake of the antioxidant nutrients vitamin C, vitamin E, and β-carotene, since high intakes of these have been associated with a reduction in the risk of certain chronic diseases. This reduction in disease risk, however, is better accomplished by consuming a diet rich in foods high in antioxidant nutrients because they are also high in health-promoting substances such as phytochemicals.

CHAPTER 10: CRITICAL THINKING: HOW TO INCREASE YOUR CALCIUM INTAKE

What changes could Laura make at breakfast to increase her calcium intake? She might consider baking muffins that contain nonfat dry milk. These could be made on weekends and frozen for a quick breakfast during the work week. She could use calcium-fortified orange juice.

What choices could Laura make to increase her calcium intake at lunch? She could have milk rather than soda as a beverage at lunch. The cola doesn't contain calcium and does contain a type of phosphorus that may speed the loss of calcium from bone. Instead of grabbing a donut for a snack, she could bring a carton of yogurt from home, and she could have milk or hot chocolate instead of tea.

How do the changes in Laura's dinner and snacks increase her calcium intake? At dinner she has selected vegetables that are richer sources of calcium, such as broccoli. She has eliminated the tea, which contains tannins that inhibit calcium absorption, and included milk, an excellent source of calcium and vitamin D. Since the type of phosphorus in the cola she drinks with her snack may have an adverse effect on calcium status, she has switched to lemon-lime soda. Fruit juice, ginger ale, and orange soda are other choices that contain almost no phosphorus.

These changes increase Laura's calcium intake to meet the RDA. How could she meet her needs if she were lactose intolerant? She could include salmon and other fish consumed with bones to increase her calcium—this would add about 180 mg of calcium. She would need to consume more vegetables that are high in calcium; 2 servings would provide about 100 mg of calcium. If she were lactose intolerant, she could not drink milk, but she may be able to tolerate small amounts of yogurt and cheeses; these could add several hundred milligrams of calcium. Another option would be calcium-fortified orange juice or calcium supplements.

CHAPTER 11: CRITICAL THINKING: IS THIS TRACE ELEMENT ESSENTIAL?

Can these results be used to establish essentiality for humans? No. They give a range of intakes at which no symptoms of deficiency or toxicity appear but do not indicate that the nutrient is essential. They have not shown that eliminating this substance from the human diet causes deficiency symptoms that can be eliminated by adding it back into the diet.

CHAPTER 11: CRITICAL THINKING: INCREASING IRON INTAKE

What dietary factors could contribute to poor iron status? Her iron intake is marginal at 12.7 mg per day compared with the RDA of 15 mg. The iron in her diet comes from plant sources that contain only nonheme iron, which is often poorly absorbed. She drinks tea, which is high in tannins, which inhibit iron absorption. The diet is low in vitamin C–rich foods, which enhance iron absorption when consumed with iron-rich foods.

What modifications could Odelia make to increase the iron content and iron bioavailability of her dinner? Beans are a good vegetarian source of iron. She could add beans to her rice. The iron content would be further increased by using iron cookware. If the food is acidic due to the addition of tomatoes or lime juice, the iron leaches more readily from the cookware. Her apple juice at dinner could be replaced with a drink that is high in vitamin C, such as grapefruit juice, which will enhance nonheme iron absorption. Tea, which contains tannins that inhibit iron absorption, could be consumed later in the evening.

CHAPTER 12: CRITICAL THINKING: INCORPORATING EXERCISE INTO YOUR LIFE

If Nicole's food intake does not increase, how long will it take for her to lose 5 pounds? One pound of body fat is equal to 3500 kcalories, so the extra 777 kcalories expended weekly is equal to about ¼ pound per week, or 1 pound every four weeks. It would therefore take her 20 weeks to lose 5 pounds. However, by increasing her exercise level Nicole may feel more energetic and as a result further increase her energy expenditure by playing more with the children and being more active over the weekends, allowing her to lose the weight more rapidly.

M

CHAPTER 12: CRITICAL THINKING: ANALYZING AN ATHLETE'S DIET

What changes would you recommend in Hector's macronutrient intake?
CARBOHYDRATE: Hector's carbohydrate intake should be increased to about 60% of energy; this will replenish the glycogen he uses up in his daily training. The added carbohydrate should come mostly from complex carbohydrates in whole grains and vegetables and naturally occurring simple sugars in fruits and milk.
FAT: His fat intake should be reduced to the recommended 30% of energy. Many of the foods he eats, such as potato chips, croissants, and pasta with cream sauce, are foods that look like good sources of carbohydrate but that also contribute a great deal of fat.
PROTEIN: His protein intake does not need to change. It is well above the RDA of 58 to 59 g per day for an adolescent male, but within the range of typical intakes in the American diet.
FIBER: His fiber intake should be increased to between 34 and 44 grams per day to meet the recommendation of 10 to 13 grams per 1000 kcalories. This can be done by adding more fresh fruits and vegetables and whole grains to his diet.

What foods could Hector change to meet these recommendations? Instead of croissants he could have pancakes, cereal, or bagels. Instead of pasta with cream sauce he could have pasta with marinara sauce or rice with stir-fried vegetables. Instead of a breaded chicken patty he could have a plain hamburger, a broiled chicken patty, or a turkey sandwich. Instead of ice cream he could have frozen yogurt, sorbet, or fresh fruit.

What are the potential risks and benefits of Hector taking the amino acid supplements and bee pollen? There is no evidence that either bee pollen or ornithine and arginine will enhance athletic performance, so they offer no benefits. Supplements of individual amino acids may inhibit the absorption of other amino acids, leading to an imbalance or a deficiency inside the body. Bee pollen can cause allergic reactions in some individuals.

CHAPTER 13: CRITICAL THINKING: MEETING THE NUTRIENT NEEDS OF PREGNANCY

Suggest some nutrient-dense snacks that would provide these. Yogurt, crackers and cheese, a hard-boiled egg, a glass of milk, a chicken leg, half a tuna or turkey sandwich.

Suggest some other sources of calcium Chevon could add to her diet. Tofu, leafy greens, sardines, canned salmon, or other fish with bones.

What foods might she choose to increase her iron intake or iron absorption? The most absorbable form of iron, heme iron, is found in animal products and is most plentiful in red meat. Although chicken and tuna contain iron, beef, which contains about twice as much, may be a better choice. Chevon should also check to make sure the hot cereal she eats at breakfast is iron fortified. She could add raisins to her cereal to further increase iron intake. She already consumes orange juice at breakfast, which will enhance nonheme iron absorption. Legumes are also a good source of iron, so adding kidney beans to her salad will increase intake.

If she breast feeds the baby, how should her intake change when she is lactating? She will need to increase her intake by about 200 kcalories above her intake for pregnancy. Some of the extra energy should come from a calcium-rich food.

CHAPTER 13: CRITICAL THINKING: HOW TO NOURISH A NEW BABY

Why should Grandma wait until Henry is four to six months old before feeding him solid food? Henry does not need solids at this age, and his gastrointestinal tract is not ready to digest them. Also, he is at risk of developing food allergies depending on her food choices.

CHAPTER 14: CRITICAL THINKING: NOURISHING A PRESCHOOLER

Suggest some foods high in iron that a four-year-old might eat. Hamburger, taco, chicken drumstick, enriched cereals, pizza, raisins.

List some foods containing wheat that Jesse must avoid. Breakfast cereals with wheat, bread, flour tortillas, cookies, cakes.

Suggest some new breakfasts Jesse can try. Cereal and milk, eggs and toast.

CHAPTER 14: CRITICAL THINKING: MEETING TEEN NEEDS

How could she modify her original diet to reduce her energy intake, provide the essential nutrients she needs, and still fit her busy schedule? She could go back to her original breakfast of cereal with milk, juice and toast with margarine. It is fairly low in energy and high in other nutrients. She could have a plain hamburger for lunch with an apple and a glass of milk but replace the chips with some carrot sticks. She could replace the pizza and cola at the mall with some low fat or nonfat frozen yogurt. At dinner she could still have a ham and cheese sandwich if she has a salad instead of potato chips.

CHAPTER 15: CRITICAL THINKING: CAN YOUR DIET KEEP YOU YOUNG?

Why is Marilyn told not to take fish oil supplements? She should avoid fish oil supplements because they inhibit the activity of vitamin K in blood clotting and so could enhance the effect of her anticoagulant Coumadin.

Can Bob and Marilyn meet their protein needs with a vegetarian diet? Yes. Vegetarian diets can provide plenty of protein. Bob and Marilyn have eliminated only meat, so they can still get high-quality protein from eggs and dairy products. If protein complementation is used, even a vegan diet will contain enough protein.

M

What micronutrients are at risk in the diets of the elderly and vegetarians? Iron and zinc are nutrients that are at risk in the elderly and in vegetarians who eliminate only meat. In the diets of vegans and the elderly, vitamin B_{12}, calcium, and vitamin D are at risk for deficiency.

CHAPTER 15: CRITICAL THINKING: DIETARY MODIFICATIONS TO MEET THE NEEDS OF THE ELDERLY

How would Shirley benefit from Meals on Wheels? This program would provide Shirley with one well-balanced meal per day. This provides nutrients and reduces the amount of cooking and shopping she needs to do for herself.

CHAPTER 16: CRITICAL THINKING: ARE THESE CHOICES SAFE?

How might raw vegetables and fruit salad become contaminated? Since the fruits and vegetables will not be cooked, bacteria that come in contact directly or via cross-contamination will not be destroyed by cooking. Both fruits and vegetables might become contaminated with fecal material in the field or during transport. If this is not washed off, it could be spread to the interior of the fruits and vegetables during cutting, and if the fruits and vegetables are left at room temperature, the bacteria will grow. These items may also become contaminated if cutting boards, knives, or other utensils used to prepare raw meats were used to cut the fruits and vegetables without washing.

After the party is over, what foods would you consider safe to keep as leftovers and what would you throw out? The fruit, raw vegetables, crackers and cheese, chips, and cookies would be the safest to keep. The cooked items that were left at room temperature for hours should be discarded. The dip that has been sitting at room temperature and dipped into by many people should be discarded.

CHAPTER 16: CRITICAL THINKING: INDIVIDUAL RISK-BENEFIT ANALYSIS

What other changes can he make that will minimize the risks associated with his family's typical diet while including foods that are beneficial? He can advise his son that he doesn't need the protein shakes but that if he wants to drink them he should use nonfat dry milk instead of raw eggs. He can

have his daughter wait for cookies to bake before tasting them. To decrease the risks associated with eating fish, he can try a wider variety of fresh and saltwater fish rather than only eating swordfish and salmon. Since the risks of eating raw fish are greater, he can limit sushi to a rare treat purchased only from a restaurant that he knows buys its fish daily and has well-trained chefs. The pesticide risks from produce are small compared with the benefits of a diet high in fruits and vegetables. To reduce the amounts of pesticides, he can buy only organic produce but must consider that it is more expensive. He can also buy more locally grown produce and keep up his summer vegetable garden.

CHAPTER 17: CRITICAL THINKING: HOW TO FEED A FAMILY ON $150 PER MONTH

What other changes could they make to reduce food costs? Commercial baby food is convenient and safe, but by pureeing portions of foods served to the rest of the family they could save about 80¢ a day; they could buy store brands rather than the more expensive brand-name products. They could buy bulk items rather than individual packages; this would reduce costs and waste from packaging.

CHAPTER 17: CRITICAL THINKING: WHAT CAN YOU DO?

What impact will the following changes Keesha makes have on the environment? Bringing her beverage in a reusable container will reduce the amount of waste she disposes of at school; composting reduces the amount of garbage sent to the dump; buying organic and locally grown produce supports the efforts of others to reduce the amount of pesticide used in growing and distributing food.

Suggest some other changes Keesha could make to reduce her impact on the environment? Keesha could buy a timer for her household thermostat and water heater. This will reduce energy usage in her home because it will allow the thermostat and water heater to be turned down during the hours when no one is home. Keesha could modify her diet to consume smaller portions of animal products. This will save energy because animal products use more energy to produce than plant products. Keesha could select range-fed beef or chicken rather than feedlot beef. This may cost more but is more environmentally sound because range-fed animals are not fed grain grown on fertile lands and they cause less pollution.

M

Absorption The process of taking substances into the interior of the body.

Accidental contaminants Substances that enter the food supply unexpectedly and are therefore not regulated as additives by the FDA.

Accutane A drug that is used orally to treat severe acne. It is derivative of vitamin A.

Acesulfame K An artificial sweetener that contains no energy and is 200 times as sweet as sugar.

Acetyl-CoA A common intermediate produced from the metabolism of carbohydrate, fat, and protein.

Acetylcholine A neurotransmitter in the brain.

Acid A substance that releases hydrogen ions (H^+) in solution.

Active transport The movement of a molecule across a cell membrane with the aid of a carrier molecule and the expenditure of energy; may occur against a concentration gradient.

Acute Effects that develop rapidly.

Adaptive thermogenesis The change in energy expenditure induced by changes in factors like ambient temperature, food intake, and emotional stress.

Adipocytes Fat-storing cells.

Adipose tissue Fat-storing tissue found under the skin and around body organs; composed of adipocytes.

Adolescent growth spurt The period of peak adolescent growth that begins at about ages 10 to 13 in girls and 12 to 15 in boys.

Adrenaline A hormone secreted by the adrenal gland in response to stress that causes changes, such as an increase in heart rate, in preparation for "fight or flight"; also called epinephrine.

Aerobic exercise Exercise such as jogging, swimming, or cycling that increases heart rate and requires oxygen in metabolism. This type of exercise improves cardiovascular fitness.

Aerobic metabolism Metabolism requiring oxygen; pyruvate is converted to acetyl-CoA, and the citric acid cycle and the electron transport chain are used to completely oxidize glucose to carbon dioxide and water and produce ATP.

Aflatoxin An extremely potent carcinogen that is produced by a mold that grows on peanuts, corn, and other grains.

Agar A polysaccharide extract of seaweed that is used in foods as an emulsifier, stabilizer, and gel.

AIDS (acquired immune deficiency syndrome) The syndrome caused by HIV infection that causes the immune system to fail, resulting in frequent recurrent infections that ultimately result in death.

Alcohol An energy-containing molecule contains 7 kcalories per gram and is made by the fermentation of carbohydrates from plant products; it is called ethanol.

Alcoholic hepatitis Inflammation of the liver caused by alcohol consumption.

Aldosterone A hormone that increases sodium reabsorption by the kidney and therefore enhances water reabsorption.

Alginate A polysaccharide extract of brown algae used in the processing of food, primarily dairy products.

Alimentary canal A hollow tube that includes the mouth, pharynx, esophagus, stomach, small intestine, large intestine, rectum, and anus; also called the gastrointestinal tract and digestive tract.

Allergen A foreign protein that stimulates an immune response.

Allergy A hypersensitive state resulting from exposure to a specific allergen; e.g., food allergy.

Alpha-linolenic acid An omega-3 fatty acid known to be essential in humans.

Alpha-tocopherol The most common and most active chemical form of vitamin E.

Alpha-Tocopherol equivalent (α-TE) The unit of measure used to express the requirements for vitamin E; equal to 1 mg of alpha-tocopherol.

Alzheimer's disease A disease characterized by progressive and irreversible loss of mental function.

Amenorrhea The absence of menstruation.

Amino acid A compound that contains a nitrogen-containing amino group and an acid group, the building block of proteins.

Amino acid pool All of the amino acids in the body that are available for protein synthesis.

Amniotic fluid The liquid in the amniotic sac that surrounds and protects the embryo and fetus during development.

Amniotic sac A fluid-filled sac surrounding the fetus that contains the amniotic fluid.

Amylopectin A plant starch that is composed of long branched chains of glucose molecules.

Amylose A plant starch that is composed of long unbranched chains of glucose molecules.

Anabolic steroid A synthetic fat soluble hormone used by athletes to increase muscle mass.

Anabolic Refers to the process by which small precursors are used to synthesize larger molecules

Anaerobic metabolism or **anaerobic glycolysis** Metabolism in the absence of oxygen. Glucose is broken down, producing 2 molecules of ATP.

Anecdotal Based on a story of personal experience, not experimental results.

Anemia A condition in which there is a reduced number of red blood cells or a reduced amount of hemoglobin.

Angiotensin II A compound found in the blood that stimulates the release of the hormone aldosterone and causes blood vessel walls to constrict.

Anisakis disease A disease caused by infection of the gastrointestinal tract with an *Anisakis* roundworm that contaminates raw fish.

Anorexia nervosa An eating disorder characterized by self-starvation, a distorted body image, and low body weight.

Antacid A drug used to neutralize acidity in the gastrointestinal tract.

Anthropometric measurement An external measurement of the body, such as height, weight, limb circumference, and skinfold thickness.

Antibiotic A substance that inhibits the growth of or destroys microorganisms; used to treat or prevent infection.

Antibody A protein produced by the immune system that destroys or inactivates foreign substances in the body.

Anticaking agent A substance added to food to prevent clumping of dry products.

Anticarcinogen A compound that can counteract the effect of cancer-causing substances.

Anticoagulant A substance that delays or prevents blood clotting.

Antidiuretic hormone (ADH) A hormone secreted by the pituitary that increases the amount of water reabsorbed by the kidneys.

Antioxidant A compound that prevents oxidative damage by donating electrons to the reactive electron-seeking compounds to inactivate them.

Anus The lower opening of the digestive tract through which the feces leave the body.

Apolipoprotein B A protein embedded in the outer shell of low-density lipoprotein (LDL) particles that binds to LDL receptor proteins on body cells.

Appetite The nonphysiological factors that signal the selection and consumption of specific foods.

Arachidonic acid An omega-6 fatty acid that can be synthesized from linoleic acid.

Arginine A nonessential amino acid found in protein.

Ariboflavinosis Riboflavin deficiency.

Arteriole A small artery that carries blood to capillaries.

Artery A blood vessel that carries blood away from the heart.

Arthritis A disease characterized by inflammation of the joints, pain, and sometimes changes in structure.

Artificial sweetener A chemically manufactured sweetener that differs from simple sugars in chemical structure and often provides little or no energy when ingested.

Ascorbic acid Vitamin C.

Aseptic processing A method that simultaneously sterilizes the food and its container during packaging.

Asparagine A nonessential amino acid found in protein.

Aspartame An artificial sweetener composed of the amino acids phenylalanine and aspartic acid.

Aspartic acid A nonessential amino acid found in protein.

Asthma A respiratory disorder characterized by wheezing and difficulty in breathing.

Atherosclerosis A type of cardiovascular disease characterized by a buildup of fatty material in the artery walls.

Atom The smallest unit of an element that still retains the properties of that element.

ATP (adenosine triphosphate) The high-energy molecule used by the body to perform energy-requiring activities.

Attention deficit hyperactive disorder A condition in children that is characterized by a high level of activity, excitability, and distractibility.

Autoimmune disease A disease that results from immune reactions that damage normal body cells.

Avidin A protein found in raw egg whites that binds biotin, preventing its absorption.

Bacteria (bacterium, singular) Tiny single-celled organisms found throughout the environment. Most are harmless or beneficial, but a few types can cause disease in humans.

Balance study A study that compares the total amount of a nutrient that enters the body with the total amount that leaves the body.

Basal metabolic rate (BMR) A measure of the minimum amount of energy that an awake but resting body needs to maintain itself.

Base A substance that accepts hydrogen ions in solution.

Bee pollen A mixture of pollen, bee saliva, and plant nectar that collects on the legs of bees; sold as an ergogenic aid.

Behavior modification A process that is used to gradually and permanently change habitual behaviors.

Benzocaine A local anesthetic used in some weight-loss products.

Beriberi A thiamin deficiency disease that is characterized by muscle weakness, loss of appetite, and nerve degeneration.

Beta-carotene (β-carotene) A pigment found in many yellow and red-orange fruits and vegetables that acts as an antioxidant in the body and is a precursor of vitamin A.

Bile A substance made in the liver and stored in the gallbladder; it is released into the small intestine to aid in fat digestion and absorption.

Bile acid An emulsifier present in bile that is synthesized by the liver and released by the gallbladder to aid in fat digestion.

Bingeing The rapid consumption of a large amount of food in a discrete period of time associated with a feeling that eating is out of control.

Bioavailability Refers to how well a nutrient can be absorbed and used by the body.

Bioelectric impedance analysis A method of assessing body composition that measures body water by directing current through the body and calculating resistance to flow.

Bioflavonoids Substances including rutin and hesperidin that are collectively referred to as vitamin P; not truly vitamins and no requirement for them has been identified in humans.

Biological value A measure of protein quality determined by comparing the amount of nitrogen retained in the body with the amount absorbed from the diet.

Biotechnology A set of techniques used to manipulate DNA for the purpose of changing the characteristics of an organism or creating a new product; also called genetic engineering.

Blood pressure The amount of force exerted by the blood against the artery walls.

Body mass index (BMI) An index of weight in relation to height that is used to compare body size with a standard; it is equal to body weight (in kilograms) divided by height (in meters squared).

Bolus A ball of chewed food mixed with saliva.

Bomb calorimeter An instrument used to determine the energy content of a food; measures the heat energy released when a food is burned.

Bovine somatotropin (bST) A hormone naturally produced by cows that stimulates the production of milk. A synthetic version of this hormone is now being produced by genetic engineering.

Bran The protective outer layers of whole grains that are concentrated sources of dietary fibers.

Brewer's yeast The type of yeast used in brewing beer; a good source of B vitamins and often used as a nutritional supplement.

Brown adipose tissue A type of fat tissue that has a greater number of mitochondria than the more common white adipose tissue; can waste energy by producing heat and is believed to be responsible for some of the change in energy expenditure in adaptive thermogenesis.

Brush border Refers to the microvilli surface of the intestinal mucosa, which contains some digestive enzymes.

Buffer A substance or substances that react with an acid or base by picking up or releasing hydrogen ions to prevent changes in pH.

Bulimia nervosa An eating disorder characterized by the consumption of large amounts of food at one time (bingeing), followed by purging behavior such as vomiting and the use of laxatives to eliminate energy from the body.

Caffeine A bitter white substance found in coffee, tea, chocolate, and other foods; a stimulant and a diuretic.

Calcitonin A hormone produced by the thyroid gland that stimulates bone mineralization and inhibits bone breakdown, thus lowering blood calcium levels.

Calorie The amount of heat required to raise the temperature of 1 g of water 1°C; equal to 4.18 joules.

Calorimetry A technique for measuring energy expenditure.

Campylobactor jejuni A bacterium common in raw milk and undercooked meat that causes food-borne illness.

Cancer A disease characterized by cells that grow and divide without restraint and have the ability to grow in different locations in the body.

Capillary A small, thin-walled blood vessel where the exchange of gases and nutrients between blood and tissues occurs.

Caprenin An artificial fat.

Carbohydrate A compound containing carbon, hydrogen, and oxygen; includes sugars, starches, and most fibers.

Carbohydrate loading A regimen of diet and exercise training designed to maximize muscle glycogen stores before an athletic endurance event.

Carbon dioxide A waste product produced by cellular respiration that is eliminated from the body by the lungs.

Carcinogen A substance that causes cells to multiply out of control, eventually resulting in cancer.

Cardiovascular Refers to the heart and blood vessels.

Cardiovascular disease A disease of the heart and blood vessels.

Caries or dental caries Cavities, or decay of the tooth enamel caused when bacteria growing on the teeth produce acid.

Carnitine A molecule that is needed to transport fatty acids and some amino acids into the mitochondria of cells.

Carotenoids Yellow-orange plant pigments, some of which have provitamin A activity and can therefore be converted into active vitamin A in the body; beta-carotene is the most active.

Carpal tunnel syndrome Numbness, tingling, weakness, and pain in the hand caused by pressure on the nerves.

Carrageenan A seaweed polysaccharide extracted from the algae Irish moss and used as a thickener mainly in dairy products.

Casein The predominant protein in cow's milk.

Cash crop A crop grown to be sold for income rather than for personal consumption.

Cassava A starchy root that is the staple of the diet in many parts of Africa.

Catabolic Refers to the processes by which large molecules are broken into smaller ones.

Catalase An iron-containing enzyme that destroys peroxides.

Cataract A disease of the eye that results in cloudy spots on the lens (and sometimes the cornea), that obscure vision.

Cell The basic structural and functional unit of life.

Cell differentiation Structural and functional changes that cause cells to mature into specialized cells.

Cell membrane The membrane that encloses the cell contents.

Cellular respiration The reactions that break down carbohydrates, fats, and proteins in the presence of oxygen to produce carbon dioxide, water, and energy in the form of ATP.

Cellulite Subcutaneous fat that has a lumpy appearance because strands of connective tissue connect it to underlying structures.

Cellulose An insoluble fiber that is the most prevalent structural material of plant cell walls.

Cephalic phase The phase of gastric secretion that is stimulated by the sight, smell, and taste of food.

Certified food coloring A food color that has been tested and certified for safety, quality, consistency, and strength of color.

Ceruloplasmin A copper-containing protein found in the blood that converts ferrous iron to the ferric form that can bind to iron-transport proteins.

Cesarean section The surgical removal of the fetus from the uterus.

Chemical bond The attractive force that links two atoms together.

Chemical score A measure of protein quality determined by comparing the amount of the most limiting amino acid in a food with that in a reference protein.

Chinese restaurant syndrome Symptoms of headache, flushing, tingling, burning sensations, and chest pain reported by some individuals after consuming MSG.

Choice grade   A USDA grade of beef with a modest amount of marbled fat.

Cholecalciferol   A form of vitamin D found in foods of animal origin; vitamin D_3.

Cholecystokinin (CCK)   A hormone that stimulates the release of enzymes from the pancreas and bile from the gallbladder.

Cholesterol   A lipid consisting of multiple chemical rings that is made only by animal cells.

Choline   A component of lecithin.

Cholic acid   A bile acid.

Chromium picolinate   A form of chromium sold as a supplement promoted to change body composition. Chromium is involved in insulin action, and supplements claim to increase lean body mass, decrease body fat, and delay fatigue. There is little evidence for their effectiveness as an ergogenic aid.

Chronic   Effects that develop slowly over a long period.

Chylomicron   A microscopic particle of dietary fat surrounded by a shell of cholesterol, phospholipids, and protein; made in the intestinal mucosal cells, it carries absorbed dietary fat into the bloodstream through the lymphatic system.

Chyme   A mixture of partially digested food and stomach secretions.

Chymotrypsin   A protein-digesting enzyme produced in an inactive form in the pancreas and activated in the small intestine, where it aids digestion.

Circulatory system   Organ system consisting of the heart, blood, and blood vessels; transports material to and from cells.

Cirrhosis   A chronic liver disease characterized by the loss of functioning liver cells and the accumulation of fibrous connective tissue.

Citric acid cycle   The stage of respiration in which acetyl-CoA is broken down into carbon dioxide and the resulting electrons are shunted to the next stage of respiration, in which ATP is produced; also called the Krebs cycle, tricarboxylic acid cycle, or TCA cycle.

Clones   Copies, often used to refer to identical copies of a gene of interest.

Clostridium botulinum   A bacterium that produces a deadly toxin and grows in a low-acid, low-oxygen environment, such as inside certain canned goods.

Clostridium perfringens   A bacterium found in meat and poultry that can cause food-borne illness.

Coagulation   Blood clotting.

Cobalamin   Vitamin B_{12}.

Coenzyme   A small organic molecule that acts as a carrier of electrons or atoms in metabolic reactions and is necessary for the proper functioning of an enzyme.

Cofactor   An inorganic ion or coenzyme required for enzyme activity.

Colic   Inconsolable crying in an infant that is believed to be due to pain from gas buildup in the gastrointestinal tract.

Collagen   A fibrous protein found in connective tissue including skin, bones, ligaments, and cartilage.

Colon   A portion of the large intestine.

Colostrum   The first milk, which is secreted in late pregnancy and up to a week after birth. It is rich in protein and immune factors.

Complete protein   A protein that provides all of the amino acids in the proper proportions required for protein synthesis.

Complex carbohydrates   Carbohydrates composed of sugar molecules linked together in straight or branching chains.

Compression of morbidity   The postponement of the onset of chronic disease such that disability occupies a smaller and smaller proportion of the lifespan.

Concentration gradient   A condition that exists when the amount of a dissolved substance is greater in one area than it is in another.

Conception   The union of sperm and egg that results in pregnancy.

Condensation reaction   A type of chemical reaction in which 2 molecules are joined to form a larger molecule and water is released.

Conditionally essential amino acid   An amino acid that is essential in the diet only if its precursor amino acid is in short supply.

Connective tissue   One of the four human tissue types; includes cartilage, bone, blood, adipose tissue, and the coverings of some organs.

Constipation   Infrequent or difficult defecation.

Control group   A group of experimental subjects that are identical to the experimental group except that no experimental treatment is undergone; used as a basis of comparison.

Coronary heart disease   A disease of the heart and blood vessels that supply blood to the heart.

Cornea   The clear, transparent fibrous outer coat of the eye.

Correlated   Two or more factors occurring together.

Covalent bond   A type of chemical bond formed when two atoms share a pair of electrons.

Creatine phosphate   A high-energy compound found in muscle that can be rapidly broken down to make ATP.

Cretinism   A condition resulting from poor maternal iodine intake during prenancy that causes stunted growth and poor mental development in the offspring.

Critical period   A time in growth and development when an organism is changing rapidly and is therefore more susceptible to harm from poor nutrition or other environmental factors.

Cross-contamination   The transfer of contaminants from one area to another.

Cross-sectional data   Information obtained by a single broad sampling of many different individuals in a population.

Crude fiber   The fiber that remains after a food has been treated with acid and base; consists primarily of cellulose and lignin.

Cyclamate   An artificial sweetener that was common in the United States in the 1960s; banned after it was found to cause cancer in laboratory animals.

Cycle of malnutrition   A cycle in which poorly nourished women give birth to low birth weight babies who are susceptible to infections that further increase their nutrient needs; the children grow into adults who cannot produce healthy offspring or contribute to a strong work force.

Cysteine   A sulfur-containing amino acid; when methionine is available in sufficient quantities, cysteine is not essential in the diet.

Cystic acne   A chronic inflammatory disease of the skin in which cysts and nodules are common and scarring may occur.

Cytoplasm   The cellular material outside the nucleus that is contained by the cell membrane.

Daily Reference Values (DRVs) A reference value established for protein and seven nutrients for which no RDA has been established. The values are based on dietary recommendations for reducing the risk of chronic disease.

Daily Value A nutrient reference value that is used on food labels to help consumers see how a food fits into the overall diet.

Deamination The removal of the amino group from an amino acid.

Dehydration A condition that results when the output of water exceeds water input, due to either low water intake or excessive loss.

Delaney Clause A clause added to the 1958 Food Additives Amendment of the Pure Food and Drug Act that prohibits the intentional addition to foods of any compound that has been shown to cause cancer in animals or humans at any dose.

Dermatitis An inflammation of the skin.

Dementia A deterioration of mental state resulting in impaired memory, thinking, and/or judgment.

Denaturation The alteration of a protein's three-dimensional structure due to a physical, chemical, or thermal process.

Dental caries The decay and disintegration of a tooth caused by acid produced by bacteria on the teeth in the presence of carbohydrate.

Deoxyribose The 5-carbon sugar that is part of DNA.

Depletion-repletion study An experiment done to determine the requirement for essential nutrients; subjects are fed a diet devoid of an essential nutrient until signs of deficiency appear, and then the nutrient is added back to the diet to a level at which deficiency symptoms disappear.

Diabetes mellitus A disorder resulting from either insufficient insulin production or decreased sensitivity of target cells to insulin; results in elevated blood glucose levels.

Diacylglycerol or **diglyceride** A molecule of glycerol with 2 fatty acids attached.

Diaphragm A muscular wall separating the abdomen from the thoracic cavity containing the heart and lungs.

Diarrhea An intestinal disorder characterized by frequent or fluid stools.

Dicumarol An anticoagulant that was isolated from moldy clover.

Diet history A dietary intake assessment method that collects information about dietary habits and patterns and combines methods such as 24-hour recall, food frequency, and food diary in order to determine an individual's typical food intake.

Diet-induced thermogenesis The increase in energy expenditure due to the digestion, absorption, metabolism, and storage of food; equal to approximately 10% of daily energy intake; also called thermic effect of food.

Dietary fiber The substances in food that are not broken down by the digestive processes in the stomach and small intestine.

Dietary Guidelines for Americans A set of nutrition recommendations designed to promote population-wide dietary changes to reduce the incidence of nutrition-related chronic diseases.

Diffusion The movement of molecules from an area of higher concentration to an area of lower concentration.

Digestion The process of breaking food into substances small enough to be absorbed into the body.

Digestive system The organ system responsible for the ingestion, digestion, and absorption of food and the elimination of food residues; includes the gastrointestinal tract as well as a number of accessory organs.

Digestive tract A hollow tube that includes the mouth, pharynx, esophagus, stomach, small intestine, large intestine, rectum, and anus; also called gastrointestinal tract or alimentary canal.

Diglyceride A molecule composed of a glycerol backbone with 2 fatty acids attached.

Dipeptide Two amino acids linked together by a peptide bond.

Direct calorimetry A method of calculating energy use by measuring the amount of heat produced by the body.

Direct food additives Substances intentionally added to food to alter their form, appearance, shelf life, or nutrient content. The amounts added and the types of food they can be added to are regulated by the FDA.

Disaccharide A sugar composed of 2 monosaccharides.

Dissociate To separate 2 charged ions.

Diuretic A drug that promotes fluid excretion.

Diverticula Sacs or pouches that protrude from the wall of the large intestine in the disease diverticulosis; when it becomes inflamed, the condition is called diverticulitis.

DNA (deoxyribonucleic acid) The genetic material that codes for the synthesis of proteins.

Docosahexaenoic acid (DHA) An omega-3 fatty acid found in fish that may be needed in the diet of newborns.

Dolomite A calcium supplement composed of ground-up limestone.

Double-blind study An experiment in which neither the study participants nor the researchers know who is in the control or experimental group.

Down syndrome A disorder caused by extra genetic material that results in distinctive physical characteristics and mental retardation.

Duodenum The first segment of the small intestine that connects to the stomach.

Eating disorder A psychological disorder affecting the regulation of food intake or energy balance.

Edema Swelling due to an accumulation of fluid in the tissues.

Eicosanoid A hormone-like compound that is made from polyunsaturated fatty acids such as arachidonic acid and eicosapentaenoic acid.

Eicosapentaenoic acid (ERA) An omega-3 fatty acid found in fish; can be synthesized from alpha-linolenic acid but may be essential in humans under some conditions.

Electrolyte A substance that separates in water to form a positively and a negatively charged ion.

Electron A negatively charged particle that orbits around the nucleus of an atom.

Electron transport chain The final stage of cellular respiration in which ATP and water are formed when electrons are passed down a chain of molecules and eventually given to oxygen.

Element   A substance that cannot be broken down into products with different properties.

Elimination diet   A diet that eliminates potential allergy-causing foods from an allergic individuals diet and then systematically adds them back one at a time.

Embryo   The stage in prenatal development that occurs between the second and eighth weeks of gestation.

Empty kcalories   Refers to foods that contribute energy but few other nutrients.

Emulsifier   A substance that can break fat into tiny droplets and suspend it in a watery fluid.

Endocrine system   Organ system composed of cells, tissues, and organs that secrete hormones to help control body functions.

Endoplasmic reticulum   A cellular organelle composed of a system of membranous tubules, channels, and sacs in the cytoplasm; rough endoplasmic reticulum has ribosomes on its outside surface; involved in the synthesis of proteins and lipids.

Endorphin   A chemical released by the brain during exercise that acts as a natural tranquilizer; may be the cause of the euphoria known as runner's high.

Endosperm   The largest portion of a kernel of grain, primarily starch, that serves as a food supply for the sprouting seed.

Endurance   The length of time one can perform a task.

Energy   The ability to do work.

Energy balance   The principle that the amount of energy consumed in the diet must equal the amount expended by the body in order to maintain a stable weight.

Enrichment   The addition of nutrients that are already present in a food to levels that meet specific government standards.

Environmental Protection Agency (EPA)   U.S. government agency responsible for determining acceptable levels of environmental contaminants in the food supply and for establishing water quality standards.

Enzyme   A substance that accelerates the rate of a specific chemical reaction within the body without being changed itself.

Epidemiology   The study of the interrelationships between health and disease rates and other factors in the environment or lifestyle of different populations.

Epiglottis   A flap of cartilage that serves as a valve during swallowing to prevent food from passing into the lung passages.

Epinephrine   A hormone secreted by the adrenal gland in response to stress that causes changes, such as an increase in heart rate, in preparation for "fight or flight"; also called adrenaline.

Epithelial tissue   One of the four human tissue types; includes the cells that form all coverings and linings of the body.

Ergogenic aid   A substance that enhances work or exercise performance.

Ergot   A toxin produced by a mold that grows on grains, particularly rye.

Esophagus   A portion of the gastrointestinal tract between the pharynx and the stomach.

Essential amino acid   An amino acid that cannot be synthesized by the human body in sufficient amounts to meet needs and therefore must be included in the diet.

Essential fatty acid   A fatty acid that must be present in the diet to maintain health because it cannot be synthesized by the human body in sufficient amounts to meet needs; includes linoleic, arachidonic, and alpha-linolenic acids.

Essential fatty acid deficiency   The condition that results when the diet does not supply sufficient amounts of the essential fatty acids.

Essential hypertension   High blood pressure that has no obvious external cause.

Essential nutrient   A nutrient that must be provided in the diet because the body either cannot make it or cannot make it in sufficient quantities to satisfy its needs.

Estimated Safe and Adequate Daily Dietary Intakes (ESADDIs)   Intakes of essential nutrients recommended when data are sufficient to estimate a range of requirements, but insufficient to develop an RDA.

Estrogen   A steroid hormone secreted by the ovaries and by the placenta that is involved in the maintenance of pregnancy and the maintenance and development of female sex organs and secondary sex characteristics.

Exchange list   A grouping of foods based on their carbohydrate, protein, fat, and energy content.

Excretory system   Organ system involved in the elimination of metabolic waste products; includes the lungs, skin, and kidneys.

Experimental controls   Factors included in an experimental design that limit the number of variables, allowing an investigator to examine the effect of only the parameters of interest.

Experimental groups or **treatment groups**   Groups of participants in an experiment who are subjected to an experimental treatment.

Extracellular fluid   The fluid located outside cells; includes fluid found in the blood, lymph, gastrointestinal tract, spinal column, eyes, joints, and tears and between cells and tissues.

Facilitated diffusion   The movement of substances across a cell membrane from an area of greater concentration to an area of lower concentration with the aid of a carrier molecule; no energy is required.

Fad bulimia   A type of bulimia that is more a trend than a psychological disorder; binge episodes are typically less dramatic and emotional than those of a true bulimic; common among teenagers and young adults who are concerned about a few extra pounds of body weight.

Failure to thrive   The inability of a child's growth to keep up with normal growth curves.

Fallopian tubes (oviducts)   Narrow ducts through which the egg travels from the ovaries to the uterus.

Famine   A widespread lack of access to food due to a disaster that causes a collapse in the food production and marketing systems.

Fasting hypoglycemia   Low blood sugar that is not related to food intake; often caused by an insulin-secreting tumor.

Fat   A lipid that is solid at room temperature; commonly used to refer to all lipids or specifically to triglycerides.

Fat soluble vitamin A vitamin that does not dissolve in water; includes vitamins A, D, E, and K.

Fat-free mass Body mass composed of all tissue except for adipose tissue.

Fatigue The inability to continue an activity at an optimal level.

Fatty acid A component of lipids that is composed of a chain of carbons linked to hydrogens with an acid group at one end.

Fatty liver The accumulation of fat in the liver.

Fatty streak A cholesterol deposit in the artery wall.

Feces Body waste, such as unabsorbed food residue, bacteria, and mucus, that is excreted from the gastrointestinal tract by way of the anus.

Fermentation A process in which microorganisms metabolize components of a food and therefore change its composition, taste, and storage properties.

Ferritin The major protein involved in iron storage.

Fertilization The union of sperm and egg to form the single cell from which an embryo develops.

Fetal alcohol effects (FAE) Also called alcohol-related birth defects (ARBD) and refers to mild symptoms such as learning disabilities, behavioral abnormalities, and motor impairments seen in the infant whose mother consumed alcohol during pregnancy.

Fetal alcohol syndrome (FAS) A characteristic group of physical and mental abnormalities that results when alcohol is consumed by the mother during pregnancy.

Fetus The developing human from the ninth week to birth.

Fiber *See* Crude fiber and Dietary fiber.

Fitness The ability to perform routine physical activity without undue fatigue.

Flexibility Range of motion.

Fluoroapatite A fluoride-containing mineral deposit in the tooth enamel that is resistant to acid.

Foam cell A cholesterol-filled white blood cell.

Food additive A substance that can reasonably be expected to become a component of a food during processing. The foods that may contain it

and the amount that may be present are regulated by the FDA.

Food and Drug Administration (FDA) U.S. government agency responsible for the safety and wholesomeness of all food except red meat, poultry, and eggs; also sets standards and enforces regulations for food labeling and for food and color additives.

Food-borne illness An illness that can be transmitted to humans through food.

Food-borne infection An illness produced by the ingestion of food containing microorganisms that can multiply inside the body and produce effects that are injurious.

Food-borne intoxication An illness produced from a food that contains a toxin.

Food diary Dietary intake assessment method in which the individual is asked to keep a record of all food and beverage consumed for a defined period.

Food disappearance study A method of determining the food use by a population in which the amount of food that leaves the marketplace is assumed to equal the amount of food used by the population.

Food frequency A dietary intake assessment method in which an interviewer obtains information about an individual's typical food consumption patterns.

Food Guide Pyramid A system of food groups developed by the USDA as a guide to the number of servings of different types of foods needed to provide an adequate diet and comply with current nutrition recommendations.

Food insecurity An inability to acquire a reliable food supply or appropriate foods in a socially acceptable way.

Food intolerance An adverse reaction to a food that does not involve the immune system.

Food jag A temporary food fixation during which a child will eat only certain foods.

Food processing Any alteration of food from the way it is found in nature.

Food self-sufficiency The ability of an area to produce enough food to feed its population.

Food shortage Insufficient food to feed a population.

Fortification The addition of nutrients to a food during processing.

Frame size An estimation of the proportion of body weight due to bone.

Free radical A highly reactive compound that seeks to steal electrons from other molecules such as DNA or unsaturated fatty acids.

Fructose A monosaccharide found in fruits and honey that is composed of 6 carbon atoms arranged in a ring structure; commonly called fruit sugar.

Galactose A monosaccharide composed of 6 carbon atoms arranged in a ring structure; when combined with glucose, it forms the disaccharide lactose.

Gallbladder An organ of the digestive system that stores bile produced by the liver.

Gastric juice A substance produced by the gastric glands of the stomach that contains pepsinogen and hydrochloric acid.

Gastric phase The phase of gastric secretion triggered by the entry of food into the stomach; involves the release of gastrin and the secretion of mucus, acid, and enzymes from the gastric glands.

Gastrin A hormone secreted by the mucosa of the stomach and duodenum that stimulates the secretion of enzymes and acid in the stomach.

Gastrointestinal tract A hollow tube consisting of the mouth, pharynx, esophagus, stomach, small intestine, large intestine, rectum, and anus in which digestion and absorption of nutrients occur; also called the alimentary canal and digestive tract.

Gastroplasty A surgical procedure that staples the lower part of the stomach, decreasing the storage capacity and consequently the amount of food that can be consumed at one time; also called stomach stapling.

Gel A jelly-like suspension of a liquid in a solid system that is semisolid in consistency.

Gelatin A protein derived from collagen that is deficient in the amino acid tryptophan.

Gene A unit of DNA that provides instruction for heritable traits.

Genetic engineering Changing the characteristics of an organism by altering the genetic material, DNA; also called gene splicing, biotechnology, or recombinant DNA.

Genetic hypothesis A hypothesis that proposes that aging is triggered by genes that disrupt cell function.

Genetics Refers to the composition of DNA or the study of inheritance.

Germ The embryo or sprouting portion of a kernel of grain; contains vegetable oil and vitamin E.

Gestation The time between conception and birth; lasts about nine months.

Gestational diabetes A consistently elevated blood glucose level that develops during pregnancy and usually resolves when the pregnancy is completed.

Ginseng An herb used in traditional Chinese medicine; claims are made that it improves athletic performance and increases sexual potency.

Glucagon A hormone produced by the pancreas that stimulates gluconeogenesis and the breakdown of liver glycogen to increase blood glucose.

Gluconeogenesis The synthesis of glucose from simple noncarbohydrate molecules.

Glucose Monosaccharide that is the primary form of carbohydrate in the blood; also called blood sugar.

Glutamic acid A nonessential amino acid that is found in protein and in MSG.

Glutathione peroxidase A selenium-containing enzyme that protects the cell from oxidative damage by degrading reactive chemical species called peroxides.

Glycemic response or **glycemic index** A measure of how quickly blood glucose levels increase after a food or combination of foods is consumed.

Glyceride The most common type of lipid; consists of one, two, or three fatty acids attached to a molecule of glycerol.

Glycerol A 3-carbon molecule that forms the backbone of triglycerides and phosphoglycerides; also used as a humectant in food.

Glycogen A carbohydrate made of many units of glucose linked together in a highly branched structure; the storage form of carbohydrate in animals.

Glycolysis A metabolic pathway in the cytoplasm of the cell that splits glucose into two molecules of pyruvate; the energy released is used to make two molecules of ATP.

Goiter An enlargement of the thyroid gland that is caused by a deficiency of iodine.

Goitrogen Any substance that interferes with the utilization of iodine or the function of the thyroid gland.

GRAS (Generally Recognized as Safe) A group of chemical additives that are generally recognized as safe based on their longstanding presence in the food supply without obvious harmful effects.

Growth hormone A hormone secreted by the pituitary gland that stimulates growth.

Guar gum A branched polysaccharide from guar plants used as an additive to increase the viscosity of food, especially candies.

Gum A plant polysaccharide and its derivatives that can dissolve in water and swell to form viscous solutions.

Gum arabic A branched polysaccharide from acacia trees; it is colorless, odorless, and tasteless, so it is used as an additive to increase the viscosity of food, especially candies.

Gum karaya A branched polysaccharide from trees; used as an additive to increase the viscosity of food, especially salad dressings, cheese spreads, and sherbets.

Gum tragacanth A branched polysaccharide from thorny shrubs that grow in the semidesert of the Near East; used as an additive to thicken foods and to stabilize emulsions.

Health claim A statement made about the relationship between a nutrient or food and a disease or health condition.

Healthy People 2000 A set of national health promotion and disease prevention objectives for the U.S. population developed by a consortium of over 300 national organizations, state health departments, and the Institute of Medicine of the National Academy of Sciences and organized through the U.S. Public Health Service.

Heart attack Condition in which an artery in the heart becomes blocked, cutting off blood flow and hence oxygen and nutrients to a segment of the heart muscle, resulting in tissue death.

Heartburn A burning sensation in the chest caused when acidic stomach contents leak into the esophagus through the gastroesophageal sphincter.

Heat cramp A muscle cramp caused by an imbalance of sodium and potassium as a result of excessive exercise without adequate fluid and electrolyte replacement.

Heat exhaustion Low blood pressure, rapid pulse, fainting, and sweating caused when dehydration decreases blood volume so much that blood can no longer both cool the body and provide oxygen to the muscles.

Heat stroke Elevated body temperature as a result of fluid loss and the failure of the temperature regulatory center of the brain.

Heimlich maneuver A procedure used to dislodge an object blocking an air passage; involves the application of sharp, firm pressure to the abdomen just below the rib cage.

Heme iron A readily absorbed form of iron found in animal products that is chemically associated with proteins such as hemoglobin and myoglobin.

Hemicellulose A insoluble fiber that is a structural component of plant cell walls.

Hemochromatosis A hereditary defect in iron metabolism that is characterized by deposits of iron-containing pigment in tissues leading to tissue damage.

Hemoglobin An iron-containing protein in red blood cells that binds to oxygen and transports it to cells.

Hemolytic anemia When there is an insufficient number of red blood cells because many have burst open.

Hemorrhoid A swelling of a large vein or veins found in the anal or rectal area.

Hemosiderin An insoluble iron-protein compound formed in the liver when the iron storage capacity of ferritin is exceeded.

Hepatic portal circulation The network of blood vessels that collect nutrient-laden blood from the digestive organs and deliver it to the liver.

Hepatic portal vein The blood vessel that delivers nutrient-laden blood from the digestive organs to the liver.

Hepatitis Inflammation of the liver.

Herbicide An agent that kills weeds.

Heterocyclic amine (HA) A class of mutagenic substances produced when there is incomplete combustion of amino acids during the cooking of meats.

High-density lipoprotein (HDL) A lipoprotein particle synthesized primarily by the liver and small intestine that picks up cholesterol so it can be eliminated from the body; low HDL cholesterol increases the risk of cardiovascular disease.

High-fructose corn syrup A sweetener made from corn syrup that is composed of approximately half fructose and half glucose.

Histamine A substance produced by cells of the immune system as part of a nonspecific response that leads to inflammation.

HIV (human immunodeficiency virus) A virus that infects cells of the immune system and eventually leads to AIDS.

Homeostasis The capacity to maintain a balanced internal body environment when conditions change.

Homocysteine A sulfur-containing amino acid that is produced from the metabolism of methionine.

Hormone A chemical messenger that is produced in one location but elicits a response at another.

Hormone sensitive lipase An enzyme present in adipose cells that responds to chemical signals by breaking triglycerides down into free fatty acids and glycerol for release into the bloodstream.

Household consumption survey A study that records the amount of food eaten by individuals in households.

Humectant A substance added to foods to retain moisture.

Hunger Internal signals that stimulate one to acquire and consume food.

Hydrochloric acid An acid secreted by the gastric glands of the stomach to aid in digestion.

Hydrogenation The process whereby hydrogens are added to the carbon double bonds of polyunsaturated and monounsaturated fatty acids, making them more saturated.

Hydrolysis A type of reaction in which a large molecule is broken into 2 smaller molecules by the addition of water.

Hydroxyapatite A compound composed of calcium and phosphorus that is deposited in the protein matrix of bone to give it strength and rigidity.

Hyperactivity Overactive, excitable, distractible behavior that is characteristic of attention deficit hyperactive disorder.

Hypercarotenemia A condition caused by a high dietary intake of carotenoids; high carotenoid levels in the blood and adipose tissue cause the skin to appear yellow.

Hypertension Elevated blood pressure.

Hypoglycemia A low blood glucose level, usually below 40 to 50 mg per 100 ml.

Hypothalamus A portion of the brain that works to maintain homeostasis and influences behaviors such as hunger and thirst.

Hypothermia A condition in which body temperature drops below normal; causes depression of the central nervous system and results in the inability to shiver, sleepiness, and eventually coma.

Hypothesis An educated guess made to explain an observation or answer a question.

Ileocecal valve The structure that separates the ileum of the small intestine from the large intestine.

Ileum The 11-foot segment of the small intestine that connects the jejunum with the large intestine.

Immunization An injection of a killed or inactivated organism into the body to stimulate the immune system to develop antibodies against the active disease-causing organism.

Implantation The process in which the zygote embeds in the uterine lining.

Incomplete protein A protein that is deficient in one or more of the amino acids required for protein synthesis in humans.

Indirect calorimetry A method of estimating energy use by the body that compares the amount of oxygen used with the amount of carbon dioxide produced.

Indirect food additives Substances that are expected to unintentionally enter foods from the environment during manufacture or from packaging. They are regulated as additives by the FDA.

Infant mortality rate The number of deaths during the first year of life per 1000 live births.

Inorganic A substance that contains no carbon atoms.

Inositol A compound that is often included in B vitamin supplements; functions as part of a phospholipid in the human brain but is not a dietary essential. Also called myo-inositol.

Insensible loss Fluid loss that is not perceived by the senses, such as evaporation through the skin and lungs.

Insoluble fiber Fiber that, for the most part, does not dissolve in water; includes cellulose, hemicellulose, and lignin.

Insulin A hormone produced by the pancreas that stimulates the uptake of glucose by body cells and stimulates the synthesis of glycogen and other macromolecules.

Insulin-dependent diabetes A disease characterized by elevated blood glucose resulting when insufficient insulin is produced by the pancreas; commonly develops during childhood; also called Type I diabetes and juvenile onset diabetes.

Integrated pest management (IPM) A method of agricultural pest control that combines nonchemical and chemical techniques.

Intermediate-density lipoprotein (IDL) A lipoprotein produced by the removal of triglycerides from VLDLs, most of which are then transformed to LDLs.

International unit (IU) A unit of measure used to express vitamin requirements.

Interstitial fluid The portion of the extracellular fluid that is located in the spaces between cells and tissues.

Interstitial space The fluid-filled spaces between cells.

Intestinal microflora The bacteria and other microorganisms that inhabit the human large intestine.

Intestinal phase   The phase of gastric secretion that is begun by the entry of food into the large intestine.

Intracellular fluid   The fluid contained inside cells.

Intrinsic factor   A protein produced in the stomach that is needed for the absorption of adequate amounts of vitamin B_{12}.

Ion   An atom or compound that has gained or lost one or more electrons, thereby acquiring an overall negative or positive charge.

Iron deficiency anemia   A condition that occurs when the oxygen-carrying capacity of the blood is decreased because there is insufficient iron to make hemoglobin and the number and size of red blood cells decrease.

Irradiation   A process whereby foods are exposed to radiation energy; causes reactions within the food that kill contaminating organisms and retard ripening and spoilage of fruits and vegetables.

Isoleucine   An essential amino acid found in protein.

Isotope   An alternative form of an element that has a different atomic mass.

Jejunum   The 8-foot-long section of the small intestine lying between the duodenum and the ileum.

Juvenile-onset diabetes   *See* Insulin-dependent diabetes.

Keratin   A hard protein that makes up hair and nails.

Keshan's disease   A heart disease that occurs in an area of China where the soil is very low in selenium.

Ketone   A molecule formed when there is insufficient carbohydrate to completely metabolize the acetyl-CoA produced from fatty acid breakdown; also called ketone body.

Ketosis   The condition that results from having high levels of ketones in the blood.

Kilocalorie (kcal)   A unit of heat that is used to measure the amount of energy provided by foods; 1 kcalorie = 4.18 kjoules

Kilojoule (kjoule)   A measure of work that can be used to express energy intake and energy output; 4.18 kjoules = 1 kcal.

Kwashiorkor   A form of protein-energy malnutrition in which only protein is deficient; characteristic of young children unable to meet their high protein needs through the available diet.

Lactase   An enzyme located in the brush border of the small intestine that breaks the disaccharide lactose into glucose and galactose.

Lactase deficiency   A deficiency of the sugar-digesting enzyme lactase, causing an inability to digest lactose in the small intestine; the lactose is digested by bacteria in the large intestine, producing acid and gas, which cause abdominal distention, flatulence, cramping, and diarrhea.

Lactation   The production and secretion of milk by the mammary gland.

Lacteal   A lymph vessel in the intestine that can accept large particles such as the products of fat digestion.

Lactic acid   An end product of anaerobic metabolism and an additive used in food to maintain acidity or form curds.

Lactitol   The sugar alcohol formed from lactose.

Lacto-ovo vegetarian   One who eats no animal flesh but eats eggs and dairy products such as milk and cheese.

Lacto-vegetarian   One who eats no animal flesh or eggs but eats dairy products.

Lactose   A disaccharide made of glucose linked to galactose that is found in milk.

Lactose intolerance   The inability to digest lactose due to a deficiency of the enzyme lactase; after consuming dairy products, symptoms such as gas and bloating may occur.

Large for gestational age   Classification for an infant weighing greater than 4 kg (8.8 pounds) at birth.

Large intestine   The portion of the gastrointestinal tract that includes the colon and rectum; some water and vitamins are absorbed and bacteria act on food residues here.

Laxative   A substance that eases the excretion of feces.

Lean body mass   The body mass attributed to nonfat body components such as bone, muscle, and internal organs; also called fat-free mass.

Leavening agent   A substance added to food that causes the production of gas, resulting in an increase in volume.

Lecithin   A phospholipid composed of a glycerol backbone, two fatty acids, a phosphate group, and a molecule of choline; often used as an emulsifier in foods.

Legume   The starchy seed of plants that produce bean pods; includes peas, beans, soybeans, and lentils.

Leptin   A protein hormone produced by adipocytes that affects energy balance by decreasing energy intake and increasing energy expenditure.

Let-down response   A reflex that is triggered by the infant's sucking; causes milk to be released from the milk ducts and flow to the nipple.

Leucine   An essential amino acid found in protein.

Life expectancy   The average length of life for a population of individuals.

Lifespan   The maximum age to which a member of a species can live.

Lignin   The substance responsible for the hard woody nature of plant stems.

Limiting amino acid   The essential amino acid that is in the lowest concentration in relation to the body's needs.

Linoleic acid   An omega-6 essential fatty acid with 18 carbons and 2 double bonds.

Lipase   A fat-digesting enzyme.

Lipid   An organic molecule, of which most types do not dissolve in water; provides energy and insulation and serves as a precursor in the synthesis of certain hormones; includes fatty acids, glycerides, phospholipids, and sterols.

Lipid bilayer   Two layers of mostly phosphoglyceride molecules that are oriented such that the fat soluble fatty acid tails are sandwiched between the water soluble phosphate-containing heads.

Lipoic acid   A coenzyme needed in the reaction that forms acetyl-CoA; not a dietary essential.

Lipoprotein   A compound containing a core of lipids surrounded by a shell of protein, phospholipid, and cholesterol.

Lipoprotein lipase   An enzyme that breaks down triglycerides into free fatty acids and glycerol; attached to the outside of the cells that line the blood vessels.

Liposuction   A procedure that suctions out adipose tissue from under the skin; used to decrease the size of local fat deposits such as on the abdomen or hips.

Locust bean gum A branched polysaccharide that is produced from the endosperm of the seed of the carob plant; used as an additive to increase viscosity in cheese products and sausages.

Longevity The duration of an individual's life.

Longitudinal data Information obtained by repeatedly sampling the same individuals in a population over time.

Low birth weight infant An infant born prematurely or at term who weighs less than 2.5 kg (5.5 pounds).

Low-density lipoprotein (LDL) A lipoprotein particle that is high in cholesterol; elevated LDL cholesterol increases the risk of heart disease.

Low-density lipoprotein receptor A protein on the surface of cells that binds to LDL particles and allows their contents to be taken up for use by the cell.

Low-input agriculture or **sustainable agriculture** Methods of producing food that leave the environment able to restore itself and continue to produce food for future generations.

Lumen The inside cavity of a tube, such as the gastrointestinal tract.

Lymph vessel A tubular component of the lymphatic system that carries fluid (lymph) away from body tissues.

Lymphatic system The organ system that includes tissues that function in the body's defense system and vessels that return excess fluid to the bloodstream and transport absorbed fats.

Lysosome A cellular organelle containing degradative enzymes.

Macrocyte A larger-than-normal mature red blood cell that has a shortened lifespan.

Macronutrient A nutrient needed by the body in large amounts; includes water, carbohydrates, lipids, and proteins.

Macular degeneration Degeneration of a structure of the eye that results in a loss of visual detail and blindness.

Major mineral A mineral needed in the diet in an amount greater than 100 mg per day or present in the body in an amount greater than

0.01% of body weight; also called macromineral.

Malnutrition Poor nutritional status resulting from a dietary intake that is either above or below that which is optimal.

Maltase An enzyme found in the brush border of the small intestine that breaks maltose into two molecules of glucose.

Maltose A disaccharide made of two glucose molecules linked together.

Mannitol The sugar alcohol formed from mannose.

Marasmus A form of protein-energy malnutrition in which a deficiency of energy in the diet causes severe body wasting.

Maturity-onset diabetes *See* Noninsulin-dependent diabetes.

Maximal oxygen consumption (VO$_2$max) The maximal amount of oxygen that can be consumed by the tissues during exercise.

Maximum heart rate The maximum number of beats per minute that the heart can attain; declines with age and can be estimated by subtracting age in years from 220.

Megaloblast A large immature red blood cell that is formed when developing red blood cells are unable to divide normally.

Megaloblastic or **macrocytic anemia** A condition in which there is a reduction in the total number of red blood cells; characterized by abnormally large immature and mature red blood cells.

Megavitamin A vitamin dose in an amount greater than ten times the RDA.

Melatonin A hormone involved in regulating the body's cycles of sleep and wakefulness. Levels decline with age. Supplements claim to boost antioxidant defenses, improve immune function and slow aging.

Menaquinone A form of vitamin K found in animals.

Menarche The onset of menstruation; occurs normally between the ages of 10 and 15.

Menopause The physiological changes that mark the end of a woman's capacity to bear children.

Menstruation The cyclic discharge of the uterine lining that, in the absence of pregnancy, occurs about every four weeks during the reproductive years of female humans.

Metabolism All of the chemical reactions that take place in a living organism.

Metallothionein A protein that binds zinc and copper in intestinal mucosal cells and limits their absorption.

Methionine An essential sulfur-containing amino acid found in protein.

Methyl group A carbon atom bound to 3 hydrogen atoms.

Micelle A droplet of lipid surrounded by bile salts in the small intestine.

Microbe An organism too small to be seen without a microscope; also called microorganism.

Microflora The microorganisms that inhabit the large intestine.

Micronutrient A nutrient needed by the body in small amounts; includes vitamins and minerals.

Microorganism An organism such as a bacterium, too small to be seen without a microscope.

Microvilli Minute projections on the cell membrane of cells lining the small intestine that increase the absorptive surface area.

Mineral An element needed by the body for structure and to regulate chemical reactions and body processes.

Miscarriage Interruption of pregnancy prior to the seventh month.

Mitochondrion (mitochondria) The cellular organelle that is the site of energy production via aerobic metabolism; the citric acid cycle and electron transport chain are located here.

Modified atmosphere packaging (MAP) A type of food packaging in which the gases inside the package have been changed to control or retard chemical, physical, and microbiological changes.

Modified starch A starch that has been treated to enhance its ability to thicken or form a gel; also called modified food starch.

Mold A multicellular fungus that secretes enzymes that decompose the food or other material on which it grows.

Molecular biology The study of cellular function at the molecular level.

Molecule A unit of 2 or more atoms of the same or different elements bonded together.

Monoacylglycerol or **monoglyceride** A molecule of glycerol with 1 fatty acid attached.

Monosaccharide A single sugar molecule, such as glucose.

Monosodium glutamate (MSG) An additive used as a flavor enhancer; made up of the amino acid glutamate bound to sodium; commonly used in Chinese food.

Monounsaturated fatty acid A fatty acid containing 1 carbon-carbon double bond.

Morbidity Diseased or disabled.

Morbid obesity A condition in which an individual's body weight is 100 pounds (45.5 kg) above desirable body weight or their body mass index is greater than 40.

Morning sickness The nausea and vomiting that affect some women during pregnancy.

Mucosa The layer of tissue lining the gastrointestinal tract and other body cavities.

Mucus A thick fluid secreted by glands in the gastrointestinal tract and other parts of the body; acts to lubricate, moisten, and protect cells from harsh environments.

Mutagen Any agent that causes a change in a cell's genetic material.

Mutation A change in DNA.

Myelin A soft white fatty substance that covers nerve fibers and aids in nerve transmission.

Myocardial infarction Heart attack.

Myo-inositol *See* Inositol.

Myoglobin An iron-containing protein in muscle cells that binds oxygen.

National Health and Nutrition Examination Survey (NHANES) An ongoing set of surveys designed to monitor the overall nutritional status of the U.S. population; combines food consumption information with medical histories, physical examinations, and laboratory measurements.

Nervous system A system of nerve cells organized in message sending, message receiving, and information processing pathways.

Net protein utilization A measure of protein quality determined by comparing the amount of nitrogen retained in the body to the amount eaten in the diet.

Neural tube A portion of the embryo that develops into the brain and spinal cord.

Neural tube defect A defect in the formation of the neural tube that occurs early in development and results in defects of the brain and spinal cord such as anencephaly and spina bifida.

Neurotransmitter A chemical substance produced by a nerve cell that can stimulate or inhibit a target cell.

Nicotinamide A form of niacin.

Nicotinamide adenine dinucleotide (NAD) A coenzyme made from niacin that transports electrons.

Nicotinamide adenine dinucleotide phosphate (NADP) A coenzyme made from niacin that is used in synthetic reactions.

Niacin equivalents (NE) Units used to measure niacin requirement that is equal to 1 mg of niacin or 60 mg of tryptophan.

Nicotinic acid A form of niacin.

Nitrogen balance When nitrogen intake is equal to nitrogen excretion.

Nitrosamine A carcinogenic compound produced by reactions involving nitrites and other molecules.

Nonessential amino acid An amino acid that can be synthesized by the human body in sufficient amounts to meet needs.

Nonheme iron A form of iron found in both plant and animal products that is not part of the iron complex found in hemoglobin and myoglobin; less well absorbed than heme iron.

Noninsulin-dependent diabetes A disease characterized by elevated blood glucose resulting from an insensitivity of the cells to the action of insulin; most commonly occurs in overweight adults; also called Type II diabetes and maturity-onset diabetes.

Nucleus In atoms it is a central core of positively charged protons and electrically neutral neutrons. In cells it is an organelle containing DNA.

Nursing bottle syndrome Extreme tooth decay in the upper teeth that results from putting a child to bed with a bottle containing milk or other sweetened liquid.

Nutrient A chemical substance in foods that provides energy, structure, and regulation of body processes.

Nutrient density A measure of the nutrients provided by a food relative to the energy it contains.

Nutrification The process of adding one or more nutrients to commonly consumed foods with the goal of adding to the nutrient intake of a group of people.

Nutrition A science that studies the interactions that occur between living organisms and food.

Nutritional assessment The use of dietary intake records, clinical measures, and laboratory measures to determine an individual's nutritional status.

Nutritional status The health of an individual as it is influenced by the intake and utilization of nutrients.

Obesity A condition that is characterized by excess body fat; defined as a body weight that is 20% or more above desirable body weight or a body mass index greater than 27.

Oil A lipid that is liquid at room temperature.

Oleic acid A monounsaturated fatty acid with 18 carbons.

Olestra An unabsorbable artificial fat made of sucrose with fatty acids linked to it. It has been approved by the FDA for use in certain snack foods.

Oligosaccharides Short chain carbohydrates containing 3 to 10 sugar units.

Omega-3 fatty acid A fatty acid containing a carbon-carbon double bond between the third and fourth carbons from the methyl end; includes alpha-linolenic acid found in vegetable oils and eicosapentaenoic acid (EPA) and docosahexaenoic acid found in fish oils.

Omega-6 fatty acid A fatty acid containing a carbon-carbon double bond between the sixth and seventh carbons from the methyl end; includes linolenic and arachidonic acid.

Opsin A protein in the retina of the eye involved in the visual cycle.

Organ A discrete structure composed of tissues organized in varying combinations that perform specialized functions in the body.

Organelle A cellular organ that carries out specific metabolic reactions.

Organic A substance that contains carbon atoms.

Organic food A food produced without the use of chemical fertilizers, pesticides, or herbicides that contains no additives.

Osmosis   The passive movement of water across a membrane to equalize the concentration of dissolved substances on both sides.

Osteoarthritis   The form of arthritis common in the elderly that is characterized by abnormalities in the joint surfaces.

Osteomalacia   A vitamin D deficiency disease in adults that causes weak bones and an increase in bone fractures.

Osteoporosis   A bone disease characterized by a reduction in bone mass that causes weak bones and an increase in bone fractures.

Overnutrition   Poor nutritional status resulting from a dietary intake in excess of that which is optimal for nutritional needs.

Overweight   Body weight greater than 10% above the desirable body weight standard.

Oviduct   *See* fallopian tube.

Ovum   The female reproductive cell.

Oxalate   An organic acid found in spinach, rhubarb, and other leafy green vegetables that can reduce the absorption of certain minerals.

Oxidation   The loss of electrons.

Oxidized LDL cholesterol   A substance formed when the cholesterol in LDLs is oxidized by reactive oxygen molecules. It is the key in the development of heroesclerosis because it is taken up by white blood cells.

Oxytocin   A hormone released by the posterior pituitary that stimulates the ejection or let down of milk during lactation.

Palmitic acid   A saturated fatty acid containing 16 carbons.

Pancreas   An organ that secretes enzymes and sodium bicarbonate into the small intestine during digestion.

Pancreatic amylase   A starch-digesting enzyme found in pancreatic juice.

Pancreatic juice   The secretion of the pancreas containing bicarbonate to neutralize acid and enzymes for the digestion of carbohydrates, fats, and proteins.

Pangamic acid   A poorly defined substance that is not a vitamin but has been sold as such by some manufacturers suggested to enhance exercise performance.

Papain   A protein-digesting enzyme found in papaya.

Parasite   An organism that lives at the expense of another without contributing to the survival of its host.

Para-aminobenzoic acid (PABA)   A chemical that is part of the folic acid molecule but alone has no vitamin activity and cannot be used by the body to synthesize folic acid; effective at blocking ultraviolet (UV) light, thus used in topical sunscreens.

Parathyroid hormone   A hormone produced by the parathyroid gland that increases blood calcium levels.

Parietal cell   A large cell in the stomach lining that produces and secretes intrinsic factor and hydrochloric acid.

Partially hydrogenated vegetable oil.   Vegetable oil that has been modified by hydrogenation to decrease the number of unsaturated bonds, therefore raising the melting point and improving the storage characteristics.

Pasteurization   The process of heating food products to a specific temperature for a specified period to kill disease-causing microorganisms.

Pathogen   An organism capable of causing disease.

Peak bone mass   The maximum amount of bone mass attained at any time in life, usually occurring in the late teens or early twenties.

Pectin   A soluble fiber found in plant cell walls that forms a gel when mixed with acid and sugar.

Peer-review   A review of the design and validity of a research experiment by scientific experts who did not participate in the research.

Pellagra   A niacin deficiency disease that is characterized by dermatitis, dementia, diarrhea, and, ultimately, death.

Pepsin   A protein-digesting enzyme produced by the stomach; secreted in the gastric juice in an inactive form and activated by the acid of the stomach.

Pepsinogen   An inactive protein-digesting enzyme produced by gastric glands and activated to pepsin by acid in the stomach.

Peptide   Two or more amino acids joined by peptide bonds.

Peptide bond   A chemical linkage between the amino group and 1 amino acid and the acid group of another.

Periodontal disease   A degeneration of the area surrounding the teeth, specifically the gum and supporting bone.

Peristalsis   The coordinated muscular contraction that moves food forward through the gastrointestinal tract.

Pernicious anemia   An anemia resulting from vitamin B_{12} deficiency; if not treated with vitamin B_{12} injections, nerve damage may result.

Peroxide   A reactive chemical that can form free radicals and cause cellular damage.

Pesticide   A substance used to prevent or decrease damage to plants from insects and microorganisms.

pH   A measure of the level of acidity of a solution.

Pharynx   The common opening of the digestive tract and the respiratory tract.

Phenylalanine   An essential amino acid that cannot be metabolized by individuals with phenylketonuria (PKU).

Phenylketone   The product of phenylalanine breakdown produced when phenylalanine cannot be converted to tyrosine; when blood levels get too high, brain damage results.

Phenylketonuria (PKU)   An inherited disease in which the body cannot metabolize the amino acid phenylalanine; if untreated, toxic by-products accumulate in the blood and cause mental retardation.

Phenylpropanolamine   A stimulant used in some weight loss aids to blunt appetite.

Phosphoglyceride   A phospholipid composed of a glycerol backbone with two fatty acids and a phosphate group attached; mixes well with both watery and oily substances and is an important component of cell membranes.

Phospholipid   A lipid containing a phosphate group.

Photosynthesis   The metabolic process by which plants trap energy from the sun and use it to make sugars from carbon dioxide and water.

Phylloquinone   The form of vitamin K found in plants.

Phytic acid (phytate)   A substance found in the husks of grains, legumes, and seeds that can bind minerals and decrease their absorption.

Phytochemicals   Chemicals found in plants that are not essential nutrients but play a role in preventing chronic disease.

Pica   The compulsive ingestion of nonfood substances such as clay, laundry starch, and paint chips.

Placebo   A fake medicine or supplement that is indistinguishable in appearance from the real thing; used to disguise the control and experimental groups in an experiment.

Placenta   An organ produced from both maternal and embryonic tissues; transfers nutrients and oxygen from the mother's blood to the growing embryo and fetus and removes wastes.

Plaque   The cholesterol-rich material that is deposited in the blood vessels of individuals with atherosclerosis; consists of cholesterol and other lipids, white blood cells, smooth muscle cells, fibrous proteins, and, eventually, calcium.

Platelets   A cell fragment found in blood that is involved in blood clotting.

Polar   Used to describe something that has a positive charge at one end and a negative charge at the other.

Polychlorinated biphenyl (PCB)   A carcinogenic industrial compound; some have found their way into the environment and subsequently the food supply; repeated exposure causes them to accumulate in biological tissues over time.

Polycyclic aromatic hydrocarbon (PAH)   A class of mutagenic substances produced during cooking when there is incomplete combustion of organic materials.

Polypeptide   A chain of 3 or more amino acids joined together by peptide bonds.

Polysaccharide   A type of complex carbohydrate containing hundreds to thousands of sugar units linked together.

Polyunsaturated fatty acid   A fatty acid containing more than 1 carbon-carbon double bond.

Postmenopausal bone loss   The accelerated loss of bone that occurs in women in the years right after menstruation stops.

Precursor   Inactive form of a substance.

Pregnancy-induced hypertension   A condition during pregnancy that is characterized by an increase in body weight, elevated blood pressure, protein in the urine, and edema. It can

be life threatening to the mother and the fetus.

Premature or preterm infant   An infant born before 37 weeks of gestation.

Premenstrual syndrome (PMS)   A syndrome of mood swings, food cravings, bloating, tension and depression, headaches, acne, and anxiety, among other symptoms, that results from the hormonal changes during the days prior to menstruation.

Preservative   A compound that prevents spoilage and extends the shelf life of a product by retarding chemical, physical, or microbiological changes.

Prime grade   A USDA grade of beef with the largest amount of marbled fat.

Progesterone   A female sex hormone needed for development and function of the uterus and mammary glands.

Programmed cell death   The death of cells at specific predictable times.

Prolactin   A hormone released from the anterior pituitary that stimulates the breasts to produce milk.

Protein   An organic molecule made up of 1 or more intertwining chains of amino acids.

Protein complementation   The process of combining proteins from different sources so that they collectively provide the proportions of amino acids required to meet human needs.

Protein efficiency ratio   A measure of protein quality determined by comparing the weight gain of a laboratory animal fed a test protein with the weight gain of an animal fed a reference protein.

Protein-energy malnutrition (PEM)   A condition characterized by wasting and an increased susceptibility to infection that results from the long-term consumption of insufficient energy and protein to meet body needs.

Protein hydrolysate   A mixture of amino acids or amino acids and polypeptides that results when a protein is completely or partially broken down by treatment with acid or enzymes.

Protein quality   A measure of the essential amino acid content of a protein relative to the essential amino acid needs of the body.

Protein-sparing modified fast   A very-low-kcalorie diet of high protein content designed to maximize loss of fat and minimize loss of protein from the body.

Prothrombin   A protein found in the blood that is essential for blood clotting.

Provitamin   A compound that the body can convert into the active form of a vitamin; also called vitamin precursor.

Psyllium   A plant product high in soluble fiber that is used in over-the-counter bulk-forming laxatives.

Puberty   The period in life characterized by rapid changes that ends in the attainment of sexual maturity.

Purging   Various methods used to rid the body of unwanted food and energy, including self-induced vomiting and the misuse of laxatives.

Pyloric sphincter   A muscular valve that helps regulate the rate at which food leaves the stomach and enters the small intestine.

Pyridoxal phosphate   The active coenzyme form of vitamin B_6.

Pyridoxamine   A form of vitamin B_6.

Pyridoxine   A form of vitamin B_6; a general name used to refer to vitamin B_6, including pyridoxal, pyridoxine, and pyridoxamine.

Pyruvate   A 3-carbon molecule produced when glucose is broken down by glycolysis.

Raffinose   An oligosaccharide found in beans and other legumes that cannot be digested by human enzymes in the stomach and small intestine.

Reactive hypoglycemia   Low blood sugar that occurs an hour or so after the consumption of high-carbohydrate foods; results from an overproduction of insulin.

Rebound scurvy   Scurvy that results because a high intake of vitamin C is abruptly stopped and the body continues to use only a portion of the vitamin C provided.

Recommended Dietary Allowances (RDAs)   Recommended intakes for nutrients to meet the needs of almost all healthy people in the United States; established by the Food and Nutrition Board of the National Academy of Sciences.

Recommended Nutrient Intakes (RNIs) Recommended intakes of nutrients established for Canadians by Health Canada.

Rectum A portion of the large intestine that connects the colon and anus.

Reference Daily Intakes (RDIs) Reference values established for vitamins and minerals that are based on the highest amount of each nutrient recommended for any adult age group by the 1968 RDAs.

Refined Refers to the process whereby the coarse parts of food are removed, leaving behind a product of more uniform composition; e.g., refined sugar.

Renin An enzyme produced by the kidney that plays a role in regulating blood pressure by aiding in the conversion of angiotensin to its active form, angiotensin II.

Rennin An enzyme produced by the stomach of infants and young children that acts on the milk protein casein to convert it to a curdy substance.

Reserve capacity The amount of functional capacity that an organ has above and beyond what is needed to sustain life.

Respiratory system Organ system including the lungs and air passageways involved in the exchange of oxygen from the environment with carbon dioxide waste from cells, by way of the bloodstream.

Resting energy expenditure (REE) or resting metabolic rate (RMR) An estimate of basal metabolic rate that is determined by measuring energy utilization after 5 to 6 hours without food and/or exercise.

Resting heart rate The number of times per minute that the heart beats in a resting state.

Resting metabolic rate (RMR) See resting energy expenditure (REE).

Retin-A A drug that is a vitamin A derivative used topically to treat acne.

Retinal The aldehyde form of vitamin A, which is needed for the visual cycle.

Retinoic acid The acid form of vitamin A, which is needed for cell differentiation, growth, and reproduction.

Retinoids The different chemical forms of preformed vitamin A: retinol, retinal, and retinoic acid.

Retinol The alcohol form of vitamin A, which can be interconverted with retinal.

Retinol-binding protein A protein that is necessary to transport vitamin A in the blood.

Retinol equivalent (RE) A unit of measure of vitamin A that is the equivalent of 1 μg of retinol.

Rhodopsin A light-sensitive compound found in the retina of the eye that is composed of the protein opsin loosely bound to retinal.

Ribose The 5-carbon sugar that is part of RNA.

Ribosome The cell organelle where protein synthesis occurs.

Rickets A vitamin D deficiency disease in children that is characterized by poor bone development due to inadequate calcium deposition.

Risk-benefit analysis When the risk of ingesting a substance is weighed against the benefits it provides in terms of production, processing, or preservation; if the risk is small and the benefits great, small amounts of this substance may be acceptable.

RNA (ribonucleic acid) The single-stranded nucleic acid that carries information in DNA from the nucleus to the cytoplasm where it is translated into a sequence of amino acids to make a protein.

Royal jelly The substance that is produced by worker bees to feed the queen; marketed as an ergogenic aid.

Saccharin An artificial sweetener that contains no energy and is used in diet products.

Saliva A watery fluid produced and secreted into the mouth by the salivary glands; contains lubricants, enzymes, and other substances.

Salivary amylase An enzyme secreted by the salivary glands that breaks down starch into smaller units.

Salivary glands The structures located internally at the sides of and below the face and in front of the ears that secrete saliva.

Salmonella A bacterium that commonly causes food-borne illness.

Satiety A feeling of fullness and a lack of desire to eat.

Saturated Refers to a fat or fatty acid in which the carbons are bound to as many hydrogens as possible and therefore contains no carbon-carbon double bonds in its structure.

Scavenger receptor A protein on white blood cells that binds to oxidized LDL cholesterol.

Scientific method The general approach of science that is used to explain observations about the world around us.

Scurvy A vitamin C deficiency disease.

Seasonal affective disorder A disorder characterized by depression and carbohydrate cravings during the fall and winter months.

Secondary lactase deficiency Lactase deficiency that occurs as a result of disease and may resolve after the disease has ended.

Secretin A hormone secreted by the mucous lining of the small intestine that stimulates the pancreas to secrete sodium bicarbonate and the liver to secrete bile into the gallbladder.

Select grade A USDA grade of beef with a medium amount of marbled fat.

Selectively permeable A membrane or barrier that will allow some substances to pass freely but will restrict the passage of others.

Semiessential amino acid An amino acid that is essential in the diet only if its precursor amino acid is in short supply.

Semivegetarian One who avoids only certain types of meat, fish, or poultry; e.g., an individual who avoids all red meat but continues to consume poultry and fish.

Serotonin The neurotransmitter that functions in the sleep center of the brain.

Settling point or **set point** A level at which body fat or body weight seem to resist change despite changes in energy intake or output.

Sickle cell anemia An inherited disease in which hemoglobin structure is altered; red blood cells containing the altered hemoglobin are sickle-shaped, rupture easily, causing anemia, and block small blood vessels, causing inflammation and pain.

Simple diffusion The movement of substances across a cell membrane from an area of greater concentration to an area of lower concentration; no energy is required.

Simple sugar Monosaccharides and disaccharides; also called simple carbohydrate.

Simplesse An artificial fat made from egg and milk proteins that contains about 1.3 kcalories per gram.

Single-blind study An experiment in which either the study participants or the investigators are unaware of who is in a control or an experimental group.

Skinfold thickness A measurement of subcutaneous fat used to estimate total body fat.

Small for gestational age A full-term infant weighing less than or equal to 2.5 kg (5.5 pounds) at birth.

Small intestine A tube-shaped organ of the digestive tract where digestion of ingested food is completed and most of the absorption occurs.

Smooth muscle Involuntary muscles that cause constriction of the gastrointestinal tract, blood vessels, and glands.

Sodium bicarbonate A compound that is part of an important buffer system in pancreatic juice and in the bloodstream.

Sodium caseinate A form of the milk protein casein that is frequently used as a food additive.

Sodium-potassium ATPase An energy-requiring protein pump in the cell membrane that pumps sodium out of the cell and potassium into the cell.

Solanine A toxic substance naturally occurring in potatoes; inhibits the action of neurotransmitters.

Soluble fiber Fiber that either dissolves or swells when placed in water; includes pectins, gums, and mucilages.

Solutes Dissolved substances.

Solution A solvent containing a dissolved substance.

Solvent A liquid in which substances dissolve.

Sorbitol A sugar alcohol formed from sorbose; used as a sweetener or humectant in food.

Sperm The male reproductive cell.

Sphincter A muscular valve that controls the flow of materials into the gastrointestinal tract.

Spontaneous abortion or **miscar-**

riage Interruption of pregnancy prior to the seventh month.

Spores A dormant state of some bacteria that is resistant to heat but can germinate to produce a new organism when environmentsl conditions are favorable.

Sports anemia A temporary decrease in hemoglobin concentration that occurs during exercise training. It occurs as an adaptation to training and does not impair delivery of oxygen to tissues.

Stabilizer A substance added to food to stabilize its consistency.

Standards of identity The regulations that define the allowable ingredients, composition, and other characteristics of foods.

Staphylococcus A bacterium, commonly found in the nasal passages, that can contaminate food and cause food-borne illness.

Starch A carbohydrate made of many units of glucose linked by a type of bond that can be broken by the human digestive enzymes.

Starchyose An oligosaccharide found in beans and other legumes that cannot be digested by human enzymes in the stomach and small intestine.

Starvation The condition that occurs when insufficient food is ingested to maintain health.

Stearic acid An 18-carbon saturated fatty acid that unlike other saturated fats does not raise blood cholesterol levels.

Steroid hormone A hormone that is made from cholesterol; includes the male and female sex hormones.

Sterol A lipid that contains multiple ring structures.

Stomach A muscular pouch-like organ of the digestive tract that mixes food and secretes gastric juice into the lumen and the hormone gastrin into the blood.

Stroke The loss of body function resulting from a blood clot or bleeding in the brain that causes brain tissue death.

Stroke volume The amount of blood pumped with each beat of the heart.

Subscapular The region just below the shoulder blade that is a common location for measuring skinfold thickness.

Subsistence crops Crops grown as food for the local population.

Sustainable agriculture *See* Low-input agriculture.

Sucrase An enzyme in the brush border of the small intestine that breaks sucrose into glucose and fructose.

Sucrose A disaccharide commonly known as table sugar that is made of glucose linked to fructose.

Sudden infant death syndrome (SIDS) The early death of unknown causes that occurs in young infants while they are asleep; also called crib death.

Sugar alcohol A sweetener that is structurally related to sugars but provides less energy than monosaccharides and disaccharides because it is not as well absorbed.

Sulfites Sulfur-containing compounds used as preservatives to prevent oxidation in dried fruits and vegetables and to prevent bacterial growth in wine.

Superoxide dismutase An enzyme that protects the cell from oxidative damage by neutralizing superoxide free radicals.

Tannin A substance found in tea and some grains that can bind certain minerals and decrease their absorption.

Taurine An amino acid that is not used in protein synthesis but is necessary for nerve function and vision and the synthesis of bile acids; made in the adult human in sufficient quantities but may be essential in premature infants; found only in animal foods.

Teratogen A chemical, biological or physical agent that causes birth defects.

Testosterone A steroid hormone secreted by the testes that is involved in the maintenance and development of male sex organs and secondary sex characteristics.

Texturizer A substance added to food to change its texture.

Theory An explanation based on scientific study and reasoning.

Thermal distress A condition resulting from the inability of the body to dissipate heat as fast as it is produced.

Thermic effect of food The increase in energy expenditure that occurs during the digestion, absorption, metabolism, and storage of food; equal to approximately 10% of daily energy intake; also called diet-induced thermogenesis.

Thiamin pyrophosphate The active coenzyme form of thiamin.

Threshold effect When a substance can be ingested without effect up to a certain amount; after that, effects increase with increasing intake.

Thyroid gland A gland located in the neck that produces thyroid hormones and calcitonin.

Thyroid hormones Hormones produced by the thyroid gland that regulate metabolic rate.

Thyroid-stimulating hormone A hormone that stimulates the synthesis and secretion of thyroid hormones from the thyroid gland.

Tocopherol The chemical name for vitamin E.

Tolerance The allowable level of pesticide residues in foods set by the EPA.

Total parenteral nutrition (TPN) A method of providing complete nutrition without use of the gastrointestinal tract by infusing a nutrient-rich solution directly into the bloodstream.

Toxic The capacity to produce injury at some level of intake.

Toxin A substance with the ability to cause harm; also called toxicant.

Trace element or **trace mineral** A mineral required in the diet in an amount less than 100 mg per day or present in the body in an amount less than 0.01% of body weight.

Trans fatty acid An unsaturated fatty acid configured such that the hydrogens are on opposite sides of the double bond; formed during the hydrogenation of oils.

Transamination The transfer of an amino group from one amino acid to a carbon skeleton to form a different amino acid.

Transferrin A protein involved in the transport of iron in the blood.

Transit time The time between the ingestion of food and the elimination from the body of the solid waste from that food.

Treatment groups See Experimental groups.

Triacylglycerols A molecule of glycerol with 3 fatty acids attached. The major form of lipid in food and the major storage form of lipid in the body; commonly called triglycerides.

Triceps Region at the back of the upper arm that is a common site for measuring skin-fold thickness.

Trichinosis The disease caused by infection with the roundworm *Trichinella spiralis* after eating undercooked contaminated pork or game meats; the juvenile form of this roundworm migrates to the muscles and causes flu-like symptoms and muscle pain and weakness.

Triglyceride See Triacylgycerols.

Trimester A term used to describe each third or three months of a pregnancy.

Tripeptide Three amino acids linked together by peptide bonds.

Tropical oil A saturated oil (coconut, palm, and palm kernel oil) that is derived from plants grown in tropical regions.

Trypsin A protein-digesting enzyme that is secreted from the pancreas in inactive form and activated in the small intestine.

Tuber The starchy underground storage organ of plants.

Tumor A growth of tissue that forms an abnormal mass that serves no physiological function.

Tumor initiator A substance that causes mutations and therefore may predispose a cell to become cancerous.

Tumor promoter A substance that stimulates a mutated cell to begin dividing.

Twenty-four-hour recall A dietary intake assessment method in which an interviewer asks an individual to recall all food and drink consumed for the past 24 hours.

Type I diabetes See Insulin-dependent diabetes.

Type II diabetes See Noninsulin-dependent diabetes.

Tyrosine A conditionally essential amino acid; when phenylalanine is available in sufficient quantities, tyrosine is not essential in the diet.

Ubiquinone A compound that transports electrons in the electron transport chain but is not essential in the diet; also called coenzyme Q.

Ulcer An open sore in the lining of the esophagus, stomach, or small intestine.

Undernutrition Poor nutritional status resulting from a dietary intake below that which is optimal to meet nutritional needs.

Underwater weighing A method for assessing body composition that involves comparing an individual's body weight while on land with his or her weight while submerged in water.

Underweight Body weight less than the desirable weight by 10% or more.

United States Department of Agriculture (USDA) U.S. government agency responsible for monitoring the safety and wholesomeness of meat, poultry, and eggs.

Unsaturated fatty acid A fatty acid that contains 1 or more carbon-carbon double bonds in its structure.

Urea A nitrogen-containing waste product used to excrete the nitrogen from protein breakdown.

Urine A fluid produced by the kidneys, consisting of wastes, excess water, and dissolved substances.

U.S. Recommended Daily Allowances (U.S. RDAs) Standard reference values for nutrients designed to be used on food labels; generally equal to the highest nutrient recommendations in any age or sex category from the published 1968 RDAs; replaced by the RDIs.

Uterus A female organ for containing and nourishing the embryo and fetus from the time of implantation to the time of birth.

Variable A factor or condition that is changed in an experimental setting.

Vegan One who avoids all food of animal origin.

Vegetarian One who eats no animal products or limited categories of animal products.

Vein A blood vessel that carries blood toward the heart.

Venule A small vein that drains blood from capillaries and passes it to larger veins for return to the heart.

Very-low-density lipoprotein (VLDL) A lipoprotein particle that transports triglycerides from the liver to other body cells.

Very-low-kcalorie diet A weight loss diet that provides fewer than 800 kcalories per day.

Villus (villi) A finger-like protrusion of the lining of the small intestine that participates in the digestion and absorption of foodstuffs.

Virus An infectious microscopic particle that depends on body cells for its nutrient, metabolic, and reproductive needs.

Vitamin An organic compound needed in the diet in small amounts to promote and regulate the chemical reactions and processes of the body.

Warfarin An anticoagulant drug that is a derivative of dicumarol; also used as rat poison.

Water A molecule composed of 2 hydrogen atoms and 1 oxygen atom; essential nutrient needed by the human body in large amounts.

Water soluble vitamin A vitamin that is soluble in water; includes the B vitamins and vitamin C.

Wear and tear hypothesis A hypothesis that proposes that the changes that occur with age result from the accumulation of cellular damage over time.

Weight cycling The cycle of repeatedly losing and regaining weight; also called yo-yo dieting.

Wheat germ oil An oil pressed from the germ of wheat that is sold as an ergogenic aid.

Whole wheat flour A flour that contains all components of the wheat kernel: the bran, the germ, and the endosperm.

Xanthan gum A plant extract used as a stabilizer in processed foods.

Xerophthalmia An eye condition resulting from vitamin A deficiency; characterized by a lack of mucus on the eye that leaves it dry and vulnerable to abrasion and infection; may lead to blindness.

Xylitol The sugar alcohol formed from xylose; used in sugarless gum.

Yo-yo diet syndrome *See* Weight cycling.

Zygote The cell produced by sperm and ovum during fertilization.

The letter "t" following a page number indicates a table.

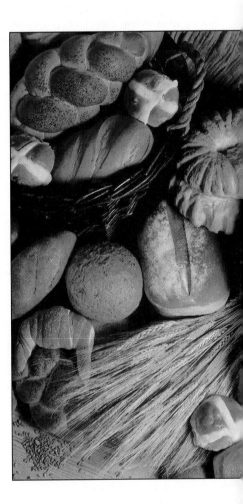

Estimated Sodium, Chloride, and Potassium Minimum Requirements of Healthy Persons[a]

Age	Weight (kg)[a]	Sodium (mg)[a,b]	Chloride (mg)[a,b]	Potassium (mg)[c]
Months				
0–5	4.5	120	180	500
6–11	8.9	200	300	700
Years				
1	11.0	225	350	1,000
2–5	16.0	300	500	1,400
6–9	25.0	400	600	1,600
10–18	50.0	500	750	2,000
>18[d]	70.0	500	750	2,000

[a] No allowance has been included for large, prolonged losses from the skin through sweat.
[b] There is no evidence that higher intakes confer any health benefit.
[c] Desirable intakes of potassium may considerably exceed these values (~3,500 mg for adults).
[d] No allowance included for growth. Valeus for those below 18 years assume a growth rate at the 50th percentile reported by the National Center for Health Statistics (Hamill et al., 1979) and averaged for males and females.

Estimated Safe and Adequate Daily Dietary Intakes of Selected Vitamins and Minerals[a]

		Vitamins	
Category	Age (years)	Biotin (μg)	Pantothenic Acid (mg)
Infants	0–0.5	10	2
	0.5–1	15	3
Children and adolescents	1–3	20	3
	4–6	25	3–4
	7–10	30	4–5
	11+	30–100	4–7
Adults		30–100	4–7

		Trace Elements[b]				
Category	Age (years)	Copper (mg)	Man-ganese (mg)	Fluoride (mg)	Chromium (μg)	Molybdenum (μg)
Infants	0–0.5	0.4–0.6	0.3–0.6	0.1–0.5	10–40	15–30
	0.5–1	0.6–0.7	0.6–1.0	0.2–1.0	20–60	20–40
Children and adolescents	1–3	0.7–1.0	1.0–1.5	0.5–1.5	20–80	25–50
	4–6	1.0–1.5	1.5–2.0	1.0–2.5	30–120	30–75
	7–10	1.0–2.0	2.0–3.0	1.5–2.5	50–200	50–150
	11+	1.5–2.5	2.0–5.0	1.5–2.5	50–200	75–250
Adults		1.5–3.0	2.0–5.0	1.5–4.0	50–200	75–250

[a] Because there is less information on which to base allowances, these figures are not given in the main table of RDA and are provided here in the form of ranges of recommended intakes.
[b] Since the toxic levels for many trace elements may be only several times usual intakes, the upper levels for the trace elements given in this table should not be habitually exceeded.

Weights and Measures

Measure	Abbreviation	Equivalent
1 gram	g	1000 milligrams
1 milligram	mg	1000 micrograms
1 microgram	μg	1/1000000 of a gram
1 nanogram	ng	1/1000000000 of a gram
1 picogram	pg	1/1000000000000 of a gram
1 kilogram	kg	1000 grams 2.2 lb
1 pound	lb	454 grams 16 ounces
1 teaspoon	tsp	approximately 5 grams
1 tablespoon	Tbsp	3 teaspoons
1 ounce	oz	28.4 grams
1 cup	c	8 ounces 16 tablespoons
1 pint		2 cups 16 ounces
1 quart	qt	2 pints 32 ounces
1 gallon	gal	64 ounces 4 quarts
1 liter	l	1.06 quarts 1000 milliliters
1 milliliter	ml	1000 microliters
1 deciliter	dl	100 milliliters
1 kcalorie	kcal	1000 calories 4.167 kilojoules
1 kilojoule	kJ	1000 joules
1 milliequivalent	mEq	

Sample Food Label
Product: Macaroni and Cheese

Nutrition Facts

Serving Size 1/2 cup (114g)
Servings Per Container 4

Amount Per Serving

Calories 260   Calories from Fat 120

	% Daily Value*
Total Fat 13g	**20%**
Saturated Fat 5g	**25%**
Cholesterol 30mg	**10%**
Sodium 660mg	**28%**
Total Carbohydrate 31g	**11%**
Dietary Fiber 0g	**0%**
Sugars 5g	
Protein 5g	

Vitamin A 4%	•	Vitamin C 2%
Calcium 15%	•	Iron

* Percent Daily Values are based on a 2,000 calorie diet. Your daily values may be higher or lower depending on your calorie needs:

		Calories:	2,000	2,500
Total Fat	Less than		65g	80g
Sat Fat	Less than		20g	25g
Cholesterol	Less than		300mg	300mg
Sodium	Less than		2,400mg	2,400mg
Total Carbohydrate			300g	375g
Dietary Fiber			25g	30g

Calories per gram:
Fat 9 • Carbohydrate 4 • Protein 4